HIGH-RISK NEWBORN INFANTS
The basis for intensive nursing care

HIGH-RISK NEWBORN INFANTS

The basis for intensive nursing care

SHELDON B. KORONES, M.D.

Professor of Pediatrics and Obstetrics and Gynecology,
University of Tennessee College of Medicine;
Director, Newborn Center, Regional Medical Center at Memphis,
Memphis, Tennessee

With a chapter by

JEAN LANCASTER, R.N., M.N.

Associate Professor of Nursing of Children, University of Tennessee
College of Nursing; Clinical Supervisor of Nurses, Newborn Center,
Regional Medical Center at Memphis,
Memphis, Tennessee

FOURTH EDITION

with 175 illustrations

The C. V. Mosby Company

ST. LOUIS • TORONTO • PRINCETON   1986

MOSBY

A TRADITION OF PUBLISHING EXCELLENCE

Editor: Barbara Ellen Norwitz
Developmental editor: Sally Adkisson

Top Graphics
Project manager: Billie Forshee
Manuscript editor: Connie Leinicke
Design: Joanne Kluba
Production: Susan Trail

FOURTH EDITION

The C.V. Mosby Company
11830 Westline Industrial Drive, St. Louis, Missouri 63146

Library of Congress Cataloging in Publication Data

Korones, Sheldon B., 1924-
   High-risk newborn infants.

   Includes bibliographies and index.
   1. Infants (newborn)—Diseases. 2. Neonatal intensive care. 3. Intensive care nursing. I. Lancaster, Jean. II. Title. [DNLM: 1. Infant, Newborn, Diseases—nursing. 2. Intensive Care Units. WY 159 K84h]
RJ254.K67 1986   618.92′01   86-2513
ISBN 0-8016-2750-8

GW/VH/VH 9 8 7 6 5 4 3 2 1   03/C/323

To

the infants
who have suffered from our past inadequacies
and to those who will benefit
from our enhanced expertise

To

Elena and **Jonathan,**
buoyant and beautiful, as they thrive
in this world, when they might have languished sadly
in the Third World of their birth

Preface

In 1972 the preface of the first edition stated that this book was not a "how-to-do-it" manual. It would describe "what to do," but more significantly, it would emphasize "why it is done." Because effectiveness of the care of sick neonates is so dependent on an understanding of rationale, this edition maintains the emphasis on "why."

Physician and nurse must function separately, but they are numerators with a common conceptual denominator. The roles of physicians and nurses were also addressed in the first edition's preface—"The book speaks to the neonatal nurse as a physician's colleague,"—to which should have then been added—"and to the physician as the nurse's co-worker."

This edition is replete with revisions. In Chapter 1 the evaluation of antepartum and intrapartum fetal status has been expanded considerably. In Chapter 2 a discussion of labor at the cellular level should provide some background for an understanding of tocolysis and the drugs that may yet be of value to effect it.

The chapter on thermoregulation has been lengthened with a discussion of body heat and transepidermal water loss in very small premature infants (birth weight less than 1000 g) who now survive in considerably greater numbers. In the chapter on birth weight and gestational age, material on body composition and body measurements for the assessment of growth has been added.

New discussions of apnea, transcutaneous oxygen measurements, and assisted ventilation will be found in the chapter on lung disorders. Furthermore, the revised ideas that concern the retinopathy of prematurity (retrolental fibroplasia) are presented here in some detail. The chapter on blood disorders has been expanded by the addition of a section on clotting and by a lengthened discussion of the complications of exchange transfusion and the prevention of Rh disease.

A new chapter on nutrition is included in this edition. It is principally concerned with parenteral and enteral nutrition of low birth weight infants. In her revision of the chapter on parent-infant relationships, Jean Lancaster has added an incisive discussion of siblings' reactions to the neonate's illness. Finally, contemporary views of the functional roles of a variety of personnel are added to the chapter on organizational aspects of neonatal intensive care units.

Thanks are due to several individuals whose indispensable roles should really be proclaimed, not just recognized. Marion Haynes prepared the manuscript. Except for the writing, she actually performed virtually all functions. Rosalind Griffin's aid in the review of galleys was pivotal. Dr. Garland Anderson, Professor and Chief, Division of Maternal-Fetal Medicine, Department of Obstetrics and Gynecology, was a supportive consultant on the maternal-fetal material. From the staff of The C.V. Mosby Company came the patience and understanding that is seldom deserved by procrastinating authors. Thus it should be known that I appreciated the pleasant, constructive plodding by Barbara Norwitz and the steadfast cooperation of Denise Lawlor, Sally Adkisson, and Connie Leinicke.

Thanks too to Susan Poo.

Sheldon B. Korones

Contents

15 Impact of intensive care on the parent-infant relationship, 407

Jean Lancaster

16 Organization and functions of a neonatal special care facility, 419

HIGH-RISK NEWBORN INFANTS
The basis for intensive nursing care

The fetus

Neonatal disorders, especially those that occur soon after birth, are usually the result of prenatal difficulties. Effective management of these illnesses requires familiarity with the intrauterine events that give rise to them. This chapter is concerned with the important aspects of fetal growth and function and the maternofetal relationships on which they depend.

THE PLACENTA: JUXTAPOSITION OF FETAL AND MATERNAL CIRCULATION

Fundamentally the placenta provides bidirectional passage of substances between the mother and the fetus, whose circulations are contiguous but separate. The placenta is comprised of a maternal contribution called the *decidua basalis* and an embryonic one called the *chorion*. The maternal tissue contains uterine blood vessels, endometrial stroma, and glands; the embryonic tissue is composed of chorionic villi anchored to the chorionic plate.

The placenta (from Latin for "flat cake") is shaped like a round biscuit. At term it is about 15% of the fetal weight, approximately 15 to 20 cm in diameter, and 2.54 cm thick. Throughout pregnancy it occupies approximately one third of the inner surface of the uterus. One side, the fetal surface, is covered by glistening amniotic membrane, which receives the umbilical cord near its center. The opposite side, the maternal surface, remains embedded in the uterine wall until it begins to separate during labor and is extruded during the third stage (Chapter 2). The placenta is composed of 15 to 28 grossly visible segments called *cotyledons* (Fig. 1-1), which are of identical structure and are separated from each other by connective tissue septa. Each cotyledon contains fetal vessels, chorionic villi, and an intervillous space. The dark red color of the placenta is a result of fetal hemoglobin rather than maternal blood, which is usually drained by the time the placenta is delivered. Thus if the placenta appears pale, the fetus was significantly anemic.

Chorionic villi, intervillous space, and placental circulation

Within a week after implantation, the embryo elaborates fingerlike projections of tissue known as the *chorionic villi*, which invade uterine endometrium at the site of implantation. They enlarge and branch considerably, becoming more deeply embedded into uterine tissue as they grow. Each of these projections is ultimately composed of an outer layer of epithelial cells (chorionic epithelium) and a connective tissue core that contains fetal capillaries. During villous invasion of the endometrium, erosion of uterine vessels and supporting tissue occurs, and as a result irregular spaces are formed in the uterine wall.

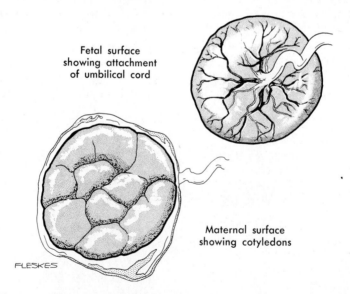

Fetal surface showing attachment of umbilical cord

Maternal surface showing cotyledons

FLESKES

Fig. 1-1. Maternal and fetal surfaces of the placenta. The cotyledons are visible on the maternal surface, which is implanted into the uterine wall. The fetal surface glistens, being covered by amnion. Branches of the umbilical vessels are on the fetal surface. (Modified from Netter: In Oppenheim, E., editor: Ciba collection of medical illustrations, vol. 2, Reproductive system, 1965.)

They are filled with maternal blood and surround the chorionic villi. These consist of the intervillous space, and the exchange of substances between maternal and fetal blood takes place at these sites. Transfer of any given substance from the maternal to the fetal circulation thus requires sequential passage from the mother's blood through the outer epithelial layer of the chorionic villus, through the connective tissue, and then through the endothelial wall of the capillary into fetal blood (Fig. 1-2). As pregnancy progresses, the villi decrease in size but increase considerably in number. This change in both size and number of villi provides a progressive increase in fetal surface area within the placenta for the greater needs of the growing fetus. The villous surface at term is estimated at 13 to 14 m², an area that is ten times greater than the total skin surface of the adult. This enhanced capacity for maternofetal exchange is further implemented by simultaneous thinning of the epithelial layer in the villus and the wells of the fetal capillary within it, thus reducing the distance between fetal capillaries and the intervillous space.

Maternal blood in the intervillous space and fetal blood in the chorionic villi, though separated, function cohesively to exchange gases between mother and fetus, to provide nutrients from mother to fetus, and to transfer waste products from fetus to mother. This spectrum of activity at a single structural site in the placenta is replaced after birth by pulmonary, gastrointestinal, and renal functions in the neonate.

Maternal blood in the uterine arteries enters the base of the *intervillous spaces* through spiral arterioles. At term there are approximately 120 arterioles supplying the placenta at points where they enter the intervillous space at its base. Spurting jets of oxygenated blood diffuse upward and laterally to surround the villi, passing out of the intervillous spaces in a deoxygenated state by way of venous orifices that are also situated at the base of the intervillous space adjacent to the spiral arteries. The direction of blood flow is normally maintained by an arteriovenous pressure gradient, that is, from higher arterial pressure to lower venous pressure (Fig. 1-3). Pressure in the spiral arteries is about 70 to 80 torr. In the draining veins it is 8 torr.

Blood leaves the fetus through two *umbilical arteries* that course through the *umbilical cord* to the placenta. Once they contact the fetal surface of the placenta, the arteries branch to supply each of the cotyledons. After continued branching and diminution in size, the vessels finally terminate in capillary loops within each chorionic villus. Villous blood receives oxygen from the maternal circulation, returns from capillary loops to venules,

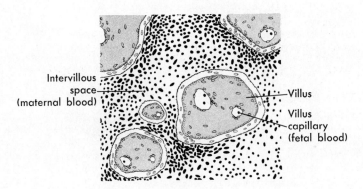

Fig. 1-2. Microscopic appearance of the villi in an intervillous space. Fetal capillaries permeate the villi, which are immersed in maternal blood within the intervillous spaces.

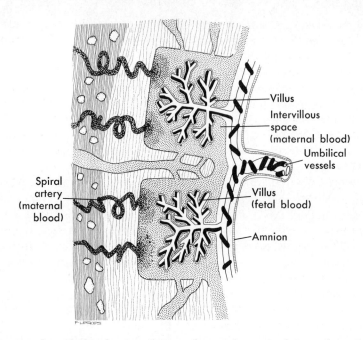

Fig. 1-3. Section through the placenta, showing the spiral arteries that supply maternal blood to the intervillous space, the branching villi immersed in the intervillous space, and the umbilical vessels that branch repeatedly to terminate as villous capillaries. (Modified from Netter: In Oppenheim, E., editor: *Ciba collection of medical illustrations*, vol. 2, *Reproductive system*, 1965.)

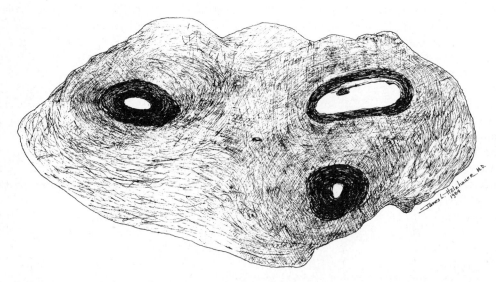

Fig. 1-4. Cross section of umbilical cord. The arteries have thick walls; the lumen of the vein is larger than those of the arteries, and its wall is thin.

and then goes to larger veins that leave each of the placental cotyledons. Coalescence of veins results in the formation of a single *umbilical vein*, which passes from the placenta through the length of the umbilical cord to the body of the fetus. A cross section of the umbilical cord reveals two thick-walled muscular arteries and one vein. The vein is noticeably larger than the arteries, although it has a considerably thinner wall (Fig. 1-4). The umbilical vessels are surrounded by a white gelatinous material called Wharton's jelly.

FETAL CIRCULATION

Two major circuits, pulmonary and systemic, comprise the circulation in the fetus as well as in the adult. A third component, the placental circuit, is peculiar to the fetus. Pulmonary circulation begins at the pulmonic valve at the origin of the main pulmonary artery, which arises from the right ventricle. It continues through the lungs and terminates at the pulmonary vein orifices in the wall of the left atrium. The systemic circulation includes all other arterial and venous channels elsewhere in the body. The placental circuit is composed of the umbilical and placental vessels as described earlier.

In any discussion of circulatory patterns a conceptual subdivision into "right" and "left" sides is often invoked. In the mature individual the right-sided circulation contains venous blood and the left side, arterial blood. Anatomically the right side begins at the venous end of capillary beds in all organs except the lungs. It continues through progressively enlarging veins to the inferior vena cava into the right atrium, to the right ventricle, into the pulmonary arteries, and finally to the pulmonary alveolar capillaries, where oxygenation occurs. Blood now continues on to the left side, which begins at the alveolar capillaries and progresses through the pulmonary veins into the left side of the heart, through the aorta to smaller arteries, and to the arterial side of capillary beds in all organs except the lungs. At the arterial side of the capillaries, blood gives up oxygen and continues to the venous side, where it reenters the right side of the circulation.

The normal mature circulation is characterized by flow of unoxygenated (venous) blood into the right side of the heart, which continues into the pulmonary circuit, where oxygenation occurs, and then returns to the left side of the heart for distribution to the rest of the body by way of the aorta. Thus the only connections between the right and left circulations are at the capillary beds in the lungs and in the capillaries of other organs of the body.

When, as in certain cardiovascular malformations, a connection between the right and left sides exists at sites other than the capillaries, an anatomic shunt is said to be present. Examples of such anomalies are persistent patency of the ductus arteriosus, arteriovenous aneurysm, and numerous malformations of the heart itself. Blood flow through an abnormal vascular channel from the venous to the arterial circulation constitutes a right-to-left shunt. Conversely, flow of blood through an anomalous channel from artery to vein is a left-to-right shunt. In either case blood enters one side of the circulation from the other before reaching the capillary bed for which it is normally destined, and the result is an admixture of oxygenated and deoxygenated blood.

Fetal circulation differs from the neonatal or adult pattern in three major respects: (1) presence of anatomic shunts, one within the heart at the foramen ovale, one immediately outside the heart in the ductus arteriosus, and another at the juncture of the ductus venosus and the inferior vena cava; (2) presence of a placental circulation; and (3) minimal blood flow through the lungs (3% to 7% of cardiac output).

The course of fetal circulation is depicted in Fig. 1-5. (The atria are *inferior* to the ventricles so that the fetal pattern of blood flow can be clearly and simply indicated.) Blood that has been oxygenated in the chorionic villi leaves the placenta through the umbilical vein, which enters the fetal abdomen at the umbilicus and then courses between the right and left lobes of the liver. Some of this blood perfuses the liver through branches of the umbilical vein, whereas the rest continues past it to the ductus venosus and empties into the inferior vena cava at a point just below the diaphragm. Blood now enters the heart through the inferior vena caval orifice, where a direct communication exists between the right and left atria (foramen ovale). Here the caval bloodstream is divided, the major portion flowing directly into the left atrium, whereas the remainder enters the right atrium to join blood from the superior vena cava, which drains the head, neck, and upper extremities. The left atrium also receives blood that has perfused the lungs from pulmonary veins, and this mixture enters successively the left ventricle, the ascending aorta, and the aortic arch, from whence most of it is distributed to the coronary arteries and the vessels of the head and upper extremities.

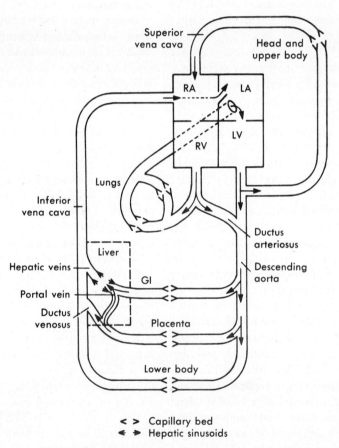

Fig. 1-5. Diagram of the fetal circulatory pathways. A portion of placental blood flows into the inferior vena cava through the ductus venosus, bypassing liver sinusoids. Another portion passes through liver sinusoids and hepatic veins into inferior vena cava. Inferior vena cavae blood flows into right and left atria; dotted arrow in right atrium indicates split flow to both atria. The small return of blood from lungs passes behind the heart into the left atrium. (From Avery, M. E., Fletcher, B. D. and Williams, R. G.: The lung and its disorders in the newborn infant, Philadelphia, 1981, W. B. Saunders Co., p. 38, as redrawn from Rudolph, A. M.: Congenital diseases of the heart, Chicago, 1974, Year Book Medical Publishers, p.1.)

The smaller quantity of blood directed to the right atrium from the inferior vena cava is added to the superior vena caval flow and enters the right ventricle and then the main pulmonary artery. Most of it is conveyed to the descending aorta through the ductus arteriosus. Some continues through the pulmonary circuit to perfuse the lungs and return to the left atrium by way of the pulmonary veins. The descending aorta bifurcates at the lower end of the body into the right and left iliac arteries. The two hypogastric arteries are branches off the latter vessels. They each course upward around the bladder and leave the abdomen through the umbilical cord, where they are called the umbilical arteries.

Admixture of blood occurs at three sites in the fetal circulation: (1) the foramen ovale, (2) from the pulmonary artery to the descending aorta through the ductus arteriosus, and (3) at the junction of the ductus venosus and inferior vena cava.

THE AMNION AND AMNIOTIC FLUID

The amnion and the amniotic cavity develop in the embryo during the first week, appearing as a small elongated sac adjacent to the dorsal embryonic surface. As the fluid-filled cavity enlarges, it spreads around the embryo in all directions and ultimately comes to surround the fetus. This cavity is traversed only by the umbilical cord, which courses from the umbilicus to its insertion into the placenta. The amniotic membrane is 0.5 mm or less in thickness and comprises five microscopic layers. Fully developed, it lines the entire inner surface of the uterine wall, except at the site of placental attachment, where it covers the fetal surface of that organ, reflects onto the umbilical cord, and completely envelops it (Fig. 1-6). The fluid that surrounds the fetus (amniotic fluid) is contained by this membrane, and when the latter ruptures at the onset of labor, the fluid is released.

Amniotic fluid accumulates progressively throughout pregnancy, attaining a volume of approximately 1 L at term (normal range: 400 ml to 1.5 L). It continuously enters and leaves the amniotic cavity in large volumes, creating a constant turnover that involves complex water and solute exchanges. Early in pregnancy, amniotic fluid is derived primarily from the amniotic membrane and probably from the fetus through the fetal skin. At approximately 16 weeks, fetal urine begins to increase the volume of amniotic fluid while fetal swallowing decreases it. Some fluid originates in the fetal lung. Egress of fluid occurs largely by absorption into the fetal bloodstream from the gastrointestinal tract, into which it gains entry as a result of repeated fetal swallowing. At term the fetus is thought to swallow 500 ml per day. Normal volumes of amniotic fluid are largely regulated by contributions of the fetal urinary tract and evac-

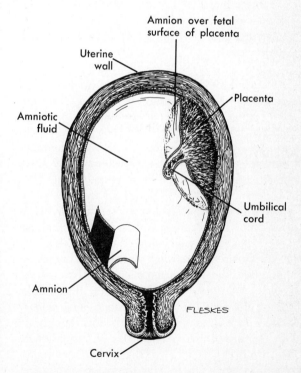

Fig. 1-6. Uterine cavity at term. The amnion lines the uterine wall. It continues over the placenta and reflects from it to envelop the umbilical cord. Amniotic fluid surrounds the fetus to fill the cavity. (Modified from Hillman, L. M., and Pritchard, J. A.; Williams obstetrics, ed. 14, New York, 1971, Appleton-Century-Crofts.)

uation through the gastrointestinal tract. Thus if the elimination of fluid is impaired, the quantity of fluid may be increased abnormally to more than 2 L. This increase is called *hydramnios*. Conversely, if little or no urine is excreted, amniotic fluid may be virtually absent or greatly reduced in quantity. This abnormality is known as *oligohydramnios*.

The elimination of fluid is impaired in any fetus who is unable to swallow, for example, a fetus with gross malformation of the brain (anencephaly, hydrocephalus). Structural obstruction to swallowing of amniotic fluid is also responsible for abnormal accumulations of volume *(hydramnios)*. These obstructions occur in high gastrointestinal malformations such as esophageal atresia and duodenal atresia. Cardiac failure of the fetus occurs in hydrops fetalis, which is also associated with hydramnios.

Hydramnios has been reported in normal fetuses who were calculated to have swallowed 700 to 800 ml of amniotic fluid in 24 hours. Presumably, then, overproduction of amniotic fluid occurred for reasons that were not identified. In contrast, three anencephalic fetuses with hydramnios were observed to have swallowed only 9, 10, and 13 ml of amniotic fluid, respectively. Thus while impairment of swallowing is accountable for a considerable number of fetuses with hydramnios, the overaccumulation of amniotic fluid can occur in the presence of normal swallowing.

If impaired swallowing restricts the outflow of amniotic fluid, obstructed micturition severely restricts the inflow. Oligohydramnios thus results from obstructed fetal micturition. Fetal urinary contribution to amniotic fluid is thus diminished or eliminated in renal agenesis or dysplasia and in urethral obstruction. Oligohydramnios (unassociated with urinary tract obstruction) is a frequent occurrence in postmaturity and fetal death.

Amniotic fluid affords a milieu that allows relatively free fetal movement. It protects the fetus from externally inflicted trauma, and it contributes to the stability of fetal body temperature. During early labor, hydrostatic forces created by uterine contractions are mediated by the fluid to aid in normal dilatation of the cervix and descent of the fetus.

MATERNOFETAL EXCHANGE OF GAS ACROSS THE PLACENTA

The placenta has a number of critical functions, but perhaps the most sensitive of all is its role as the fetus' lung. The juxtaposition of maternal and fetal circulations at the placental site, with separation of each circulatory unit by a relatively thin membrane, provides the structural basis for exchange of gases between mother and fetus. The diffusion of gases across placental membranes is similar to gas diffusion across cellular membranes in any other organ of the body. Although the placenta functions as a lung for the fetus, the obvious and fundamental difference is that it accommodates the exchange of gases from one individual's circulation to another. The placenta is not as efficient as the lung, yet it is effective for this purpose; gas diffusion in the placenta is only one fiftieth as efficient as in the postnatal lung.

Fetal respiration occurs by transfer of oxygen from maternal blood in the intervillous space to fetal blood in the villous capillaries and by release of carbon dioxide in the opposite direction from fetus to mother. The flow of these gases depends on their respective partial pressures in maternal and fetal blood and by unimpeded fetal and maternal blood flow in the placenta for maintenance of normal pressure relationships.

Gases have a tendency to expand, and they exert measurable pressure in the process. This pressure is expressed in torr (mm Hg). Thus pressure exerted by gases in the atmosphere at sea level is 760 torr. In any mixture of two or more gases, the pressure exerted by each of them is called their *partial pressure*. The sum of the partial pressures of each constituent gas in a mixture is the total pressure exerted by that mixture. The expression symbolizing partial pressure of a gas is written P preceding its chemical formula. The partial pressures of oxygen and of carbon dioxide are written as PO_2 and PCO_2. (This terminology is utilized routinely in reports from clinical and research laboratories.)

Assuming normal placental blood flow, the differences in the partial pressures of gases (PO_2, PCO_2) that exist between maternal and fetal blood determine the direction in which these gases move. Gases are transferred in response to pressure gradients, that is, from a higher pressure to a lower one. Tissues intervening between the maternal and fetal circulations (normally 3.5 to 5.5 μm in total thickness) seem to offer more resistance to the movement of oxygen than to carbon dioxide; the diffusion rate of carbon dioxide is 20 times greater than that of oxygen. Table 1-1 gives PO_2 and PCO_2 values of fetal blood in the umbilical artery, maternal blood in the intervillous space, and fetal blood in the umbilical vein as reported by a number of investigators. The acquisition of oxygen and the surrender of carbon dioxide by fetal blood are indicated in the alterations of PO_2 and PCO_2 that result from the exchange of gases with maternal blood in the intervillous space. The influence of partial pressure gradients can be appreciated by noting, in Table 1-1, that a higher maternal PO_2 in the intervillous space moves oxygen into the fetal circulation to raise PO_2 from 16 torr in the umbilical artery to 29 torr in blood returning to the fetus by way of the umbilical vein. The flow of oxygen is therefore from mother to fetus. The direction of carbon dioxide transfer is from fetus to mother because PCO_2 in the intervillous space (38 torr in maternal blood) is lower than in the umbilical artery (46 torr in fetal blood); thus carbon dioxide moves from fetus to mother with a resultant diminution of PCO_2 in the umbilical vein (42 torr) compared with that in the umbilical artery (46 torr).

Maintenance of these pressure gradients depends on normal maternal blood gas levels and normal blood flow in the placenta.

During labor, contractions increase intrauterine pressure, and placental blood flow diminishes. Possibly as a compensatory device during contractions, blood volume is increased in the intervillous space to make more blood available for gas

Table 1-1. Mean quantitative changes in fetal blood gases resulting from fetomaternal exchange*

	PO_2 (torr)	PCO_2 (torr)
Umbilical artery (blood from fetus)	16	46
Intervillous space (maternal blood)	40	38
Umbilical vein (blood to fetus)	29	42

*Based on data from Seeds, A. E.: Pediatr. Clin. North Am. **17**:811, 1970.

exchange. Accumulation of blood results from greater compression of the veins that drain the intervillous space than the spiral arteries that supply it. Veins are more readily compressed than arteries because their walls are thinner. This phenomenon theoretically minimizes impairment of gas exchange during contractions. Normal exchange of gases resumes during intervals of uterine relaxation. Experimental data from rhesus monkeys and sheep indicate that the decrement in placental perfusion is almost proportional to the magnitude of increased amniotic fluid pressure during a contraction. Diminished placental blood flow impedes the rate of maternofetal gas exchange; impaired fetal oxygenation is the most significant result of this phenomenon. Clinical observations in humans indicate that intact fetal survival during labor seems to depend on a balance between the forces generated by uterine contractions to expel the fetus, and the extent to which placental blood flow (and oxygen transfer) is interrupted by these forces. The normal fetus apparently tolerates the changes in blood flow that occur during contractions, but if uteroplacental perfusion is marginal or insufficient (as in maternal hypertension or other maternal vascular diseases), contractions may precipitate fetal distress.

A number of disorders other than maternal hypertension may hamper gas exchange at the intervillous space. Thus severe pneumonia, asthma, congestive heart failure, and apnea during convulsions (epilepsy, eclampsia) may result in maternal hypoxemia that endangers the fetus. Impairment of blood flow to the intervillous space may occur as a consequence of maternal shock or congestive heart failure. Local impediment to placental perfusion may result from abnormally intense and frequent uterine contractions during labor or from compression of the inferior vena cava by the overlying heavy uterus when the mother is supine (supine hypotension syndrome).

FETAL GROWTH

Growth is constant from the embryonic period to approximately 36 gestational weeks. Daily increment in weight is greatest between 32 and 36 weeks. Afterward, weight gain continues but at a diminished rate, presumably as a function of limited uterine size and diminished effectiveness of the placenta in the transmission of nutriment to the fetus. After the neonate's loss of extracellular fluid during the several days that follow birth, weight gain resumes to approximate the intrauterine rate.

Growth of the fetus involves an increase in the number of cells (hyperplasia) and an increase in their size (hypertrophy). Growth progresses through three stages: (1) hyperplasia, (2) hyperplasia and hypertrophy, and (3) predominant hypertrophy. Embryonic growth is largely hyperplastic; hypertrophy becomes increasingly prominent later in pregnancy. Growth may be impeded during any or all of these progressive stages, resulting in different types of growth failure. Thus the number of cells may be diminished, although their size remains relatively normal, cell size rather than quantity may be reduced, or both size and number may be diminished. The net result is subnormal size and weight of affected organs. These effects depend on the stage of growth during which an insult is inflicted. For example, intrauterine rubella infection, which occurs early in pregnancy, produces a severe reduction in the quantity of cells in many organs. On the other hand, the effects of toxemia, which often appear

late in pregnancy, are characterized by a significant reduction in cell size, although cell number is relatively normal. All these changes have been produced in pregnant animals that were starved at various stages of pregnancy. Interference with cellular proliferation (hyperplastic growth) may cause a permanent diminution in the quantity of cells, although impaired hypertrophy is apparently reversible to some extent if proper feeding is instituted after birth. There is evidence that these phenomena may also be operative in humans. The human brain continues to grow by cellular proliferation (hyperplasia) for at least 8 postnatal months after 40 gestational weeks. Postnatal malnutrition impairs this process. Data from animal studies and clinical observations of human infants suggest that permanent limitation of growth does indeed occur.

The characteristics of normal cellular growth are of importance in understanding the abnormalities of birth weight and size that are peculiar to prematurity and intrauterine growth retardation. A more detailed discussion of fetal growth is presented in Chapter 5.

EVALUATION OF FETAL STATUS

During the past two to three decades, techniques for assessment of fetal health have revealed a number of fetal attributes that previously could only be identified after birth. Before the 1960s, perinatal loss and fetal health attracted little professional concern; according to the traditional view, "it was meant to be" or "you can have another." In recent years the capacity to define several important parameters of fetal well-being has changed all that; the fetus is now a patient. The state of fetal health can be usefully estimated. Before the late 1960s, for example, cardiac status was barely surmised by applying a stethoscope to the maternal abdomen. Now fetal cardiac activity can be demonstrated intrapartum and antepartum during moments of fetal movement or during mild uterine contractions. Heart rate patterns warn of fetal incapacity to withstand labor or of marginally adequate oxygenation that may progress to severe distress. For a number of years fetal assessment has also entailed quantitative determinations of certain components of amniotic fluid for the diagnosis of genetic disorders, for the estimation of the severity of maternofetal blood incompatibility, and for the determination of levels of surfactant to assess pulmonary maturity. Ultrasound techniques have put the fetus in direct view so that fetal maturity can be estimated, gross malformations identified, abnormal growth patterns revealed, and placental location delineated. Using ultrasound, needle placement during amniocentesis is in direct view of the operator. Antepartum procedures have now broken through the myometrial barrier; the signs of impaired fetal health have become increasingly demonstrable.

During labor, fetal assessment largely depends on electronic fetal heart rate monitoring and sampling of fetal blood from the scalp for pH determinations. The following discussions present reliable procedures for intrapartum and antepartum assessment of fetal health.

Intrapartum assessment of fetal status: electronic fetal heart rate monitoring

The advent of fetal heart rate monitoring is a historic milestone that was largely responsible for an awakened interest in fetal assessment and for stimulating the development of maternal-fetal medicine as a designated subspecialty. Fetal heart rate monitoring during labor is now so pervasive that in the United States delivery suites are considered inadequately equipped if a fetal heart rate monitor is not in place. Even though there is persistent dissension among a few thoughtful investigators who question the real value of fetal heart rate monitoring during labor, most are convinced that monitoring has diminished the incidence of adverse fetal outcomes. Fetal heart rate monitoring identifies distress that is otherwise imperceptible. Some day intrapartum monitoring will be unnecessary, but only when precise antepartum assessment can identify with certainty all those fetuses whose intact survival will be

threatened by parturition. Antepartum procedures are not yet that precise, nor do they have the capacity to identify all fetuses at risk. Opinions also differ in regard to the type of pregnancy for which intrapartum monitoring is appropriate. Some contend that all patients should be monitored during labor; others would limit monitoring to specific disorders that are known to be associated with suboptimal outcomes.

That labor is a stressful experience even to normal fetuses has been appreciated for a number of years, but a normal fetus has the wherewithal to emerge unscathed and to recover rapidly. In contrast, an unhealthy fetus may become asphyxiated during normal labor.

Fetal oxygenation is crucial. It depends on several factors, principally uteroplacental and umbilical blood flow, maternal oxygenation, and the avid affinity of intact fetal erythrocytes for oxygen. Alteration of uteroplacental blood flow is the most frequent cause of fetal hypoxia. Electronic heart rate monitoring reveals the cardiac responses that are characteristic of hypoxic stress and thus identifies the fetus who is in jeopardy.

Fetal heart rate monitoring during labor provides continuous displays of cardiac activity on one channel of a recorder, and uterine motility on the other. The most reliable method entails placement of a spiral metal electrode into the fetal scalp to record cardiac activity, and transcervical insertion of an intrauterine catheter to record pressure changes generated by contraction and relaxation of the uterus. This direct monitoring procedure requires ruptured membranes and some degree of cervical dilatation. The procedure is thus invasive. It is an *internal* modality for recording fetal heart rate and uterine contractions simultaneously. *External methods* are alternatively utilized, but they are less informative. During external monitoring of fetal cardiac activity, ECG electrodes are placed on the maternal abdomen. The mother's cardiac activity is obliterated electronically; the resultant record demonstrates greater detail of fetal cardiac activity than any other external device. External recording of uterine activities is feasible with a tocodynamometer. This device is strapped onto the maternal abdominal wall; it responds to the periodic tightness generated by contractions. Resultant recordings reveal the frequency and duration of contractions, but they cannot quantitate pressure changes. Another disadvantage of the tocodynamometer is the supine position that is required for its fixation to the abdomen.

Components and configurations of fetal heart rate patterns. The internal (direct) fetal heart monitor records rate and rhythm of the fetal heart beat and the frequency and quantitative intensity of uterine contractions. These two tracings are recorded simultaneously; a temporal relationship between cardiac and uterine activities is then interpreted from the resultant recording. Continuous tracings display "baseline fetal heart rate," which indicates cardiac activity between uterine contractions as well as episodic (periodic) variations that indicate cardiac activity during uterine contractions *(early or late deceleration)* or in response to compression of the umbilical cord *(variable deceleration)*. Furthermore, *heart rate variability* is critically significant in all these patterns of cardiac activity.

Baseline fetal heart rate. Normal fetal heart rate varies between 120 and 160 beats per minute *when the uterus is not in contraction*. The rate often swings between these two limits with a tendency toward sustained higher rates in the more immature fetus. When these limits are violated for less than two minutes the temporary change is called an "acceleration" (increased rate) or a "deceleration" (diminished rate). Baseline fetal heart rate changes include tachycardia (over 160 beats per minute) or bradycardia (less than 120 beats per minute).

Tachycardia is most frequently associated with maternal fever. Occasionally, in the presence of chorioamnionitis, fetal tachycardia precedes the appearance of maternal fever. Drugs such as parasympathetic blocking agents (atropine) or sympathomimetic agents (ritodrine) increase heart rate by disrupting the balance between parasym-

pathetic and sympathetic control of cardiac activity. Parasympathetic blockers impede impulses of the vagus nerve. Cardiac rate thus increases because parasympathetic activity is depressed and sympathetic activity predominates. Sympathomimetic drugs such as ritodrine or epinephrine cause an increased rate by imitation of sympathetic nerve activity. Maternal *hyperthyroidism* also causes fetal tachycardia.

Extreme fetal tachycardia (200 to 300 beats per minute) may be paroxysmal or sustained. It is usually attributable to *supraventricular tachycardia*. Persistence of these extreme elevations may lead to cardiac failure and fetal hydrops.

Tachycardia may be associated with chronic hypoxia. Gradually developing fetal distress is widely recognized as a serious cause of elevated baseline heart rate in which decreased heart rate variability occurs uniformly (see below). Transient tachycardia may be observed during recovery from acute fetal distress that itself was associated with bradycardia before recovery. This form of transient tachycardia is associated with diminished variability.

Fetal movements are frequently associated with transient accelerations in heart rate. Sustained fetal activity may be associated with protracted elevation of baseline heart rate. In such circumstances, heart rate variability may be increased or unchanged, rather than decreased as in the case of chronic hypoxia.

Bradycardia is most often the first response of the fetus to abrupt onset of hypoxemia. This is a reflex bradycardia caused by increased vagal nerve activity resulting from hypoxemic stimulation of chemoreceptors in the wall of the aortic arch. This type of bradycardia appears suddenly and is usually associated with normal or occasionally increased variability. Recognition and remedy of the cause of acute hypoxemia (supine hypotension syndrome, for example) is followed by restoration of a normal heart rate pattern. These are the situations in which rebound tachycardia (see above) often follows recovery from acute hypoxemia.

The most sinister causes of bradycardia are late manifestations of chronic hypoxemia or, occasionally, persistence of acute onset hypoxemia. The myocardium is hypoxic; reflex slowing of the heart as described previously is not operative. Baseline rate falls below 100 beats per minute and variability is absent or diminished. The heart rate tracing loses its normal serrated configuration; now it is a flat line or it may barely wiggle. Fetuses so affected are usually hypotensive and extremely acidotic.

Beta-adrenergic blocking agents such as maternally administered propranolol may produce diminished fetal heart rate by depressing sympathetic activity and thus allowing predominance of vagal (parasympathetic) activity. Paracervical block, using a local anesthetic, is a well-known cause of bradycardia. Two mechanisms are postulated. Most often, uterine vasoconstriction occurs in response to injection of the local anesthetic. Diminished placental perfusion produces abrupt onset hypoxemia and reflex bradycardia. Less frequently, a high fetal blood level of the anesthetic agent depresses myocardial activity directly. High fetal blood levels may occur whether or not inadvertent direct injection into the fetus occurred during the paracervical block procedure.

Sustained bradycardia occurs in congenital heart block. Congenital cardiac anomalies are frequent when the heart block is complete, infrequent in the presence of milder forms (first or second degree) of heart block.

Fetal heart rate variability. The interval between each heart beat of the normal fetus varies constantly. The usual cardiac monitor used for intensive neonatal care "averages out" these differing intervals and simply displays a rate in beats per minute. In reality, when measured from the peak of one R wave to the next, the intervals between each pair of beats are of differing duration. When the heart rate is calculated separately from each of these intervals, the result is a change in the calculated rate in beats per minute, based on the duration of each interval. These differing intervals are seen on a tracing in a sawtooth configuration that indicates beats per minute. When the line rises, the calculated heart rate has increased for that *isolated interval*. When the line falls slightly, the calculated heart rate for the succeeding interval has decreased slightly. The interval between the first pair of beats was shorter than the second; based on that one interval between R waves, calculated rate in beats per minute was greater than the second interval. The shorter the interval between R waves, the higher the calculated rate in beats per minute for that particular interval. These differences from one electronically indicated heart beat to the next are called "beat-to-beat variability" or "short-term variability." When a tracing is unwavering, having lost its sawtooth configuration, beat-to-beat variability has disappeared.

The second type of ongoing variation in heart rate is called *long-term variability*. It is measured by changes in the calculated rate over a one-minute period, rather than the single interval between adjacent R waves. Long-term variability is characterized by changes in rate that occur two to six times per minute. These changes may range in magnitude from 5 to 15 beats per minute. Long-term variability is seen as an undulating line that rises and falls. The tracing produced by combined short-term and long-term variabilities is a serrated line that rises and falls recurrently several times each minute.

Early deceleration. Early deceleration produces a wave form that is a mirror image of the rising wave form caused by elevations in intrauterine pressure during contractions. Early decelerations are seen in a uniform repetitive U-shaped pattern (Fig. 1-7). Diminished heart rate occurs simultaneously with increased intrauterine pressure. The nadir of the heart rate tracing corresponds temporally to the peak of the intrauterine pressure tracing. Heart rate slowing is usually commensurate with the force of uterine contraction. The fetal heart rate rarely declines below 110 beats per minute. Early decelerations are observed only with cephalic presentations, and they

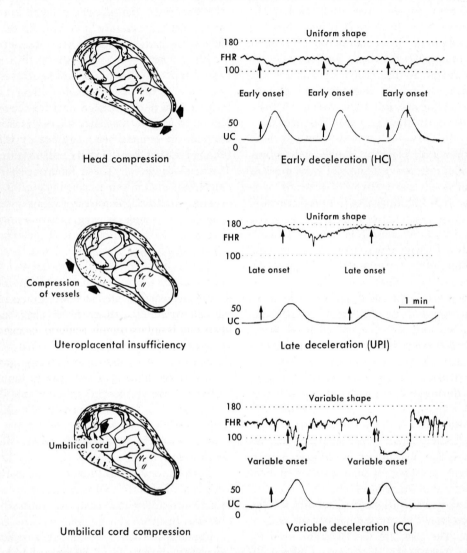

Fig. 1-7. The three major patterns of decelerated fetal heart rates. Note the relationship of onset and end of bradycardia to increased intrauterine pressures (contractions). *FHR,* Fetal heart rate; *UC,* uterine contraction; *HC,* head compression; *UPI,* uteroplacental insufficiency; *CC,* cord compression. See text for full explanation. (From Hon, E.H.: An introduction to fetal heart rate monitoring, Los Angeles, 1973, University of Southern California Press.)

appear characteristically after cervical dilatation approaches 6 or 7 cm. These decrements in fetal heart rate are believed to be associated with head compression during uterine contractions. The resultant rise in fetal intracranial pressure transiently diminishes perfusion to the brain. The reflexes that ensue apparently cause parasympathetic (vagus) overactivity. The result is a slowing of the fetal heart rate. The totally reflex nature of these decelerations is suggested by experimental data in which slowed rates were prevented by injection of atropine, thereby blocking impulses from the vagus nerve. Early accelerations are not associated with fetal or neonatal morbidity, or with alterations in fetal blood pH that might indicate distress (acidosis). This pattern is considered a normal response to uterine contractions. The hallmark of the early deceleration is its occurrence in synchrony with the elevation of intrauterine pressure.

Late deceleration. The configuration of the late deceleration tracing is identical to that described for early deceleration, that is, heart rate decreases and intrauterine pressure increases, but the timing differs. Late deceleration in heart rate occurs 10 to 30 seconds after onset of elevated pressure from uterine contractions. The peak of the uterine contraction curve appears a number of seconds prior to the trough of the fetal heart rate deceleration. Late decelerations occur with each uterine contraction. The extent of decrement in rate corresponds to the intensity of uterine contractions. Late decelerations may be of *reflex* origin or they may occur as a result of *direct myocardial hypoxia*. The latter is a sinister sign of fetal difficulty. In either category, late decelerations are indicative of fetal hypoxia resulting from diminished placental blood flow during uterine contractions. The effect of diminished placental perfusion on fetal heart rate is mediated by the resultant decline in fetal arterial oxygen tension. The delayed appearance of heart rate deceleration reflects the time interval between uterine contraction and the decline in arterial oxygen tension. Correspondingly, the delayed restitution of normal heart rate

reflects the time period between relaxation of the uterus, increased placental perfusion, and restoration of normal arterial oxygen tension. Late decelerations of reflex origin, while indicative of temporary fetal distress during uterine contractions, are considerably less troublesome than the decelerations that result from myocardial hypoxia. The patterns that indicate reflex origin are characterized by persistence of fetal heart rate variability, at least during intervals of uterine relaxation. In most instances heart rate variability is retained during the period of deceleration as well. The fetal stress of late decelerations that are of reflex origin are often remediable by change in maternal position when supine hypotension syndrome is identified, or by administration of 100% oxygen to the mother through a tightly fitted mask. Reflex late deceleration is also associated with the administration of excessive oxytocin. It may thus be relieved by curtailing or eliminating its use. The fetus with late decelerations and a normal variability pattern in the baseline fetal heart rate is not extremely acidotic, or may in fact have a normal scalp pH.

Late decelerations associated with myocardial hypoxia are more ominous than reflex late decelerations. This pattern is caused by hypoxic depression of myocardial activity as well as the reflex mechanism previously described. It occurs in fetuses who are marginally oxygenated or who have experienced prolonged distress. These are the fetuses who cannot tolerate normal labor. These circumstances are most often encountered in the presence of maternal vascular disease and placental insufficiency.

Late decelerations of either variety indicate abnormal gas exchanged in the maternal-placental-fetal unit. The problem may be acute and remediable as in the reflex type, or it may be chronic and life-threatening as in myocardial hypoxia. Fundamentally a reduction has occurred in intervillous blood flow to a level that the fetus can tolerate because fetal hypoxia has supervened. The fetal heart rate tracing therefore detects a sign of illness that has its origin in a variety of maternofetal abnormalities. The fetus is a patient in whom abnormal cardiac activity has been identified electronically and then interpreted clinically as a serious sign of illness.

Variable deceleration. Variable deceleration is more frequently encountered during labor than any other type of deviation from baseline heart rate patterns. It has been observed in approximately 50% of fetal monitoring records. These decelerations are regularly characterized by a dip in fetal heart rate, but this is the only characteristic common to all of them. They vary considerably in duration, extent, and configuration. Most begin and end abruptly, and they are unrelated to uterine contractions. Variable decelerations are due to cord compression. Abrupt decline from and restoration to normal heart rates within a short period of time probably indicates a reflex origin. Deceleration thus occurs in response to parasympathetic activity that some believe is a direct result of cord compression. Others have postulated that the placenta receives almost 50% of total fetal blood volume, and that compression of the cord diminishes flow to the placental circuit, increasing fetal blood volume and raising blood pressure. The resultant stimulation of baroreceptors releases vagal discharge to abruptly slow the heart rate.

Variable decelerations entail a broad spectrum of clinical significance. When decelerations of reflex origin occur in an otherwise normal fetus, the short episodes of cord compression are of little consequence. The benign nature of these changes can be ascertained by observing that baseline heart rate and variability are preserved despite abrupt changes in cardiac rate. Variable decelerations are sometimes signs of existing or impending severe asphyxia. Compression of the cord alters maternofetal gas exchange to some extent however momentary the disruption may be; the fetus may be endangered when these episodes occur with excessive frequency or if they are protracted. Oxygen deprivation and accumulation of CO_2 are then inevitable. Evidence of fetal distress is observed in diminution or loss of heart rate variability, acceleration in baseline heart rate during intervals between decelerations, or by gradual rather than abrupt onset of decreased heart rate associated with a slow return to normal. Furthermore, when marginal oxygenation from deficient placental perfusion preexists, recurrent and protracted variable decelerations impose sufficient fetal jeopardy to warrant rapid obstetric intervention. The administration of oxygen to the mother and changes in her position are of no avail in eliminating variable decelerations.

Complications of fetal heart rate monitoring. Several complications of direct invasive fetal heart rate monitoring have been recorded, including maternal infection, neonatal infection, and maternal and neonatal soft tissue injury.

The status of maternal infection as a complication of invasive fetal heart rate monitoring is controversial. Although it is logical to expect that an invasive catheter that is passed into the uterine cavity through a contaminated field is likely to introduce infection in at least some instances, the variables that have influenced outcomes of numerous studies have precluded clear conclusions. Thus maternal infection during direct monitoring is also influenced by such factors as the length of membrane rupture, cesarean section, predisposal to infection, and high risk for any reason. Numerous published studies have differed so widely in their conclusions that it is impossible to be certain that monitoring causes a significant increase in the incidence of maternal infection.

The risk of neonatal infection is real but small. The most common site of infection is the scalp, as might be expected, from invasive attachment of an electrode. The most common implicated organisms are *Escherichia coli* and group B β-hemolytic *Streptococcus*. The incidence of scalp abscesses varies among a number of reports from 0.1% to 5.4%. These infections are not usually serious. However, a few serious infections have been reported, such as osteomyelitis of the skull and septicemia. Usually these have been caused by group B β-hemolytic *Streptococcus* organisms.

Maternal soft tissue injury is largely restricted to uterine perforation and its sequelae. The incidence of this complication is not known, but the possibility of occurrence is real. Uterine perforation may be asymptomatic, but on the other hand, intraperitoneal bleeding and abscess have been reported. An infected hematoma of the broad ligament has also been observed.

Fetal and neonatal hemorrhage from the scalp has been noted on several occasions. Significant bleeding from the scalp following the laceration of an artery during the insertion of the needle has been observed. Additionally, bleeding may occur from the scalp of a fetus or neonate in the presence of an inherited or acquired coagulation defect. Thus bleeding is possible in a fetus or infant whose mother has or has had thrombocytopenic purpura. It is also possible in infants who are at risk for inherited coagulation defects (hemophilia). Invasive fetal heart rate monitoring should be avoided when family history indicates the possibility of a bleeding diathesis. The inadvertent attachment of a scalp electrode at inappropriate sites has also occurred occasionally. Electrodes have been applied to an eyelid and to a posterior fontanelle with drainage of cerebrospinal fluid from the site of attachment for 3 days.

The incidence of all these complications is low. In some instances they are the result of ineptness of the operator. In other instances, such as fetal infections, they are probably unavoidable.

Fetal scalp pH for intrapartum assessment of fetal status

The technique of sampling and the parameters for interpretation of fetal blood pH were introduced in the 1960s at about the same time that electronic fetal heart rate monitoring was described. The two procedures combined probably represent the best methods available for intrapartum estimation of fetal health. Fetal blood sampling is complementary and supplementary to heart rate monitoring. It is indicated in a variety of clinical circumstances, all of which are likely to be associated with fetal hypoxia.

Fetal acid-base balance and blood gas content depend on the status of gas exchange across the placenta. When fetal-placental exchange is disrupted for any reason, blood oxygen tension falls, carbon dioxide tension rises, and pH falls. Usually, disruption of gas exchange is the result of inadequate placental blood flow. The disorders most frequently associated with diminished placental perfusion are preeclampsia, maternal hypotension due to supine hypotension syndrome, hemorrhage, anesthesia, umbilical cord compression, and hyperactive uterine contractions in response to excessive use of oxytocin. The decline in pH is a consequence of fetal attempts to maintain energy needs by metabolizing glycogen to glucose in hypoxic circumstances. Thus the validity of pH determination is based on the biochemical changes that occur in response to fetal hypoxia. In the presence of oxygen deprivation, anaerobic metabolism of glucose supervenes and lactic acid production increases considerably. The result is metabolic acidosis (a lowered pH). Appearance of metabolic acidosis is the ultimate biochemical expression of significant hypoxia. It has been reasoned, therefore, that a low pH usually suggests significant fetal hypoxia. These changes can be demonstrated and usefully applied to fetal management during labor by sampling capillary blood from the presenting fetal part, usually the scalp. The pH, rather than the blood gas content, has been found to correlate with intrauterine status and with the infant's condition at birth because blood gas changes have a tendency to be transient. Several studies have established the comparability of fetal capillary blood pH with that of the umbilical vessels; the collection of capillary blood from the presenting part is thus a valid sampling procedure. The technique is simple, and undesirable side effects are infrequent. Excessive bleeding from the scalp may rarely occur in utero and postnatally as well, requiring sutures to the incision after birth. Compression of the collection site usually controls bleeding. Scalp abscess has also been reported as a complication.

Fetal blood pH is normal when it is above 7.25,

abnormal when it is below 7.20. Between 7.20 and 7.25 the possibility of progressive acidosis is likely. This must be explored with repeated samples at intervals of 20 to 60 minutes.

Maternal acidosis influences fetal pH significantly. A fetal pH below 7.20 may be the direct result of maternal acidosis rather than fetal hypoxia. It is thus important to determine the acid-base status of the mother simultaneously with the fetal blood pH. Low maternal pH is a consequence of protracted labor and inadequate fluid therapy. Acidosis in the mother may be asymptomatic, yet produce fetal pH below 7.20. Maternal alkalosis from hyperventilation during labor may mitigate the fall in pH that would otherwise occur with fetal hypoxia.

In the presence of normal fetal heart rate tracings, blood sampling is of no value. A normal heart rate pattern indicates a healthy fetus in virtually all who are monitored. There are few diagnostic procedures of greater validity, and there is thus no need for further pursuit of evidence of pathology. On the other hand, abnormal fetal heart rate tracings leave much to be desired insofar as specificity is concerned. They often occur in normal fetuses. A considerable number of infants are delivered in vigorous condition, their abnormal tracings notwithstanding. Verification of the difficulty suggested by abnormal tracings, and assessment of its extent, are often feasible with determinations of fetal blood pH.

Antepartum assessment of fetal status: electronic fetal heart responsiveness

A substantial interest in antepartum evaluation of fetal cardiac activity became apparent in the early 1970s. Emphasis was placed on the assessment of fetal heart rate patterns in response to artificially induced uterine contractions. Oxytocin was generally used for this purpose. The test was known as the oxytocin challenge test (OCT), and was later renamed the contraction stress test (CST). Several years later it became apparent that nonstress testing was a promising alternative to the contraction stress test. Impetus for nonstress

testing came from the observation that in healthy fetuses, movement was regularly associated with acceleration of heart rate. Cardiac accelerations associated with fetal movements in the nonstressed state were subsequently reported to be as efficacious in identifying a healthy fetus as the oxytocin challenge test had been. Since that time a number of studies have evaluated cardiac accelerations, fetal movements, and several other responses in the nonstressed state. The nonstress test has therefore virtually replaced the oxytocin challenge test as a primary procedure for antepartum assessment of fetal health. The oxytocin challenge test requires a hospital setting with the administration of intravenous solutions and oxytocin, as well as well-trained personnel for close observation during the procedure. On the other hand, the nonstress test is simple and noninvasive. It can be staged in the obstetrician's office. As with so many other antepartum and intrapartum diagnostic procedures, the nonstress test is an excellent predictor of favorable outcome in healthy fetuses, but identification of the sick fetus is often equivocal. The oxytocin challenge test is currently recommended only when results of nonstress testing suggest that the fetus is other than normal. The oxytocin challenge test is therefore appropriate for a small percentage of all patients who require antepartum fetal heart rate assessment. Some investigators are convinced that the oxytocin challenge test has no place in antepartum fetal assessment.

The nonstress test. The nonstress test records the reaction of the fetal heart to fetal movement, and occasionally to spontaneous uterine contractions. It detects the fetal capacity to increase heart rate in response to muscular movement. A reactive heart is one in which the rate increases in association with fetal movement. The nonreactive heart is one that does not accelerate or accelerates poorly and infrequently during fetal body movements. The nonstress test also records the frequency of fetal movements with or without accelerations of heart beat. Results are classified as *reactive* (normal healthy fetus), *nonreactive* (abnormal, potential fetal distress), or *suspicious* (neither normal nor abnormal with certainty). The quantitative criteria by which these categorizations are established have varied from one study to another. The variations in criteria involve duration of observation, number of fetal movements within a defined time frame, the number of accelerative episodes, and the number of beats per minute during the acceleration.

In most instances, a test of 20 to 40 minutes duration is recommended. The fetus is classified as *reactive* if a minimum of four fetal movements have been demonstrated within 20 minutes and heart rate has increased at least 10 beats per minute. The baseline heart rate should be within the normal range, and some investigators believe that the amplitude of long-term variability should be at least 10 beats per minute. The record of a *nonreactive* fetus indicates no fetal movement and no increase in heart rate during the period of observation. Long-term variability is considerably diminished or absent; the baseline heart rate may or may not be outside of the normal limits. The results of nonstress testing are classified as *suspicious* when there is fetal movement, but fewer than four episodes are observed in the 20 minutes of testing, or if acceleration of the heart is consistently less than 10 beats per minute.

A *reactive* test indicates a 99% chance of fetal survival within the week following the test. A *nonreactive* pattern is not as specifically predictive as the reactive one. Studies on the outcome of fetuses with nonreactive patterns are hampered by a compelling necessity to intervene with additional tests and active treatment when indicated. In most instances the fetus with a nonreactive pattern will survive labor, but the incidence of abnormal outcomes is considerably greater.

The procedure entails placement of the mother in a recumbent position with the left hip elevated. This may be accommodated in a reclining chair for comfort, either in the hospital or in the office. A heart monitor is attached to the maternal abdomen: fetal activity is perceived by the mother and recorded electronically or by an observer who is standing by. Studies on the accuracy of maternal identification of fetal movements indicate that the mother is correct in identifying approximately 85% of movements recorded electronically. The temporally related recording of fetal heart rate and fetal movement is then analyzed for one of the three diagnostic categories.

A reactive result requires repeat nonstress testing weekly thereafter. If the test is nonreactive, an oxytocin challenge test may be recommended. The suspicious record must be evaluated again within 24 hours, utilizing another nonstress test or an oxytocin challenge test.

Contraction stress test (CST) (oxytocin challenge test [OCT]). A contraction stress test is indicated in a small percentage of antepartum patients who require fetal heart rate assessment. This test is generally used for fetuses whose cardiac activity was unequivocally nonreactive during a nonstress test.

The test is based solely on the fetal cardiac reaction to uterine contractions. During actual labor a uterine contraction decreases blood flow in the intervillous space. If placental reserve is adequate, a normal fetus will not be stressed significantly, since diminished blood flow in the intervillous space does not impair oxygen supply. The fetal heart rate patterns will thus be normal. If, however, placental circulation is marginal or impaired in the resting state, decreased blood flow in the intervillous space during uterine contractions will diminish fetal oxygen supply. The resultant stress is reflected in a fetal heart rate pattern of *late deceleration*.

The oxytocin challenge test imposes conditions on the fetus that are similar to labor by stimulating a series of uterine contractions with oxytocin. During the procedure, fetal heart heart is recorded externally for 15 to 30 minutes in the maternal resting state. Oxytocin is then administered intravenously to the mother at a constant rate of approximately 0.5 mU/min, after which it is gradually increased until three firm uterine contractions occur within 10 minutes. The test is *positive* (indicating impending fetal danger during labor) if at least two episodes of *late deceleration* are produced. The test is *negative* (normal) if the fetal heart rate is stable and there is no evidence of deceleration.

If the test is *negative*, one may be assured that in 99% of patients tested, fetal death will not occur within a week after the test was administered. A *positive* contraction stress test indicates a 50% chance of poor fetal outcome. Poor outcome for these purposes is defined as perinatal death, a low Apgar score at 5 minutes, or the appearance of late decelerations during monitoring in actual labor.

Indications for antepartum nonstress tests. Antepartum nonstress testing is performed on selected patients. The prospect of testing all women has been commented on in the literature; indirect evidence seems to warrant large-scale study of the value of nonstress tests for all patients. For the present, patients who require antepartum assessment are those with high-risk factors such as postdates, history of stillbirths, chronic hypertension and pregnancy-induced hypertension, diabetes mellitus, and intrauterine growth retardation. The earliest tests are performed at 26 to 28 weeks of gestation. Early testing implies an intent to intervene in behalf of a better fetal outcome.

Antepartum evaluation of fetal movements

Fetal movements have been the subject of intense clinical study for the past several years. A number of studies have demonstrated good correlation between normal fetal activity and a reactive (normal) nonstress test. Particular attention has been paid to monitoring of fetal motion in high-risk pregnancies. In any circumstances an active fetus is usually a healthy one. However, data on fetal movements is not sufficiently refined to justify intervention in a pregnancy based on motion studies alone. There is, however, sufficient information to suggest that fetal inactivity should be considered a warning that requires further investigation.

Three types of gross fetal motions have been reported. The fetus may *roll and rotate*. This involves the entire fetal body and evokes a definite maternal perception of activity. *Simple movements*, which involve both trunk and extremity, are also rather forceful. The third type has been called *high-frequency movement*. It involves either the chest wall (fetal breathing movements) or an isolated extremity, and is often described as a "weak kick" by the mother.

Movements are visible as early as the seventh gestational week, when the embryonic body moves in a smooth vermicular fashion. Twitching of the body and head is seen at 8 weeks. Limb movement is more coordinated at 10 weeks, and the initial stages of coordinated movements combining the head, trunk, and limbs are first evident at 12 weeks. Maternal perception of fetal movement occurs between 16 and 20 weeks. Various investigators have defined quantities of movements during specific time periods as representative of minimal acceptable activity. Regardless of parameters, investigators who have identified fetal inactivity have found that 50% of affected fetuses are distressed or stillborn at the time of delivery.

The fetus has active periods that alternate with intervals of rest. The active state in a fetus, or wakefulness, is termed REM (rapid eye movement) sleep. During these periods the fetus moves, heart rate variability is evident, and breathing movements occur frequently. The regular association between fetal trunk motion and heart rate acceleration is well documented. Non-REM sleep is a quiet resting state during which body movements and fetal heart rate accelerations are minimal or absent. Resting-active cycles are of 60 to 75 minutes duration. The period of rest generally lasts 30 minutes. Accurate interpretation requires awareness of normal sleep states if misinterpretation of recordings is to be avoided.

Several techniques are used to detect and record movements of the fetus. The simplest technique involves maternal perception and recording of fetal movement. Maternal perception is accurate in approximately 85% of instrumentally recorded fetal motion. In fact, maternal perception has been observed in 100% of fetal motions involving propulsive lower limb and trunk movements as visualized by ultrasound. Another technique utilizes real-time ultrasonography to detect a number of details such as fetal respiratory movements and fetal hand-to-face contact. Most ultrasonographic visualizations are limited to periods of 10 to 30 minutes duration. Interpretations may be confounded by physiologic rest periods that exceed test intervals. An alternative technique involves electromechanical devices to detect fetal movements indirectly by recording changes in the configuration of the uterus and abdominal wall. The tocodynamometer has been found to be particularly useful for the monitoring of fetal movements. The pressure changes that result from fetal activity are detected from abdominal wall motion and are categorized by duration and amplitude.

In the future, refinement of observations on fetal neuromotor behavior will provide data that enhances the accuracy of health assessment. Patterns of fetal responses to various stimuli can then be interpreted for the determination of fetal status. Ultimately examination of the fetus will entail a number of items that in combination will provide a basis for identification of illness.

Amniotic fluid analysis for pulmonary surfactant

Lecithin-sphingomyelin ratio (L/S ratio). In the fetal lung, fluid is secreted into the alveoli, and it is ultimately deposited into amniotic fluid after migration up the respiratory tract and out the glottic opening into the posterior pharynx. This secretion contains surfactant, a complex substance composed of several phospholipids, which lowers surface tension forces of alveolar walls (Chapter 8). This function is indispensable for initial opening of the alveoli during the first breath and for prevention of subsequent alveolar collapse (atelectasis). Deficiency of surfactant results in the widespread atelectasis that characterizes hyaline membrane disease. The demonstration, in am-

niotic fluid prenatally, of sufficient surfactant to preclude hyaline membrane disease postnatally is one of the most helpful and reliable of all intrauterine tests for fetal maturity. This procedure actually indicates the maturational status of fetal lungs, that is, the capacity of the lungs to accommodate normal ventilation after birth. There is no consistent relationship between fetal weight, age, and pulmonary maturity. Up to 10% of mature fetuses have been reported to have low L/S ratios, whereas normal ratios have been reported in premature fetuses.

The principal constituent of surfactant is lecithin. Its presence in relation to sphingomyelin is expressed as a ratio that usually changes predictably as pregnancy progresses. Two other phospholipids, while present in considerably smaller quantities than lecithin itself, are essential for effective function of surfactant. These substances are called *phosphatidyl glycerol (PG)* and *phosphatidyl inositol (PI)*. They are important in the diminution of surface-active forces because they stabilize lecithin in the surfactant layer that lines the alveoli. The presence of PG indicates lung maturity. It appears at 36 weeks gestation, increasing gradually thereafter. It is the most dependable of the known indicators of lung maturity, even in diabetic pregnancies (types A, B, C). PG is not present in blood, vaginal secretions, or meconium. It is found only in pulmonary surfactant and semen.

Surface-active lecithin appears in amniotic fluid at 24 to 26 weeks of gestation, at which time concentrations are slightly above those of sphingomyelin. Before this time, very little lecithin is measurable; afterward, lecithin increases while sphingomyelin concentration remains relatively unchanged. Surfactant is secreted into the alveolar spaces at approximately 26 to 27 weeks gestation. Between 30 and 32 weeks, lecithin concentrations rise slightly to 1.2 times greater than that of sphingomyelin (L/S ratio = 1.2). At 35 weeks an abrupt rise in lecithin to at least twice the concentration of sphingomyelin (ratio = two or more) signifies pulmonary maturity; this virtually assures that hyaline membrane disease will not occur after birth. Fig. 1-8 depicts the quantitative changes of lecithin and sphingomyelin. It illustrates that the relationship between lecithin and sphingomyelin in amniotic fluid provides a basis for the assessment of fetal pulmonary maturity.

L/S ratios correlate well with gestational age in normal pregnancies. In high-risk pregnancies the correlation is not so straightforward. Lung maturity, as indicated by the L/S ratio, may occur early or late in gestation, depending on the existing maternal disorder. For example, a 3300 g infant at 38 weeks of gestation has been reported with a ratio of only 0.75, whereas a 920 g infant at 28 weeks had a normal mature ratio. The older and larger infant had severe hyaline membrane disease, but the smaller infant did not. The boxed

material on p. 23 lists maternal diseases that have been shown to alter the normal developmental schedule of pulmonary maturity, that is, the attainment of an L/S ratio of two or more was either accelerated (pulmonary maturity before 35 weeks) or delayed (pulmonary maturity after 35 weeks). Maternal conditions associated with accelerated development of pulmonary maturity are generally those that cause diminished maternal blood flow to the placenta and therefore an impairment, to some extent, of oxygen transport to the fetus. The resultant fetal distress apparently increases the blood level of corticosteroid, which triggers elaboration of surfactant in type II alveolar cells.

Numerous other variables may affect the outcome of predictions of pulmonary maturity based on the L/S ratio. Some have already been demonstrated, and extensive investigation will no

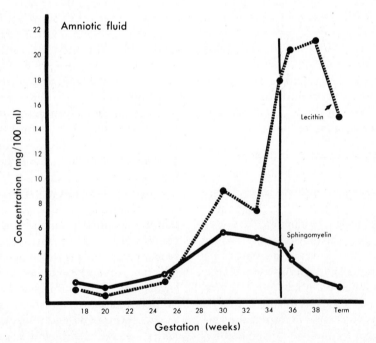

Fig. 1-8. Lecithin (broken line) and sphingomyelin (solid line) concentrations plotted against gestational age. L/S ratio rises to 1.2 at 28 weeks, and to 2 or more at 35 weeks, indicating little chance of hyaline membrane disease postnatally. (From Gluck, L., Kulovich, M. V., Borer, R. C., Jr., et al: Am. J. Obstet. Gynecol. **109:**440, 1971.)

doubt identify others. The presence of maternal blood in amniotic fluid tends to lower the L/S ratio. Thus a mature ratio in bloody fluid is a valid result; an immature ratio may be artifactual. The presence of meconium in amniotic fluid affects reliable results in an unpredictable fashion; it may either raise or lower the L/S ratio from its true value by a mechanism that is not understood. In some instances a ratio of two or more may be

---

DISORDERS ASSOCIATED WITH ALTERATION FROM NORMAL TIME OF APPEARANCE OF MATURE L/S RATIO*

Appearance of mature ratio before 35 gestational weeks (accelerated maturation)

Maternal conditions
    Toxemia (early onset)
    Hypertensive renal disease
    Hypertensive cardiovascular disease
    Sickle cell disease
    Narcotic addiction
    Diabetes, class D, F, R (Chapter 11)
    Chronic retroplacental hemorrhage
    Hyperthyroidism
    Corticosteroids, aminophylline
    Maternal infections
    Placental insufficiency
    Parabiotic twinning—donor (small) twin
Fetal disorders
    Prolonged rupture of membranes

Appearance of mature ratio after 35 gestational weeks (delayed maturation)

Maternal condition
    Diabetes, class A, B, C (Chapter 11)
    Chronic glomerulonephritis
Fetal condition
    Rh disease, particularly with hydrops fetalis
    Smaller of identical twins (nonparasitic)

---

*Modified from Gluck, L.: Clin. Obstet. Gynecol. **21**:547, 1978.

associated with postnatal hyaline membrane disease because of events that transpire after collection of the sample. Thus among 425 pregnancies observed in one study, 13 infants whose ratios were normal, nevertheless, had respiratory distress after birth. Twelve of these babies had a low Apgar score (less than 7) at 5 minutes, reflecting intrauterine and/or intrapartum stress that occurred subsequent to the L/S ratio determination. This acute distress may have impaired surfactant activity and therefore induced the occurrence of hyaline membrane disease.

Prolonged rupture of membranes is believed by many to be associated with a significant diminution in the incidence of hyaline membrane disease. The data indicate that this association is prevalent when membranes have ruptured 48 to 72 hours or longer prior to delivery. Apparently prolonged rupture of membranes results in an elevated level of corticosteroids in fetal blood, which stimulates production of surfactant earlier in gestation.

As data accumulate, new insights will evolve regarding accuracies and errors in the predictive value of the ratio. This amniotic fluid analysis is currently indispensable as an aid in deciding whether the fetus of a high-risk pregnancy is safer inside or outside the uterus. A ratio of two or more reliably predicts the absence of hyaline membrane disease with only occasional inaccuracy. On the other hand, a ratio of less than two does not predict the occurrence of hyaline membrane disease as reliably as does a ratio greater than two predict its absence. A mature ratio accurately predicts the absence of hyaline membrane disease in approximately 98% of cases. On the other hand, a ratio of less than two (immature) has been reported to be associated with hyaline membrane disease in only 40% to 80% of fetuses tested. Apparently the lower the ratio, the more likely the occurrence of hyaline membrane disease.

Shake test. The shake test, or foam test, is a simple procedure that attempts to correlate mature or immature L/S ratios with the presence or absence of foam in prepared samples of amniotic fluid. The sample is mixed with ethanol and shaken for 15 seconds; a reading is made 15 minutes later. The test depends on the ability of lecithin to create a stable foam in ethanol. A positive result is produced by a complete ring of bubbles at the surface that persists for 15 minutes. It appears to be a reliable indication of pulmonary maturity. Hyaline membrane disease has rarely followed a positive foam test. The absence of foam suggests that hyaline membrane disease will occur, but such absence is not as reliably predictive as the low L/S ratio itself. Therefore the shake test is a good screening procedure for maturity (positive for foam), but in the absence of foam, an L/S ratio should be performed.

Antepartum biochemical tests for fetal well-being and fetal maturity

Amniotic fluid. Amniotic fluid is withdrawn simply and safely by amniocentesis, which entails insertion of a needle through the abdominal and uterine walls into the amniotic cavity. Amniocentesis has been performed as early as the twelfth gestational week. Amniotic fluid components can be usefully analyzed for the severity of erythroblastosis (Rh incompatibility), for predictions of hyaline membrane disease (see discussion of L/S ratio), for certain chromosomal disorders, congenital anomalies, and inborn errors of metabolism. Although the complications of amniocentesis are uncommon, a variety of them have been reported. These include abortion, maternal hemorrhage, infection, fetal puncture wounds, laceration of the fetal spleen, damage to placental and umbilical vessels, and sudden death from fetal exsanguination.

Bilirubin. Determination of bilirubin in the amniotic fluid is valuable for assessment of the severity of Rh disease. Bilirubin is derived from the breakdown of red blood cells (Chapter 10), and it is present at certain levels in normal amniotic fluid. Peak levels are attained between 16 and 30 weeks of gestation, and steady decline thereafter usually culminates in its disappearance by 36 weeks. In most instances there is no bilirubin in amniotic fluid beyond 36 weeks of gestation. This finding is variable, however, and bilirubin determination is thus not valuable for estimations of fetal maturity. If, as in fetal erythroblastosis, an excessive rate of hemolysis occurs, bilirubin levels in amniotic fluid rise abnormally. These values are plotted on a graph that delineates three zones of fetal involvement (mild, moderate, and severe), depending on the bilirubin concentration. If the results indicate severe disease, an intrauterine transfusion or an immediate termination of pregnancy may be indicated. If moderate involvement is present, repeated frequent determinations are required to monitor the course of fetal hemolysis. Values falling into the zone of mild involvement contraindicate intrauterine transfusion or interruption of pregnancy because postnatal management (exchange transfusion or phototherapy) is effective. Determination of amniotic fluid concentration of bilirubin for fetal maturity is an obsolete procedure because there is such wide variation in results.

Creatinine. It has long been known that levels of creatinine in the amniotic fluid increase with gestational age, and in the past the test was useful in assessment of fetal maturity. It is no longer performed because of the superiority of ultrasonography and because the test is difficult to interpret. Creatinine in later pregnancy is derived from fetal urine. It is excreted through the kidneys across the glomeruli, which increase substantially in number during the third trimester. Thus it was reasonable to expect that creatinine levels would rise steadily as pregnancy progressed. In normal pregnancies 1.6 to 1.8 mg/dl of creatinine was thought to indicate gestational age of 36 or 37 weeks in approximately 95% of patients. However, the usefulness of this determination for the estimation of fetal age is limited in complicated pregnancies involving impaired maternal renal function. In such circumstances maternal creatinine crosses the placenta and maternal creatinine retention is reflected as a high level in the amniotic fluid. The lack of specificity of the test and the availability of superior modalities for estimation of fetal age have made creatinine determinations obsolete.

Cytology. This test for assessment of fetal maturity is also obsolete. It depended on the demonstration of certain quantities of lipid containing cells. These cells are exfoliated from fetal skin into amniotic fluid in increasing numbers as term is approached. Gestational age was then estimated according to a percentage of fat-stained cells. The technique of staining itself altered results unpredictably, and variations between laboratories caused difficulty in standardization.

Other tests

Estriol determinations. Estriol, a major metabolite of estrogen, is found in relatively large quantities in maternal urine during the latter half of pregnancy. The fetal contribution to maternal urinary estriol concentration is ten times as great as the maternal contribution. Estriol was thought to be a valuable indicator of fetal health because its synthesis requires a normal placenta and fetal adrenal cortex. From the placenta it crosses into the maternal blood and eventually is excreted through the kidneys. Intact function of both the fetal adrenal and the placenta are required for excretion of normal quantities of estriol. Because ultimate excretion of estriol also requires maternal metabolic activity in the liver, the gastrointestinal tract, and the kidneys, estriols were thought to be a test of the entire maternal-fetal-placental unit. Determinations were most commonly performed on maternal urine, which had to be collected over a period of 24 hours. Plasma determinations were studied in an attempt to simplify collections and eliminate normal diurnal variations, but difficulties in interpretation of results diminished enthusiasm for this approach. Determination of estriol is not considered a useful modality for assessment of fetal status. Occasionally it may be contributory in diabetic pregnancies, but biophysical (electronic) fetal monitoring must also be used. The frequency of spurious low levels of estriol is considerable. From studies on the predictive value of estrogen assays, fetuses at risk are not reliably identified. In most instances the overlap between normal and abnormal values is too extensive for clinical applications. Only a few institutions use estriol determinations for assessment of fetal well-being, and they do so on few patients.

Human placental lactogen (HPL). HPL is a hormone produced in the human placenta by the syncytiotrophoblast. Its production first appears at 20 to 40 days after implantation. Serum levels rise gradually until 37 weeks of gestation; a slight decline occurs thereafter. It was thus expected that maternal HPL levels would increase in relation to placental growth during pregnancy. Abnormalities of pregnancy associated with large placentas then might be identified by increased HPL levels. This is generally true in multiple pregnancy, Rh disease, and suboptimally controlled maternal diabetes mellitus. HPL has been studied extensively for assessment of placental function and, therefore, fetal well-being. Correlations have been inconsistent, and in no instance has there been a recommendation that therapeutic decisions be based solely on HPL values. The high hopes for HPL determinations in early reports have not been realized. Furthermore, electronic fetal heart rate monitoring is considerably more effective in identifying fetal hazard, while ultrasonography provides more information relative to fetal growth. Contemporary opinion is that HPL determinations provide little information about fetal status. The test is not generally used.

α-Fetoprotein. α-Fetoprotein is the major protein of fetal serum. It is a glycoprotein similar to albumin in molecular weight and structure. In the fetus, serum levels peak at 13 to 15 menstrual weeks, at which time concentrations are approximately 3 mg/ml. Levels in the amniotic fluid rise in parallel with those of fetal serum, but at 0.01 of the concentration. In maternal serum, low concentrations (in nanograms) gradually rise with advancing gestational age; peak levels occur at 34 gestational weeks.

The principal clinical application of α-fetoprotein concentrations is the identification of neural tube defects, including anencephaly, encephalocele, and spina bifida. These malformations are the result of disrupted closure of the embryonic neural tube. Closure begins in the cervical region of the spinal cord and continues cephalad and caudad simultaneously until complete, at which time the neural tube is totally covered by ectoderm (skin). Closure of the entire neural tube occurs by 28 days after conception; neural tube defects are thus present by that time. An open neural tube causes α-fetoprotein to leak across exposed membranes into amniotic fluid from fetal blood. In the vast majority of cases, elevations of amniotic fluid α-fetoprotein over five standard deviations from the normal mean are indicative of the malformation. Normally a diminution of α-fetoprotein concentration in amniotic fluid occurs during the second trimester. Designation of abnormal values is critically dependent on accurate assessment of gestational age. Furthermore, amniotic fluid α-fetoprotein is significantly elevated in other conditions that include congenital nephrosis, omphalocele, cystic hygroma associated with Turner's syndrome, gastrointestinal tract obstructions, and sacrococcygeal teratomas. The presence of fetal blood in amniotic fluid also elevates levels. If the presence of fetal blood can be excluded, abnormal levels usually indicate neural tube defect or one of the other malformations previously mentioned.

Determination of maternal levels of the fetal protein may provide a basis for mass screening. Discussions of the feasibility and usefulness of mass screening have been ongoing for several years. The abnormal implications of an elevated level are crucially dependent on accurate gestational age data. This would be a particularly troublesome source of error in mass screening. Furthermore, elevated levels occur in fetal death, fetomaternal bleeding, and multiple gestations. When high concentrations are identified, amniocentesis and ultrasonographic evaluation of fetal morphology must be performed.

Meconium in amniotic fluid

The intestine of the term infant contains 200 to 600 g of meconium. Meconium is viscous and sticky, and it varies in color from greenish brown to black. It contains cells from the skin, alimentary tract, lanugo, and vernix caseosa. Meconium may contain blood group substances or it may give a positive result for occult blood under normal circumstances. This is apparently a result of the ingestion of maternal blood or perhaps from clinically inconsequential oozing of alimentary tract vessels. Normal meconium contains little protein because the fetal proteolytic enzymes digest it. In dry weight, the bulk of meconium is composed of mucopolysaccharides, which are the residue of mucous secretions from intramural glands in the alimentary tract. Meconium contains 1 mg of bilirubin per gram of wet weight. If in the term infant there are approximately 200 g of meconium in the intestine, it can be surmised that 200 mg of prenatally excreted bilirubin is available for absorption from the intestinal tract as a contribution to neonatal physiologic hyperbilirubinemia. In 99.8% of normal term infants, the first passage of meconium occurs by 48 hours of age.

Although the literature recurrently cites a study that demonstrated enhanced bacterial growth in amniotic fluid that contains meconium in a concentration over 1%, the clinical significance of this observation has not been proved. Furthermore, experimental data have demonstrated that meconium does not diminish the tensile strength of amniotic membranes, and it therefore does not predispose to early membrane rupture.

The incidence of meconium staining, taken from a number of studies, has ranged from 0.5% to 10.9% of all births. Five to ten percent is probably a realistic estimate. In utero passage of meconium occurs preponderantly at term or past term; rarely earlier than 34 gestational weeks. During the course of amniocentesis for genetic counseling, several investigators have reported meconium-stained amniotic fluid during the second trimester in 1% to 2% of patients studied, but spectrophotometric analysis reveals that the discoloration is usually a result of old blood. It is generally believed appropriate to evaluate fetal status by ultrasound if meconium-stained fluid is recovered from an amniocentesis in the second trimester.

Meconium released by the fetus is generally considered a response to hypoxia. That meconium-stained fluid is present in a substantial number of deliveries of normal infants has been recognized for a long time. The incidence of fetal asphyxia in the presence of meconium-stained amniotic fluid has not been determined since the association was reported in 1954. The hypothesized mechanism of meconium release involves increased peristalsis accompanied by relaxation of the anal sphincter in response to hypoxic fetal stress. The most direct postnatal consequence of meconium release into amniotic fluid is the *meconium aspiration syndrome* (see Chapter 8). Some particles of meconium are drawn into the respiratory tract in utero; most aspiration occurs during the first breaths after birth. The resultant postnatal distress is often sufficiently severe to require mechanical ventilatory support. Prolonged illness is not unusual; occasionally death ensues.

Presence of meconium in the amniotic fluid of an apparently healthy infant may indicate transient intrauterine hypoxia that is of no significance to the infant's status at birth. The staining of fetal tissue (nails, skin, umbilical cord) is thought to indicate meconium passage 4 to 6 hours or more prior to delivery. In vitro, vernix suspended in meconium has been noted to stain yellow in 12 to 14 hours. Meconium is often passed by fetuses in the breech presentation even though they have not experienced hypoxic stress.

Amniotic fluid analysis in genetic counseling

The performance of amniocentesis is a pivotal procedure in the overall process of genetic counseling. Amniocentesis for inherited disease states is an end point that follows assiduous family histories, physical examinations with appropriate laboratory studies of parents, and detailed frank discussions in regard to psychosocial ramifications of the genetic counseling procedure. In the presence of demonstrated fetal abnormalities, some parents elect to terminate pregnancy, while others do not. The importance of inherited disease in perinatal outcomes has been amplified in the past decade because of the availability of diagnostic technology, and the diminution of fetal and neonatal deaths from nongenetic causes. Thus the percentage contribution to death rates by inherited diseases has increased as the number of deaths from other causes has diminished.

For the most part, analysis of amniotic fluid for determination of genetic disease states devolves on culture of the cells suspended in the fluid. In the late 1950s the first application of cellular studies demonstrated fetal sex by the presence or absence of sex chromatin bodies. In the middle 1960s amniotic fluid cells could be grown in tissue culture in sufficient numbers for karyotypic analysis and for biochemical studies. Amniocentesis is performed for suspected chromosomal disorders if one of the parents is a known carrier, if maternal age is advanced, if there is a history of previous offspring with a trisomy, or if the mother is a known carrier of X-linked disease. To this listing one would also add birth of a previous child with a neural tube defect. Advanced maternal age is probably the most frequent reason for amniocentesis, the most prominent indication being the established higher incidence of Down's syndrome (trisomy 21). Advanced age is variably defined between 35 to 37 years.

Among the X-linked genetic disorders, only three uncommon abnormal states are specifically verifiable by biochemical analysis of the cells as well. For the remainder, (for example, hemophilia) specific involvement of the fetus cannot be demonstrated. For the majority of X-linked disorders, identification of a male merely indicates a 50% chance of fetal involvement.

To date, approximately 200 inborn errors of metabolism have been identified in terms of their specific biochemical deficiencies. These disease states can be diagnosed by biochemical analysis of amniotic fluid cells. Inborn errors of metabolism comprise approximately 10% of total prenatal diagnoses of genetic disorders. Amniocentesis for inborn errors of metabolism requires definite identification of an affected family member, or heterozygote designation of both parents if the disease is an autosomal recessive one. For a few of these diseases, mass programs of heterozygote screening have been initiated in recent years. An archetypical example is Tay-Sachs disease among Ashkenazi Jews. The gene frequency for Tay-Sachs disease in this population is approximately 1 in 27, which is 100 times more frequent than in non-Jews. Screening programs have used blood specimens, and some couples have been identified as carriers at risk for an affected infant. Screening programs require knowledge that there is a significantly increased gene frequency in the population to be screened. Thus sickle cell disease can be identified in carriers among those of African, Arab, Mediterranean, or Indo-Pakistani derivation. β-Thalassemia is identifiable in couples of Mediterranean, Southeast Asian, or Indo-Pakistani descent. Insofar as demonstration of biochemical abnormalities in cultured amniotic fluid cells is concerned, any metabolic disorder that can be diagnosed using fibroblasts after birth can ordinarily be identified prenatally from amniotic fluid cells.

Ultrasound and the visible fetus

With the introduction of ultrasound for visualization of the pregnant uterus, an impressive array of observations became available for the first time. Diagnostic ultrasound has virtually replaced radiography. Ultrasound uses high-frequency sound waves beyond human audibility, projects them at target organs, and records their rebound (echo) on a transducer that converts the mechanical energy into an image on a screen (Fig. 1-9). Sound waves beyond 20,000 cycles/second (MHz) are inaudible by the human ear. Those that

are utilized in ultrasonography usually range between 2 to 5 MHz. They are transmitted from a scanner in direct contact with the maternal abdominal wall. The waves penetrate tissues of varying density at different depths and, depending on the tissue density encountered, part of the transmitted waves are returned (reflected) to the scanning instrument. It is the reflected waves, of differing intensities, that are recorded and projected as dots on the screen, which in the aggregate compose the fetal and uterine image. Ultrasound images are static or dynamic. *Static ultrasound* projects a single image. When ultrasound produces an image of a target in motion, movements are recorded as they transpire. This is *real-time ultrasound*. It is the most frequently used form of dynamic imaging in perinatal medicine. Fetal anatomy, body movements, and organ motion (for example, the heart) can be evaluated routinely during pregnancy with the use of high-resolution real-time scanners. It is also a safe diagnostic modality in contrast to x-rays. Sound waves of high intensity can damage tissue, but only at levels of intensity that are considerably higher than those used in diagnostic procedures.

Ultrasound studies provide information on fetal maturity, multiple gestations (Fig. 1-10), fetal death, fetal position (Fig. 1-11), the course of fetal growth, amniotic fluid volume, placental position, and a growing number of congenital anomalies. It is used to visualize insertion of catheters for fetal transfusions into the peritoneal space and for guidance during the performance of amniocentesis.

Pregnancy is identifiable as early as 5 weeks past the last menstrual period. At this time the gestational sac is visible as a group of dense circular echoes (white images on the screen). The embryo is visible at 6 or 7 weeks. Measurement of crown-rump length at 8 to 13 weeks predicts within 5 days the expected date of delivery (Fig. 1-12). Estimation of gestational length is more accurate at this time than at any other. Later in pregnancy, between 12 and 26 weeks, measurements of the fetal biparietal diameter (BPD) are

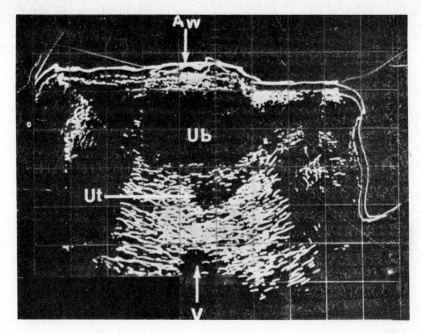

Fig. 1-9. Normal nonpregnant structures, transverse scan. *Aw*, Abdominal wall; *Ub*, urinary bladder; *Ut*, uterus; *V*, vertebral body. The urinary bladder and uterus are non–echo-producing structures. The vertebra is an inverted U. (From Thompson, H. E.: Clin. Obstet. Gynecol. **17:**1, 1974.)

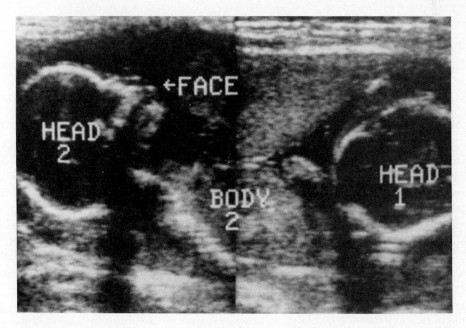

Fig. 1-10. Twins. (Courtesy Dr. George Flinn, Methodist Hospital, Memphis, Tenn.)

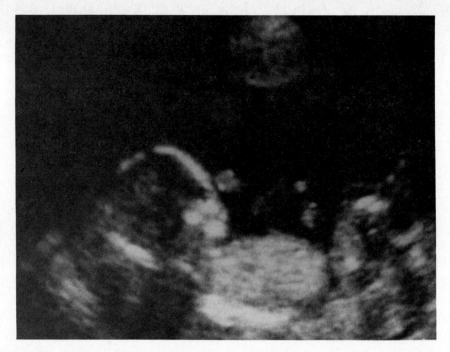

Fig. 1-11. Fetus in breech position. (Courtesy Dr. George Flinn, Methodist Hospital, Memphis, Tenn.)

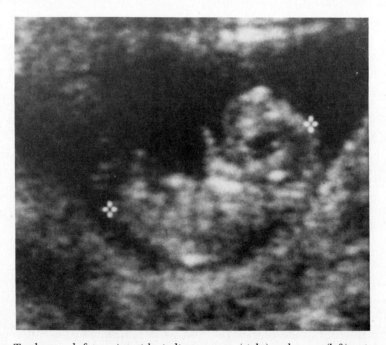

Fig. 1-12. Twelve-week fetus. Asterisks indicate crown (right) and rump (left) points of measurement. (Courtesy Dr. George Flinn, Methodist Hospital, Memphis, Tenn.)

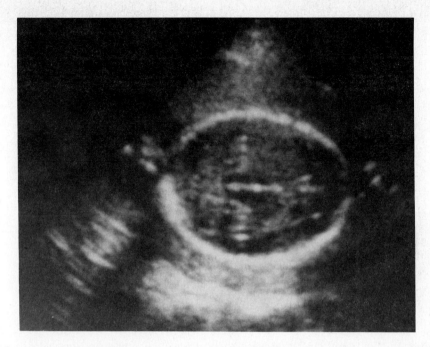

Fig. 1-13. Sonogram of skull at 24 gestational weeks. The midline echogenic streak indicates proper level for measuring biparietal diameter. (Courtesy Dr. George Flinn, Methodist Hospital, Memphis, Tenn.)

well correlated with fetal maturity (Fig. 1-13). The rate of head growth diminishes after 26 weeks, and normal increments in head size no longer correlate with the passage of time. Measurement of the length of the calcified femur is thought to predict gestational age within 1 week, if measurement is obtained by the end of the twenty-third gestational week. Growth of the femur is variable afterwards, and there is no correlation between its length and fetal age. The value of femoral length for estimation of gestational age is not firmly established.

Ultrasound is helpful in the diagnosis of intrauterine growth retardation. The most common ultrasonographic approach involves calculation of the head-abdomen ratio (H/A ratio). This entails measurement of the BPD and the circumference of the abdomen at the level of umbilical vein in-sertion into the abdominal wall. Early in pregnancy the head-abdomen ratio is larger than late in pregnancy. In the third trimester cumulative glycogen deposits in the liver, increased muscle mass, and deposition of subcutaneous fat in the abdominal wall contribute to increased girth of the abdomen. In the third trimester, abdominal circumference exceeds the head size; the H/A ratio is lowered. The girth of the abdomen should exceed that of the head in the last trimester. If abdominal measurements are less than head measurements, intrauterine growth retardation of the head-sparing type (see Chapter 5) is likely. The usefulness of these morphometric measurements depends on an accurate estimation of gestational age. Without this information, head-abdomen measurements are of little use.

A growing number of congenital anomalies are

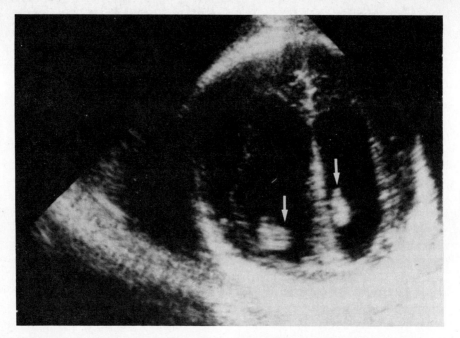

Fig. 1-14. Severe dilatation of lateral ventricles in a hydrocephalic fetus. Arrows indicate a choroid plexus in each ventricle. (Courtesy Dr. George Flinn, Methodist Hospital, Memphis, Tenn.)

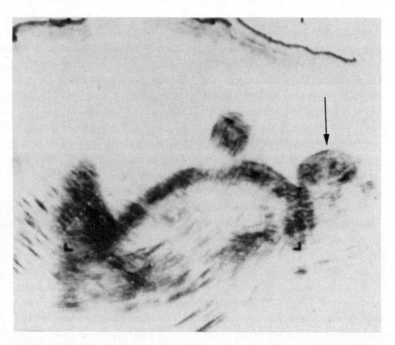

Fig. 1-15. Anencephalic fetus. Arrow indicates diminutive head. (Courtesy Dr. George Flinn, Methodist Hospital, Memphis, Tenn.)

identifiable by ultrasound examination. In the central nervous system the major anomalies that have been identified are hydrocephalus (Fig. 1-14), anencephaly (Fig. 1-15), microcephaly, and neural tube defects. The appearance of a mass at the anterior or lateral neck suggests cystic hygroma or giant hemangioma. Several types of congenital heart disease have also been identified by expert ultrasonographers. Gastrointestinal obstructions at virtually all levels are readily seen by ultrasound. Polyhydramnios is often associated with obstructions high in the gastrointestinal tract. *Omphalocele* is identified by the presence of abdominal viscera within the umbilical cord. *Gastroschisis* is identified by bowel loops and liver that float outside the fetal body in amniotic fluid. Limb deformities are readily apparent. Kidneys can be visualized from the fourteenth or fifteenth gestational week onward. Enlargement, cystic malformations, and agenesis have been identified by ultrasound. Fetal sex determination is also feasible when genitals become visible.

The pervasive use of diagnostic ultrasound has radically changed the nature of obstetric practice. Growth, function, and anatomy of the fetus are now in view (Fig. 1-16). Body movements and cardiac activity are clearly visible. The most promising potential of diagnostic ultrasound is in the accumulation of data on normal fetal growth and development. Observations on neuromuscular development are already accumulating. Fetal body movement in response to stimuli and respiratory movements are likewise being studied. Recently the response to auditory stimuli has been revealed in more detail. Fetal responses to acoustic stimuli had been recognized years ago. The recorded end points were the startled changes in fetal activity, not unlike those observed during hearing screening procedures in the nursery. Heart rate accelerations were also observed

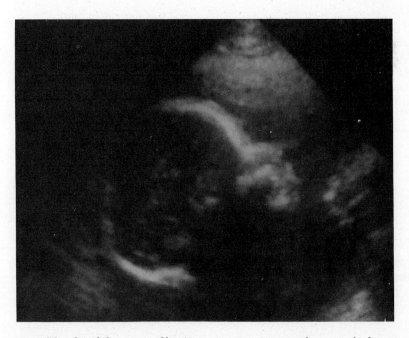

Fig. 1-16. Fetal head and face in profile. (Courtesy Dr. George Flinn, Methodist Hospital, Memphis, Tenn.)

in response to acoustic stimuli. With real-time ultrasonography, eye-blinks (auropalpebral reflex) have been observed in response to specific vibroacoustic stimulation. A few fetuses responded at 24 to 25 weeks of age. After 28 weeks, all of them responded with clearly identifiable facial movements. The major contribution of ultrasonography to the welfare of perinatal patients will be the studies of fetal behavior that it implements.

HIGH-RISK PREGNANCY

Neonatal intensive care programs have diminished mortality and incidence of brain damage among survivors, but much if not most of their activity could be eliminated by optimal delivery of prenatal care. Usually the sick neonate is a distressed fetus whose mother's vulnerability to perinatal misadventure could have been identified in at least 60% of cases. The ideal medi-

---

ANTEPARTUM MATERNAL FACTORS THAT INDICATE HIGH RISK
FOR ADVERSE FETAL OUTCOME

Previous pregnancy misadventure

Grand multiparity (more than five pregnancies)
Cesarean section
Midforceps delivery
Prolonged labor
Fetal loss before 28 weeks (two such)
Fetal loss after 28 weeks
Premature infant
Postterm infant (42 weeks or over)
Abnormal fetal position
Polyhydramnios
Multiple pregnancy
Neonatal death
Infant over 4.5 kg at birth
Fetal or neonatal exchange transfusion
Congenital anomalies
Bleeding in second or third trimester
Toxemia, eclampsia

Abnormalities of reproductive anatomy

Uterine malformation
Incompetent cervix
Small bony pelvis

Metabolic and endocrine disorders

Family history of diabetes
Gestational diabetes
Diabetes
Thyroid disorder
Hyperparathyroidism

Cardiovascular disorders

Toxemia
Chronic hypertension
Rheumatic heart disease
Congenital heart disease
Congestive heart failure

Renal disorders

Chronic glomerulonephritis
Acute pyelonephritis
Acute cystitis
Renal insufficiency

Hematologic disorders

Sickle cell disease
Rh sensitization
Anemia (hemoglobin less than 10 g)
Idiopathic thrombocytopenic purpura

Other factors

Age: Under 16 or over 35 years
      Over 30 years (primipara)
Weight: Less than 45 kg or more than 90 kg
Syphilis
Tuberculosis
Hereditary CNS disorder
Epilepsy
Drug addiction
Smoking
Alcoholism
Maternal malnutrition

cal facility for the management of reproductive events is not a neonatal center nor an obstetric center, but it is rather a *perinatal center* capable of providing continuous care for the well-known biologic continuum that is composed of conception, gestation, labor, birth, and neonatal life.

Identification and special care of patients at high risk early in pregnancy have constituted a fruitful approach to the diminution of perinatal misadventure. The high-risk pregnancy is characterized by one or more maternal conditions that impose considerable hazard to intact survival of the fetus or newborn infant. A list of the most common antepartum factors that identify such pregnancies is presented in the boxed material. A similar but more extensive tabulation of maternal disorders and their associated fetal or neonatal effects is presented in Chapter 2.

Preselection is most effectively accomplished early by considering the historic factors with which a woman enters gestation.

Neonatal mortality is lowest if the mother is between 20 and 30 years of age. The risk of poor outcome is considerably increased below 16 and over 40 years of age. Neonatal mortality and morbidity are significantly greater among diabetic gravidas. Prematurity, stillbirth, and low birth weight for gestational age (Chapter 4) are considerably more common among mothers with toxemia and hypertensive cardiovascular disease. Neonatal thyroid difficulty is more often associated with maternal thyroid disorder as a consequence of treatment than as a result of the maternal dysfunction itself. Previous Rh sensitization increases the possibility that an erythroblastotic infant will result from the current pregnancy. Hydramnios may be associated with congenital malformations of the gastrointestinal tract or the brain. It is also common in diabetic pregnant women. Bleeding during the second and third trimesters usually follows disruption of placental attachment, which then poses a serious threat to fetomaternal gas exchange. Multiple pregnancy (twins, triplets) may be fraught with difficulty because at least one of the twins is often delivered from the breech position or is retarded in the rate of intrauterine growth. Excessive cigarette smoking (consumption of more than 20 cigarettes daily) is associated with an increased incidence of low birth weight. Rubella is responsible for severe congenital anomalies and for other tissue changes that are usually incompatible with survival or with a normal postnatal course (Chapter 13). Maternal hyperparathyroidism may cause severe hypocalcemia in the neonate. Idiopathic thrombocytopenic purpura often results in severe thrombocytopenia in the fetus and newborn.

Although these are only some of the conditions that impose a high risk on pregnancy, they involve the majority of high-risk gravidas. In separating these special pregnancies from the uncomplicated ones, it becomes possible to refer a relatively small number of patients (among whom the bulk of perinatal deaths occur) to medical centers that are equipped and staffed to manage them. There remain the unanticipated events for which preparation is difficult, such as the sudden appearance of complications during labor or delivery in a previously uneventful pregnancy or the first occurrence of premature labor, fetal loss, and neonatal death. Nevertheless, with optimal prenatal management, perinatal mortality can be reduced considerably. This has been demonstrated repeatedly in organized programs of prenatal and postnatal care.

BIBLIOGRAPHY

Abramovich, D.R.: Fetal factors influencing the volume and composition of liquor amnii, J. Obstet. Gynaecol. Br. Comm. **77:**865, 1970.

Abramovici, H., Brandes, J. M., Fuchs, K., and Timor-Tritsch, I.: Meconium during delivery: a sign of compensated fetal distress, Am. J. Obstet. Gynecol. **118:**251, 1974.

Amarose, A. P., Wallingford, A. J., and Plotz, E. J.: Prediction of fetal sex from cytologic examination of amniotic fluid, N. Engl. J. Med. **275:**715, 1966.

Aubry, R. H., and Pennington, J. C.: Identification and evaluation of high-risk pregnancy: the perinatal concept, Clin. Obstet. Gynecol. **16:**3, 1973.

Behrman, R. E., Parer, J. T., and de Lannoy, C. W.: Placental growth and the formation of amniotic fluid, Nature **214:**678, 1967.

Birnholz, J. C., and Benaceraff, B. R.: The development of human fetal hearing, Science **222**:516, 1983.

Bryan, P. J., and Jassani, M. N.: Antenatal ultrasound. In Fanaroff, A. A., and Martin, R. J., editors: Behrman's neonatal-perinatal medicine, St. Louis, 1983, The C.V. Mosby Co.

Clements, J. A., Platzker, A. C. G., Tierney, D. F., et al.: Assessment of the risk of the respiratory distress syndrome by a rapid test for surfactant in amniotic fluid, N. Engl. J. Med. **286**:1077, 1972.

Collea, J. V., and Holls, W. M.: The contraction stress test, Clin. Obstet. Gynecol. **25**:707, 1982.

Cook, L. N., Shott, R. J., and Andrews, B. F.: Fetal complications of diagnostic amniocentesis: a review and report of a case with pneumothorax, Pediatrics **53**:421, 1974.

Cruikshank, D. P.: Amniocentesis for determination of fetal maturity, Clin. Obstet. Gynecol. **25**:773, 1982.

Desmond, M. M., Lindley, J. E., Moore, J., and Brown, C. A.: Meconium staining of newborn infants, J. Pediatr. **49**:540, 1956.

DeVoe, S. J., and Schwarz, R. H.: Determination of maturity and well-being using maternal and amniotic fluids. In Gruenwald, P., editor: The placenta, Baltimore, 1975, University Park Press.

Fox, H. E., and Hohler, C. W.: Fetal evaluation by real-time imaging, Clin. Obstet. Gynecol. **20**:339, 1977.

Fuchs, F.: Volume of amniotic fluid at various stages of pregnancy, Clin. Obstet. Gynecol. **9**:449, 1966.

Gibbons, J. M., Jr., Huntley, T. E., and Corral, A. G.: Effect of maternal blood contamination on amniotic fluid analysis, Obstet. Gynecol. **44**:657, 1974.

Gluck, L.: Evaluating functional fetal maturation, Clin. Obstet. Gynecol. **21**:547, 1978.

Gluck, L., Kulovich, M. V., Borer, R. C., Jr., et al.: Diagnosis of the respiratory distress syndrome by amniocentesis, Am. J. Obstet. Gynecol. **109**:440, 1971.

Gluck, L., Kulovich, M. V., Eidelman, A. I., et al.: Biochemical development of surface activity in mammalian lung. IV. Pulmonary lecithin synthesis in the human fetus and newborn and etiology of the respiratory distress syndrome. Pediatr. Res. **6**:81, 1972.

Golbus, M. S., and Stephens, J. D.: Prenatal diagnosis of chromosomal abnormalities and neural tube defects, Clin. Perinatol. **6**:245, 1979.

Goldstein, A. S., Fukunaga, K., Malachowski, N., and Johnson, J. D.: A comparison of lecithin/sphingomyelin ratio and shake test for estimating fetal pulmonary maturity, Am. J. Obstet. Gynecol. **118**:1132, 1974.

Goodlin, R. C.: Amniotic fluid. In Care of the fetus, New York, 1979, Masson Publishing Co.

Goodlin, R. C.: Why fetal monitoring? Sem. Perinatol. **5**:105, 1981.

Goodlin, R. C., and Clewell, W. H.: Sudden fetal death following diagnostic amniocentesis, Am. J. Obstet. Gynecol. **118**:285, 1974.

Hertz, R. H., and Jarrell, S. E.: Estimation of the placental function and reserve. In Fanaroff, A. A., and Martin, R. J., editors: Behrman's neonatal-perinatal medicine, St. Louis, 1983, The C.V. Mosby Co.

Heymann, M. A.: Biophysical evaluation of fetal status. In Creasy, R. K., and Resnik, R., editors: Maternal-fetal medicine—principles and practice, Philadelphia, 1984, W. B. Saunders Co.

Hobbins, J. C.: Assessment of fetal maturity and well-being. In Warshaw, J. B., and Hobbins, J. C., editors: Principles and practice of perinatal medicine, Menlo Park, Calif., 1983, Addison-Wesley Publishing Co., Inc.

Hon, E. H.: An introduction to fetal heart rate monitoring, New Haven, Conn., 1969, Hearty Press, Inc.

Hon, E. H.: Detection of asphyxia in utero—fetal heart rate. In Gluck, L., editor: Intrauterine asphyxia and the developing fetal brain, Chicago, 1977, Year Book Medical Publishers, Inc.

Ianniruberto, A., and Tajani, E.: Ultrasonographic study of fetal movements, Sem. Perinatol. **5**:175, 1981.

James, L. S., Morishima, H. O., Daniel, S. S., et al.: Mechanism of late deceleration of the fetal heart rate, Am. J. Obstet. Gynecol. **113**:578, 1972.

Jepson, J. H.: Factors influencing oxygenation in mother and fetus, Obstet. Gynecol. **44**:906, 1974.

Kochenour, N. K.: Estrogen assay during pregnancy, Clin. Obstet. Gynecol. **25**:659, 1982.

Kubli, F.: Antepartum monitoring of fetal heart rate. In Beard, R. W., and Nathanielsz, P. W.: Fetal physiology and medicine—the basis of perinatology, New York, 1984, Mercel Dekker, Inc.

Lavery, J. P.: Nonstress fetal heart rate testing, Clin. Obstet. Gynecol. **25**:689, 1982.

Ledger, W. J.: Complications associated with invasive monitoring, Sem. Perinatol. **2**:187, 1978.

Liley, A. W.: Intrauterine transfusion of foetus in haemolytic disease, Br. Med. J. **2**:1107, 1963.

Lind, J., Stern, L., and Wegelius, C.: Human foetal and neonatal circulation, Springfield, Ill., 1964, Charles C. Thomas, Publisher.

Mahoney, M. J.: Prenatal diagnosis of inborn errors of metabolism, Clin. Perinatol. **6**:255, 1979.

Manning, F. A.: Ultrasound in perinatal medicine. In Creasy, R. K., and Resnik, R., editors: Maternal-fetal medicine—principles and practice, Philadelphia, 1984, W. B. Saunders Co.

Manning, F. A., Morrison, I., Lange, I. R., and Harman, C.: Antepartum determination of fetal health: composite biophysical profile scoring, Clin. Perinatol. **9**:285, 1982.

Martin, C. B.: Regulation of the fetal heart rate and genesis of FHR patterns, Sem. Perinatol. **2**:131, 1978.

Mendez-Bauer, C., Poseiro, J. J., Arellano-Hernandez, G., et al.: Effects of atropine on the heart rate of the human fetus during labor, Am J. Obstet. Gynecol. **85**:1033, 1963.

Miller, F. C., and Paul, R. H.: Intrapartum fetal heart rate monitoring, Clin. Obstet. Gynecol. 21:561, 1978.

Naeye, R. L.: Structural correlates of fetal undernutrition. In Waisman, H. A., and Kerr, G., editors: Fetal growth and development, New York, 1970, McGraw-Hill Book Co.

Nathan, D. G., Alter, B. P., and Orkin, S. H.: Prenatal diagnosis of hemoglobinopathies, Clin. Perinatol. 6:275, 1979.

Nelson, N. M.: Respiration and circulation before birth. In Smith, C. A., and Nelson, N. M., editors: The physiology of the newborn infant, Springfield, Ill., 1976, Charles C. Thomas, Publisher.

Nesbitt, R. E. L., Jr.: Prenatal identification of the fetus at risk, Clin. Perinatol. 1:213, 1974.

Parer, J. T.: Fetal heart rate. In Creasy, R. K., and Resnik, R., editors: Maternal-fetal medicine—principles and practice, Philadelphia, 1984, W. B. Saunders Co.

Patrick, J.: Fetal breathing and body movements. In Creasy, R. K., and Resnik, R., editors: Maternal-fetal medicine—principles and practice, Philadelphia, 1984, W. B. Saunders Co.

Paul, R. H.: The evaluation of antepartum fetal well-being using the nonstress test, Clin. Perinatol. 9:253, 1982.

Potter, E. L.: Bilateral absence of ureters and kidneys, Obstet. Gynecol. 25:3, 1965.

Pritchard, J. A.: Deglutition by normal and anencephalic fetuses, Obstet. Gynecol. 25:289, 1965.

Pritchard, J. A.: Fetal swallowing and amniotic fluid volume, Obstet. Gynecol. 28:606, 1966.

Queenan, J. T.: Polyhydramnios and oligohydramnios. In Fanaroff, A. A., and Martin, R. J., editors: Behrman's neonatal-perinatal medicine, St. Louis, 1983, The C. V. Mosby Co.

Rayburn, W. F.: Antepartum fetal assessment—monitoring fetal activity, Clin. Perinatol. 9:231, 1982.

Resnik, R.: Phospholipid analysis of amniotic fluid. In Creasy, R. K., and Resnik, R.: Maternal-fetal medicine—principles and practice, Philadelphia, 1984, W. B. Saunders Co.

Roopnarinesingh, S.: Amniotic fluid creatinine in normal and abnormal pregnancies, Obstet. Gynaecol. Br. 77:785, 1970.

Rudolph, A. M.: Oxygenation in the fetus and neonate—a perspective, Sem. Perinatol. 8:158, 1984.

Rudolph, A. M., Itskovitz, J., Iwamoto, H., et al.: Fetal cardiovascular responses to stress, Sem. Perinatol. 5:109, 1981.

Sabbagha, R. E., Tamura, R. K., and Socol, M. L.: The use of ultrasound in obstetrics, Clin. Obstet. Gynecol. 25:735, 1982.

Sadavosky, E.: Fetal movements and fetal health, Sem. Perinatol. 5:131, 1981.

Saling, E.: Blood chemistry as a method of detection of fetal distress. In Wood, C., and Walter, W. A. A., editors: Fifth World Congress of Gynecology and Obstetrics, Sydney, 1967, Butterworth & Co. (Australia), Ltd.

Seeds, A. E.: Maternal-fetal acid-base relationships and fetal scalp-blood analysis, Clin. Obstet. Gynecol. 21:579, 1978.

Sorokin, Y., and Dierker, L. J.: Fetal movement, Clin. Obstet. Gynecol. 25:719, 1982.

Stocker, J., Mawad, R., Deleon, A., and Desjardins, P.: Ultrasonic cephalometry, Obstet. Gynecol. 45:275, 1975.

Thompson, H. E.: Evaluation of the obstetric and gynecologic patient by the use of diagnostic ultrasound, Clin. Obstet. Gynecol. 17:1, 1974.

Varner, M. W., and Hauser, K. S.: Current status of human placental lactogen, Sem. Perinatol. 5:123, 1981.

Varner, M. W., and Hauser, K. S.: Human placental lactogen and other placental proteins as indicators of fetal well-being, Clin. Obstet. Gynecol. 25:673, 1982.

Winick, M.: Malnutrition and brain development, New York, 1976, Oxford University Press.

Wood, C.: Fetal scalp sampling: its place in management, Sem. Perinatol. 2:169, 1978.

CHAPTER 2

Fetal and neonatal consequences of abnormal labor and delivery

The condition of an infant at birth is determined by numerous antecedent factors such as genetic endowment, maternal health before and during gestation, maternal complications of pregnancy, development of the embryo, growth of the fetus, and the course of labor and delivery. This chapter addresses the fetal effects of labor and delivery, normal and abnormal. Although some of the abnormal conditions have their inception well before the onset of labor (placenta previa, for example), they are discussed here because they affect the birth process so profoundly. Maternal medical disorders such as diabetes, toxemia, or infectious diseases are considered elsewhere in relation to their associated neonatal abnormalities. However, Table 2-1 lists a majority of ma-

Text continued on p. 46.

Table 2-1. Maternal abnormalities and associated fetal and neonatal disorders

Maternal factors	Fetal, neonatal disorders
Antepartum	
Metabolic	
Diabetes mellitus	Prematurity*
	Hyaline membrane disease
	Hyperbilirubinemia
	Hypoglycemia
	Macrosomatia
	Hypocalcemia
	Renal vein thrombosis
	Polyhydramnios
	Congenital anomalies
	Intrauterine growth retardation
Gout	Hyperuricemia (transient, asymptomatic)
Malnutrition	Intrauterine growth retardation
Porphyria	Porphyrinuria (transient, asymptomatic)
Endocrine	
Addison's disease	Prematurity
	Intrauterine growth retardation
Chronic hypoparathyroidism	Hyperparathyroidism (intrauterine and postnatal)
Primary hyperparathyroidism	Neonatal tetany (hypocalcemia)
	Hypomagnesemia
Thyroid	
Goiter (nontoxic)	Goiter
Hyperthyroidism (untreated)	Hyperthyroidism (goitrous or nongoitrous)
Hyperthyroidism (treated)	Goiter (nontoxic)
	Hyperthyroidism (goitrous or nongoitrous)
	Hypothyroidism (goitrous or nongoitrous)
Hypothyroidism	CNS defects
	Hypothyroidism
Cardiac	
Congestive failure	Prematurity
	Asphyxia†
Hypertensive cardiovascular disease	Asphyxia
	Intrauterine growth retardation
Pulmonary	
Asthma (intractable) or any disorder associated with hypoxemia and hypercapnia	Asphyxia
	Prematurity
	Intrauterine growth retardation
Gastrointestinal	
Regional ileitis	Prematurity
Renal	
Polycystic kidney disease	Polycystic kidney disease
Chronic glomerulonephritis	Prematurity
	Intrauterine growth retardation
	Asphyxia

*Prematurity = gestational age less than 37 completed weeks.
†Asphyxia = hypoxemia, hypercapnia, low pH.

Continued.

Table 2-1. Maternal abnormalities and associated fetal and neonatal disorders—cont'd

Maternal factors	Fetal, neonatal disorders
Antepartum—cont'd	
Neurologic	
Myasthenia gravis	Myasthenia gravis
Status epilepticus	Asphyxia
Hematologic	
Blood incompatibility (Rh, ABO, other)	Erythroblastosis fetalis
Idiopathic thrombocytopenic purpura	Idiopathic thrombocytopenia purpura (transient)
Leukemia (acute)	Prematurity
Megaloblastic anemia	Hazards of abruptio placentae
Sickle cell anemia	Low birth weight
	Intrauterine growth retardation
	Abruptio placentae
	Fetal loss
Anemia (iron deficiency)	Low birth weight, prematurity
Skin	
Pemphigus	Bullae (transient)
Neoplastic	
Hodgkin's disease	Hodgkin's disease
Ovarian tumors (complicated)	Prematurity
Collagen disease	
Lupus erythematosus (acute)	Systemic lupus erythematosus
Lupus erythematosus (subacute)	Syndrome of congenital heart block, fibroelastosis, fibrosis of liver, spleen, kidney, adrenals
Infection (antepartum or intrapartum)	
Viral	
Coxsackie	Coxsackie infection (encephalomyocarditis)
Cytomegalic inclusion disease	Cytomegalic inclusion disease
Hepatitis (SH)	Neonatal hepatitis
Herpesvirus infection	Herpesvirus infection
Measles	Measles
Mumps	?Congenital anomalies
Poliomyelitis	Poliomyelitis
Rubella	Congenital rubella syndrome
Smallpox	Smallpox
TRIC agent (cervicitis)	Inclusion blennorrhea
Vaccinia (primary vaccination)	Generalized vaccinia
Varicella	Varicella
Western equine encephalomyelitis	Western equine encephalomyelitis
Protozoan	
Candidiasis (vaginal)	Thrush
Malaria	Malaria
Toxoplasmosis	Toxoplasmosis
Trypanosomiasis	Trypanosomiasis

Prematurity = gestational age less than 37 completed weeks.
Asphyxia = hypoxemia, hypercapnia, low pH.

Table 2-1. Maternal abnormalities and associated fetal and neonatal disorders—cont'd

Maternal factors	Fetal, neonatal disorders
Bacterial	
Acute pyelonephritis	Prematurity
	Bacterial infections
Enteropathogenic *E coli* (carrier)	Diarrhea (enteropathogenic *E coli*)
Gonorrhea	Gonorrheal infection (usually ophthalmia)
Listeriosis	Listeriosis
Pneumococcal meningitis	Pneumococcal meningitis
Salmonellosis	Salmonellosis
Septicemia (any organism)	Septicemia (any organism)
Shigellosis	Shigellosis
Syphilis	Congenital syphilis
Tuberculosis	Tuberculosis
Typhoid fever	Typhoid fever
Obstetric and gynecologic	
Amputated cervix	Prematurity
Incompetent cervix	Prematurity
Toxemia	Prematurity
	Intrauterine growth retardation
	Hypoglycemia
	Hypocalcemia
	Aspiration syndrome
	Polycythemia
	Asphyxia
Pharmacologic	
Alcohol (IV or oral)	Hypoglycemia
Alcohol (chronic alcoholism)	Fetal alcohol syndrome
	Low birth weight
	Developmental delay
	Microcephaly
	Small palpebral fissures
	Maxillary hypoplasia
	Cardiac anomaly (ventricular septal defect, patent ductus arteriosus)
	Abnormal palm creases
Aminopterin and amethopterin	Multiple anomalies
	Abortion
	Intrauterine growth retardation
Ammonium chloride	Acidosis
Amphetamines	Transposition of great vessels
Androgen (methyl testosterone)	Masculinization of females
	Advanced bone age
Barbiturates	Withdrawal syndrome
	Diminished sucking
	Diminished serum bilirubin

Prematurity = gestational age less than 37 completed weeks.
Asphyxia = hypoxemia, hypercapnia, low pH.

Continued.

Table 2-1. Maternal abnormalities and associated fetal and neonatal disorders—cont'd

Maternal factors	Fetal, neonatal disorders
Antepartum—cont'd	
Pharmacologic—cont'd	
Cephalothin	Direct Coombs' positive test
Chlorambucil	?Renal agenesis
Chlorothiazides	Thrombocytopenia
	Salt and water depletion
Chloroquine	?Retinal damage
	Death
	Mental retardation
Chlorpromazine	Depression
	Lethargy
	Extrapyramidal dysfunction
Chlorpropamide	Hypoglycemia
	Increased fetal wastage
Cigarette smoking	Intrauterine growth retardation
	Increased neonatal hematocrit
Diazepam (Valium)	Hypothermia
Dicumarol	Fetal hemorrhage and death
Diphenylhydantoin (Dilantin)	Hypoplastic phalanges
	Diaphragmatic hernia
	Cleft lip
	Coloboma
	Pulmonary atresia
	Patent ductus arteriosus
Estrogen	Masculinization of females
	Carcinoma of vagina and cervix (years later)
	Advanced bone age
Ethchlorvynol (Placidyl)	Irritability, jitteriness (withdrawal symptoms)
Hexamethonium bromide	Paralytic ileus
Insulin shock	Death
Intravenous fluid (copious, hypotonic)	Hyponatremia
	Convulsions
	Edema
Isoxsuprine (and some other betamimetic tocolytics)	Hypoglycemia
	Hypocalcemia
	Ileus
	Hypotension
	Death
Lithium	Lithium toxicity (cyanosis, hypotonia)
	Cardiac anomalies (especially Ebstein's)
Lysergic acid diethylamide	Chromosome damage
Magnesium sulfate	Hypermagnesemia
	CNS depression
	Peripheral neuromuscular blockage

Prematurity = gestational age less than 37 completed weeks.
Asphyxia = hypoxemia, hypercapnia, low pH.

Table 2-1. Maternal abnormalities and associated fetal and neonatal disorders—cont'd

Maternal factors	Fetal, neonatal disorders
Meperidine (Demerol)	Placental vasoconstriction
	CNS and respiratory depression
Mepivacaine, lidocaine, other "amides"	Bradycardia
	Convulsions
	Apnea
	Death
	Depression
	Tachycardia
	Flaccidity
	Metabolic acidosis
	Hypoxemia
Methimazole	Goiter
Morphine, heroin, methadone	Withdrawal symptoms (tremors, dyspnea, cyanosis, convulsions, death)
	Intrauterine growth retardation
	Lower serum bilirubin
Naphthalene (mothballs)	Hemolytic anemia (in G-6-PD deficiency)
Nitrofurantoin	Hemolytic anemia (in G-6-PD deficiency)
Nortriptyline	Urinary retention (bladder)
Pentazocine (Talwin)	Neonatal depression
Potassium iodide	Goiter
Prilocaine	Methemoglobinemia; others as in mepivacaine
Primaquine	Hemolytic anemia (in G-6-PD deficiency)
Progestins	Masculinization of female infants
	Advanced bone age
Propranolol	Low Apgar scores
	Bradycardia
	Hypoglycemia
Propoxyphene (Darvon)	Hyperactivity
	Sweating
	Convulsions
	Withdrawal symptoms
Propylthiouracil	Goiter
Quinine	Thrombocytopenia
	Abortion
Radioactive iodine	Hypothyroidism
	Thyroid destruction
Reserpine	Obstructed respiration due to nasal congestion
	Lethargy
	Bradycardia
	Hypothermia
Salicylates	Neonatal hemorrhage due to platelet dysfunction
Sedatives (excessive during labor)	CNS depression and respiratory distress

Prematurity = gestational age less than 37 completed weeks.
Asphyxia = hypoxemia, hypercapnia, low pH.
Continued.

Table 2-1. Maternal abnormalities and associated fetal and neonatal disorders—cont'd

Maternal factors	Fetal, neonatal disorders
Antepartum—cont'd	
Pharmacologic—cont'd	
Steroids (adrenocortical)	Increased incidence of fetal death
	Adrenal suppression
	Accelerated fetal lung maturation
	?Cleft palate
Streptomycin	Deafness, eighth nerve damage
Stilbestrol	Adenocarcinoma of vagina in adolescents
Sulfonamides (long-acting)	Kernicterus at low bilirubin levels
Tetracyclines (after first trimester)	Tooth stain, enamel hypoplasia (primary teeth)
	Temporary inhibited linear growth (premature infants)
Thalidomide	Phocomelia and other anomalies
	Death
Tolbutamide (Orinase)	Thrombocytopenia, bilirubin displacement from albumin, hypoglycemia
Vitamin D (excessive)	?Hypercalcemia (supravalvular aortic stenosis, mental retardation, osteosclerosis)
Vitamin K (excessive)	Hyperbilirubinemia
Warfarin	Mental retardation
	Optic atrophy
	Hemorrhage
	Fetal death
Intrapartum	
Cord pathology	
Inflammation	Bacterial infection
	Umbilical vein thrombosis (asphyxia)
Meconium staining	Asphyxia
Prolapsed cord	Asphyxia
Single umbilical artery	Congenital anomalies
	Intrauterine growth retardation
True knot	Asphyxia
Velamentous insertion, vasa previa	Intrauterine blood loss
Rupture of normal cord (precipitous delivery), varices, aneurysm	Intrauterine blood loss
Fetal membrane, amniotic fluid	
Amnion nodosum	Renal agenesis
	Severe obstructive uropathy (bilateral)
	Intrauterine parabiotic syndrome (small twin)
Amnionitis	Infection, usually bacterial
Early membrane rupture	Bacterial infection
	Prematurity
	Prolapsed cord

Prematurity = gestational age less than 37 completed weeks.
Asphyxia = hypoxemia, hypercapnia, low pH.

Table 2-1. Maternal abnormalities and associated fetal and neonatal disorders—cont'd

Maternal factors	Fetal, neonatal disorders
Meconium stain (fluid or membranes)	Asphyxia
	Aspiration syndrome
	Pneumonia
Oligohydramnios	Postmaturity
	Renal agenesis and dysplasia
	Polycystic kidney
	Urethral obstruction
	Intrauterine parabiotic syndrome (small twin)
	Fetal death
Polyhydramnios	High gastrointestinal obstruction
	Spina bifida
	Hydrocephalus
	Anencephaly
	Achondroplasia
	Hydrops fetalis
	Intrauterine parabiotic syndrome (large twin)
Placenta	
Placenta previa	Prematurity
	Asphyxia
	Prolapsed cord
	Intrauterine blood loss
Abruptio placentae	Prematurity
	Asphyxia
	Intrauterine blood loss
Fetomaternal transfusion	Intrauterine blood loss (chronic or acute)
	Asphyxia
Incision during cesarean section	Intrauterine blood loss (acute)
Placental insufficiency	Asphyxia
	Intrauterine malnutrition
Multilobed placenta (rupture of communicating vessels)	Intrauterine blood loss (acute)
Complications of labor	
Breech delivery	Asphyxia
	Intracranial hemorrhage
	Visceral hemorrhage (adrenal, kidney, spleen)
	Spinal cord trauma
	Brachial plexus injury
	Bone fracture (clavicle, humerus, femur)
	Epiphyseal injury (proximal femur or humerus)
	Characteristic posture
	Edema, ecchymosis of buttocks, genitalia, and lower extremities

Prematurity = gestational age less than 37 completed weeks.
Asphyxia = hypoxemia, hypereapnia, low pH.

Continued.

Table 2-1. Maternal abnormalities and associated fetal and neonatal disorders—cont'd

Maternal factors	Fetal, neonatal disorders
Intrapartum—cont'd	
Complications of labor—cont'd	
Face and brow presentation	Edema, ecchymosis of face
	Asphyxia
	Characteristic posture (head retraction)
Transverse presentation	Asphyxia, trauma
Precipitate delivery	Asphyxia, trauma
	Intracranial hemorrhage
Prolonged labor	Asphyxia, trauma
	Bacterial infection
Uterine inertia	Hazard of prolonged labor
Uterine rupture	Asphyxia
Uterine tetany	Asphyxia
Shoulder dystocia	Asphyxia
	Brachial plexus injury
	Fractured clavicle
	Fractured humerus
Manual version, extraction	Asphyxia
	Bone fractures
	Brachial plexus injury, spinal cord trauma
Forceps (high or mild)	Asphyxia
	Cephalhematoma
	Intracranial hemorrhage
Multiple gestation	Asphyxia (usually second twin)
	Prematurity
	Intrauterine growth retardation
	Intrauterine parabiotic syndrome (fetofetal transfusion)
	Hypoglycemia (smaller twin)
	Congenital anomalies
	Bacterial infection (first or both twins)

Prematurity = gestational age less than 37 completed weeks.
Asphyxia = hypoxemia, hypercapnia, low pH.

ternal disorders and the fetal or neonatal effects they are known or presumed to produce.

NORMAL LABOR

A review of normal labor is essential for an understanding of the abnormalities that play a role in fetal or neonatal difficulties. The classic division of labor into three stages is as follows:

First stage: Cervical dilatation is initiated with the first contraction and ends when the cervix is completely dilated.

Second stage: Fetal expulsion begins when the cervix is completely dilated and ends with birth of the infant.

Third stage: Placental expulsion starts after birth of the baby and terminates with delivery of the placenta.

Before considering each stage of labor, a discussion of uterine contractions is appropriate.

Gross characteristics of uterine contractions

Contractions provide the force necessary for descent of the fetus; they accentuate differentiation of the uterine wall into upper and lower segments, and they bring about dilatation and effacement of the cervix (see later discussion). During the first stage, intrauterine pressure ranges from 20 to 50 torr. At these pressures the cervix seems to dilate easily. During the second stage, with the addition of conscious maternal expulsive efforts (bearing down), pressures may rise to 70 torr. At the onset of the first stage of labor, contractions appear every 10 minutes, increasing in frequency to every 1 or 2 minutes during the second stage. They normally last for 30 to 90 seconds. Alternation of contraction and relaxation is indispensable to fetal well-being because the flow of blood through the intervillous space is greatly impeded during a contraction, returning to normal during relaxation. The significance to the fetus of abnormally long and vigorous contractions is thus apparent; that is, sustained reduction of placental blood flow impairs maternofetal gas exchange, and fetal hypoxia may ensue.

As labor proceeds, increasing differentiation of the uterine wall into a thick muscular superior segment and a thin inferior one (Fig. 2-1) assures that most of the force produced by contractions emanates from the upper segment. The lower one remains relatively passive and distensible. This arrangement is essential if fetal descent is to be accomplished. If the entire uterine wall were as thick and muscular as the upper segment, the force of each contraction would be applied to the fetus equally from all sides rather than from above. The fetus would get nowhere. Also, as will be seen in the description of the first stage, the cervix would neither efface nor dilate.

First stage of labor. As the upper and lower segments become more sharply differentiated

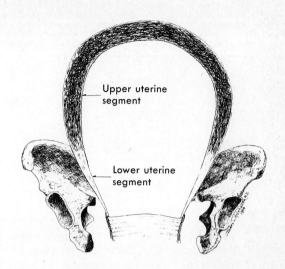

Fig. 2-1. Upper (dark shading) and lower uterine segments are shown delineated from each other. Most of the force that propels the fetus originates from the thick muscular upper segment. (Modified from Hellman, L. M., and Pritchard, J. A.: Williams obstetrics, ed. 14, New York, 1971, Appleton-Century-Crofts.)

with each contraction, cervical effacement (thinning) and dilatation progress gradually. At the onset of labor, the cervical wall is approximately 2 cm in thickness, surrounding a thin canal of equal depth. Fully effaced at the end of the first stage, the wall of the cervix is only a few millimeters thick. It becomes incorporated into and indistinguishable from the uterine wall of the lower segment. Fully dilated, the cervical canal becomes a shallow, wide orifice that is 10 cm in diameter (Fig. 2-2). The canal becomes wider and thinner as the wall of the cervix retracts to become part of the uterine wall. Thinning and widening of the cervix occurs in response to downward pressure on the fetus that is provided by repeated contractions. Most of the effacement is accomplished during the early part of the first stage, when dilatation is minimal. Later, with effacement almost complete, dilatation progresses more rapidly to completion, marking the onset of the second stage (Fig. 2-3).

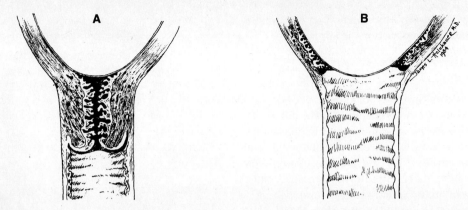

Fig. 2-2. Effacement and dilatation of the cervix. **A,** Appearance of the cervix before onset of labor. The cervical canal is only a few millimeters wide. **B,** Appearance of the cervix late in labor. The cervix is effaced and dilated, having been drawn upward and incorporated into the wall of the lower uterine segment. The cervical canal has widened to approximately 10 cm. (Modified from Hellman, L. M., and Pritchard, J. A.: Williams obstetrics, ed. 14, New York, 1971, Appleton-Century-Crofts.)

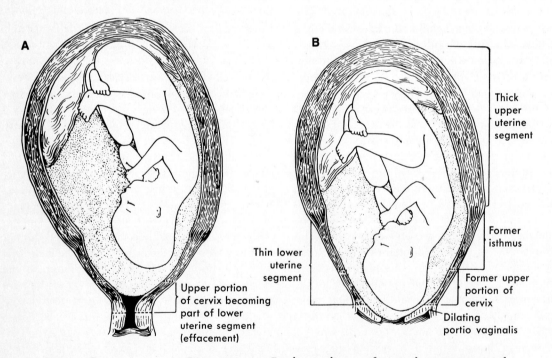

Fig. 2-3. Pregnant uterus. **A,** Late pregnancy. Bracket marks part of cervix that is incorporated into lower uterine segment during effacement. **B,** During labor. Effacement is complete, and dilatation is in progress. Upper segment is thicker, whereas lower segment is longer and thinner. (From Reid, D. E., Ryan, K. J., and Benirschke, K.: Principles and management of human reproduction, Philadelphia, 1972, W. B. Saunders Co.)

Second stage of labor. Although variations are numerous, significant descent of the fetus usually does not occur until the cervix is completely dilated. During the second stage, fetal descent is brought about not only by uterine contractions but also by periodic increases of intraabdominal pressure. The latter is accomplished by the mother during voluntary contraction of abdominal muscles and fixation of the diaphragm. Maternal oversedation may reduce or eliminate voluntary cooperation.

As fetal descent proceeds, the head rotates to accommodate to the contour of the bony pelvis and thus is normally delivered face downward. Delivery of the shoulders is accomplished when the unextruded body rotates 90 degrees to change their internal position from a horizontal to an anteroposterior one. The face is now turned to one side (Fig. 2-4). The anterior (upper) shoulder is delivered first, then the posterior (lower) shoulder, and rapidly thereafter, the rest of the body. The cord is cut by the operator after extrusion of the body, the proximal end remaining attached to the undelivered placenta while the distal segment is attached to the infant.

Third stage of labor. After birth of the baby, the placenta separates and is extruded by continued contractions that pry it loose from its attachment to the uterine wall. There is thus a smooth transition from intrauterine placental respiration in a liquid environment to extrauterine pulmonary respiration in a gaseous one. If extensive separation of the placenta occurs during the first or second stage, the reduction of surface area available for gas exchange produces hypoxia, which cannot be relieved until the head is delivered.

Cellular characteristics of uterine contractions

Throughout pregnancy the myometrium and cervix are progressively prepared for the onset of contractions in the regulation of uterine motility. The expulsion of a normal fetus requires orderly progress of uterine activity once labor has begun. Intense research has been in progress for a number of years in an attempt to understand the physiologic factors that comprise normal labor. It follows, therefore, that efforts to control the onset of labor and its progress have also been intense, particularly in recent years. There are several reasons for therapeutic intervention. First, the fetus may be compromised by uterine contractions. Contractions must therefore be halted and Ce-

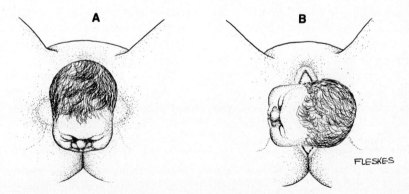

Fig. 2-4. Rotation of the shoulders prior to delivery. **A,** The head has just been delivered. The shoulders are in a horizontal direction. **B,** Ninety-degree rotation of the entire body has now placed the shoulders in a vertical (anteroposterior) direction while the face has turned to one side. (Modified from Hellman, L. M., and Pritchard, J. A.: Williams obstetrics, ed. 14, New York, 1971, Appleton-Century-Crofts.)

sarean section contemplated. Second, early onset of labor and premature birth is the major source of perinatal morbidity and mortality. Therefore labor must be postponed to allow fetal maturation. Third, delayed onset of labor (postdatism) causes retention of a fetus in utero and jeopardizes intact survival. Myometrial contractions and cervical ripening must therefore be stimulated. In these varying circumstances, therapeutic interference is desirable; effective therapy directly depends on an understanding of normal labor. Without such an understanding, delineation of the factors that may have gone awry would not be possible.

Myometrium. The myometrium consists of billions of smooth muscle cells and a supporting web of interstitial (connective) tissue. During pregnancy the uterus changes dramatically in contour and in size, compared to its nongravid state. In the absence of pregnancy, the uterus weighs approximately 60 g with a volume capacity of 10 ml. At term, average uterine weight is 1000 g and average capacity is 5000 ml. Early in pregnancy the uterus is flame-shaped. By the end of the first trimester it becomes globular. It retains a spherical shape until term, at which time it is somewhat oval in contour. Soon after the onset of pregnancy and under the influence of estrogen, the synthesis of protein increases remarkably. As a consequence, individual fibers of the myometrium ultimately become ten times longer and three times wider as the fetus and placenta grow. The cytoplasm (sarcoplasm) of muscle cells contains filaments of protein (myofilaments) that bring about cell contractility and are ultimately responsible for contraction of the uterine wall. Each cell also contains a labyrinthine arrangement of tubules (sarcoplasmic reticulum) that remains in contact with the inner surface of the cell membrane (sarcolemma). These tubules store calcium ions, which are critical to the intracellular contractile process. In response to sodium and potassium exchange across the cell membrane, calcium is drawn into the cell from outside and from the sarcoplasmic reticulum (reservoir tubules) as well. Concentration of calcium thus increases within

the sarcoplasm; activation of the myofilaments now becomes possible. In response to reversed exchange of sodium and potassium across the cell membrane, calcium recedes out of the cell to the interstitial tissue and into its intracellular reservoir, the sarcoplasmic reticulum. With reduced calcium concentration in sarcoplasm, the cell must now relax. Myometrial cells are unable to contract unless the concentration of calcium in sarcoplasm is increased. This is the rationale for preliminary trial of "calcium blockers," which can inhibit the passage of calcium into the cytoplasm and thus forestall cellular contractility.

The coordination of uterine contractions requires structures to accommodate communication between cells. These develop in the form of "gap junctions" close to the onset and during progress of labor. In providing intercellular communication, the gap junctions synchronize the function of billions of myometrial cells. Gap junctions enlarge and increase in number as term approaches.

In essence, the contractility of myometrial cells seems to be governed by exchanges of sodium and potassium within and without the cell, which in turn promote influx of calcium into the sarcoplasm, thus raising calcium concentration within the cell. Increased calcium concentration promotes the activity of myofilaments that exert contractile activity. In the aggregate, contractility of individual cells is orchestrated by gap junctions so that the uterine wall contracts in synchrony to propel the fetus downward.

The activity of the myometrium is influenced by certain pharmacologic and hormonal agents. Estrogens promote contractility of the myometrial cell. The precise mechanism has not yet been identified. Progesterone depresses uterine contractility. It is generally believed, but not yet proved, that progesterone is responsible for a relatively quiet uterus during pregnancy, and that a diminution in its concentration associated with a rise in estrogens may trigger the onset of labor. In numerous studies, however, plasma progesterone has not been shown to decrease close to term. Recent investigations suggest that the concentration of progesterone may be regulated within the uterus itself, and that these changes are not reflected in plasma concentration. There is further conjecture that the number of receptor sites for estrogen, located on the surface of cells, increases as term is approached. The myometrial cells thus become more sensitive to unchanged plasma levels of estrogen. The same may be said for oxytocin. Circulating levels of oxytocin have not been shown to increase during labor, but it is hypothesized that the number of oxytocin receptors increases, thereby rendering myometrial cells more sensitive to its presence. It is also of interest that the concentration of oxytocin receptors is higher in the upper body of the fundus than in the lower, less contractile segment of the uterus and cervix. Thus the principal influence on the initiation of labor seems to be an elevated estrogen-progesterone ratio, with increased production of receptors for estrogen and oxytocin. Increased intracellular calcium concentrations activate myofilaments for contractility; intercellular communications are conducted through gap junctions.

Prostaglandins also play an active role in the contractile process. The mode of action is unknown. Prostaglandins have been found elevated in the amniotic fluid and blood of patients in labor and in spontaneous abortions. These are considerably elevated over levels found during all other stages of pregnancy when the uterus is comparatively quiet. Induction of labor and therapeutic abortion is feasible with prostaglandins. Further evidence of their activity has been demonstrated in the action of prostaglandin inhibitors like indomethacin, which abolish or diminish uterine contractions. The use of indomethacin has been limited by its possible harm to the fetus.

Cervix. Early in the first stage of labor, dilatation of the cervix proceeds at a slow pace (latent phase), while later the cervix dilates at a considerably accelerated rate (active phase). Cervical dilatation becomes more rapid when the cervix is capable of reacting to increased uterine pressure created by myometrial contractions. At that time the "reaction point" is reached, and dilatation proceeds with relative rapidity. This occurs in nulliparous women at approximately 4 cm dilatation, and in multiparous women at about 3 cm. Swelling and softening of the cervix is called "ripening."

The structure of the cervix differs considerably from that of the uterine wall. There is considerably less smooth muscle tissue, more collagen, and connective tissue ground substance. Softening of the cervix accommodates dilatation and effacement (thinning), and softening primarily results from changes in collagen and connective tissue and from water retention within the cervix itself. Connective tissue ground substance becomes more prominent as labor proceeds, and collagen fibrils become swollen and fragmented. Certain enzymes are apparently responsible for the breakdown of protein and collagen, which is thought to be fundamental to cervical ripening.

The activities of the myometrium and the cervix must be coordinated as labor progresses. The uterine wall must become more active as the cervix relaxes. Both functions appear to be regulated by the same or similar hormonal mechanisms. While the precise nature of cervical maturation is far from defined, a number of active substances have been suggested. These include relaxins, prostaglandins, and the estrogen-progesterone ratio. Search for the common mechanism that controls uterine contractions and cervical dilatation continues with intensity, but when explanations do materialize, the ultimate benefits of intervention will then require documentation.

Fetal effects of uterine contractions

The relationship between fetal status and progress of labor is discussed in Chapter 1 as these relate to antepartum and intrapartum fetal heart rate monitoring. The principal stress exerted by labor on a fetus is interference with placental perfusion. The healthy fetus can tolerate the oxygen deficit that occurs during normal contractions; when the uterus relaxes, placental perfusion increases and fetal arterial PO_2 is restored. Fetal health during labor depends on sufficient uterine activity for expulsion on the one hand, and minimal interference with fetal oxygenation on the other. The effect of labor is sensitively influenced by fetal status. Maternal vascular disease associated with placental hypoperfusion enhances fetal vulnerability to the forces of labor even when contractions are normal. The fetus has been nurtured by marginally acceptable placental perfusion prior to the onset of labor. If the maternal disorder has also caused fetal growth retardation, the effects of labor may be even more troublesome. Antepartum fetal heart rate monitoring is designed to detect these phenomena. In another category of abnormality, excessive uterine contractions associated with diminished periods of relaxation may sufficiently disrupt maternofetal gas exchange to cause fetal asphyxia, even in a previously normal pregnancy.

DYSTOCIA (DIFFICULT LABOR)

Prolongation of labor resulting from mechanical factors is called dystocia. Precise time limits for the normal duration of labor are difficult to fix. However, it is generally agreed that the combined length of the first and second stages should not exceed approximately 20 hours and that the second stage itself is abnormal if it surpasses 2 hours in primiparas and 1 hour in multiparas. If labor is prolonged, perinatal mortality and morbidity increase because (1) separation of the placenta during the second stage is more likely, and severe fetal hypoxia may ensue; (2) compression of the cord is more likely, and it causes profound fetal hypoxia because blood flow in the umbilical vessels is obstructed; and (3) the incidence of intrauterine bacterial infection rises sharply as labor becomes more protracted, especially if the amniotic membranes have ruptured early (Chapter 12).

Dystocia may be caused by one or more of the following factors: (1) uterine dysfunction (inertia), which involves abnormal contractions of uterine muscle; (2) abnormal presentation, excessive fetal size, or congenital anomalies (such as hydrocephalus), which obstruct fetal descent during the

birth process; (3) abnormal size or shape of the birth canal, which impedes fetal passage (contracted pelvis); or (4) fetal macrosomia.

Uterine dysfunction

Uterine dysfunction may be hypotonic (weak contractions) or hypertonic (excessive contractions and muscle tone). The former, which is by far the most common variety, is usually caused by impairment of normal fetal descent (contracted pelvis or abnormal fetal presentation). In some labors hypotonic dysfunction is caused by overdosage of anesthetic and analgesic agents. This type of dysfunction generally appears during the latter part of the first stage. Progressive dilatation of the cervix is retarded or halted, and contractions weaken or cease altogether. Dangers of prolonged labor to the fetus were described earlier.

The hypertonic variety of dysfunction is infrequent. It appears early in the first stage of labor. Contractions are inordinately painful and sustained. Progress of labor is either slowed or nonexistent. In these circumstances, fetal hypoxia results from impaired placental blood flow from continuously increased intrauterine pressure. The effects of diminished placental blood flow on maternofetal gas exchange are discussed on pp. 9 and 51.

Contracted pelvis

An abnormal contour of the bony pelvis often involves a constricted birth passage that impedes normal descent of the fetus; complete obstruction is a rare phenomenon. Pelvic contraction occurs in approximately 5% of white women and in about 15% of black women. Pelvic size may be diminished in the anteroposterior diameter, the transverse diameter, or both. The slowed fetal descent caused by a narrow birth canal causes hypotonic uterine dysfunction and prolonged labor. The fetal dangers of protracted labor have already been enumerated, but in addition, trauma often occurs as a consequence of pressure exerted by the bony pelvis on a tightly fitting fetal part. For instance, cephalopelvic disproportion may cause molding of the fetal head, which is characterized by a misshapen skull, usually in the anteroposterior dimension. Occasionally pressure marks on the scalp are also seen at the point of contact with the maternal sacrum. In the extreme, a depressed fracture that is grossly visible as an indentation in the surface of the skull may result from excessive pressure against the bony pelvis.

Abnormal fetal presentation

The normal vertex presentation (head first) occurs in 95% of all deliveries. Abnormal presentations include breech, face, brow, and shoulder. Breech deliveries occur in approximately 4% of all births whereas other abnormal presentations occur in 1% of all births.

Face and shoulder presentations can in themselves prolong labor by impeding fetal passage, even if the pelvis is normally constituted. Breech presentations do not in themselves prolong labor unless pelvic narrowing is also present.

Face presentations are not common. They are more likely to occur when the maternal pelvis is contracted, when maternal abdominal musculature is lax (in multipara), and when the fetus is large. Characteristically the head is drawn back so that the occiput almost touches the upper spine. The resultant misfit of the head in the birth canal usually precludes normal passage, and delivery may be considerably delayed. At birth, facial edema and ecchymosis impart a characteristically grotesque appearance, which disappears in about a week (Fig. 2-5). Just as it was in utero, the head is held backward as the infant lies in the crib. Fetal and neonatal mortality are increased severalfold, primarily because of the hypoxic effects of prolonged labor and trauma.

A shoulder presentation occurs when the fetus lies transversely across the pelvis (transverse lie).

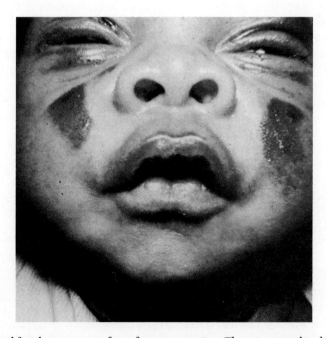

Fig. 2-5. Typical facial appearance after a face presentation. There is generalized swelling, most pronounced in the upper lip. Ecchymoses and abrasions are the result of birth trauma.

In this position the long axis of the body is perpendicular to the axis of the birth canal; the head is on one side of the pelvis and the buttocks on the other, with one shoulder up and the lower one protruding through the cervical orifice (shoulder presentation). Prolongation of labor is inevitable because fetal passage is obstructed. A considerable degree of obstetric skill is required for correction of a transverse lie; if correction fails, the only alternative is delivery by cesarean section. Shoulder presentations increase in frequency with multiparity. It is thus ten times more frequent in women with parity of four than during first pregnancies. Placenta previa and contracted pelvis may shift fetal position to a transverse one.

BREECH PRESENTATION

The breech position does not in itself impede progress of labor unless pelvic size is diminished. Depending on the part of the body that presents at delivery, breech presentations may occur in one of three varieties. In *frank breech* the buttocks are the presenting part, the lower extremities being flexed upward against the body. In a *complete breech* the buttocks and lower extremities present simultaneously, since the latter are not flexed upward but are approximately on the same plane as the buttocks. *Footling (incomplete) breech* refers to presentation of the feet and legs first, the buttocks later (Fig. 2-6).

The fetal and neonatal hazards of breech delivery are trauma, asphyxia, and prematurity. As a consequence, perinatal mortality may be increased four to ten times over vertex deliveries. The most serious traumatic event is intracranial hemorrhage. In vertex deliveries, the oncoming head may be slowed because of cephalopelvic disproportion. Since labor is still in an early stage, a decision to perform a cesarean section is timely as well as effective in avoiding head trauma. In breech deliveries, however, difficulty in descent of the head cannot be appreciated early in labor— at least not until the hips and shoulders have already been delivered. It may then be too late for a cesarean section. Sustained compression of the head during attempts to extract it often causes trauma and hemorrhage resulting from torn cerebral veins. The outcome is either lethal or permanent crippling. Spinal cord injury is also more common than in vertex presentations because stretching of the vertebral column occurs as traction is applied to the body during the anxious moments that precede delivery of the head. Hemorrhage into the abdominal viscera may occur, particularly in the adrenals and kidneys, and occasionally in the spleen. It may be caused by pressure exerted by the hands of the obstetrician while grasping the flanks of the infant's exteriorized body and in an attempt to extract the head under difficult circumstances. Other injuries include

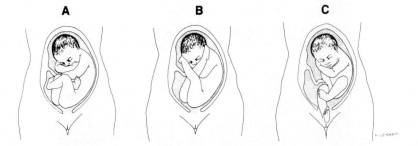

Fig. 2-6. Breech presentations. **A,** Complete breech: the legs, feet, and buttocks present simultaneously. **B,** Frank breech: only the buttocks are born first because the hips are maximally flexed, placing the thighs against the abdomen. **C,** Footling breech: one or both feet appear first.

brachial plexus palsy (p. 68), fractures of the humerus and femur (p. 65), and rupture of a distended bladder.

Compression of a prolapsed cord (p. 57) may cause severe asphyxia. This is twenty times more common in complete and footing (incomplete) breech than in vertex deliveries. It is only three times more frequent in frank breech presentations because the buttocks effectively occlude the cervical orifice and the cord is thus prevented from advancing. Placenta previa is an important cause of breech presentation, and in itself often leads to asphyxia. Separation of the placenta well before delivery of the head deprives the fetus of its only source of oxygen.

Persistent hyperextension of the neck in utero is an infrequent association of breech presentation. This unusual position may be detected by abdominal palpation, which reveals the fetal head to be drawn backward, as in opisthotonos. Ultrasound or x-ray examination confirms the suspicion. If hyperextension persists into the onset of labor and vaginal delivery is attempted, 25% of such fetuses will suffer transection of the spinal cord at the cervical level, which results in severe permanent disability or in death. Delivery by cesarean section consistently avoids the spinal cord injury.

ABNORMAL PLACENTAL IMPLANTATION AND SEPARATION
Placenta previa

Placenta previa is the result of abnormal implantation of the fertilized egg. Normally implantation is in the thick muscular wall of the upper uterine segment; in placenta previa it is misplaced in the lower uterine segment. Depending on the proximity of the placenta to the cervical os, three types are recognized (Fig. 2-7). Total placenta previa completely covers the cervical orifice. Partial placenta previa occludes the cervical orifice incompletely. In the third type, called low implantation of the placenta, the placental edge barely encroaches on the margin of the cervical aperture. Although these placental positions may

impede or totally block fetal passage, the most frequent causes of fetal and neonatal jeopardy are early placental separation and premature onset of labor. In early placental separation, fetal asphyxia occurs because the surface area available for maternofetal gas exchange is dangerously reduced. Even when fetal asphyxia is averted by expert management, perinatal mortality remains high because of the increased incidence of prematurity.

The hemorrhage that follows early placental separation is painless; it may cause maternal shock. Blood loss does not often occur before the end of the second trimester. Hemorrhage may first appear at the onset of labor. Occasionally cleavage also occurs through the fetal side of the placenta, and acute hemorrhage causes fetal shock that is clearly recognizable at birth (Chapter 9).

The placenta separates early because it is tenuously attached to the thin lower uterine wall. As pregnancy and labor proceed, the wall of the lower segment becomes progressively thinner. The placental attachment is thus easily disrupted before its time; hemorrhage and premature onset of labor are the result.

Placenta previa is effectively identified by ultrasound with 95% accuracy. Other methods are either less accurate or more troublesome.

Abruptio placentae (placental abruption)

Premature separation of a normally implanted placenta is called abruptio placentae. If the placenta separates at its margin, blood drains toward the cervix between the uterine wall and the amniotic membrane, ultimately becoming visible as vaginal bleeding. Approximately 80% of abruptions are of this marginal variety. If separation of the placenta is limited to its central portion while the margin remains intact, a more sinister situation exists because a considerable amount of blood loss may occur before it is recognized. In both instances the major fetal hazards are asphyxia (because of reduced gas exchange surface) and prematurity (because abruptio placentae stimulates early onset of labor). As in placenta previa, sep-

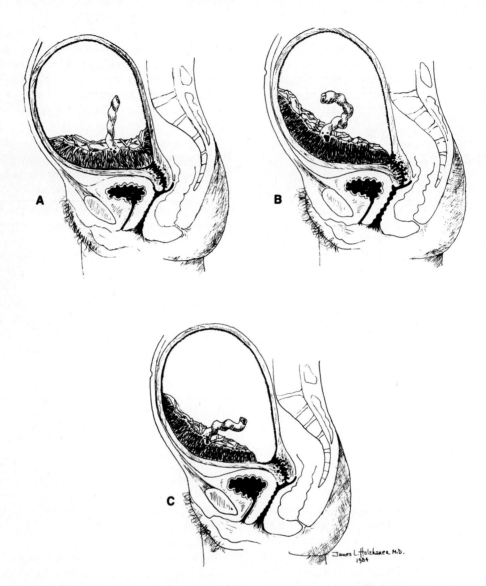

Fig. 2-7. Placenta previa. **A,** Total: the cervical outlet is completely occluded by the placenta, **B,** Partial: the placenta does not completely block the cervical outlet. **C,** Low implantation: the cervical outlet is not obstructed. (Modified from Netter: In Oppenheim, E., editor: Ciba collection of medical illustrations, vol. 2, Reproductive system, 1965.)

aration may cause hemorrhage from the fetal side of the placenta to produce neonatal shock at birth or soon thereafter (Chapter 9).

IMPAIRED BLOOD FLOW THROUGH THE UMBILICAL CORD

The umbilical vessels may be partially or completely occluded by compression of the cord. Prolapse of the cord involves visible protrusion through the cervical opening in advance of the presenting fetal part. Compression occurs when the cord is trapped between a fetal part and the bony pelvis or the dilated cervix. The same mechanism is operative in occult prolapse, which involves compression by a presenting fetal part but without visible protrusion of the cord through the cervix. Transient compression in utero without prolapse occurs frequently throughout pregnancy and is usually, but not always, innocuous. If fetal heart rate is monitored, these evanescent episodes of compression are marked by periods of deceleration that are unrelated to uterine contractions (variable deceleration). If these episodes are frequent and protracted, the fetus is in danger of severe asphyxia.

Prolapse of the cord, occult or obvious, is a dangerous complication that may cause complete depletion of fetal oxygen within 2½ minutes if the compression is not relieved. Prolapse is most common in breech delivery, multiple gestation, premature rupture of membranes, and transverse lie.

A cord wrapped around the fetal neck or body is generally harmless, but occlusion of umbilical circulation may occur if the cord is stretched in the extreme.

FETAL ASPHYXIA: RELATIONSHIP TO OBSTETRIC ABNORMALITIES

Fetal distress is often caused by diminution in the flow of oxygen from mother to fetus. The factors that inhibit oxygen transfer from mother to fetus simultaneously reduce the transfer of carbon dioxide from fetus to mother. These factors include maternal hypoxia, disrupted uteroplacental circulation, placental dysfunction, impaired blood flow through the umbilical cord, or an intrinsic fetal disorder. The most common cause of fetal asphyxia is impairment of maternal blood flow through the intervillous space.

Biochemical characteristics of asphyxia

Fetal asphyxia implies reduction in P_{O_2} (hypoxia), elevation of P_{CO_2} (hypercapnia), and lowering of blood pH (acidosis). The acidosis is called *mixed* because it comprises respiratory and metabolic components (Chapter 7). Respiratory acidosis is characterized by an accumulation of carbon dioxide in the blood that renders it more acid than normal (low pH). Metabolic acidosis refers to a low pH that follows accumulation of organic acids (Chapter 7). In the presence of asphyxia, these acids (principally lactic acid) are the end products of an abnormal process that must produce glucose at low levels of oxygen. This process is called *anaerobic glycolysis* because the breakdown of glycogen (principal source of glucose) transpires in the presence of hypoxia. Hypoxia thus causes metabolic acidosis because it forces anaerobic glycolysis. If the asphyxiated fetus were properly oxygenated by removing the cause of impaired gas exchange, P_{CO_2} would also diminish (eliminating respiratory acidosis), and the production of lactic acid would decline because glycogen breakdown could then proceed aerobically. Thus the concern with suboptimal oxygenation of the fetus is directed not only to the cellular damage caused by lack of oxygen but also to the difficulties of the resultant acidosis.

The initial fetal cardiovascular response to impaired gas exchange is caused by a gradual or precipitous fall in arterial oxygen tension. The heart rate drops at first and then rises temporarily, only to fall again as asphyxia progresses. An initial increase in blood pressure for the first few minutes is apparently a response to a surge in catecholamine release. The rise in blood pressure is also temporary; it falls progressively after several minutes. PCO_2 rises gradually, and pH drops progressively. In fetal lambs, the initial compensatory reactions cease after 4 minutes. At this time heart rate falls, blood pressure decreases, and acidosis worsens.

Signs of fetal asphyxia

Optimally, fetal asphyxia should be anticipated by antepartum heart rate tests (see Chapter 1). During labor, asphyxia is suggested by the presence of meconium in amniotic fluid, by changes of cardiac rate, and by sampling fetal scalp blood. Meconium-stained fluid is observable only when membranes rupture or when amniocentesis is performed. Alterations in heart rate are detectable by fetal heart rate monitoring. Asphyxial blood gas and pH changes are demonstrated by determinations on fetal scalp blood.

Specific maternal abnormalities associated with fetal asphyxia

A number of maternal disorders produce fetal vulnerability to asphyxial episodes. The detection of this vulnerability and the hypoxia that results from it have been discussed in Chapter 1. Maternal disorders that jeopardize the fetus are, with few exceptions, easily identified. The significance of the important ones and the mechanisms by which they endanger the fetus must be understood by all who care for sick neonates. The future of optimal perinatal care will largely depend on the obstetrician's (or perinatologist's) capacity to identify fetal compromise as early in its course as possible. Alertness to fetal hazard will usually depend on identification of maternal difficulty.

Maternal hypoxia deprives the fetus of oxygen by reducing oxygen tension in the blood that perfuses the placenta. The maternofetal PO_2 gradient is thus reduced or eliminated, and fetal oxygen deprivation follows. *Maternal vascular disease* may reduce placental blood flow so that the amount of oxygen delivered to the fetus is significantly reduced. Specific conditions that pro-

duce maternal hypoxia are (1) acute asthma, (2) severe pneumonia, (3) low environmental oxygen tension at high altitudes, (4) apnea associated with convulsive episodes of idiopathic epilepsy or eclampsia, (5) depressed ventilation caused by oversedation, (6) disturbed oxygen-carrying ability of hemoglobin resulting from carbon monoxide poisoning or hemolytic anemia, (7) diminished blood flow to all maternal organs (including the placenta) that characterizes congestive heart failure, (8) vasoconstrictive states associated with toxemia and essential hypertension, and (9) maternal hypotension from any cause, such as septic shock, traumatic hemorrhage, or the inferior vena cava syndrome (supine hypotension syndrome). The inferior vena cava syndrome results from pressure exerted on the inferior vena cava by the uterus when the mother is supine for long intervals. Venous return to the heart thus is impeded. A change in maternal position removes the obstruction to blood flow. The result of vascular occlusion is diminished perfusion of the intervillous space and reduced fetal oxygen supply. Low maternal blood pressure may also be associated with improperly managed conduction anesthesia (spinal, epidural, caudal, or saddle). Systolic blood pressures below 80 torr impair perfusion of the intervillous space.

As described previously, placenta previa and abruptio placentae reduce placental gas exchange in another way. A considerable reduction in the surface area available for oxygen diffusion results from the placental separation that characterizes both of these conditions. Furthermore, considerable maternal blood loss may cause hypotension and impair perfusion of the intact portion of the placenta.

The disorders mentioned above originate on the maternal side of the placenta. On the fetal side, and often unrelated to maternal status, the most frequent cause of fetal oxygen deprivation is compression of the cord, which may reduce blood flow to and from vessels in the chorionic villi. In the extreme the two arteries and the vein may be compressed. When less pressure is applied to the cord, the vein may be more occluded than the arteries because venous walls are thinner and more easily compressed, whereas the thicker walls of the arteries are more resistant to external pressure. Fetal asphyxia also results from cardiac failure in utero (hydrops fetalis) and from fetal hypotension associated with hemorrhage or drugs.

NEONATAL AFTERMATH OF FETAL ASPHYXIA

During asphyxial episodes in utero, reduced quantities of oxygen are delivered to tissues. Tissue hypoxia is the result of diminished perfusion (ischemia), diminished blood oxygen content (hypoxemia), or both. Fetal hypoxemia may occur as a consequence of several disrupted functions. First, the occurrence of maternal hypoxemia causes diminished oxygen transfer across the placenta. Hypoxemia in the mother is inherent in generalized seizures, cardiac failure, or shock. In these circumstances fetal hypoxemia is produced despite preexistent normal placental function. Second, and most frequently, fetal hypoxemia is caused by hypoperfusion of the placenta in maternal vascular diseases such as hypertension or advanced diabetes. In these circumstances the fetus is hypoxic despite the fact that the mother herself is well oxygenated. Abnormal placental function impairs oxygen diffusion to the fetus. Third, hypoxemia occurs when severe fetal anemia reduces oxygen content of blood. This phenomenon is operative in hemolytic anemia resulting from severe Rh incompatibility, or in hemoglobinopathies exemplified by α-thalassemia.

Theoretically hypovolemia causes tissue hypoxia when perfusion is impaired even in the presence of normal blood oxygen content. In the presence of poor perfusion, however, oxygen content of the blood usually falls precipitously.

Hypovolemia is a consequence of cord prolapse or a cord that is tightly wound around the neck (nuchal cord). Each of these conditions impedes

Table 2-2. Diving reflex: redistribution of blood flow

Increased flow to	Decreased flow to
Heart	Intestine
Brain	Kidneys
Adrenals	Lungs
	Peripheral vessels

venous return from the placenta to diminish fetal blood volume. Compressive forces occlude the umbilical vein more completely than the artery because the venous wall is substantially thinner.

Fetal hypoxemia may be accompanied by hypercapnia and metabolic acidosis. This is fetal asphyxia. The cardiovascular response to asphyxia should be interpreted as an attempt to survive. The redistribution of blood that characterizes this response provides remarkable increments in blood flow to the brain, the myocardium, the adrenals, and the placenta. Commensurately, blood flow must diminish in the lungs, the gastrointestinal tract, the kidney, and elsewhere throughout the body. There is a discernible purpose in the design of this response. It attempts to maintain tissue oxygen supply by increasing perfusion to the organs needed most for immediate survival. Increased flow of fetal blood to the placenta is an effort to acquire maximum quantities of available oxygen. In monkeys, blood flow to the brain increases twofold; a greater proportion perfuses the brain stem where cardiorespiratory functions are regulated. The altered distribution of blood is termed the "diving reflex," a response that was identified in mammals like the seal who dives into water and remains for protracted periods.

The postnatal sequelae of fetal asphyxia are largely a consequence of the redistribution of blood during activation of the diving reflex (Table 2-2). Multiple organ systems are affected simultaneously. The resultant clinical entities are usually identifiable. Organ system involvement in the aftermath of fetal asphyxia is as follows:

Brain
  Hypoxic-ischemic encephalopathy
  Periventricular/intraventricular hemorrhage
Lung
  Respiratory distress syndrome (increased severity)
  Meconium aspiration
  Pulmonary edema
Cardiovascular
  Persistent fetal circulation (PFC)
  Myocardial ischemia
  Tricuspid insufficiency
  Congestive heart failure
Renal
  Renal insufficiency resulting from acute tubular
    necrosis and cortical necrosis
Gastrointestinal
  Necrotizing enterocolitis
Hematologic
  Disseminated intravascular coagulopathy (DIC)
  Thrombocytopenia
  Leukopenia, neutropenia, increased immature
    neutrophiles (shift left)
Metabolic
  Metabolic and mixed acidosis
  Hypoglycemia
  Hypocalcemia
  Hypomagnesemia

Brain damage

The sites of asphyxial damage in the brain are largely determined by fetal maturity. In the full-term infant the resultant clinical entity is *hypoxic-ischemic encephalopathy* (see Chapter 14), which is characterized by neuronal necrosis principally in the cerebral cortex and basal ganglia. Affected areas are boundary zones between segments of brain supplied by separate arteries ("watershed" regions). Alternatively, an entire region of the brain supplied by a single artery may be affected. The most severe involvements affect wider and deeper areas such as the thalami and brain stem.

In the preterm infant, lesions produced by fetal asphyxia are most often hemorrhagic. They occur in the subependymal matrix and in the ventricles of the brain (see Chapter 14). The entity is termed *periventricular-intraventricular hemor-*

rhage. Another type of lesion is known as *periventricular leukomalacia*. It is an infarct, a focal area of softening at sites that are peripheral to the periventricular region. This type of damage affects preterm and term infants as well.

Lung problems

Hypoxia of pulmonary tissue affects airways, adjacent tissues, and blood vessels. The specific effects on blood vessels are described in the next paragraph. The diving reflex diminishes pulmonary blood flow from 7% of cardiac output to 3% or less by virtue of pulmonary vasoconstriction. Parenchymal tissue is thus deprived of oxygen. In premature fetuses whose nutritional requirements for the development of pulmonary tissue are high, extensive cell damage occurs. The epithelial cells of alveolar walls are particularly vulnerable. Damaged capillaries leak fluid into interstitial tissue and alveoli. In alveoli this transudate forms hyaline membranes when postnatal breathing is initiated. *Hyaline membrane disease* (respiratory distress syndrome) is more severe when intrauterine asphyxia has occurred (see Chapter 8).

Meconium aspiration syndrome is a major pulmonary sequela of fetal asphyxia. Plugged airways produce atelectasis and regional emphysema. The ratio of alveolar air movement and blood flow through alveolar capillaries (V/Q ratio) is disrupted. The meconium aspiration syndrome is often life-threatening, requiring mechanical ventilatory support. Having passed meconium when asphyxiated, the fetus gasps and aspirates it. The pathogenesis of the syndrome is discussed in Chapter 8.

Cardiovascular threats

Changes in the pulmonary vasculature and in the myocardium are the principal cardiovascular threats to survival. Normally pulmonary arterioles of the fetal lung are relatively constricted, imposing a high resistance to blood flow through the lung that will lessen considerably during the first few breaths after birth. Successful establishment of respiration depends on dilatation of constricted pulmonary vessels. When the fetus is asphyxiated, dilatation does not occur to a normal extent; high resistance to blood flow is maintained. This is called the *"persistent fetal circulation" (PFC) syndrome* because the fetal pattern of cardiopulmonary blood flow has not changed with initiation of respiratory effort after birth. Resistance to flow remains high, pulmonary artery pressure does not diminish, and right-to-left shunts across the foramen ovale and ductus arteriosus are maintained. This persistent fetal arrangement is life-threatening to the neonate.

Myocardial ischemia is sometimes sufficiently severe to cause congestive heart failure. The chest film depicts cardiac enlargement, and the electrocardiogram is often diagnostic. Occasionally myocardial ischemia is associated with *necrosis of the anterior papillary muscle* in the right ventricle. The chordae tendineae are attached to this muscle at one end, and to the tricuspid valve at the other. When papillary muscle contracts poorly during systole, the tricuspid valve remains patent so that blood is regurgitated from the right ventricle back to the right atrium. A murmur at the lower left sternal border is sufficiently characteristic to suggest *tricuspid insufficiency* (tricuspid regurgitation).

Renal insult

Acute tubular necrosis is the result of hypoxic damage to renal parenchyma. Hypoxia and ischemia follow diminished renal perfusion, which is inherent to the diving reflex. Parenchymal cells are swollen and edematous when the insult is mild or moderate. Signs of impaired renal function are generally confined to oliguria (less than 1.0 ml/kg/hr). If parenchymal damage is severe, necrosis of the renal cortex or segmental infarction give rise to anuria. Most of these infants do not survive, but the outlook is not necessarily hopeless. Blood urea nitrogen and serum creatinine levels are elevated in both moderate and severe disease. The urine contains protein, red cells, and casts.

Gastrointestinal disease

During asphyxia, blood flow to the gastrointestinal tract is considerably diminished. Although documentation is not available, a number of authors believe that fetal asphyxia imposes vulnerability to *necrotizing enterocolitis (NEC)*. NEC occurs in 3% to 5% of admissions to intensive care nurseries. It is primarily a disease of premature babies, although involvement of term infants is not rare. It is often sufficiently severe to require surgical resection of the bowel. Death occurs in approximately 25% of affected infants. Necrotizing enterocolitis generally becomes apparent between the fifth and twelfth days of life, and with few exceptions, after the baby has been fed. It is characterized by ischemia and infection of gut wall. Perforation requires bowel resection. The gastrointestinal vulnerability produced by asphyxial circulatory inadequacy has not been explained.

Hematologic sequelae

Disseminated intravascular coagulopathy (DIC) is an occasional sequela to fetal asphyxia. It comprises thrombocytopenia, increased degradation of fibrin products, and diminution of clotting factors. Sometimes only thrombocytopenia is apparent. DIC and thrombocytopenia are usually transient phenomena.

Changes in peripheral blood leukocyte counts are similar to those that indicate bacterial infection. Leukopenia (less than 4,000 or 5,000/mm³) and immature neutrophil quantities in excess of 16% of total neutrophils are typically associated with both asphyxia and infection. In the presence of infection these abnormalities persist or worsen for a few days. In contrast, when an infant has been asphyxiated in utero, the tendency for reversion to normal is evident within 12 to 24 hours.

Metabolic disturbances

The hallmark of severe asphyxia is *metabolic acidosis*, which is the result of increased production of lactic acid by anaerobic glycolysis. Elevated PCO_2 levels also contribute to a lowered pH.

Hypoglycemia is frequent in asphyxiated infants who do not receive intravenous dextrose soon after birth. During asphyxia, glycogen is rapidly depleted by anaerobic glycolysis. Release of norepinephrine during asphyxia further contributes to hypoglycemia by promoting accelerated peripheral utilization of glucose.

Hypocalcemia is commonly associated with perinatal asphyxia. The mechanism is unknown. Low serum calcium concentrations (less than 7 mg/dl) do not cause seizures during the first 48 to 72 hours of life. If seizures occur, they are a result of hypoxic brain injury. Severe hypocalcemia produces changes in the electrocardiogram that reveal abnormal myocardial function associated with dysrhythmia. Diminished concentrations of serum magnesium occasionally accompany hypocalcemia for reasons as yet undetermined.

TRAUMA OF LABOR AND DELIVERY

Although trauma to the fetus may be inevitable in certain abnormalities of labor and delivery, skillful obstetric manipulation may often avoid or minimize it. Traumatic lesions of the neonate are listed below. Most of them are mild and transient. Occasionally they cause permanent disability; they rarely cause death.

Mechanical injuries to the fetus
Skin, subcutaneous tissue
  Caput succedaneum
  Cyanosis and edema of buttocks, upper or lower extremities
  Diffuse scalp subgaleal hemorrhage
  Subcutaneous fat necrosis (pressure necrosis)
  Abrasion of the skin
  Petechiae and ecchymoses of the skin
Skull
  Molding
  Fracture (linear or depressed)
  Cephalhematoma
Long bone fractures
  Clavicle
  Humerus
  Femur
Central nervous system
  Hemorrhage into brain substance
  Subdural hematoma
  Spinal cord injury
Ocular
  Subconjunctival (scleral) hemorrhage
  Retinal hemorrhage
  Rupture of inner membrane of cornea (Descemet's)
Peripheral nerves
  Brachial plexus injury
  Diaphragmatic paralysis (phrenic nerve injury)
  Facial paralysis
Hemorrhage into abdominal organs
  Liver
  Spleen
  Kidney
  Adrenals
Rib fracture

Physical signs of trauma

Skin, subcutaneous tissue. *Caput succedaneum* is a localized edematous swelling of the scalp caused by sustained pressure of the dilating cervix against the presenting part. Venous return from the affected area is thus obstructed, and edema results. The swelling is most pronounced in prolonged labor. It disappears in several days and is of no pathologic significance.

Edema and cyanosis of the buttocks and extremities are produced by obstructed venous return from pressure of the presenting part against the dilating cervix in abnormal presentations. Swelling of the buttocks and genitals may thus be severe in frank breech deliveries. In footling breech the lower extremities are involved (Fig. 2-8); in complete breech the buttocks and lower extremities are simultaneously affected. The upper extremity is involved in shoulder presentation from a transverse lie.

Diffuse scalp subgaleal hemorrhage is an infrequent occurrence that involves bleeding into the entire scalp or a major portion of it. Loss of blood may be life-threatening. The most severe bleeding is associated with failure to administer vitamin K at birth or with other abnormalities of the clot-

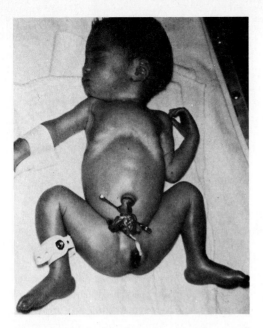

Fig. 2-8. Double footling breech, with edema and cyanosis of legs and feet, considerably more on left than right. Note frog leg position and absence of molding of head.

ting process that are unrelated to vitamin K deficiency, such as hemophilia. Coagulopathy has been reported in approximately 30% of affected infants. Hemoglobin levels may fall as low as 3 or 4 g/100 ml. Immediate simple transfusion is lifesaving. Scalp hemorrhage is cumulative over the first 24 to 48 hours. Tremendous swelling of the scalp extends over the forehead and behind the ears, and a characteristic blue discoloration is seen through the overlying skin. The scalp swelling is not limited by suture lines as in cephalhematoma. The life-threatening nature of this condition requires its early recognition. Swelling of part of the scalp and blue discoloration of the skin are the earliest signs that indicate a need for immediate attention.

Subcutaneous fat necrosis is a localized lesion produced by pressure against the bony pelvis or by forceps. It may also occur if the infant is slapped vigorously in attempts to stimulate the onset of respiration. The area of pressure necrosis varies in size, is sharply limited by distinct margins, and is always firm. The overlying skin remains intact and is occasionally blue or red. Subcutaneous fat necrosis may not be apparent for a number of days after birth. The lesion resolves in a few days to several weeks and is of no pathologic significance. It occurs most often in the face but also over the back and shoulders, arms, thighs, and buttocks.

Abrasion of the skin may be caused by application of forceps, pressure of an involved part against the bony pelvis, or careless handling of the infant after birth. The abraded area may serve as a portal of entry for infection.

Petechiae and ecchymoses of the skin are purple discolorations caused by hemorrhage into the superficial skin layers. By definition, petechiae are pinpoint in size, and ecchymoses are larger areas that resemble the common bruise. These skin lesions may result from severe systemic infections, but more commonly they are the result of direct injury or of pressure that obstructs the venous return from a presenting part. The resultant increase in back pressure ruptures capillaries, and skin hemorrhage ensues. Hemorrhage into the skin thus may indicate difficult labor and delivery, severe infection, or a clotting defect. It is also common in small premature infants in whom extensive bruising is evident, presumably as a function of capillary fragility. These small infants regularly develop hyperbilirubinemia from breakdown of extravasated blood.

Skull. *Molding of the head* is usually present to some degree in almost all vertex presentations. The contour of the head may be minimally distorted or grotesquely misshapen. Molding is caused by gradual shaping of the head as it accommodates to the contours of the bony and soft parts of the birth canal during labor. It is more severe in dystocia caused by contracted pelvis and in primiparous women. Usually the distortion is characterized by flattening of the anterior half of the head, with gradual rise to an apex at the pos-

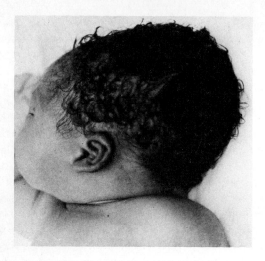

Fig. 2-9. Commonest type of molding, characteristic of vertex presentation.

terior half, and an abrupt drop at the occiput (Fig. 2-9). Schaffer has described the severely molded head as reminiscent of the drawings of Egyptian queens. The normal spherical shape of the cranium is gradually restored in 2 or 3 days. There is no valid evidence to suggest that subsequent brain dysfunction is associated with molding, but in the most severe cases the suspicion is inescapable.

Skull fractures (Fig. 2-10) may be linear or depressed. They must occur in parietal bones. Linear fractures are asymptomatic unless the force that produces them also ruptures underlying blood vessels to produce subdural hematoma or contusion of the brain. Depressed fractures are often self-correcting, but they may require surgical elevation if the depressed bone compresses underlying brain tissues. These fractures may result from high forceps or midforceps application, or from severe contraction of the pelvis associated with prolonged labor.

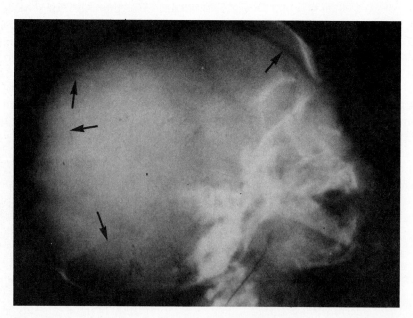

Fig. 2-10. Linear skull fractures (arrows) are straight radiolucent lines as opposed to sutures, which are linear but irregular and sometimes serrated.

Cephalhematoma is a collection of blood from ruptured blood vessels situated between the surface of the parietal bone and its tough, overlying periosteal membrane. It is usually unilateral, but occasionally bilateral (Fig. 2-11). Within 24 to 48 hours an obvious swelling develops beneath the scalp over one or both parietal bones. Rarely the occipital bone is involved, and even more rarely, the frontal bone is affected. A cephalhematoma is delineated by definite margins. It does not cross suture lines, being limited to an area overlying a single bone by firm attachment of the periosteum to the edges of that bone. In contrast, the margins of caput succedaneum and subgaleal hemorrhage are indistinct, and the swelling usually crosses suture lines. Cephalhematoma disappears gradually in several weeks, sometimes sooner. In 5% to 24% of affected infants, x-ray examinations re-veal a linear skull fracture beneath it. There are no known abnormal sequelae, whether or not a linear fracture is present. Occasionally, however, and particularly if the lesion is bilateral, hyper-bilirubinemia may result from breakdown of the accumulated blood (Chapter 10).

Long bone fractures. *Fractures of the clavicle and humerus* (Fig. 2-12) are the most common long bone fractures. The clavicle is affected far more frequently than the humerus. Each of these injuries is produced during difficult delivery of a shoulder or upper extremity in vertex or in breech deliveries. The incidence of trauma increases with birth weight. They are thus more frequent among infants who weigh over 4 kg. Clavicular fracture is usually detectable during movement of the shoulder when a snapping sensation is palpable over the involved bone. Spontaneous movement

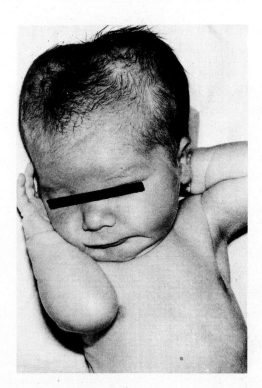

Fig. 2-11. Bilateral cephalhematoma over the parietal bones.

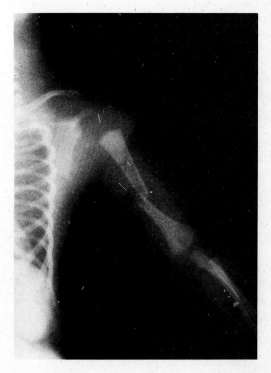

Fig. 2-12. X-ray film of fractured humerus, after difficult breech delivery.

of the upper extremity may not be restricted, and the Moro response may be normal. Fracture of the humerus is suspected by diminished motion of the extremity, by pain on passive movement, and often by a grossly visible deformity. Attempts to elicit a snap are contraindicated. Spontaneous motion of the involved extremity is diminished, and forced movement is painful. Reduced motion and pain are especially prominent in fractures of the humerus.

Fracture of the femur is an infrequent injury generally associated with breech deliveries. Swelling of the thigh and severely restricted spontaneous motion of the extremity are characteristic findings. Occasionally the involved thigh is blue because of associated hemorrhage into muscle and subcutaneous tissue.

Central nervous system. *Intracranial hemorrhage* is a common event in sick newborns, particularly in the premature infant. Intracranial hemorrhages are due to trauma, hypoxia, or both. *Subdural hemorrhage* and *subarachnoid hemorrhage (primary)* are primarily caused by trauma. *Periventricular-intraventricular hemorrhage* is usually the result of asphyxia. The discussion in this chapter is concerned with intracranial hemorrhages principally caused by trauma.

Subdural hemorrhage is a collection of blood in the subdural space that results from tears in the dura and the veins that permeate it. The dura is the toughest and most external of the three membranes that envelop the brain; the other two are deep to the dura and are called the arachnoid and the pia mater. Subdural hemorrhages are produced by stretching and tearing of veins that permeate the dural membrane. The resultant collection of blood may or may not produce clinical signs, depending on the location and the extent of the hemorrhage. Subdural hemorrhages are traumatic by virtue of head compression and elongation in the anteroposterior diameter, with consequent stretching of dural veins. This process can best be visualized by compressing an air-filled balloon on two opposed surfaces and noting the degree of expansion in the uncompressed diameter. The dura stretches during a similar process. Skull compression is most dangerous when relatively abrupt. Abrupt compression occurs during precipitate labor and delivery (less than 2 to 3 hours duration). Occasionally the same type of compressive stress is imposed when high forceps or midforceps are applied inaccurately. Most subdural hemorrhages occur over the cerebral hemispheres where bridging veins (between dura and venous sinuses) are torn. This type of subdural hemorrhage is virtually exclusive to term infants; premature babies have not yet developed bridging veins. Subdural hemorrhage also occurs in the posterior fossa from tears in the tentorium cerebelli. The tentorium cerebelli extends into the cranial vault and stretches across the posterior portion of the skull, separating the cerebral hemispheres above from the cerebellum below. It contains large venous sinuses. When they are torn, blood accumulates in the infratentorial space (posterior fossa) to rapidly compress the brain stem. This is a lethal process. Laceration of the tentorium is the most severe type of subdural hemorrhage.

Accumulations of subdural blood over the surfaces of the cerebral hemispheres are clinically identifiable soon after birth or not until several days later. As blood accumulates in the subdural space, the telltale signs of increased intracranial hemorrhage become evident. They include separation of skull sutures and tense bulging of the anterior fontanelle. Convulsions, coma, and repeated vomiting are characteristic. Untreated, this type of subdural hemorrhage may cause death. The subdural collections are generally bilateral, and they are almost invariably associated with blood in the subarachnoid space. Asymptomatic, unidentified small subdural bleeds are probably frequent, judging from common occurrence as an incidental finding at autopsies of term infants.

Subarachnoid hemorrhage (primary) is often asymptomatic. It is called *primary* subarachnoid hemorrhage when unassociated with other hemorrhage in the brain, such as the subdural or periventricular-intraventricular types. Primary subarachnoid hemorrhage is largely a traumatic disorder of term infants. In symptomatic babies, seizures are usually noted between the second and third day of life. As a rule, these seizures are generalized; occasionally they are focal. It is our experience that affected infants are otherwise in good health. Between seizures, spontaneous activity, color, and feeding performance are normal. The disorder is most often self-limited. Confirmation of the diagnosis requires computed tomography (CT scan) because the subarachnoid hemorrhage is not discernible by intracranial ultrasound.

Spinal cord injury is a rare event that is virtually restricted to breech deliveries. It is inflicted by forcible traction applied to the legs during the last phase of breech extraction when the head remains to be delivered. The spinal cord itself is relatively inelastic and does not comply to stretching, whereas the vertebral column is compliant. Since the spinal cord is fixed to the vertebral column, stretching or rotation of the latter results in tears of the cord or rupture of vessels within it. Transection of the cord causes permanent damage. A degree of recovery, sometimes complete, may follow edema, hemorrhage, or ischemia. Cord injury is frequently unassociated with dislocation or fracture of the vertebrae. X-ray films of the spine may be normal. In some instances vertebral fracture or dislocation is indeed evident on film, and reduction is urgently required for the relief of cord compression and maximal restoration of function. The type of paralysis that results depends on the level at which the cord is injured. Trauma to the lumbar area is most common, producing paralysis of the lower extremities, bladder, and anal sphincter. Laceration in the cervical region may cause total paralysis below the neck, including the muscles of respiration.

Spinal cord injuries present three types of clinical signs. In one, there is stillbirth or death shortly after delivery. In another, survival is only for a short period. These infants are in spinal shock. They have respiratory depression, and the pathologic picture of their lungs simulates hyaline membrane disease. Neurologic abnormalities depend on the level of injury. The intercostal or abdominal muscles may be paralyzed; the upper or lower extremities may be similarly involved. Affected areas of the body are insensitive to pain or touch. The third type is characterized by long-term survival with transient or permanent paralysis, usually of the lower limbs. Some surviving infants may be extensively affected from the neck down, thus involving paralysis of respiratory muscles, extremities, the anal sphincter, and bladder. Long-term postneonatal care is complex and stressful, requiring mechanical respiratory support, and bladder and bowel function hygiene. Pneumonia and urinary tract infections are inevitable.

Ocular. *Subconjunctival (scleral)* and *retinal hemorrhages* are caused by rupture of capillaries from increased intracranial pressure during the birth process. Ophthalmoscopy reveals flame-shaped and round hemorrhages in the retina. Retinal hemorrhage has been noted in as many as 20% of apparently normal full-term infants. With rare exception, there is no residual visual im-

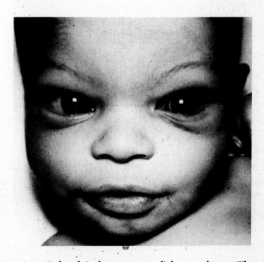

Fig. 2-13. Scleral (subconjunctival) hemorrhage. There were no sequelae.

pairment. The hemorrhages generally disappear by 5 days of age. Subconjunctival hemorrhage (into the sclera) imparts a striking external appearance to the eyes, which in the extreme are bright red except for the iris and pupil (Fig. 2-13) Abnormal sequelae to these lesions have not been documented. They clear within several days after birth.

Rupture of corneal membrane (Descemet's) may be the result of forceps injury. The healing process involves formation of a persistent white opacity called a *leukoma*. Edema of cornea occasionally occurs from normal pressure during the birth process. The resultant corneal haziness disappears in several days.

Peripheral nerves. *Brachial plexus injuries.* The brachial plexuses are formed by nerves from the fifth cervical through the first thoracic spinal roots (C-5 through T-1). They are situated at the anterolateral bases of the neck just above the lateral portions of each clavicle. Peripheral nerves that supply the muscles of the upper extremities emanate from the brachial plexuses. Injury thus causes some degree of paralysis of the upper extremity on that side. This rather common occurrence is related to a traumatic delivery. Paralysis of an upper extremity is usually partial, rarely complete. In vertex deliveries, it results from stretch injury to the brachial plexus when the operator laterally flexes the head excessively toward one of the shoulders, thus damaging the brachial plexus on the opposite side. It also occurs during breech deliveries when the extruded body is flexed laterally just prior to delivery of the head. Usually the involved nerve trunks become edematous; this condition resolves within days or weeks, and the paralysis clears. Paralysis is permanent when trauma causes irreversible discontinuity of nerve trunks.

Brachial plexus injuries can be suspected at a glance. It occurs in two forms. One type *(Erb's paralysis)* involves the nerve trunks of the brachial plexus that emanate from its *upper spinal roots* (C-5, C-6). It is by far the most common variety, primarily producing variable degrees of

paralysis of the shoulder and arm muscles. Spontaneous activity of that extremity is reduced. The arm is held close to the body. and the elbow is straightened, in contrast to that of the opposite, unaffected arm. When the baby is lifted and held in the supine position, the affected extremity is limp whereas the normal one is held in a flexed position. In eliciting of the Moro reflex, the paralyzed arm responds little or none at all, but the fingers extend almost normally. Involvement is primarily at the shoulder and arm and not in the hand muscles. Fig. 2-14 shows a baby at rest who has Erb's paralysis. The diagnosis can be suspected at a glance. The involved extremity is

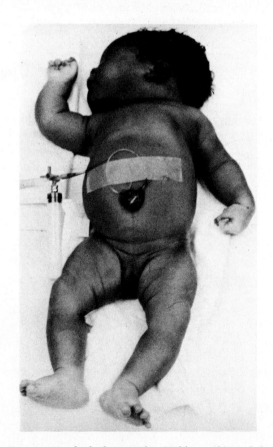

Fig. 2-14. Brachial plexus palsy (Erb's paralysis), left. Diagnosis can be suspected at a glance. See text for complete description.

straight; the opposite one is flexed. Both fists are closed. If the hand muscles of the paralyzed extremity were affected, the fingers would not be fisted. The Moro reflex of such an infant is illustrated in Fig. 2-15. Held supine, the involved left upper extremity is limp; it dangles (Fig. 2-15, *A*).

The Moro reflex is characterized by partial movement of the paralyzed extremity; the baby raises it partially from the original position. The opposite member responds with full motion (Fig. 2-15, *B*). Furthermore, the fingers of the left hand are partially extended.

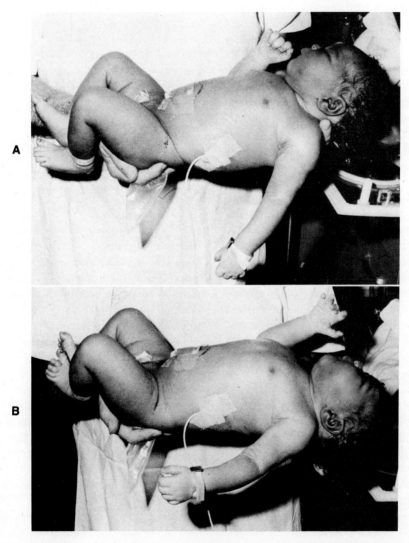

Fig. 2-15. Response to Moro reflex of infant with left brachial plexus palsy. **A,** Baby held supine, with left arm dangling. **B,** When head is dropped, left arm responds weakly, right arm completely. Note the position of fingers before Moro reflex and later.

The remarkable progress of obstetric practice in the past several years has made brachial plexus injuries relatively rare. The few that we now encounter are not extensive; many are barely discernible. These mildly affected infants are large. Their Moro response varies little, if any, from normal. However, the injury is in fact identifiable by holding the baby supine, as shown in Fig. 2-15, for approximately one minute. The affected upper extremity will ultimately dangle, even though an abnormal Moro response is not clearly discernible. The dangling response is probably the most reliable clinical indication of brachial plexus injury.

An infant with the second type of brachial plexus injury, *Klumpke's paralysis*, is shown in Fig. 2-16. This variety involves the nerve trunks that originate from the *lower spinal roots* that supply the brachial plexus (C-7, T-1). Involvement is therefore in the hands. Fig. 2-16 shows an unusually affected infant, with bilateral wrist drop. The fingers are relaxed, not fisted as is normal. This baby's Moro reflex was characterized by active motion of the shoulder and arm. The upper extremities are extended and abducted normally; the wrists and fingers remained flaccid.

Facial paralysis occurs as frequently in normal deliveries as in traumatic ones. It results from pressure on the facial nerve at a point just posterior to the lower part of the ear lobe, where it lies close to the surface. This pressure is exerted against the maternal bony pelvis during labor or by forceps that are applied inaccurately.

At rest, the facial palsy may escape notice. The palpebral fissure on the affected side is open while the opposite member is closed. The forehead and the nasolabial fold on the same side are flattened compared to the unaffected side of the face.

Facial paralysis is more easily detected when the infant cries. The entire face on the paralyzed side is immobile, and the palpebral fissure remains open. The muscles on the functional side of the face contract, the eye closes, the lips deviate toward the normal side, and the forehead fails to wrinkle. Facial paralysis usually disappears spontaneously in a few days.

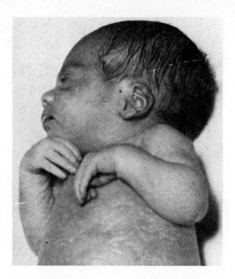

Fig. 2-16. Brachial plexus palsy (Klumpke's paralysis). Note bilateral wrist drop, relaxed fingers.

Paralysis of the diaphragm (phrenic nerve injury) usually occurs in association with brachial plexus injury, rarely by itself. It is caused by the same forces that are implicated in brachial plexus palsy, but with additional involvement of the phrenic nerve at its origin from the cervical portion of the spinal cord. The phrenic nerve receives fibers from the third, fourth, and fifth cervical nerves (C-3 through C-5). Because the phrenic nerve is the only one that innervates the diaphragm, respiratory distress may be severe. The lung on the affected side fails to expand completely. The diagnosis of diaphragmatic paralysis is strongly suggested in an infant who has respiratory distress and a paralyzed upper extremity. Whether or not the upper extremity is paralyzed, the signs of respiratory distress are those of diaphragmatic immobility. The infant will appear to have chest retractions with each inspiration; scrutiny indicates primary involvement of the affected side of the chest. Breath sounds are diminished on the involved side because diaphragmatic motion is limited and atelectasis has occurred. The point of maximal cardiac auscultation is displaced because the mediastinum has shifted toward the

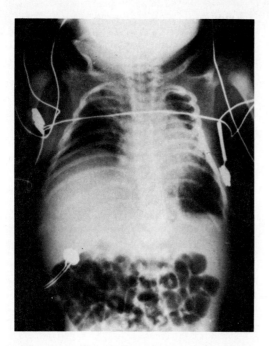

Fig. 2-17. X-ray film of chest showing right diaphragmatic paralysis associated with brachial plexus palsy on same side. Note inordinate height of right diaphragm and partial atelectasis of the upper lobe of the right lung.

unaffected side. X-ray films of the chest usually reveal the paralyzed diaphragm to be abnormally high (Fig. 2-17). Ultrasound examination reveals deficient mobility of the affected side of the diaphragm.

Hemorrhage into abdominal organs. The *liver* is more susceptible to injury than any of the abdominal organs. Injury is most likely in the presence of severe liver enlargement (as in Rh disease, congenital nonbacterial infections), particularly in large babies. Most often, the liver parenchyma is focally crushed during the inflicted trauma, and the resultant oozing of blood collects beneath the tough membrane that envelops the liver to form a subcapsular hematoma. Blood collects beneath the capsule gradually, over a period of 24 to 72 hours, before illness is apparent. The infant is pale because of anemia; the liver seems to enlarge progressively, and in some infants a distinct large mass (the hematoma) is palpable. At some point during the accumulation of blood, the liver capsule ruptures abruptly. Now, without containment, hepatic bleeding becomes brisk. Shock and cyanosis appear rapidly, and abdominal distention is severe. Often, the blood in the peritoneal space imparts a bluish hue to the abdominal skin, occasionally also involving the scrotum. Liver trauma is most often caused by excessive pressure to the costal margin during delivery or vigorous resuscitation. Less frequently a laceration involves the capsule and parenchyma simultaneously. Some infants escape rupture of the capsule when tamponade increases sufficiently as blood accumulates, to eliminate parenchymal ooze. The subcapsular hematoma then resolves; liver enlargement, or the palpable hepatic mass, recedes.

Since affected infants often have a disorder of blood coagulation, this must be identified rapidly. Blood transfusion is lifesaving. Surgical repair of the liver trauma is definitive.

The *spleen* ruptures far less frequently than the liver. In most instances, enlargement of the spleen is present as a consequence of disorders such as syphilis, Rh disease, or one of the nonbacterial intrauterine infections. An enlarged spleen is considerably more fragile than an enlarged liver. Rupture occurs directly from trauma; blood does not accumulate beneath the capsule. Loss of blood into the peritoneal space produces the same clinical signs of hypovolemia that were described for rupture of the liver. Whole blood transfusion must be given immediately. Surgical repair is urgent and definitive.

Small focal hemorrhage in the *adrenals* is asymptomatic, often first perceived months or years later when an x-ray film of the abdomen reveals calcifications. Adrenal hemorrhage is most likely to occur in large babies during a dystocic labor when trauma is inflicted. It is probably most common in breech deliveries. These injuries are also more frequent in the presence of syphilis, Rh disease, and neuroblastoma.

Massive adrenal hemorrhage usually produces a flank mass and sometimes also a bluish discoloration of overlying skin. Hemorrhage rarely extends into the peritoneal space because the adrenals are retroperitoneal. Blood may seep downward to surround the kidneys, and they may thus seem to be enlarged to palpation.

Signs of adrenal insufficiency are infrequent. These include vomiting and diarrhea, hypoglycemia, and early hypokalemia soon followed by hypernatremia. In the extreme, shock, seizures, and coma ensue. Without signs of impaired adrenal function, the hemorrhage itself produces pallor and cyanosis, flank masses, and occasionally fever. Surgery may not be necessary unless the blood loss is particularly copious. Restoration of blood volume and treatment of adrenal insufficiency are essential.

MULTIPLE BIRTHS

Perinatal mortality among twins is two or three times greater than among singletons. Therefore the presence of multiple gestation should be detected as early as possible, and the remainder of the pregnancy should be managed with the high risk in mind. The overriding cause of neonatal mortality in twins is prematurity. Other complications of pregnancy, labor, and delivery that occur with increased frequency include placenta previa, premature separation of the placenta, prolapsed cord, and abnormal presentations (especially breech) (Table 2-1). The increased incidence of fetal and neonatal abnormalities is also attributable to congenital malformations, intrauterine growth retardation (Chapter 5), fetofetal (twin) transfusion syndrome (Chapter 11), hypoglycemia (Chapter 9), and intrauterine bacterial infection.

Approximately one third of all twins born in the United States are identical; the remainder are fraternal. Identical twins originate from a single ovum (monovular or monozygous); they are thus of the same sex, and they resemble each other closely. Fraternal twins are derived from the separate fertilization of two ova (biovular or dizygous). They may not be of the same sex, and they do not necessarily resemble each other. In approximately half the cases, fraternal twins are of the same sex. Perinatal mortality is higher among identical twins.

Twinning is more frequent in blacks (approximately 1 in 70 births) than in whites (1 in 80 births). It is least frequent in Orientals. The widely held belief that twin pregnancies are familial applies only to biovular (fraternal) twins. Genetic and ethnic factors do not influence the incidence of identical twins. Multiple gestation appears to increase in frequency as maternal age and parity advance.

BIBLIOGRAPHY

Adamsons, K., and Joelsson, I.: The effects of pharmacologic agents upon the fetus and newborn, Am. J. Obstet. Gynecol. **96:**437, 1966.

Alstalt, L. B.: Transplacental hyponatremia in the newborn infant, J. Pediatr. **66:**985, 1965.

Bancalari, E., and Berlin, J. A.: Meconium aspiration and other asphyxial disorders, Clin. Perinatol. **5:**317, 1978.

Benirschke, K.: Origin and clinical significance of twinning, Clin. Obstet. Gynecol. **15:**220, 1972.

Bhagwanani, S. G., Price, H. V., Laurence, K. M., and Ginz, B.: Risks and prevention of cervical cord injury in the management of breech presentation with hyperextension of the fetal head, Am. J. Obstet. Gynecol. **115:**1159, 1973.

Brann, A. W., and Schwartz, J. F.: Central nervous system disturbances. In Fanaroff, A. A., and Martin, R. J., editors: Behrman's neonatal-perinatal medicine, St. Louis, 1983, The C. V. Mosby Co.

Bresnan, M. J., and Abroms, I. F.: Neonatal spinal cord transection secondary to intrauterine hyperextension of the neck in breech presentation, J. Pediatr. **84:**734, 1974.

Bronsky, D., Kiamko, R. T., Moncado, R., et al.: Intrauterine hyperparathyroidism secondary to maternal hypoparathyroidism, Pediatrics **42:**606, 1968.

Cannell, D., and Veron, C. P.: Congenital heart disease in pregnancy, Am. J. Obstet. Gynecol. **85:**744, 1969.

Challis, J. R. G., and Mitchell, B. F.: Hormonal control of preterm and term parturition, Sem. Perinatol. **5:**192, 1981.

Cosmi, E. V.: Drugs, anesthetics and the fetus. In Scarpelli, E. M., and Cosmi, E. V., editors: Reviews in perinatal medicine, Baltimore, 1976, University Park Press.

Desmond, M. M., et al.: The relation of maternal disease to fetal and neonatal disorders, Pediatr. Clin. North Am. **8:**421, 1961.

Ertel, N. H., Reiss, J. S., and Spergel, G.: Hypomagnesium in neonatal tetany associated with maternal hypoparathyroidism, N. Engl. J. Med. **280:**260, 1969.

Faix, R. G., and Donn, S. M.: Immediate management of the traumatized infant, Clin. Perinatol. **10:**487, 1983.

Fitzhardinge, P. M.: Complications of asphyxia and their therapy. In Gluck, L.: Intrauterine asphyxia and the developing fetal brain, Chicago, 1977, Year Book Medical Publishers, Inc.

Forman, A., Andersson, K-E., and Ulmsten, U.: Inhibition of myometrial activity by calcium antagonists, Sem. Perinatol. **5**:288, 1981.

Goodlin, R. C.: Care of the fetus, New York, 1979, Masson Publishing.

Goodwin, J. W., Godden, J. O., and Chance, G. W., editors: Perinatal medicine, Baltimore, 1976, The Williams & Wilkins Co.

Guillozet, N.: The risks of paracervical anesthesia: intoxication and neurological injury of the newborn, Pediatrics **55**:533, 1975.

Huszar, G.: Biology and biochemistry of myometrial contractility and cervical maturation, Sem. Perinatol. **5**:216, 1981.

Hutchen, P., and Kessner, D. M.: Neonatal tetany: diagnostic lead to hyperparathyroidism in the mother, Ann. Intern. Med. **61**:1109, 1964.

Jones, W. S., and Martin, E. B.: Thyroid function in pregnancy, Am. J. Obstet. Gynecol. **101**:898, 1968.

Klein, R. B., Blatman, S., and Little, G. A.: Probable neonatal propoxyphene withdrawal: a case report, Pediatrics **55**:882, 1975.

Mangurten, H. H.: Birth injuries. In Fanaroff, A. A., and Martin, R. J., editors: Behrman's neonatal-perinatal medicine, St. Louis, 1983, The C. V. Mosby Co.

McKay, R. J., and Lucey, J. F.: Medical progress: neonatology, N. Engl. J. Med. **270**:1231, 1964.

Mizrahi, A., and Gold, A. P.: Neonatal tetany secondary to maternal hyperparathyroidism, J.A.M.A. **190**:155, 1964.

Nathenson, G., Cohen, M. I., Litt, I. F., and McNamara, H.: The effect of maternal heroin addiction on neonatal jaundice, J. Pediatr. **81**:899, 1972.

Niebyl, J. R.: Prostaglandin synthetase inhibitors, Sem. Perinatol. **5**:274, 1981.

Palmer, R. H., Quellette, E. M., Warner, L., and Leichtman, S. R.: Congenital malformations in offspring of a chronic alcoholic mother, Pediatrics **53**:490, 1974.

Resnik, R.: Gestational changes of the reproductive tract and breasts. In Creasy, R. K., and Resnik, R., editors: Maternal-fetal medicine—principles and practice, Philadelphia, 1984, W. B. Saunders Co.

Rumack, B. H., and Walravens, P. A.: Neonatal withdrawal following maternal ingestion of ethchlorvynol (Placidyl), Pediatrics **52**:714, 1973.

Seeds, E. A.: Adverse effects on the fetus of acute events in labor, Pediatr. Clin. North Am. **17**:811, 1970.

Shearer, W. T., Schreiner, R. L., and Marshall, R. E.: Urinary retention in a neonate secondary to maternal ingestion of nortriptyline, J. Pediatr. **81**:570, 1972.

Soyka, L. F.: Prenatal exposure to stilbestrol and adenocarcinoma of the female genital tract: the pediatrician's responsibility, Pediatrics **55**:455, 1975.

Sutherland, J. M., and Light, I. J.: The effect of drugs on the developing fetus, Pediatr. Clin. North Am. **12**:781, 1965.

Volpe, J. J., and Koenigsberger, R.: Neurologic disorders. In Avery, G. B., editor: Neonatology—pathology and management of the newborn, Philadelphia, 1981, J. B. Lippincott Co.

Wallenburg, H. C. S.: Human labour. In Boyd, R., and Battaglia, F. C., editors: Perinatal medicine, London, 1983, Butterworths International Medical Reviews.

Yaffe, S. J., and Catz, C. S.: Drugs and the intrauterine patient. In Aladjem, S., editor: Risk in the practice of modern obstetrics, ed. 2, St. Louis, 1975, The C. V. Mosby Co.

Zelson, C., Lee, S. J., and Pearl, M.: The incidence of skull fractures underlying cephalhematomas in newborn infants, J. Pediatr. **85**:371, 1974.

CHAPTER 3

Evaluation and management of the infant immediately after birth

I have long been convinced that primary evaluation and care of infants at birth should be delegated to an appropriately trained neonatal nurse who can consult a qualified physician when the need arises. Contemporary therapeutic regimens have created a need for skilled personnel to care for infants in the delivery room during the first minutes after birth and in the nursery thereafter. Salvage of increasing numbers of jeopardized infants occurs in hospitals that utilize these regimens properly. However, their application has not been sufficiently widespread because of a lack of skilled personnel. The physician performing a delivery is preoccupied with the mother and yet must turn from her to help the distressed baby; or a pediatrician must be summoned, perhaps from some distance, only to arrive after the issue has been resolved unhappily. Obviously the continuous presence of someone who is adept and knowledgeable is essential for the care of all infants, especially the sick ones; wasted minutes are crucial to survival and to the preservation of intact central nervous system function. The trained neonatal nurse can play a vital role in solving these problems.

NEONATAL ASPHYXIA

The neonate may become asphyxiated by a sudden turn in events during the second stage of labor or immediately after birth, despite preexisting normal status. Examples of abrupt occurrences are cord compression, fetal dystocia, and acute hemorrhage. Alternatively, neonatal asphyxia is no more than a continuum of intrauterine events. Most often neonatal asphyxia is the visible culmination of disorders that began in utero, only to be compounded by subsequent misadventures during labor and after delivery. Fetal asphyxia is discussed in Chapter 2. In essence, the fetus is asphyxiated as a result of maternal hypoxia, or placental dysfunction even in the presence of normal maternal oxygenation, or intrinsic fetal difficulties such as severe anemia. The neonatal factors generally complicate the preexisting ones. Thus mechanical obstruction of the airway by meconium will impair extrauterine oxygenation in a neonate who has already experienced asphyxia in utero. Similarly, surfactant-deficient lungs of premature infants will not expand sufficiently in response to initial respiratory efforts, thus precluding normal extrauterine oxygenation. This serious postnatal handicap takes a greater toll if the baby was hypoxic in utero.

Delivery room management should protect the normal infant from misadventure, and it should rectify the defective functions that threaten the intact survival of others. Decisions must be made rapidly; remedial action must follow promptly. Effectiveness varies directly with the provider's fund of knowledge. Therefore physiology of the normal first breaths (Chapter 8) and the pathophysiology of fetal asphyxia (Chapter 2) must be understood and applied to the situation at hand. One cannot know what is best to do unless one knows why it must be done.

EVALUATION: THE APGAR SCORE

In 1952 Dr. Virginia Apgar introduced a simple straightforward scoring system for the clinical evaluation of infants at birth. A total score ranging from 0 to 10 is assigned; the more vigorous the infant, the higher the score. The procedure is best performed by an impartial nurse who is not directly involved with delivery of the infant and is primarily concerned with the postnatal status. This method of evaluation provides a grossly quantitative expression of the infant's condition that is well correlated with prenatal events and the postnatal course.

Procedure for scoring

Table 3-1 presents the components of the Apgar scoring system. A score of 0 to 2 is assigned to each item. The total of the five individual assessments is the Apgar score. A total score of 0 to 3 represents severe distress, 4 to 6 signifies moderate difficulty, and 7 to 10 indicates absence of stress or only the mildest difficulty. Evaluations are ordinarily conducted at 1 and 5 minutes after delivery of the entire body. One minute was chosen as the optimal time for the first score because experience has indicated that maximal depression occurred at that time. The 5-minute score correlates more closely with neurologic status at 1 year of age than does the score at 60 seconds.

Table 3-1. Apgar scoring chart

Sign	Score 0	Score 1	Score 2
Heart rate	Absent	Slow (below 100)	Over 100
Respiratory effort	Absent	Slow, irregular, hypoventilation	Good Crying lustily
Muscle tone	Flaccid	Some flexion of extremities	Active motion, well flexed
Reflex irritability	No response	Cry Some motion	Vigorous cry
Color	Blue, pale	Body pink Hands and feet blue	Completely pink

Most babies score 6 or 7 at 1 minute and 8 to 10 at 5 minutes after birth. If a score of 7 or less is assigned at 5 minutes, assessment should be repeated at 10 minutes. The individual components are evaluated as follows.

The *heart rate* is just as sensitive an indication of hypoxia after birth as it is in utero. A rate below 100 beats per minute is associated with severe asphyxia. The heart rate should be counted for at least 30 seconds. If a stethoscope is not available at the moment, palpation of the umbilical cord at its junction with the skin of the abdomen is also reliable for counting. In fact, pulsations of the cord are normally visible at this location. The heart rate is the most important of the five evaluated items. A score of 2 is assigned if the heart rate exceeds 100, a value of 1 is given if it is below 100, and if no heartbeat is detected, the score is 0. If it is less than 100 beats per minute, an urgent need for resuscitation exists.

Respiratory effort is next in importance to heart rate. Regular respirations and a vigorous cry merit a score of 2. If respirations are irregular, shallow, or gasping, a score of 1 is appropriate, whereas 0 indicates complete absence of any respiratory effort (apnea).

Muscle tone refers to the degree of flexion and the resistance offered to straightening the extremities. The normal infant's elbows are flexed, and his thighs and knees are drawn up toward the abdomen (flexed hips). In addition, some degree of resistance is encountered when one attempts to extend the extremities. This normal muscle tone is assigned a score of 2. At the other extreme, an asphyxiated infant is limp. There is no resistance to straightening of the extremities, nor is there any semblance of flexion at rest. This state of muscle tone is scored 0. Muscle tone that is intermediate between the normal and limp asphyxiated states is given 1 point.

Reflex irritability is judged by the infant's response to flicking the sole of the foot. If he cries, a score of 2 is given. If he only grimaces or cries feebly, a score of 1 is given. If there is no response, the score is 0.

Color evaluation is directed to the presence or absence of pallor and cyanosis. Only a few infants are completely pink; they are assigned 2 points. Most babies are given a score of 1 because normally their hands and feet are blue, whereas the rest of the body is pink (acrocyanosis). Only 15% of all infants score 10 at 1 minute because of the high incidence of acrocyanosis. Pallor and cyanosis over the entire body is scored 0.

Relationship of Apgar scores to arterial pH and clinical depression

As the score declines, pH usually diminishes and clinical depression of the infant becomes increasingly severe. The scores provide a sound basis for the management of neonates immediately after birth, and the resuscitative procedures that are described later are based on them. There are, however, three notable exceptions to the close relationship between the Apgar score and blood pH: (1) A low score may be associated with a normal or slightly diminished pH if the infant is depressed as a consequence of maternal anesthesia; (2) a relatively high score may be associated with a low pH in small-for-dates infants who have suffered chronic marginal intrauterine hypoxia; and (3) a normal score may accompany a low pH as a result of maternal acidosis.

Relationship of Apgar scores to birth weight and neonatal mortality

Systematic observations on thousands of infants have clearly demonstrated a relationship between Apgar scores and birth weight, time of scoring, neonatal mortality, and neurologic status at 1 year of age.

The increased prevalence of stress among low birth weight infants is indicated by the incidence of low scores. In 57% of infants who weigh 1500 g or less, the 1-minute scores are 0 to 3, whereas these low scores occur in only 5% of infants over 3000 g. Vigor at birth is far more common among larger babies; scores of 9 and 10 occur in 52% of them, whereas in small infants only 4% score similarly.

The status of most infants improves between the 1- and 5-minute scores. Fewer babies are in a precarious state at 5 minutes than at 1 minute. In the *Collaborative Perinatal Study*, observations on 17,000 infants revealed that at 1 minute 7% scored 0 to 3, and at 5 minutes 2% scored similarly. The same trend toward improvement is indicated by the incidence of higher scores. At 1 minute 79% scored 9 or 10, and at 5 minutes 95% achieved the same scores. Because improvement between 1 and 5 minutes occurs in a substantial number of infants, the later scores are generally more reliable for the prediction of death during the first 28 days of life (neonatal mortality), and of abnormal neurologic status at 1 year.

The risk of death is increased if the 5-minute Apgar score is low. In the absence of an intensive care program, death can be expected during the neonatal period in 50% of all infants with a 5-minute score of 0 or 1, and the vast majority of these babies expire within the first 48 hours of life. Low birth weight enhances this risk considerably. For instance, among babies under 2000 g who score 0 to 3 at 5 minutes, approximately 80% die during the neonatal period, but among infants over 2500 g with the same scores the mortality is 15%. The vast majority of these deaths occur during the first 2 postnatal days.

These data were compiled in the era that immediately preceded contemporary intensive care of the neonate. Although mortality and morbidity have improved, the relative predictive value of lower scores for more ominous outcomes is probably unchanged. Death of low-scored infants may be up to fifteen times more frequent than in those whose scores are high.

Relationship of Apgar scores to neurologic status at 1 year of age

The link between later brain dysfunction and perinatal distress is also convincingly demonstrated in data from the *Collaborative Perinatal Study*. A close relationship was evident between low birth weight, low Apgar scores at 5 minutes, and an increased incidence of neurologic abnormali-

Table 3-2. Percentage of neurologic abnormality at 1 year according to 5-minute Apgar score and birth weight*

Birth weight (grams)	5-minute Apgar scores		
	0-3	**4-6**	**7-10**
1001 to 2000	18.8%	14.3%	8.8%
2001 to 2500	12.5%	4.6%	4.0%
Over 2500	4.3%	4.2%	1.4%

*Modified from Drage, J. S., and Berendes, H.: Pediatr. Clin. North Am. **13:**635, 1966.

ties at 1 year of age. That hypoxia around the time of birth may well be lethal can be appreciated from the correlation of low scores with increased neonatal mortality. A low 5-minute score indicates persistence of asphyxia. Thus if a distressed infant with a low score survives, his chances of brain damage are considerably greater than they would have been if he had scored normally. This is reflected in statistical data that relate birth weight and Apgar scores to 1-year outcomes. Birth weight exerts the same sort of influence on 1-year outcome as on neonatal mortality. Table 3-2 is taken from data compiled by the *Collaborative Perinatal Study*. With identical scores, the frequency of neurologic abnormalities at 1 year increases as birth weight diminishes. At identical birth weights, the frequency of abnormalities increases as the Apgar score declines. Together the effects of weight and score reinforce each other. Thus of all the groups in the table the smallest infants with the lowest scores are most likely to have brain damage (18.8%), whereas the largest babies with the highest scores are least likely to be affected (1.4%).

The diminished incidence of neurologic deficit among surviving infants that has occurred since the advent of intensive care is well documented. The results described above have thus undoubtedly improved, but the influence of low scores and low birth weight on poor outcome is probably unchanged.

Value of Apgar scores

The quality of neonatal care has improved as a result of the Apgar score. Perhaps the most important contribution of the procedure is that it requires scrutiny of the baby immediately after birth. Thorough evaluation of heart rate, respiration, muscle tone, reflex response, and color was not performed systematically prior to the introduction of scoring. The value of the procedure is so well established that it is unquestionably negligent to omit it. Aside from its predictive value, the score identifies high-risk infants who urgently require resuscitation. It also provides a universally understood quantitative expression of the infant's condition. It further enables statistical assessment of a hospital's perinatal practices and the level of risk in the population it serves. The procedure is simple, but it requires conscientiousness and skill if its purposes are to be fulfilled. The most accurate results are obtained when a knowledgeable nurse executes the scoring.

MANAGEMENT: ROUTINE CARE AND RESUSCITATION OF DISTRESSED INFANTS

Information regarding resuscitative procedures is presented with full awareness that too few nurses have been taught to use them and with the distinct conviction that many infants would be saved if more nurses could do so. The procedures cannot be learned from a printed page. These descriptions are like a map; real familiarity with the terrain is gained only after traveling the road, but the itinerary must be known beforehand. Resuscitation and its rationale must first be read about and then performed with proper supervision.

Care of normal infants
(Apgar score 7 to 10)

There is often a moment of suspense, sometimes tension, when birth is imminent as the top of the baby's head first becomes visible. *The events that follow birth have their origins in those that preceded it.* If the history is known in detail, and if labor and delivery have been followed closely, many of the infant's potential difficulties can be anticipated, and they have already been discussed in some detail. Although most babies are normal and have no difficulties, they nevertheless must be supported by a few simple procedures.

After delivery of the entire body, the operator holds the head downward as suction is applied to the nostrils and oropharynx with a bulb syringe. The cord is cut and clamped, and the nurse takes the baby in charge. The infant is placed in a 15-degree Trendelenburg position on a table supplied with radiant heat emanating from above. The importance of providing environmental warmth to minimize loss of body heat cannot be overemphasized. Control of body temperature (thermoregulation) is discussed in detail in Chapter 4. At birth, a major cause of heat loss is the evaporation of amniotic fluid that covers the infant's skin. The infant must therefore be dried rapidly, preferably by another individual, while the neonatal nurse removes oropharyngeal secretions with a bulb syringe if they have reaccumulated.

The 1-minute Apgar score should now be performed, and if the result is 7 to 10, resuscitative therapy is unnecessary. The infant should be observed on a warmed table until the 5-minute Apgar score is assigned, and for a least an additional 5 minutes thereafter. During the interval after the 5-minute Apgar score, the nurse should examine the infant. Auscultation of the chest will ascertain proper position of the heart and normal air exchange. The head and body surfaces are scrutinized for trauma and for obvious congenital anomalies. Spontaneous movement of the extremities is observed for indications of weakness or paralysis. The abdomen is palpated for masses and for enlargement of the liver, spleen, or kidneys. The genitalia are examined for normal sexuality. Each of the shoulders is moved while a finger is placed over the clavicle. A crunching sensation (crepitus) betrays a fracture. Normal findings of the physical examination and their variants are presented in detail in Chapter 6.

At some time prior to transfer of the infant to the nursery, the cord is cut again, leaving a stump approximately 1 inch in length to which a clamp is applied. Before the clamp is applied, the cut surface should be examined closely for the normal number of vessels (two arteries and one vein). The presence of only one artery suggests one or more major congenital malformations. The cut edges of the arteries are seen as two white papular structures, which usually stand out slightly from the surface. The vein is larger, often gaping so that the lumen and thin wall are readily discernible (Fig. 1-4). A drop of silver nitrate or an antibiotic preparation is then placed in each eye for prophylaxis against gonorrheal infection. The eyes should not be irrigated thereafter. In some communities antibiotic drops are preferred for this purpose.

A complete record of labor, delivery, and postnatal events must accompany the infant on transfer to the nursery. The condition should be reported verbally to the physician in charge before the nurse leaves the delivery room with the baby. The nursery should have already been notified of the infant's anticipated arrival.

Care of moderately depressed infants (Apgar score 4 to 6)

Moderately depressed infants are limp, cyanotic or dusky, and dyspneic. Respirations may be shallow, irregular, or gasping. The heart rate is normal, however, and there is at least a fair response to flicking of the sole. Management entails the same regimen described for normal infants during the first minute after birth, but if effective spontaneous respiration is not established thereafter, ventilatory support is essential. The urgency for this support is indicated by continued cyanosis and flaccidity. Initially a laryngoscope is inserted. The larynx is visualized, and

suction is applied through a catheter attached to a De Lee trap. The De Lee trap is operated by suction from the operator's mouth. This procedure, under direct visualization of the larynx, assures removal of blood clot, particles of meconium and vernix, and thick mucus. The suction catheter is withdrawn, and a curved plastic airway is inserted between the tongue and palate to prevent the base of the tongue from falling backward over the glottic opening of the larynx. Oxygen is then administered through a tightly fitting face mask attached to a hand-operated bag that receives 100% oxygen and delivers it to the infant in high concentrations. At our hospital we have used the Penlon mask-and-bag apparatus with satisfaction. The chest rises with each squeeze of the bag if oxygen is delivered adequately. Further ascertainment is obtainable if an assistant listens to each lung with a stethoscope for the presence of breath sounds. If color and respirations have not improved after 1 minute or the heart rate falls below 100 beats per minute at any time, endotracheal intubation is urgently indicated (see following discussion). If the mask-and-bag procedure is effective, the heart rate quickens or does not decline, spontaneous respiration begins within 1 minute, and cyanosis should disappear. When the baby begins to breathe, free-flowing oxygen should be supplied.

Care of severely depressed infants (Apgar score 0 to 3)

Gentle swiftness is the essence of resuscitation of profoundly depressed infants. Their woeful state is instantly recognizable. They are blue and limp, and they make little or no attempt to breathe. The heart rate is less than 100 beats per minute, if it is at all present; preliminary suction of the upper airway and a vigorous flick of the sole are of no avail. The Apgar score is 0 to 3. This evaluation should consume no more than a few seconds. The experienced observer recognizes the gravity of the situation without consciously scoring the infant's status. Suction and endotracheal intubation under direct visualization with a laryngoscope are the only procedures that can save an infant in such straits. Generally, once oxygen is delivered to the lungs, the response is gratifying. Improvement may be noted in seconds, although frequently intubation must be maintained for 10 minutes or longer. The heartbeat returns; if it is present initially, the rate quickens and the sounds are louder and sharper. With the return of more effective cardiac function, the baby becomes pink, and some spontaneous muscle activity may appear. If heart activity is absent after 3 or 4 insufflations, external cardiac massage is mandatory. Occasionally, after cardiac activity is restored, intravenous administration of sodium bicarbonate and dextrose is essential because hypoxia causes metabolic acidosis and it may also produce hypoglycemia as a result of rapid depletion of glycogen store (Chapter 11). The details of resuscitation follow.

Equipment

Laryngoscope (pencil handle with attached Miller size 0 premature or size 1 infant blade). The adequacy of the light source must be ascertained during periodic routine checks of all equipment when not in use.

Endotracheal tubes. Some operators prefer Cole endotracheal tubes with metal stylet to prevent kinking. These tubes are tapered at the distal end (sizes 10, 12, or 14). We prefer untapered Portex tubes in sizes ranging from 2.5 mm to 4 mm. We avoid metal stylets because of the trauma they may cause during intubation.

De Lee trap. A De Lee trap is preferred for suction, which should be applied by the operator's mouth. Wall suction in delivery rooms is traumatic to neonates because it is far too forceful. If wall suction is used, it must be modulated by a regulator to a level no greater than 120 torr.

Bag resuscitator. This bag is attached to the inserted endotracheal tube. It receives 100% oxygen from a wall source or from a tank. Infant masks are usually supplied with this apparatus but are of no value in resuscitation of severely depressed infants.

Procedure for ventilation by tracheal intubation

1. The infant should be supine, with a flattened, rolled towel to support the upper back at the level of the shoulders.

2. The baby's head is held with the right hand; the face looks upward. The laryngoscope is held in the left hand with the blade attachment downward.

3. The blade is slipped past the right corner of the mouth for a distance of approximately 2 cm along the right side of the oral cavity. In so doing, the blade is moved toward the midline, thus displacing the tongue to the left side of the oral cavity.

4. The tip of the blade is advanced slightly so that it comes to rest in a wedge-like space (the vallecula), which is situated between the epiglottis and the base of the tongue (Fig. 3-1). A slight upward tilt of the tip of the blade now exposes the opening of the larynx (glottis). The glottis is more easily seen if slight downward pressure is applied externally to the larynx by the hand that holds the laryngoscope, or by an assistant. As now viewed, the following structures are identifiable from above downward (anterior to posterior): the base of the tongue, the blade placed in the vallecula, the epiglottis, the glottis, the esophageal opening, and the posterior hypopharyngeal wall (Fig. 3-2). The epiglottis is a valuable landmark because it is sometimes visible when the glottis is not. The epiglottis appears as an arched rim of pink tissue, which often tapers to a rounded point so that it resembles a diminutive tongue. If it is visible and the glottis is not, the operator need only tilt the laryngoscope slightly so that the tip of the blade moves upward. The glottic opening is thus revealed as a black vertical slit. If obstructed by fluid and particulate matter, the slit is discerned with difficulty. Suction is necessary to clear the area and to evacuate unseen material that may fill the trachea as well. The suction catheter should be advanced through the glottis to clear the trachea prior to insertion of an endotracheal tube.

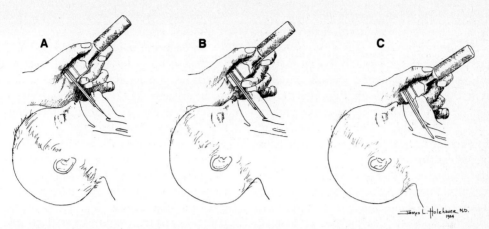

Fig. 3-1. A, Position of laryngoscope blade prior to insertion into the vallecula. **B,** Blade tip resting in vallecula directly above the epiglottis. **C,** Misplaced blade inserted into the esophagus.

5. If spontaneous respirations do not immediately follow the removal of fluid and particulate matter, an endotracheal tube is introduced through the glottis. If a straight tube such as the Portex is used, insertion past the glottis should not exceed 1 to 1.5 cm. Remove the laryngoscope cautiously while holding the tube in place. Oxygen may now be delivered through a bag (Penlon) attached to the endotracheal tube. The bag is abruptly squeezed and released at a rate approximating 40 times per minute. If the bag is grasped in the palm of the hand and squeezed with all five fingers, pressures in excess of 60 to 70 cm H_2O are delivered, and pneumothorax may ensue. By squeezing with the thumb, index, and middle fingers only, safer and usually effective pressures of 25 to 35 cm H_2O are delivered. A manometer attached to the bag effectively indicates peak inspiratory pressures. Sometimes higher pressures are required initially for adequate lung expansion, necessitating use of the entire hand for bag compression. As insufflation proceeds, absent or minimal chest movement indicates inadequate peak inspiratory pressure or malposition of the tube. If the endotracheal tube has been inserted too deeply, it will pass directly into the right main stem bronchus. Delivery of oxygen is therefore

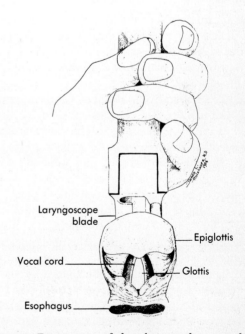

Fig. 3-2. Direct view of the glottis and surrounding structures after the blade tip is inserted into the vallecula.

confined to the right lung, and insufflation causes expansion in the right chest, with little or no visible excursion on the left. This discrepancy can be determined more accurately by an assistant who listens with a stethoscope. Breath sounds are absent on the left, whereas on the right they are loud and clear. This being the case, the endotracheal tube should be withdrawn slightly until breath sounds are equal on each side of the chest.

External cardiac massage

1. If the heartbeat has not returned after three or four insufflations, external cardiac massage must be instituted immediately. It should be performed by an assistant, leaving the primary operator free to manage ventilation. When downward pressure is applied at the left margin of the lower sternum, the heart is compressed (systole); when the pressure is released, the heart is dilated (diastole).

2. The index and middle fingers are placed at the appropriate spot and abruptly pressed downward and released. The total downward displacement of the chest wall should not exceed 1 in. Excessive vigor may cause a laceration of the liver with severe blood loss.

3. It is imperative to maintain cardiac massage and ventilation. This is accomplished by alternating the two maneuvers. The heart is compressed two or three times (at a rate approximating 120 times per minute), after which a breath of oxygen is supplied. The two procedures should never be performed simultaneously, since the pressure applied during cardiac massage may rupture a lung that is simultaneously inflated by artificial ventilation. Pneumothorax and pneumomediastinum may ensue.

4. If cardiac massage is effective, the femoral or temporal artery pulses are palpable in synchrony with depression of the sternum. Cardiac compression should be discontinued every 30 to 60 seconds to detect the presence of spontaneous cardiac activity.

5. When a regular heartbeat is discerned, cardiac massage may be discontinued. Assisted ventilation may be discontinued when spontaneous respiration appears.

Correction of metabolic acidosis. The asphyxiated neonate is by definition, hypoxemic, hypercarbic, and acidotic. Metabolic acidosis is the result of lactic acid accumulation from anaerobic glycolysis during hypoxemia; retention of CO_2 results in respiratory acidosis. To correct acidosis during the resuscitative procedure, the pervasive practice for well over a decade has entailed the administration of sodium bicarbonate by rapid intravenous infusion in the delivery room. Now, well-controlled studies have led to the conclusion that this practice requires revision—the fact is, sodium bicarbonate therapy is only exceptionally necessary and is contraindicated for the correction of acidosis during resuscitation. Contemporary evidence also demonstrates that bicarbonate for the acidosis that accompanies hyaline membrane disease is rarely indicated and that it is often dangerous.

Rapid infusion of alkali for resuscitation in the delivery room is, as a rule, contraindicated because:

1. Bicarbonate is changed in the blood to CO_2 and water. Its beneficial effect thus depends on the efficient elimination of CO_2 by the lungs. If bicarbonate is given when the elimination of CO_2 is impaired, the P_{CO_2} rises significantly and the pH actually falls as a result of the bicarbonate therapy.

2. Rapid administration of alkali, particularly if undiluted, raises serum osmolality to the high levels (over 320 milliosmoles). Hyperosmolar blood damages the normally tough blood-brain barrier at the capillaries. Subsequent rupture of the capillaries is the most frequently encountered mechanism in the development of periventricular hemorrhage in premature infants.

Bicarbonate is often used to reduce the metabolic acidosis that persists after the resuscitative procedure. The data clearly demonstrate the acidosis in these circumstances is not usually corrected and that PCO_2 rises. If correction does occur, the process is no more rapid in infants who are given bicarbonate than in infants who receive only dextrose water.

Sodium bicarbonate therapy should thus be a rare event. If it must be utilized, the bicarbonate should be diluted two to five times with water for injection. Addition of five parts of water results in an isotonic solution that can be rapidly injected into an asphyxiated infant. A typical dose would then entail infusion of 10 to 15 ml/kg, which is likely to be effective for the hypotension that is a frequent component of asphyxia. *Sodium bicarbonate is indicated only if there is no response to assisted ventilation. This lack of response is characterized by persistence of bradycardia (less than 100 beats per minute) and hypotension.*

If intravenous medication is an urgent need, rapid access is accomplished by inserting a catheter into the umbilical vein. The catheter is passed into the umbilical vein for distances varying from 5 to 9 cm, depending on the size of the baby. The distal end of the catheter should never be open to room atmosphere because a deep gasp may cause the entry of a significant quantity of air into the heart. A three-way stopcock thus should be attached at the distal end of the fluid-filled catheter for administration of sodium bicarbonate by syringe and for slow infusion of 10% dextrose solution afterward. The umbilical vein should be abandoned as soon as possible in favor of a peripheral vein if continued intravenous administration of fluid is necessary. An infusion pump must be used to maintain the appropriate flow rate.

Maintenance of body heat. Provision of external heat is indispensable if optimal results are to be derived from the resuscitative procedures just described. The implications of low body temperature are discussed in Chapter 4. Evaluation and management of all infants must be performed on a table that is supplied by an overhead source of radiant heat. Without it, the response to resuscitation is delayed, diminished, or absent. The prevention of heat loss is also crucial during transfer of the baby to the nursery. The severely depressed infant should be moved in an incubator that is equipped with a battery-operated heat source and an independent oxygen supply. If this equipment is not available, double-layered plastic bags that are designed to minimize heat loss may be used. These transparent bags fit snugly over the infant. The two layers are separated by large, multiple, self-contained air bubbles. If these bags are unavailable, the baby should be wrapped in a warmed blanket and transferred rapidly. A stocking cap (over the head) effectively diminishes loss of body heat.

Errors commonly committed during resuscitation

With so many procedures to be performed and with so little time in which to accomplish them, it is no wonder that errors are sometimes committed even by experienced personnel, not to mention the mistakes of the uninitiated and untrained. Perhaps the most fundamental of all errors is the attempt to resuscitate with little knowledge of rationale and with ignorance of the physiologic processes that have gone awry. The quality of performance increases directly with an understanding of rationale.

Specific errors in technique should be recognized if they are to be avoided or quickly corrected. The most frequent error during laryngoscopy is passage of the blade beyond the epiglottis into the esophageal opening, which is round or oval rather than slitlike and vertical (Fig. 3-2). At this point one is peering into the esophagus while the glottic slit is concealed above the blade. The blade should be withdrawn slowly while pointing the tip slightly upward. The glottis and the epiglottis soon fall into full view just beneath the laryngoscope blade. If, on the other hand, the blade tip is placed short of its goal, very slight advancement will position it in the vallecula.

Often an operator extends the baby's head in the erroneous assumption that intubation is facilitated, when in fact such positioning virtually precludes success. One frequently observes an operator with one hand on the chin, pulling it backward to extend the head while the laryngoscope is being inserted. The resultant stretching of the neck projects the larynx upward (anteriorly) so that it is hidden by the base of the tongue. It also tends to close the glottis. In these circumstances the tip of the blade is invariably directed into the esophagus, and even when it is withdrawn gingerly, the larynx will not drop into view while the head is maintained in extension. Rather than pull the chin backward, one should place the head in a neutral position.

Trauma is always a hazard when a metallic instrument is swiftly introduced into soft tissues. Lacerations and bruises of pharyngeal and laryngeal structures may result from rough insertion of the laryngoscope. Injury to the larynx is particularly serious because the airway may be occluded by the resultant edema or hemorrhage.

Another frequently committed error, previously mentioned, is insertion of the endotracheal tube too deeply into the trachea. The bifurcation of the trachea into two main stem bronchi is such that the right bronchus is almost a direct continuation of the trachea, whereas the left one branches from it at a sharper angle. Thus overinsertion of the tube almost invariably places it in the right main stem bronchus; ventilation is restricted to the right lung, and the left lung remains unventilated. Detection and correction of this error have already been described.

In the anxiety of the moment, the operator often inadvertently insufflates at a needlessly rapid rate, sometimes over 100 times per minute. The optimal rate is 40 to 50 times per minute. Also, if a bag-and-tube arrangement is used, the operator should be certain that the bag is connected to a source of oxygen; otherwise only room air (20% oxygen) will be delivered, and although it may sometimes be effective, higher oxygen concentrations are usually an urgent requirement.

Several additional factors require mention. Secretions may accumulate in the pharynx while endotracheal ventilation is in progress. Before removing the tube, suction should be applied to evacuate the secretions. Failure to provide ambient (surrounding) heat is a gross error. Every delivery room must be equipped with a heating apparatus.

The use of central nervous system stimulants such as caffeine, nikethamide (Coramine), and pentylenetetrazol (Metrazol) has no place in resuscitative procedures. The latter two drugs are particularly dangerous. The most effective stimulator of respiration is oxygen. Initial efforts to resuscitate the newborn must be concerned exclusively with delivery of oxygen to the lungs. Certain pharmacologic agents are sometimes indicated, but only for purposes other than central nervous excitation. Thus the use of narcotic antagonists is essential in drug-induced respiratory depression caused by maternal narcotic overdosage. Naloxone hydrochloride (Narcan) is given if fetal depression from maternal narcosis is caused by morphine, meperidine (Demerol), dihydromorphone (Dilaudid), and methadone.

SUMMARY

The extent of resuscitative procedures varies from the simple provision of free-flowing oxygen by mask to insufflation through an endotracheal tube, depending on the severity of depression. The Apgar score is an excellent indication of the infant's status and the type of resuscitation required. All babies need a clear airway and warmth. The establishment of spontaneous respiration is the most important and immediate goal of resuscitation; failure to prevent loss of body heat and to correct acidosis may prolong the time to complete recovery, or preclude it. The ultimate goal of resuscitation is not only immediate survival of the baby but also the prevention of central nervous system dysfunction during the years after birth.

BIBLIOGRAPHY

Apgar, V.: The newborn (Apgar) scoring system, Pediatr. Clin. North Am. **13**:645, 1966.

Apgar, V., and James, L. S.: The first sixty seconds of life. In Abramson, H., editor: Resuscitation of the newborn infant, ed. 3, St. Louis, 1973, The C. V. Mosby Co.

Berendes, H., and Drage, J. S.: Apgar scores and outcome of the newborn, Pediatr. Clin. North Am. **13**:635, 1966.

Desmond, M. M., Rudolph A. J., and Philtaksphraiwan, P.: The transitional care nursery, Pediatr. Clin. North Am. **13**:651, 1966.

Eidelman, A. I., and Hobbs, J. F.: Bicarbonate therapy revisited—a study in therapeutic revisionism, Am. J. Dis. Child. **132**:847, 1978.

James, L. S.: Emergencies in the delivery room. In Fanaroff, A. A., and Martin, R. J., editors: Behrman's neonatal-perinatal medicine, St. Louis, 1977, The C. V. Mosby Co.

James. L. S., and Apgar, V.: Resuscitation procedures in the delivery room. In Abramsom, H., editor: Resuscitation of the newborn infant, ed. 3, St. Louis, 1973, The C. V. Mosby Co.

Moya, F., James, L. S., Burnard, E. D., and Hanks, E. C.: Cardiac massage in the newborn infant through the intact chest, Am. J. Obstet. Gynecol. **84**:798, 1962.

Phibbs, R. H.: Delivery room management of the newborn. In Avery, G. B., editor: Neonatology—pathophysiology and management of the newborn, Philadelphia, 1981, J. B. Lippincott Co.

Shanklin, D. R.: The influence of placental lesions on the newborn infant, Pediatr. Clin. North Am. **17**:25, 1970.

CHAPTER 4

Thermoregulation

THERMOREGULATION IN THE NEONATE: IMPORTANCE OF HEAT BALANCE

Maintenance of an optimal thermal environment is one of the most important aspects of effective neonatal care, and without knowledge of the basic principles of thermoregulation, it cannot be provided consistently. However, with the facts at hand, cold stress can be prevented, and many of the riddles that arise daily can be solved. For example, why did a premature infant in our nursery continue to lose body heat even though the air temperature in his incubator constantly registered 33.3° C (92° F) on two thermometers? Why did this same infant fail to gain weight optimally despite an adequate caloric intake? The answers: Heat loss occurred because the incubator walls were chilled by a continuous blast of cold air from a window air conditioner that was only inches away. Weight gain was poor because the energy of metabolism was partially diverted to the compensatory production of body heat in preference to the laying down of new tissue. To one of our informed nurses the solution was simple: the baby must be moved across the room in his incubator, away from the air conditioner. The basis for that decision and other aspects of heat balance are discussed in some detail in the following pages.

The association of low body temperature with lower survival rates was observed in 1900 by the French neonatologist Pierre-Constant Budin, who was probably the first such physician on record. In his observation, only 10% of neonates survived if body temperatures were 32.5° to 33.5° C (90.5° to 92.3° F); 77% survived at temperatures between 36° and 37° C (96.8° and 98.6° F). The significance of this early observation was not appreciated until about 40 years later, when modern inquiries began. A voluminous literature continues to accumulate. The complex problem of maintaining an appropriate environment for small, sick neonates is not yet completely solved. However, sufficient data are on hand to permit provision of a thermal environment that minimizes the morbidity and mortality that are directly or indirectly due to cold stress.

The human being is homeothermic (Greek: *homoios* = similar, *thermē* = heat); that is, the organism can maintain its body temperature within narrow limits in spite of gross variations in environmental temperatures. In contrast, animals such as the turtle are poikilothermic (Greek: *poikilos* = variable, *thermē* = heat). Their body temperatures vary widely in response to environmental changes. In humans, normal deep-body (core) temperature is maintained within very narrow limits; it does not vary more than 0.3%. This is contrasted to the more variable limits of blood sugar, which may fluctuate 50% normally, and to hydrogen ion concentrations (pH), which vary from 10% to 20% within normal limits.

Heat is produced by the metabolic processes that provide energy. Body heat is thus a by-product of metabolism. Normal temperature is maintained only if there is a balance between the generation of heat and its dissipation. In large animals, body surface is comparatively small for body weight; they therefore dissipate heat at a relatively slow rate. The rate of heat loss is further reduced by a thick layer of subcutaneous fat and a copious coat of fur. The resultant tendency to retain heat is the basis for considerable difficulty in maintaining thermal equilibrium during physical activity, when heat production is markedly increased. These animals are vulnerable to hyperthermia; dissipation of heat is the most important aspect of their thermoregulatory function. On the other hand, in small animals, body surface is disproportionately large for body weight; insulation is meager. In these animals, excessive heat loss is an ongoing threat to the maintenance of normal body temperature; they are thus vulnerable to hypothermia. The most important aspect of their thermoregulatory function is the conservation of heat.

Thermal balance is maintained by regulation of heat loss and heat production. Perhaps the most frequently encountered example of heat imbalance at any age is fever, in which heat is produced in excess of the capacity to dissipate it. Core (rectal) temperature thus rises. In neonates, particularly smaller ones, heat loss is excessive by adult standards despite a capacity for reasonably effective heat production. Hypothermia is therefore the principal problem of heat balance in the newborn infant. The tendency to lose heat rapidly at ordinary room temperature is often a threat to survival, particularly for small babies who are ill.

BODY TEMPERATURE OF THE FETUS

A number of direct measurements have demonstrated that, at term, fetal core temperature is 0.5° C (0.9° F) higher than maternal core temperature. Fetal temperature is 37.6° to 37.8° C (99.7° to 100.0° F). It had been previously believed that fetal and maternal temperatures were equal, that the mother's heat maintained the body temperature of the fetus. It is now known that, at term, the fetal metabolic processes produce sufficient heat to maintain the body temperature at a higher level than the mother's. An ongoing need to dissipate fetal heat is thus required. Some is lost through the skin to the amniotic fluid, but the major site of heat loss is the intervillous space in the placenta. Heat is transferred from fetal capillaries in chorionic villi to the slightly cooler maternal blood within the intervillous space. It has been estimated that the total surface area of chorionic villi is greater than the fetus' body surface. In addition, blood is an effective vehicle for heat transfer from the body core to the surface; its rapid flow through the villi delivers a significant quantity of heat to the large villous surface. By this mechanism the placenta is normally capable of dissipating virtually all the heat produced by fetal metabolism. Normal flow of heat from fetus to mother may be reversed when the mother is febrile. Furthermore it is possible that in the presence of impaired placental perfusion, the fetus may lose heat more slowly.

Based on this thermal relationship between mother and fetus, speculation on two well-known clinical events is in order. The first concerns the extremely poor status of infants at birth whose mothers are severely febrile at the time of delivery. This may be attributable to an increased demand for oxygen in the febrile fetus beyond that which is available. The possibility of brain damage at high body temperatures may also contribute to the infant's stress. The second clinical event is benign. It is not uncommon for a mother to shiver for some time postpartum, beginning immediately after the birth of her baby. The transfer of heat from her fetus has contributed a significant portion of her body heat and she has thus become accustomed to a reduced need to generate her own heat. An important thermal source is eliminated when her infant is born, and she now shivers to rapidly generate heat in response to the abrupt deprivation that follows the baby's birth. It may thus be speculated that her shivering is no different from that which is expected on a cold day—at a football game, for instance.

HEAT LOSS IN THE NEONATE

Thermal equilibrium is present when the rate of heat generation equals the rate of heat loss. If more heat is produced than is lost, heat storage ensues—body temperature rises. If more heat is lost than is generated, body temperature declines. Thus the normal organism must continuously lose heat to a variable extent, depending on the rate of thermogenesis within the body and the thermal factors outside it (the environment). The heat that is produced by metabolic activity must be transferred from the core of the body to the surface; dissipation then continues from body surface to environment. The difference in temperature between the warmer *body core* and the cooler *body surface* is the *internal thermal gradient* (ITG). The difference in temperature between the *body surface* and the *environment* is the *external thermal gradient* (ETG). The smallest premature

infants are handicapped by the greatest heat losses and the most limited capacity for thermogenesis. Recent evidence suggests that at gestational ages less than 30 weeks, immature infants actually approach a state of poikilothermy; body temperature rises and declines in response to environmental changes in the same direction.

Neutral thermal environment refers to a relatively narrow range of environmental temperatures in which an infant can maintain normal body temperature with the least thermogenic activity. In neonates, thermogenic activity is largely a function of metabolic rate, which in turn entails oxygen consumption. Thermogenic activity has thus been measured in terms of quantitative changes in oxygen consumption. The normal term infant consumes oxygen at a rate of 5 ml/kg/min. If oxygen consumption is not shown to increase, metabolic rate (and therefore thermogenesis) has not increased. The *neutral thermal environment* has been defined experimentally as the range of ambient temperature within which oxygen consumption is lowest while normal body temperature is maintained. If the lower limit of the neutral environment is violated, oxygen consumption increases; thermogenesis is activated. If the upper limit of the neutral environment is violated, dissipation of heat in response to the environmental warmth is triggered; oxygen consumption rises. The range of temperature that defines a neutral environment is narrowest at the lowest gestational ages. The range of temperature is considerably wider at term.

The concept of a neutral thermal environment is difficult to apply clinically. An infant's response to the environment and the multiple thermal components of that environment involve complex measurements that are impractical in clinical circumstances. The thermal environment is multifactorial, comprising air temperature, ambient humidity, movement of air, and the temperature of objects close to but not in contact with the body, such as incubator walls. Furthermore, these multiple determinants of environmental temperature are unsteady; they change frequently. Procedures for the estimation of an infant's thermal status in a clinical setting must be accurate and simple. Characterization of the complex thermal environment, and an infant's response to it, is a research endeavor that requires team effort. The estimation of an infant's thermal status for clinical management in the nursery is discussed later in this chapter.

The internal thermal gradient (the body)

The neonate's anatomy predisposes to loss of heat to the environment. Thermal balance is more precarious in newborns than in older individuals, particularly in infants weighing less than 2000 g. The newborn's normal capacity for heat production in itself presents no problems except in very low birth weight infants. The crucial issue is heat loss, which is largely a function of the ratio of body surface to body weight. The larger the surface in relation to body mass, the greater the opportunity to dissipate heat to the environment. At birth the term infant is only 5% of adult body weight; yet his body surface is 15% of the adult's. The neonate has three times more body surface per kilogram of body weight than the adult. The discrepancy between weight and body surface is even greater for low birth weight infants. A larger surface area provides more extensive exposure to the environment, thus promoting more heat loss. Loss of heat per unit of body weight is four times greater in the term newborn and five times greater in a 1500 g premature infant than in the adult. This loss of heat is the principal source of the neonate's difficulty with maintaining thermal balance.

An equally important anatomic handicap to conservation of body heat is the paucity of subcutaneous fat, especially in infants who weigh less than 2000 g. Heat is thus more readily transferred from the core of the body to the skin (ITG). Deep body temperature is generally higher than surface (skin) temperature. Since a gradient exists between the core and the surface, constant transfer of heat occurs in that direction. Heat is transferred from core to surface by conduction from tissue to adjacent tissue. This transfer is normally impeded in the presence of a substantial layer of subcutaneous fat; it is accelerated if the fat layer is minimal. Because small infants are poorly insulated, they lose core body heat to the skin more readily than term infants. The gradient from core to surface is generally less in preterm babies than in those born at term. In the smallest preterm infants, skin and core temperatures approximate each other. This is an important consideration in choosing sites for taking body temperatures.

The flow of heat along the ITG is also a function of blood flow from the core to subcutaneous tissues. The quantity of heat delivered depends on the amount of blood that flows to the skin and the thickness of the subcutaneous fat. Fat is a heat-retaining tissue; its capacity to conduct heat (thermal conductivity) is considerably lower than that of other tissues. It is a critical impediment to the transmission of heat to the environment; the thicker the layer of fat, the more effective the insulation. Considerably less heat is lost from blood vessels if they permeate a thick subcutaneous fat layer, as in a term infant. The surface vasculature of a premature baby is prominently visible through the skin because of the virtual absence of subcutaneous fat and the diminished thickness of the epidermis. These blood vessels are immediately beneath the uppermost skin layer and therefore lose heat more readily to the environment.

Posture influences the rate of heat loss. Flexion of the extremities should theoretically reduce heat loss by decreasing the amount of surface area exposed to the environment. Normal posture after birth varies with gestational age. The tendency for flexed extremities increases as gestational age advances. At birth the normal term infant has not yet completely relinquished the fetal position; a substantial degree of flexion of the extremities is evident. In contrast, the small premature infant lies flat on the mattress by virtue of the hypotonicity that characterizes preterm gestational ages. In terms of thermal balance, the premature infant has a neuromuscular as well as an anatomic disadvantage. Furthermore, hypotonicity is exaggerated when central nervous system depression is imposed by perinatal asphyxia. Increased exposure of skin surface in these flaccid states enhances heat loss by convection, radiation, and evaporation. In adults the spread-eagle posture entails a 61% increase in exposed surface area compared to a fetal position. Similar data are not available for neonates, and the relationship of heat loss to posture has not been measured.

In summary, the loss of heat from the skin to the environment is increased in low birth weight babies because the skin surface is relatively large; loss of heat from deep body layers to the skin is greater because the insulating layer of fat is thin and the distance from core to surface is short. Therefore the smaller the infant, the greater the thermal losses to the environment. The handicaps of body size and surface persist, though they diminish as gestational and postnatal ages advance. The well-trained nurse is constantly aware of these factors because they affect survival and the rapidity of recovery from asphyxia; they influence the effectiveness of therapy for respiratory distress, and may also alter the rate of weight gain.

The external thermal gradient (the environment)

The difference between skin temperature and environmental temperature is the *external thermal gradient*. Physical factors in the environment that determine the extent of this gradient are air temperature and movement of air (velocity), temperature of surrounding surfaces that may be in contact with the body or apart from it, and relative humidity of ambient air. Each of these factors determines the amount of heat that is transferred between the body and the environment by four modalities: *convection*, *radiation*, *evaporation*, and *conduction*. Although they are discussed in the context of heat loss, the first three methods may also be involved in heat gain.

Convection. Convection involves a flow of heat from the body surface to cooler surrounding air. The rate of loss by convection depends on ambient (surrounding) temperature and the velocity of air-

flow. A rapid flow of air enhances heat loss. Ideal ambient temperature in the incubator reduces convective heat loss only, having no significant effect on the loss of heat by radiation or evaporation (Fig. 4-1).

Radiation. Radiant loss involves transfer of body heat to cooler *solid* surfaces in the environment that are *not in contact* with the baby (incubator walls). Thermal dissipation increases as these solid objects become colder or closer to the body. *Radiant heat loss is independent of ambient temperature in the incubator*. It was by this mechanism that inordinate heat loss occurred in the premature infant mentioned earlier. The incubator wall that was closest to the air conditioner was cold, and as a result the baby continuously lost heat to the wall by radiation despite the high temperature of incubator air, which minimized only convective heat loss. Thus even if the temperature of ambient air is high, significant loss may occur by radiation if the incubator walls are inordinately cool. This loss is a common phenomenon at ordinary room temperature, and especially during the winter in inadequately insulated nurseries in which babies are placed close to windows. It is also frequent in air-conditioned nurseries when the vents release concentrated drafts of cool air directly onto incubators (Fig. 4-2).

Evaporation. Evaporative heat loss occurs during conversion of a liquid to a vapor because thermal energy is used in the process.

Heat is lost by evaporation of insensible water loss, visible sweat, and moisture from the respiratory tract mucosa. Insensible water loss (IWL) occurs by evaporation from the skin and in exhaled gases. Evaporation from the skin is transepidermal water loss (TEWL). Approximately 0.6 calories are lost for each gram of water evaporated. Evaporation, and thus the rate of heat loss, is increased when humidity is low. At birth a considerable amount of thermal dissipation occurs by evaporation, especially in air-conditioned delivery rooms with low humidity. Because the infant is covered with amniotic fluid, he loses a considerable amount of heat as the fluid evaporates. This

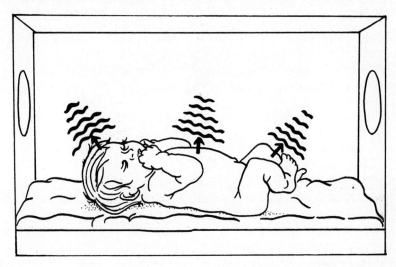

Fig. 4-1. *Convective loss* is indicated here as transfer of heat from body surface to cooler ambient air in the incubator.

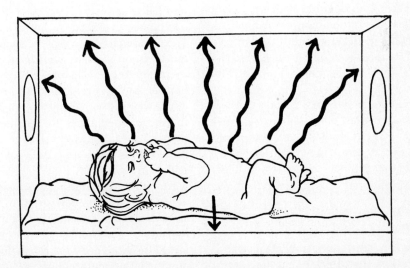

Fig. 4-2. *Radiant loss* is shown as transfer of heat from body surface directly to cooler incubator wall, regardless of the temperature of air within the incubator. *Conductive loss* is shown as heat transfer to mattress in direct contact with body surface.

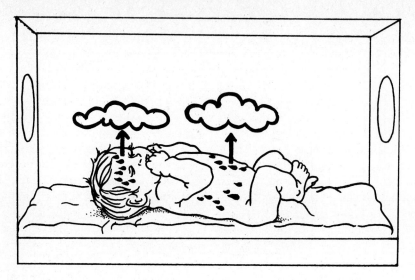

Fig. 4-3. *Evaporative loss* is depicted in the conversion of skin water to vapor. Heat consumed in this process is lost from the body surface.

mode of heat loss is readily minimized when the baby is dried immediately with a warm towel. Another practical consideration with respect to evaporative heat loss is the timing of the first bath after arrival in the nursery. Whether term or premature, neonates should not be bathed until the body temperature is stable at normal levels (Fig. 4-3).

Conduction. Conductive loss of body heat occurs during *direct contact* of the skin with a cooler *solid* object. Placement of a naked infant on a cold table, or the cold mattress of an unprepared incubator, would thus promote conductive heat loss (Fig. 4-2).

The tiny infant: heat balance and water loss

Recently an increased survival of infants whose birth weight is less than 1000 g (or whose gestational age is below 30 weeks) has attracted considerable attention to the unique problems of heat and water balance in tiny infants. Maintenance of optimal body temperature in tiny infants has not been consistently successful. The thermal handicaps of neonates are most severe in the tiny ones whose core and skin temperatures are often suboptimal despite high incubator temperatures or continuous overhead output of infrared energy. With increased survival of the smallest infants and more opportunity to wrestle with problems of their care, the critical role of evaporative heat loss has become apparent. In addition, there is evidence that the tiny infant can muster little if any thermogenic effort for the maintenance of body temperature. It has even been suggested that these babies need to be "incubated in much the same way as eggs."*

Ambient temperatures required for maintenance of rectal temperatures at 37° C (98.6° F) are dependent on infant size, the capacity of thermogenesis, and the rate of transepidermal water loss (TEWL). TEWL increases in magnitude as gestational age and size diminish. At birth weights of less than 1000 g (or gestational age less than 30 weeks), suppression of heat loss by radiation

*Wheldon, A. E., and Hull, D.: Incubation of very immature infants. Arch. Dis. Child. **58:**504, 1983.

and convection in incubators does not sustain normal body temperature. Evaporative losses are relatively unchanged in these circumstances, and these losses exceed the tiny infant's capacity to generate heat. A familiar clinical situation arises from these physiologic difficulties. A baby below 800 g is housed in an incubator and covered with a Plexiglas heat shield. Incubator temperature is maintained at higher than usual levels to eliminate convective losses; the plastic heat shield is in place to eliminate radiant losses. Nevertheless, rectal temperatures remain unacceptably low because evaporative loss of heat exceeds the capacity to produce it. The problems of thermal balance in tiny infants are largely attributable to huge transepidermal water losses.

TEWL is a function of skin maturity. The smaller the baby at birth, the more permeable the skin to outward diffusion of water. In essence, the skin of immature babies is incapable of retaining moisture. It is thus said to be less resistant to diffusion of water to the environment. Resistance to water diffusion becomes more effective as the superficial layer of the epidermis, the *stratum corneum*, matures. The stratum corneum is composed of dry, compact cells that resist water diffusion more efficiently than the deeper layers of epidermal cells because of a fibrous protein called *keratin*. This substance in the stratum corneum is probably the major barrier to diffusion of water through skin. The appearance of the skin of tiny babies at birth is a familiar one. The stratum corneum is not yet developed; keratin has not been produced. The skin is thin and moist; the vascular pattern beneath it is clearly visible. Yet, after 2 or 3 weeks (sooner under radiant warmers), the epidermis of tiny infants appears similar to that of term infants. Apparently extrauterine existence accelerates maturation of the premature infant's skin. Whether this is associated with keratin formation has yet to be shown. Commensurate with the apparent epidermal maturation within 3 weeks (in incubators), the magnitude of transepidermal water loss in tiny babies is diminished to quantities typical in term babies.

The pattern of postnatal diminution of TEWL varies with gestational age. At birth, initial water loss is lowest at term; and slightly higher at 34 to 37 weeks. After 4 hours the rate of water loss is approximately halved in term babies. At gestational ages of 30 to 33 weeks, water losses through the skin at birth are considerably higher. Furthermore, diminution of water loss does not occur until the beginning of the second week in these moderately small infants. In tiny babies (less than 30 weeks gestation), the magnitude of water loss through the skin is huge, and diminution does not occur for 2 or 3 weeks after birth.

The rate of transepidermal evaporation differs from one region of the body to another in addition to the variations of gestational and postnatal age. In tiny infants the highest losses are from the abdomen; the next highest are from the back and the extremities. Surprisingly, the lowest losses have been measured from the forehead and face. Even the naked eye can perceive as much; skin of the face and forehead has a thicker appearance than that of the abdomen. As babies grow older, losses from all surface areas diminish, except for the palms and soles, where they increase. In term infants, water loss is proportionately greater from the palms and soles, but this is of no apparent clinical significance.

These findings indicate an urgency in diminishing the TEWL of tiny infants. The special considerations of altered microenvironment for all neonates apply with greatest emphasis to the smallest of them. Reports that indicate superiority of one procedure over another must be interpreted in terms of gestational and postnatal ages. A technique that diminishes TEWL at 35 weeks may not be successful at 28 weeks, because so much water is lost so quickly it cannot be contained.

HEAT PRODUCTION: RESPONSE TO COLD STRESS

The homeothermic animal maintains core temperature within a narrow range by virtue of a capacity to produce heat continuously and, when challenged by a cold environment, to conserve it and increase its production. On the other side of the balanced thermal equation, homeothermy also entails a capacity to minimize heat production and to increase the rate of dissipation.

As environmental temperature falls, the homeothermic animal enhances heat production by four mechanisms: (1) voluntary increase in skeletal muscle activity, (2) involuntary rhythmic contractions of skeletal muscle that may be grossly imperceptible but can be demonstrated by electromyograms, (3) involuntary rhythmic contractions that are grossly visible (shivering), and (4) nonshivering thermogenesis. (The neonate rarely shivers.)

The human neonate, when exposed to cold, conserves heat by constricting blood vessels in the skin; attempts to maintain body temperature within a narrow range are activated by increasing the production of heat. Effectiveness of insulation is increased by limiting the flow of blood to the body surface. This neonatal function is as efficient as the adult's, but the neonate's small body size and large ratio of surface to weight make maximal effectiveness impossible.

In a heat-losing environment, newborn infants increase the rate of heat production by increasing metabolic rate, a process called nonshivering thermogenesis. It is operative in both term and premature infants, although heat production is less active in the latter. The term infant who is exposed to cold can increase the thermogenic rate two and one-half times over the resting state, to a level that almost equals the adult's. At gestational ages of 30 weeks and less, the capacity to generate heat on demand is apparently limited.

Heat production is increased in proportion to the fall in environmental temperature. The metabolic response is thus greater, for instance, in a room temperature of 21.1° C (70° F) than in 26.6° C (80° F). Neonates have the capacity to generate heat from the moment of birth, although the response is not as effective during the first 24 hours of life as it is afterward. Of direct clinical interest

is the experimental observation that responses to environmental cold occur before there is any drop in core (rectal) temperature. Furthermore, when the environment warms, the rate of heat production diminishes, and this change also occurs prior to a change in core temperature. The infant's thermal activity is therefore increased or decreased with no demonstrable relationship to rectal temperature. Rather, thermogenic activity is stimulated by the response of thermal nerve endings (receptors) in the skin. Heat production becomes elevated when average *skin temperature* declines to 35° to 36° C (95.0° to 96.8° F).

Heat production in the adult who is exposed to cold stress involves involuntary muscle activity (shivering) and increased metabolic rate (nonshivering thermogenesis). In contrast, the nondepressed neonate becomes restless and hyperactive when first exposed to cold, but this form of voluntary muscle activity is not a significant source of heat. This has been shown by the administration of curare (which paralyzes skeletal muscle); the metabolic response to cold stress is not diminished despite the resultant absence of muscle activity. The neonate does not shiver when chilled, but in the adult these involuntary tremors are a significant source of heat. Thus nonshivering thermogenesis appears to be the only mechanism available for increasing heat production in the cold-stressed newborn infant.

Nonshivering thermogenesis refers to the heat that is produced by a metabolic rate (and therefore a rate of oxygen consumption) that is minimal in an ideal thermal environment or increased in a cold one. In the neonate, enhancement of heat production must involve a hypermetabolic state that requires increased oxygen consumption. Obviously a severely depressed hypoxic infant can ill afford the oxygen cost of cold stress. Heat is produced as a by-product of the accelerated chemical reactions that occur at a cellular level when metabolic rate increases. The neonate's brain, liver, and perhaps skeletal muscle are important thermogenic organs. Augmented rates of metabolism at these sites probably contribute in some measure to increased heat production, but the major source of heat that is produced by nonshivering thermogenesis is *brown fat*. Direct evidence for the significant role of this tissue has been derived from animal experiments. There is also considerable evidence to support its role in human neonates. There are no data that precisely define the contribution of brown fat to the total metabolic response to cold stress (nonshivering thermogenesis). In the newborn rabbit, brown fat is known to account for two thirds of this total response. For human neonates the estimate is 90%.

In the early 1960s it became apparent that metabolic activity in brown fat was considerably greater than in white fat. The belief that this tissue was unique to animal hibernators was dispelled by its demonstration in nonhibernating animals, principally in neonates. Its distribution is widespread in the human fetus and neonate. It accounts for approximately 1.5% of total body weight. The largest deposits are posterior cervical, axillary, suprailiac, and perirenal. Deposits of intermediate size are found in the interscapular region, the axillae, and in the area around the trapezius and deltoid muscles. Relatively small masses are located in the anterior mediastinum just above and behind the sternum, between the esophagus and trachea, in the intercostal areas and anterior abdomen, and along the aorta. Probably smaller deposits exist between groups of skeletal muscle fibers throughout the body. Thus brown fat distribution is such that it forms a sort of vest around the thorax (axillary, interscapular, trapezial, deltoid, anterior mediastinal, and intercostal regions) and a collar around the neck (posterior cervical region around the jugular veins and carotid arteries).

The cells of brown fat differ considerably from those of white adipose tissue. The brown fat cell contains a central nucleus; numerous mitochondria and small lipid inclusions are dispersed throughout the cytoplasm. The white fat cell contains a peripheral nucleus and only a single, large

fat globule. The color of brown fat is easily distinguished from white fat distributed throughout the body. The buff to reddish-brown color is imparted by a copious blood supply, dense cellular content, and profusion of nerve endings. Brown fat is densely innervated by sympathetic nerves, which seem to furnish the stimulus for its enhanced metabolism during cold stress by releasing norepinephrine. These nerve endings are seen by electron microscopy to terminate in direct contact with brown fat cell membranes.

Primitive brown fat cells first appear at 26 to 30 weeks of gestation. The tissue mass continues to enlarge as late as the third to the fifth postnatal week, unless significant cold stress intervenes and depletes it. It ordinarily disappears some weeks after birth. Exposure to cold, acutely or over protracted periods, tends to deplete the stores. Tissue from autopsied babies who were clothed and kept in room air at only 21.1° to 26.6° C (70° to 80° F) is considerably depleted in comparison to tissue of infants who were managed in incubators as warm as 33.9° to 35° C (93° to 95° F).

Norepinephrine is released from sympathetic nerve endings. It is currently thought to be the principal mediator of *nonshivering thermogenesis*. When norepinephrine is infused intravenously into the neonate, oxygen consumption increases by 60%, indicating induced hypermetabolism. That enhanced production of norepinephrine occurs in response to cold stress is indicated by its increased excretion in urine at these times. Norepinephrine stimulates fat metabolism in brown adipose tissue. It activates lipase, which breaks down intracellular fat to form triglycerides. Triglycerides are subsequently hydrolized to form glycerol and nonesterified fatty acids (NEFA). Oxidation of NEFA within the brown fat cell is a heat-producing reaction. Presumably, at this point in the metabolic chain of triglyceride breakdown, brown fat responds to a demand for increased heat production that is initially perceived by thermal sensors in the skin. The by-product of this increased chemical activity is a relatively bountiful amount of heat, which is then applied directly to blood that perfuses the tissue mass. Warmer skin temperatures have been recorded over subcutaneous deposits of brown fat during periods of cold stress, suggesting the tissue's thermogenic role in such circumstances.

In summary, the neonate reacts to cold stress by conserving heat (peripheral vasoconstriction) and by generating it in increased quantities on demand. This is accomplished primarily by the enhancement of metabolism; the principal metabolic source of additional heat is brown fat. On the other hand, the neonate responds to excessive warmth by increasing the dissipation of heat. This is accomplished by dilatation of peripheral (skin) vessels and by augmentation of evaporative losses from visible sweat and insensible water. Reactions to thermal challenges in the environment are initiated by thermal receptors in the skin, of which those of the face are the most sensitive and responsive. *Thus peripheral vasoconstriction and nonshivering thermogenesis (as well as vasodilatation and increased water loss) become active even though there is no change in core (rectal) temperature.* This is the essence of adaptation to changing environmental temperature—peripheral stimulation activates vasomotor and metabolic processes to control the balance of heat, thereby protecting the stability of body temperature at the core.

This relatively well-defined mechanism for maintaining heat balance is not as neatly operative in tiny infants whose gestational age is below 30 weeks. At least during the first or second week after birth, their capacity to generate heat is likely to be significantly diminished in comparison to their older counterparts. It is estimated that between the gestational ages of 26 and 30 weeks, maximum heat production is 35 to 40 kcal/kg/day—considerably lower than in infants of more advanced gestational age. The problem for tiny infants is compounded by the overwhelming heat loss associated with massive loss of water from the skin, which has been estimated to occur at a cost of 40 kcal/kg/day.

Impaired response to cold stress

The neonate's capacity to respond to cold stress may be impaired by several factors. Hypoxia is among the most important of these. In babies who suffer from hyaline membrane disease, or hypoxia for any reason, the metabolic response to cold is limited when arterial P_{O_2} is 45 to 55 torr, and it is abolished at 30 torr. In normal infants, these arterial oxygen tensions are produced by breathing gas mixtures that contain 12% and 8% oxygen, respectively.

Other factors that impair the response to cold include intracranial hemorrhage, severe cerebral malformations, and symptomatic hypoglycemia. Infants in deep sleep, when exposed to cold, at first respond suboptimally until they awaken several minutes later. This observation and the limitation of response associated with severe central nervous system abnormalities suggest that the stimulus to heat production depends on intact brain function. Anencephalic infants, for example, do not increase heat production in lowered environmental temperatures; yet their brown fat stores are completely normal. Interference with the response to cold by symptomatic hypoglycemia may thus be rooted in disrupted function of the central nervous system.

Protracted cold stress seems to deplete brown fat stores, and when this depletion is severe, it is hypothesized that effective thermogenic capacity is eliminated. Infants who have died of "neonatal cold injury" were noted to be virtually devoid of brown fat.

RESPONSE TO HYPERTHERMIA

In an inappropriately warm environment, the rate of heat loss must increase; within physiologic limits, the neonate dissipates heat effectively. All infants, regardless of gestational age, respond to external heat by dilatation of peripheral vessels and by enhancement of evaporative heat loss.

The quantity of heat delivered to the skin from deep body tissues depends on vasomotor reactions in the skin itself. Less heat is delivered to the skin (and thus less is lost from the body surface) when external temperatures are low because skin vessels constrict and blood flow is diminished. This vasomotor response is particularly pronounced in the hands and feet. When external temperature is inordinately high, skin vessels dilate, blood flow increases, and more heat is delivered to the skin and lost from the body surface. Vasodilatation is also most pronounced in the hands and feet where more heat is lost per square centimeter of surface then elsewhere. In addition, the neonate dissipates more heat by increasing evaporative losses. This is accomplished by enhanced insensible water loss and by visible perspiration. Visible sweat is first seen at approximately 30 to 32 weeks (conceptional age) when it appears on the forehead and temples. It soon appears on the chest, and by approximately 34 to 36 weeks, sweating also occurs on the lower extremities. The premature infant is less capable of visible perspiration than the term infant; this phenomenon is probably a function of the immaturity of sweat glands.

The factors responsible for the rapid rate of heat loss in neonates (more body surface per gram of weight and minimal subcutaneous fat) also tend to increase the rate of heat gain in excessively warm environments. In the premature infant the development of hyperthermia is incredibly rapid when equipment is mismanaged or neglected. Core temperature of 41.1° C (106° F) may occur in a very short time; the smaller the infant, the shorter the time. Severe hyperthermia culminates in death or in gross brain damage in the surviving infant.

CONSEQUENCES OF COLD STRESS

The principal difficulties that beset a cold-stressed baby are hypoxemia, metabolic acidosis, rapid depletion of glycogen stores, and reduction of blood glucose levels. The newborn responds to chilling by increasing his metabolic rate, which inherently entails augmented oxygen consumption. Lowered oxygen tension is apparently related to diminished effectiveness of ventilation, which is a consequence of pulmonary vasocon-

striction caused by the release of norepinephrine that occurs in response to cold stress. Breakdown of glycogen to glucose now proceeds under hypoxic circumstances, and the alternate chemical pathway (anaerobic glycolysis) that must be utilized dissipates glycogen at approximately 20 times the normal aerobic rate. Hypoglycemia ensues. Furthermore, anaerobic glycolysis generates extra lactic acid, and now metabolic acidosis appears. In babies with intrauterine malnutrition, hypoglycemia is more likely in the presence of cold stress because glycogen stores are already diminished at birth (Chapter 11). These phenomena are also more pronounced in babies who are inadequately oxygenated because of ventilatory difficulty or as a result of some other disorder. The significance of an optimal thermal environment for such infants is therefore critical. Relentless monitoring is required if normothermia is to be maintained or restored.

Oxygen deprivation itself impairs or abolishes the metabolic response to chilling, thus depriving the infant of the principal source of heat. It may contribute to the abrupt drop in body temperature that occurs in normal infants at birth, since low oxygen saturation is the rule. There is evidence to indicate that thermogenesis is impaired at an arterial PO_2 of 45 torr or less. The infant with severe hyaline membrane disease may thus require higher environmental temperatures to maintain body heat, presumably because thermogenesis is handicapped by oxygen deprivation.

During the nursery stay, protracted failure to provide an optimal thermal environment may impair weight gain. This was described in the example cited earlier in this chapter. Experiments with human infants indicate, however, that in most instances increased caloric intake can compensate for energy diverted from the growth process to the production of heat.

THERMAL MANAGEMENT IN
THE DELIVERY ROOM

All babies lose body heat to some extent during the moments immediately after birth. Vigorous, full-sized babies usually experience little adversity as a result, but low birth weight infants, depressed or not, are in noteworthy danger. Metabolic acidosis, hypoxemia, and hypoglycemia can be expected in most severely cold-stressed infants.

The fall in core (rectal) and skin temperatures is most rapid immediately after birth. In the usual air-conditioned delivery room, if no countermeasures are applied, deep body temperature of the normal term infant falls 0.1° C (0.2° F) per minute; skin temperature declines 0.3° C (0.5° F) per minute. The total drop in deep body temperature may be as great as 2° to 3° C (3.6° to 5.4° F). A dramatic decrease in skin temperature occurs within 10 seconds of exposure to room air. Scalp temperature has been noted to fall from 36° to 34° C (96.8° to 93.2° F) in those few seconds. As other parts of the body are delivered, similarly rapid changes may occur. This high rate of thermal dissipation is largely attributable to the anatomic factors that have been previously described; the relatively large body surface/body weight ratio and the meager deposit of subcutaneous fat are critical. An inappropriately cold environment accentuates the

difficulty. The resultant rapid rate of heat loss cannot be fully compensated, even if the infant's metabolic response is unimpaired. In normal infants the metabolic response to cold is somewhat limited during the first few minutes of life because of low arterial oxygen tensions that often persist for 10 or 15 minutes after birth. The observed hypoxemia is comparable to that of an infant who breathes only 15% oxygen. Thermal loss is more accentuated as birth weight declines and as respiratory distress increases. Contemporary standards thus require rational measures to minimize heat loss in normal term babies and especially in those who are small and depressed.

The modalities by which heat is lost in the delivery room, and their relative significance, must be known to all who care for infants during the moments that follow birth. The baby is drenched in amniotic fluid when delivered in a cool room with moderately low humidity. A substantial amount of heat is immediately lost to the cold environment by evaporation. This loss can be minimized by drying the baby with a warm towel or blanket. After drying is done, loss by convection and radiation must be minimized. Thus the

Table 4-1. Equivalent Celsius and Fahrenheit temperature reading*

Celsius degrees	Fahrenheit degrees	Celsius degrees	Fahrenheit degrees
0	32.0	31	87.8
21	69.8	32	89.6
22	71.6	33	91.4
23	73.4	34	93.2
24	75.2	35	95.0
25	77.0	36	96.8
26	78.8	37	98.6
27	80.6	38	100.4
28	82.4	39	102.2
29	84.2	40	104.0
30	86.0	41	105.8

*For values between centigrade degrees listed, add 0.18 F for each 0.10 C.
EXAMPLE:
  30.5° C = 86.0 plus 5 × 0.18 = 0.9 = 86.90° F.
  35.7° C = 95.0 plus 7 × 0.18 = 1.26 = 96.26° F.

baby may be dried and then wrapped in a warm blanket and kept in room air, dried and placed in an incubator, or dried and placed on an open radiant heater. Any of these methods of management is acceptable. If resuscitation is required, the open table is mandatory for adequate accessibility to the infant. There should be one such table in every active delivery room.

In a study that evaluated several methods of thermal management in the delivery room, infants who remained wet in room air experienced a mean decline in rectal temperature of 2.1° C (3.8° F) and a mean fall in skin temperature of 4.6° C (8.3° F) within 30 minutes after birth. In contrast, those who were dried and placed nude under a radiant heater experienced the least fall in core temperature of only 0.7° C (1.3° F) and a decrease in skin temperature of 0.8° C (1.5° F). Wet babies placed under radiant heat had a 60% greater drop in core temperature than those who were dried before being placed under radiant heat. Simply drying and wrapping infants in warm blankets also diminished their heat loss considerably. Thermal losses were as much as 65% lower in such babies than in those who were not dried and were left nude in room air. Fig. 4-4 is a graphic representation of the decline in skin temperatures after birth according to the various methods of thermal management that were studied. Fig. 4-5 presents the effects of these methods on simultaneously recorded rectal temperatures. During 30 minutes of observation, both skin and rectal temperatures diminished least in those babies who were dried using a warm blanket and placed under radiant heat. The importance of drying and warming is apparent. Dry babies who were wrapped in blankets had somewhat lower skin and core temperatures than the dry radiated infants, but the drop in skin temperature at 1 minute was followed by an abrupt rise within 5 minutes, presumably after the babies were wiped dry. In these same infants, core temperatures were only slightly lower than in the dried and radiated ones. In normal term babies these decrements in temperature are probably of little clinical significance; they are not a contraindication to family-oriented delivery rooms.

In essence, optimal thermal management requires immediate drying and placement under a radiant heater. Drying and placement in an incubator that is warmed at 32° to 35° C (90° to 95° F) is satisfactory. Simply drying and wrapping in a warm blanket is not acceptable for low birth weight infants.

Under any circumstances, failure to dry is negligent; allowing a wet, nude baby to remain in room air is callous.

A certain amount of heat loss is physiologic. Indeed, cold stimuli are probably essential to the initiation of extrauterine respiratory function. Stimuli from thermal skin sensors are transmitted to the reticular formation (respiratory center) in the medulla oblongata, and thence down the phrenic nerve to stimulate contraction of the diaphragm. Experiments with lambs have demonstrated convincingly that delivery into warm fluid, simulating intrauterine conditions, impairs or precludes the onset of respiration. Furthermore, alternate gradual cooling and warming of a water bath in which term newborn lambs are immersed results in stimulation of respiratory activity at the cool temperatures and cessation of respiratory activity at the warm ones. Human infants who are delivered by cesarean section into a warm bath cease to breathe. Some cold is therefore necessary, but too much is hazardous. Purposeful exaggeration of physiologic cold stimuli cannot be justified by available evidence, nor can delivery into a warm water bath.

Ambient temperature in the delivery room should be 25.5° C (78° F), which is not excessively cool for the infant or uncomfortably warm for the mother. The radiant heater should be utilized only for stressed infants whose accessibility must be assured for effective treatment. The normal term infant can safely be placed prone on the mother's chest immediately after cutting the cord and drying the skin. Skin contact between mother and infant should be assured, but a blanket folded into several layers must cover the baby's back.

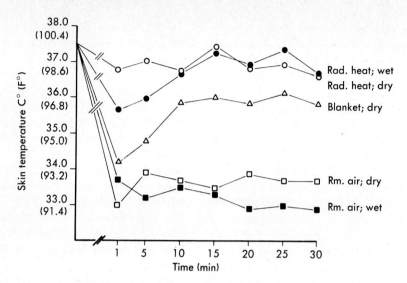

Fig. 4-4. Decline in skin temperature during 30 minutes following birth according to five different methods of thermal management. Babies who were dried and placed on a radiant heat bed maintained their body temperature best. (Modified from Dahm, L. S., and James, L. S.: Pediatrics 49:504, 1972.)

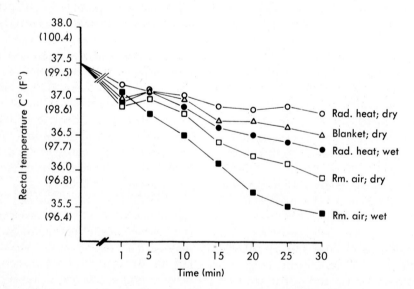

Fig. 4-5. Simultaneously recorded rectal temperatures from babies in the same study as in Fig. 4-4. Note that the decline in rectal temperatures was considerably slower than in skin temperatures shown in Fig. 4-4. See "Clinical Assessment and Management of the Infant's Thermal Status" on p. 107 and "Heat Production" on p. 93. (Modified from Dahm, L. S., and James, L. S.: Pediatrics 49:504, 1972.)

The skin of the maternal chest is sufficiently warm to provide heat by conduction to her infant; the covering blanket minimizes heat loss by convection and radiation. A radiant heater over mother and baby during the moments of their exciting first contact is thus an unnecessary technologic intrusion.

Radiant heaters effectively prevent excessive heat loss while treatment of a distressed infant is in progress. They are indispensable for the management of asphyxiated babies. A skin sensor for servocontrol of the heat source is not essential during resuscitation.

Transfer of a resuscitated infant to the nursery or to the intensive care unit requires the use of a transport incubator that is heated by power from its own portable battery. A nursery incubator that has no portable power source for the continuous provision of heat is totally inadequate for transport within the hospital. In such incubators, radiant and convective heat losses during transport are sufficient to cause significant cold stress, depending on the ambient temperature of hospital corridors and the duration of transport.

THERMAL MANAGEMENT IN THE NURSERY

By adult standards the neonate's *thermal stability* is restricted, not so much by an inability to produce heat, as by a propensity for losing it. Thermal management in the nursery attempts to provide conditions that are as close as possible to the baby's *neutral thermal environment*. At the very least, the *control range* of environmental temperature must be maintained. Definitions of these terms follow in subsequent paragraphs.

Thermal stability is the capacity to oppose changes in body heat content caused by the loss or gain of heat that results from exchange with the environment. Heat production and heat conservation that is effected by constriction of surface blood vessels tend to prevent diminution of core temperature caused by dissipation of body heat to the environment. The functions of production and conservation are critical for maintenance of thermal stability in any patient at any age. Thermal stability also requires effective dissipation of heat by vasodilatation, sweating, and rapid breathing to prevent elevation of core temperature resulting from heat gain from the environment or to a hypermetabolic state (fever due to infection). The net effect of activities that bring about the production and conservation of heat on one hand, and dissipation on the other, is the maintenance of a normal core temperature within narrow limits. This is *thermal stability*.

A *neutral thermal environment* provides conditions that permit maintenance of normal core temperature at a minimal rate of oxygen consumption in a resting subject. In the nursery, determination of the components of each infant's neutral thermal environment is not particularly practical; at least four factors are involved: temperature of surrounding air, temperature of surrounding radiant surfaces, velocity of ambient air flow, and relative humidity.

The *control range of environmental temperature* defines the upper and lower limits of environmental temperatures in which the body can effectively regulate heat loss or gain. The lower limit of the control range for nude adults is 0° C (32° F); for the term infant, the lower limit is 20° to 23° C (68° to 73° F). The smaller the infant and the more meager the subcutaneous fat insulation, the narrower the range of environmental temperature (control range) in which heat balance can be maintained.

Provision of a warm microenvironment

Intensive care of neonates almost always requires nudity of the patient. Historically, when the baby was stripped of diapers, shirts, and blankets, monitoring and therapy became feasible as never before. The problems of thermoregulation that resulted, however, have since preoccupied the neonatologist as have few other facets of total infant care.

Since demonstration of the close relationship between abdominal skin temperature and oxygen consumption, it has been the usual practice of intensive care units in this country to automatically adjust the thermal environment in response to changes in skin temperatures as they are registered over the epigastrium. Oxygen consumption (and therefore metabolic rate) is minimal at an abdominal skin temperature of 36.5° C (97.7° F). When skin temperature increases to 37.2° C (98.9° F), oxygen consumption increases by 6%; when skin temperature declines to 35.9° C (96.6° F), oxygen consumption also increases, but by 10%. Thus the temperature of the skin signals the presence of a metabolic response. It reflects a change in the environment that requires increased metabolic activity to preserve normal core temperature. A drop in skin temperature usually indicates a heat-losing environment that requires warming.

Normal full-term infants can generally maintain heat balance in an open bassinet when the room temperature is 23.9° to 25.5° C (75° to 78° F) if they are clothed with diaper and shirt, covered with some sort of cotton blanket, and have not been placed in a high velocity of airflow. Sick infants of any size and low birth weight infants in any state of health, especially those below 2000 g, require a controlled microenvironment for maintenance of normal core temperature. The term infant acquires maximal thermal stability for age several hours after delivery, although the baby's ability to increase metabolic rate in response to cold stress has been demonstrated as early as 15 minutes after birth. Small infants require variable lengths of time for development of a maximal metabolic response, sometimes as long as several weeks. Infants who weigh less than 1500 g are particularly handicapped because of minimal insulation and a large ratio of body surface to weight.

Incubators. Controlled microenvironments are commonly provided by incubators in which the temperature of circulating air is either manually adjusted or automatically controlled (servocontrolled). Air temperature is most frequently servocontrolled by a thermal sensor attached to the skin. The effectiveness of available incubators is almost totally dependent on warm ambient air, which minimizes convective heat losses. Evaporative losses can be diminished by choosing to humidify the incubator air. This is accomplished by passing heated air over a reservoir of water situated beneath the deck on which the infant lies. Heated incubator air is filtered from room air, drawn in by fans that force air over heaters of varying size, and then passing it into the infant chamber. Depending on the manufacturer, heated air enters the chamber by various patterns, but in all incubators it is exhausted into room air. Insofar as protection from airborne infection is concerned, the pattern of air intake and exhaust isolates the infant, but not the infant's neighbors. The incubator is protective, but other infants are exposed to its exhausted air unless they too are in incubators. Isolation from airborne infection in any room is only possible when all infants are in incubators.

Most incubators in use today are single-walled. The single wall permits significant radiant heat

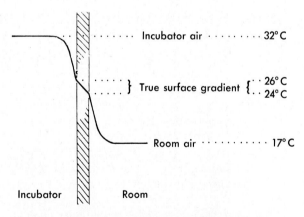

Fig. 4-6. Temperature of incubator wall at 24° to 26° C (75.2° to 78.8° F) is approximately midway between incubator air temperature of 32° C (89.6° F) and nursery air temperature of 17° C (70° F). Radiant loss from body surface increases as temperature of incubator wall decreases as a result of air temperature in the nursery. (Modified from Hey, E. N., and Mount, L. E.: Arch. Dis. Child. **42:**75, 1967.)

loss. Temperature of the wall is midway between room air and incubator air (Fig. 4-6). The cooler the nursery, the cooler the incubator walls, and thus the greater the rate of radiant heat loss. *Heat loss by radiation is independent of the temperature of incubator air*. The clinical significance of radiant heat loss varies inversely with temperature of an incubator wall and the size of the baby. In most situations, radiant heat loss can be compensated by diminution of convective loss. This occurs automatically by servocontrol, which raises the temperature of incubator air. Radiant heat loss can be virtually eliminated by surrounding the baby with an inner plastic shield, which becomes the primary surface to which heat is transferred by radiation. Temperature of the shield walls approximates ambient incubator temperature; the skin-to-wall temperature gradient is minimized, thereby reducing radiant heat loss.

Double-walled incubators are commercially available. They are constructed of a two-layered plastic wall separated by a compartment of air. The inner surface of the inside layer is protected from cool nursery air by the outside layer, and by circulating warm air in the compartment between layers. The temperature of the inner wall is close to ambient incubator temperature. Published reports on the effectiveness of double-walled incubators are contradictory. The most recent study, utilizing partitional calorimetry, demonstrated no significant difference in *total heat loss* between a single- or double-walled incubator. Partitional calorimetry separately measures the rate of body heat loss by each of the three principal routes of heat exchange: evaporation, radiation, and convection. The study found that in infants whose skin temperature was servocontrolled at 36.5° C, radiant heat loss was indeed dimin-

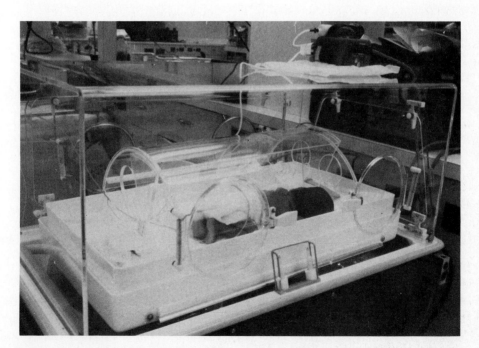

Fig. 4-7. Radiant losses are diminished by a cylindrical plastic heat shield ("igloo") in the incubator. Surrounding air warms igloo walls, thereby minimizing the temperature gradient between body surface and primary radiant surface. Half of the curved wall slides backward over the remaining half to provide convenient accessibility to the baby.

ished, but convective heat loss increased. Diminished radiant loss was effected by a warm inner wall, but with reduced radiant loss a lower servocontrolled air temperature induced increased convective loss. Evaporative loss did not differ between types of incubator. The double wall did not reduce oxygen consumption, insensible water loss, or metabolic heat production. It did reduce skin-to-wall temperature gradient, but it augmented the skin-to-air gradient. Since infant heat balance was similar in both incubators, there seems to be no advantage in using double-walled incubators.

As long as radiant heat loss can be compensated by diminished convective losses, the infant has no thermal difficulty. In the smallest sick infants, however, radiant dissipation is often critical. Among the limitations of available incubators, excessive radiant loss is an important consideration in situations that impose thermal risk.

The provision of humidity is also a disadvantage of available incubators. Water in a reservoir beneath the deck of the incubator is stagnant; it thus becomes a medium for the growth of "water bugs," most notably *Pseudomonas aeruginosa* (Chapter 12). Humidification is indispensable for management of tiny infants in incubators. Water should be changed frequently, at least every 8 hours.

Thermometers for display of incubator temperature are generally remote from the infant. Readings are lower than the actual temperature of air immediately surrounding the infant. If incubator air, rather than skin, is used to servocontrol ambient temperature, the skin probe can be hung from the incubator roof so that it is just above the infant. Adjustment of the set point is made by the same mechanism as for skin temperature.

Incubator temperature is servocontrolled by a gradual (partial) increase or decrease in heat output in response to changes in skin temperature. The set point for activation of the heater is 36.5° C (97.7° F). In the partial response device, heat output diminishes gradually as skin temperature rises above the set point, and it increases gradually as skin temperature falls. The gradual response tends to minimize fluctuations in incubator temperature that characterized the previously pervasive all-or-none mechanism. Partial response was introduced because an increased incidence of apneic episodes was observed with abrupt rise or fall of ambient temperatures. Most of the apneic episodes were related to sudden elevations.

The need for frequent entry through portholes presents another difficulty inherent to the use of incubators. The temperature drops precipitously, but warming is slow. Entry into the incubator causes a sudden drop in temperature that persists protractedly after withdrawal and closure of portholes.

Cold drafts from air-conditioning vents should not strike directly on incubator walls; nor should incubators be near cold windows. Recurrent or relentless cold stress caused by large radiant heat losses can thus be avoided.

Water in reservoirs is required for only a small number of infants, and if the reservoir is utilized, water should be changed frequently, preferably every 8 hours.

With a heat-sensing probe on the abdomen, the infant should never be prone, since the resultant false registration of high skin temperature diminishes or eliminates activation of the heater. The result may be a very cold baby.

Heat gain is possible from protracted exposure of the incubator to sunlight from a window. Serious elevation of core temperature may ensue. Oxygen consumption increases in response to hyperthermia. The metabolic penalties are similar to those of hypothermia and are often even more dangerous.

Radiant warmers. The open bed provides indispensable accessibility for resuscitation during acute emergencies and for sustained management of gravely ill infants. The need for accessibility has increased since radiant warmers first became pervasive in the 1970s. Diagnostic procedures at the bedside are more numerous; monitoring equipment has proliferated. Tiny infants now survive in larger numbers, and the nursery stay of nonsurvivors is longer. These are the infants who require a type of management that now entails a broader array of procedures than were available in the past. Mounting progress and passing time have enhanced the urgency of continuous accessibility.

The radiant warmer provides heat in the form of infrared energy from an overhead source. Wavelength emissions are in the "far infrared" range (greater than 2.0 μ); this avoids damage to the eye. Wavelengths in the "near infrared" spectrum (0.7 to 2.0 μ) are injurious to the cornea and retina. The source of heat is sufficiently high to be unobtrusive to personnel yet close enough to the infant to be effective. The emission of infrared energy is focused for minimal dissemination beyond the bed.

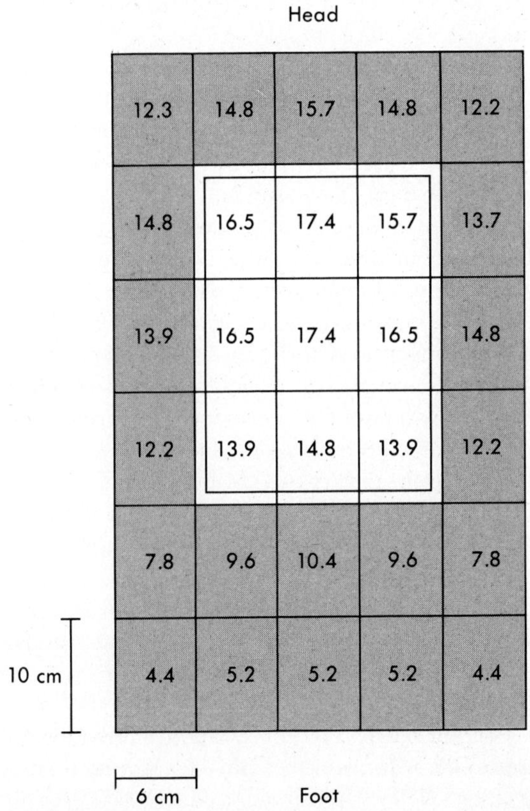

Delivery of infrared energy to the table surface varies from one section to another. Fig. 4-8 demonstrates the distribution of radiant energy (in mW/cm^2) over the surface of an Air Shields Infant Care System. The framed central area delineates the area in which maximal energy is delivered. The precipitous fall in energy delivered outside the delineated area is noteworthy.

Quantity and duration of infrared energy are determined by a sensing probe that is fastened to the abdominal skin. The probe must be covered with a reflective foam pad to prevent spurious registration of high temperatures from the direct effect of radiant heat on the sensor. Without a probe cover, the baby would remain hypothermic. The sensor, warmed directly by radiant heat rather than by abdominal skin, signals discontinuation of heat output. The probe is heated, but the baby remains cold.

In closed incubators the heat source is convective; for open warmers, the heat source is solely radiant. The major route of heat loss in an incubator is radiation; for the open warmer it is convection. Evaporative heat loss is common to both devices; it is significantly greater under radiant warmers. Loss of heat by convection is substantial on radiant warmers because air currents in the nursery are relentless. Total exposure to air movement also enhances evaporative losses.

The principal disadvantage of the radiant warmer is its well-known effect on transepidermal water loss (TEWL), which is considerably greater than in the incubator. Measured quantities of lost water vary from one study to another, but greater loss in radiant heat is unequivocally demonstrated in all reports. Most of these reports have analyzed water loss for infants grossly grouped above or below 1500 g; in some reports, comparisons are also made between those two groups and term babies. Recently, additional published data have

Head

Fig. 4-8. Variations in delivery of power density (mw/cm²) plotted on the deck of an Air Shields radiant warmer. The framed central area is most radiodense for maximal heat delivery. (From Baumgart, S.: J. Pediatr. **99:**948, 1981.)

specifically concerned infants whose weights are below 1 kg (or 30 weeks gestation). The measured amounts of water lost on radiant beds has reportedly varied from 25 ml/kg/24 h to 84 ml/kg/24 h in study populations of mixed gestational and postnatal ages. However, in infants between 0.66 kg and 1.00 kg, mean water loss is as high as 126 ml/kg/24 h. These are *averages* for a *group* of infants studied. In individual infants, losses can be as high as 160 ml/kg/24 h. Evaporative losses of water and heat are a major threat to the survival of tiny infants (below 1000 g). Insensible water loss increases as body size, gestational age, and postnatal age decrease. In addition, more radiant energy is required to maintain the body temperature of these smallest infants. Aside from body proportion and age, available data also suggest that infrared energy itself promotes evaporation from the skin. We know that exposure to infrared energy increases skin blood flow, but the relationship of increased perfusion to enhanced TEWL has not been explained. The propensity to lose more water on radiant warmers as gestational age decreases is a function of body size, surface area, and maturity of skin. Keratin in the stratum corneum is thought to be an effective barrier to water diffusion, and immature skin is devoid of it for variable periods after birth.

The obvious answer to large volumes of water loss for tiny infants is the administration of large volumes of intravascular fluid. Unfortunately, that solution is not completely effective, and it creates new difficulties of equal gravity. Personal communications from numerous sources tell of infants who need 300 ml/kg/day or more. The logistics of administration and the electrolyte imbalances that result from these voluminous infusions compound the difficulties of management. Large volumes of water often cause severe hyperglycemia and hypernatremia, depending on the concentrations of glucose and sodium administered. Water balance is not consistently achieved.

Radiant warmers and heat shields. Plastic shields reduce water and heat losses. One report suggested a Plexiglas shield that was subsequently shown to be unpredictably effective under radiant warmers. Furthermore, Plexiglas is virtually opaque to infrared energy; effectiveness, if any, would depend on a slow, gradual accumulation of heat in the walls of the shield. During the interval of accumulation, cold stress may develop in a tiny infant because only minimal amounts of infrared energy are delivered through Plexiglas. Alternatively, a thin sheet of plastic (a thermal blanket over the baby) effectively diminishes water loss and increases body temperature. These blankets, directly applied to the skin of infants, invariably produce denuded areas that ooze blood and fluid, often becoming infected. By diminishing air velocity, the thermal blanket minimizes convective and evaporative heat loss. As a consequence, radiant power requirements for the maintenance of normal skin temperature are reduced.

Since the mid-1970s we have used a heat shield composed of plastic walls and covered by a thin plastic film (Fig. 4-9). The polyvinyl chloride film does not contact skin. Walls of the shield are in two sections to permit an easy telescope type of adjustment for infant length. Semilunar openings along the bottom margins permit passage of ventilator connections and other support apparatus. With the use of these shields, insensible water loss (TEWL was not measured specifically) was reduced by 51% and radiant energy requirements by 59%. Air velocity has not been measured, but the virtually complete enclosure provided by this shield presumes a significant reduction, if not elimination, of air turbulence. With the shield in place, air temperature close to the baby was 4.4° C higher than it was when the shield was removed. Vapor pressure within the shield was significantly higher than with the shield in place. Gestational ages of the 12 study babies ranged from 30 to 34 weeks; birth weight varied from 0.92 to 1.65 kg. The shield is effective. It is easily removed for accessibility; it causes little if any inconvenience in the performance of procedures. While it is effective at the gestational ages and weights that were studied, the shield is not entirely satisfactory for infants under 750 g. A dif-

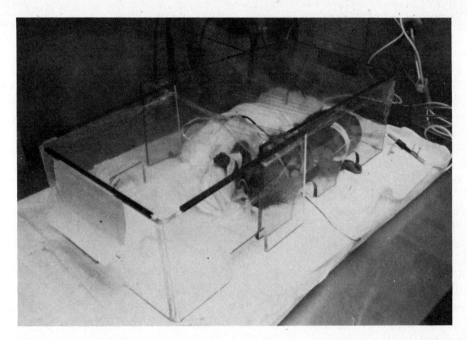

Fig. 4-9. The walls of these "windshields" are 8 inches high. Two separate three-sided structures surround upper and lower halves of the baby for convenient accessibility. They are covered with disposable thin plastic sheets similar to Saran Wrap. Insensible water loss is diminished because normal skin temperature of babies can be maintained using half the quantity of radiant energy required in the absence of these covers.

ferent device for these tiny infants is under investigation.

Clinical assessment and management of the infant's thermal status

The major concern in assessment and management of body temperature is maintenance of normal heat balance at the lowest level of oxygen consumption. Metabolic rate increases rapidly in response to cold stress that is sensed by thermal receptors in the skin, particularly those over the face. The response does not await a drop in core temperature to become activated. Rather, to support core temperature, it is triggered early and rapidly by a change in the environment that is sensed by the skin. Rectal temperature may therefore be normal in the cold-stressed baby because metabolic hyperactivity compensates suc-

cessfully for thermal losses. (Compare Figs. 4-4 and 4-5.) The increased metabolic rate is triggered by environmental changes that are perceived by thermal receptors in the skin. *When rectal temperature becomes subnormal, the thermal battle is lost; the baby cannot generate enough heat to maintain normal core temperature.*

Body temperature is taken from the rectum, axilla, or skin. The rectal temperature is assumed to be equivalent to core temperature, but even when properly taken, it is only an approximation. Experimentally, the esophagus or the tympanic membrane are the most reliable sites for true core temperature. These sites are obviously impractical in a clinical setting. Rectal temperature approximates core temperature, depending on the depth of thermometer insertion. The more deeply the temperature probe is inserted, the higher the temperature recorded, until a depth of 10 cm is reached. Obviously, this is also impractical in a clinical setting. The difference between inserting a thermistor to a depth of 1 cm and 5 cm into the rectum can be in excess of 1.5° C (approximately 2.0° F). Insertion of a mercury thermometer for rectal temperature should be at a depth of 2 cm. The depth of insertion should be standardized so that readings are comparable. The thermometer must be in place 5 minutes for accurate recording.

The axilla has often been recommended as an acceptable alternative to the rectum for taking body temperature. Axillary temperatures are indeed reliable for close estimation of rectal temperature taken at a depth of 2 cm. In both term and preterm infants there is less than 0.10° C (0.18° F) difference between the two sites. These differences are not clinically significant. These data are based on temperatures taken with mercury-in-glass thermometers kept in place for 5 minutes for a stabilized reading.

Skin temperatures are essential for infants who are maintained in a controlled thermal environment (incubator or radiant warmer). When servocontrol is utilized, the skin temperature set point is generally kept at 36.5° C (97.7° F). In unusual circumstances, particularly for tiny babies, the skin temperature set point must sometimes be slightly higher to achieve acceptable axillary or rectal temperature. The approximate range of normal axillary temperature for the preterm infant is 36.2° C to 37.3° C (97.2° F to 99.1° F).

Available data unequivocally demonstrate that thermal sensors of the face are more influential in activating increased metabolism than other nerve endings in the skin elsewhere over the body. When the environment is well heated below the neck, a baby whose facial environment is cool will react as if cold stressed. The practical importance of this observation relates to oxygen administration. *It is mandatory that oxygen supplied to a head hood be warmed.* Ambient temperature within the hood should be monitored and maintained at levels equal to the incubator. Furthermore, cold oxygen should not be blasted onto an infant's face through a face mask or tube for protracted periods.

A significant quantity of heat is lost from the respiratory tract, particularly in infants who are tachypneic. Oxygen must be warmed and humidified, particularly for intubated babies. Dry oxygen causes significant evaporation from the extensive mucosal surface that lines the respiratory tract, and heat loss by this modality can be significant.

Whether they are nurses, physicians, or attendants in any capacity, the neonate's best caretakers are his most protective ones. Unflagging attention to the environmental requirements of optimal heat balance is the essence of such protectiveness. In respect to temperament, training, continuous presence, and sphere of activity, no one is better equipped to perform this function than the neonatal nurse. Furthermore, if the nurse fails to perform it, quite likely no one else will.

BIBLIOGRAPHY

Abrams, R. M.: Thermal physiology of the fetus. In Sinclair, J. C., editor: Temperature regulation and energy metabolism in the newborn, New York, 1978, Grune and Stratton, Inc.

Adamsons, K., Jr.: The role of thermal factors in fetal and neonatal life, Pediatr. Clin. North Am. **13**:599, 1966.

Adamsons, K., Jr., and Towell, M. E.: Thermal homeostasis in the fetus and newborn, Anesthesiology **26**:531, 1965.

Adamsons, K., Jr., Gandy, G. M., and James. L. S.: The influence of thermal factors upon oxygen consumption of the newborn human infant, J. Pediatr. **66**:495, 1965.

Anagnostakis, D., Economou-Mavrou, C., Agathopoulas, A., and Matsaniotis, N.: Neonatal cold injury: evidence of defective thermogenesis due to impaired norepinephrine release, Pediatrics **53**:24, 1974.

Anonymous by request: Comment; speed of rewarming after postnatal chilling, J. Pediatr. **85**:551, 1974.

Aynsley-Green, A., Robertson, N. R. C., and Rolfe, P.: Air temperature recordings in infant incubators, Arch, Dis. Child. **50**:215, 1975.

Baumgart, S.: Radiant energy and insensible water loss in the premature newborn infant nursed under a radiant warmer, Clin. Perinatol. **9**:483, 1982.

Bell, E. F., and Rios, G. R.: A double-walled incubator alters the partition of body heat loss of premature infants, Pediatr. Res. **17**:135, 1983.

Bruck, K.: Temperature regulation in the newborn infant, Biol. Neonate **3**:65, 1965.

Bruck, K.: Heat production and temperature regulation. In Stave, U., editor: Perinatal physiology, New York, 1970, Plenum Publishing Corp.

Cross, K. W., and Stratton, D.: Aural temperature of the newborn infant, Lancet **2**:1179, 1974.

Dahm, L. S., and James, L. S.: Newborn temperature and calculated heat loss in the delivery room, Pediatrics **49**:504, 1972.

Day, R., Curtis, J., and Kelly, M.: Respiratory metabolism in infancy and in childhood, Am. J. Dis. Child. **65**:376, 1943.

Day, R. L., Caliguiri, L., Kamenski, C., et al.: Body temperature and survival of premature infants, Pediatrics **34**:171, 1964.

Doyle, L. W., and Sinclair, J. C.: Insensible water loss in newborn infants, Clin. Perinatol. **9**:453, 1982.

Fanaroff, A. A., Wald, M., Gruber, H. S., and Klaus, M. H.: Insensible water loss in low birth weight infants, Pediatrics **50**:236, 1972.

Fitch, C. W., and Korones, S. B.: Heat shield reduces water loss, Arch. Dis. Child. **59**:886, 1984.

Glass, L., Silverman, W. A., and Sinclair, J. C.: Effect of the thermal environment on cold resistance and growth of small infants after the first week of life, Pediatrics **41**:1033, 1968.

Hahn, P., and Skala, J. P.: Nonshivering heat production in the newborn. In Scarpelli, E. M., and Cosmi, E. V., editors: Reviews in perinatal medicine, New York, 1978, Raven Press.

Harned, H. S., Jr., and Ferreiro, J.: Initiation of breathing by cold stimulation: effects of change in ambient temperature on respiratory activity of the full-term fetal lamb, J. Pediatr. **83**:663, 1973.

Hey, E. N.: The relation between environmental temperature and oxygen consumption in the newborn baby, J. Physiol. **200**:589, 1969.

Hey, E. N., and Mount, L.: Temperature control in incubators, Lancet **2**:202, 1966.

Hey, E. N., and Mount, L. E.: Heat losses from babies in incubators, Arch. Dis. Child. **42**:75, 1967.

Hull, D., and Smales, O. R. C.: Heat production in the newborn. In Sinclair, J. C., editor: Temperature regulation and energy metabolism in the newborn, New York, 1978, Grune and Stratton, Inc.

Kajtar, P., Jequier, E., and Prod'hom, L. S.: Heat losses in newborn infants of different body size measured by direct calorimetry in a thermoneutral and a cold environment, Biol. Neonate **30**:55, 1976.

Levison, H., Linsao, L., and Swyer, P. R.: A comparison of infra-red and convective heating for newborn infants, Lancet **2**:1346, 1966.

Marks, K. H., Lee, C. A., Bolan, C. D., and Maisels, M. J.: Oxygen consumption and temperature control of premature infants in a double-wall incubator, Pediatrics **68**:93, 1981.

Mayfield, S. T., Bhatia, J., Nakamura, K. T., et al.: Temperature measurement in term and preterm neonates, J. Pediatr. **104**:271, 1984.

Mestyan, J., Jarai, I., Bata, G., and Fekete, M.: The significance of facial skin temperature in the chemical heat regulation of premature infants, Biol. Neonate **7**:243, 1964.

Motil, K. J., Blackburn, M. G., and Pleasure, J. R.: The effects of four different radiant warmer temperature set-points used for rewarming neonates, J. Pediatr. **85**:546, 1974.

Oliver, T. K., Jr.: Temperature regulation and heat production in the newborn, Pediatr. Clin. North Am. **12**:765, 1965.

Perlstein, P. H.: Part 2. Physical environment—the thermal environment (temperature and survival). In Fanaroff, A.A., and Martin, R. J., editors: Behrman's neonatal-perinatal medicine, St. Louis, 1983, The C. V. Mosby Co.

Perlstein, P.H., et al.: Apnea in premature infants and incubator-air-temperature changes, N. Engl. J. Med. **282**:461, 1970.

Perlstein, P. H., Hersch, C., Glueck, C. J., and Sutherland, J. M.: Adaptation to cold in the first three days of life, Pediatrics **54**:411, 1974.

Robinson, R. O., and Jones, R.: Advantages of overhead radiant heaters, Proc. Roy. Soc. Med. **70**:209, 1977

Rutter, N., and Hull, D.: Water loss from the skin of term and preterm babies, Arch. Dis. Child. **54**:858, 1979.

Sauer, P. J. J., Dane, J. H., and Visser, H. K. A.: New standards for neutral thermal environment of healthy very low birthweight infants, Arch. Dis. Child. **59**:18, 1984.

Sauer, P. J. J., and Visser, H. K. A.: Commentary: The neutral temperature of very low-birth-weight infants, Pediatrics, **74**:288, 1984.

Scopes, J. W.: Metabolic rate and temperature control in the human baby, Br. Med. Bull. **22**:88, 1966.

Scopes, J. W., and Ahmed, I.: Range of critical temperatures in sick and premature newborn babies, Am. J. Dis. Child. **41**:417, 1966.

Silverman, W. A.: Diagnosis and treatment; use and misuse of temperature and humidity in care of the newborn infant, Pediatrics **33**:276, 1974.

Silverman, W. A., et al.: The oxygen cost of minor changes in heat balance of small newborn infants, Acta Paediatr. Scand. **55**:294, 1966.

Silverman, W. A., and Sinclair, J. C.: Temperature regulation in the newborn infant, N. Engl. J. Med. **274**:146, 1966.

Silverman, W. A., Zamelis, A., Sinclair, J. C., and Agate, F. J.: Warm nape of the newborn, Pediatrics **33**:984, 1964.

Sinclair, J. C.: Heat production and thermoregulation in the small-for-date infant, Pediatr. Clin. North Am. **17**:147, 1970.

Sinclair, J. C.: Metabolic rate and temperature control. In Smith, C. A., and Nelson, N. M., editors: The physiology of the newborn infant, Springfield, Ill., 1976, Charles C Thomas, Publisher.

Stephenson, J. M., Du, J. N., and Oliver, T. K., Jr.: The effect of cooling on blood gas tensions in newborn infants, J. Pediatr. **76:**848, 1970.

Swyer, P. R.: Heat loss after birth. In Sinclair, J. C., editor: Temperature regulation and energy metabolism in the newborn, New York, 1978, Grune and Stratton, Inc.

Wheldon, A. E., and Hull, D.: Incubation of very immature infants, Arch. Dis. Child. **58:**504, 1983.

Wheldon, A. E., and Rutter, N.: The heat balance of small babies nursed in incubators and under radiant warmers, Early Human Develop. **6:**131, 1982.

Williams, P. R., and Oh, W.: Effects of radiant warmer on insensible water loss in newborn infants, Am. J. Dis. Child. **128:**511, 1974.

Wu, P. Y. K., and Hodgman, J. E.: Insensible water loss in preterm infants: Changes with postnatal development and non-ionizing radiant energy, Pediatrics **54:**704, 1974.

Yashiro, K., Adams, F. H., Emmanouilides, G. C., and Mickey, M. R.: Preliminary studies on the thermal environment of low-birth-weight infants, J. Pediatr. **82:**991, 1973.

Yeh, T. F., Voora, S., Lilien, L. D., et al.: Oxygen consumption and insensible water loss in premature infants in single-versus double-walled incubators, J. Pediatr. **97:**967, 1980.

CHAPTER 5

Significance of the relationship of birth weight to gestational age

Until the early 1960s birth weight was considered the most reliable index of an infant's maturity. If an infant weighed less than 2500 g, he was assumed to be premature; if his weight exceeded 2500 g, he was considered mature. This approach implied that intrauterine growth rates were similar for all fetuses and that birth weight could thus be utilized as an accurate expression of gestational age. However, a considerable amount of data have accumulated to demonstrate the inaccuracy of this assumption. Regardless of birth weight, an infant is in fact premature if he is born before term. Birth weight less than 2500 g simply indicates that growth was incomplete, whether due to a short gestational age, impairment of intrauterine growth, or both. These separate considerations of weight (for assessment of growth) and gestational age (for assessment of maturity) have resulted in a more meaningful classification in which important biologic correlates are identifiable.

INTRAUTERINE GROWTH
Significance of physical measurements

Fetal and neonatal growth are a continuum; they are not separate unrelated phenomena. The influence of intrauterine events and growth patterns on postnatal growth will become apparent in discussions presented in this chapter.

Fetal growth rate is dependent on two categorical factors: (1) intrinsic fetal growth potential and (2) the limitations of intrauterine environment, both normal and abnormal. Intrinsic growth potential is genetically established with fertilization, or it may be influenced early in pregnancy by intrauterine infection. Intrauterine environment is a function of the maternal circulatory pattern, which comprises the fetal "growth support system" that provides nutrients and accommodates gas exchange at the intervillous space. Deviations from normal are therefore attributable to (1) impaired fetal potential due to genetic abnormalities at conception, or early acquisition of intrauterine infection; and (2) impairment of the growth support system as a result of maternal hypertension, pregnancy-induced hypertension,

advanced diabetes, and other maternal disorders. Even in normal pregnancies the growth support system becomes limited as term approaches. These normal limitations ultimately influence fetal growth rate.

Weight. Weight is the most frequently performed measurement for assessment of growth status because it is accurate and easily obtained. It is also the most sensitive indicator of day-to-day changes. Weight is a summary value; in the aggregate, it reflects changes in the content of protein, fat, and water and in the growth of the brain and skeleton. Other important components of physical growth can be indicated more specifically. Thus head circumference is used for growth of the brain and total body length (crown-heel) for skeletal growth.

A well-defined pattern of intrauterine weight gain, particularly during the third trimester, has evolved from studies of several populations. Despite variations, the overall pattern suggests that fetal growth potential is normally unrestricted during most of pregnancy. It progresses in a linear fashion until late in the third trimester when limitations of the growth support system can no longer sustain the preexisting growth rate. The fetus continues to grow, but at a significantly slower rate. In normal singletons, growth is linear from the twenty-eighth to the thirty-sixth or thirty-ninth week, at which time the limitations imposed by uterine size and an aging placenta limit the *rate* (velocity) of weekly growth (Fig. 5-1). The limitations of intrauterine environment are exemplified in decreased growth velocity of twin fetuses. In contrast to singletons, decreased growth rate begins as early as 30 weeks. In triplets and in quadruplets this phenomenon is accentuated, occurring at 28 and 26 weeks, respectively (Fig. 5-2). As in singletons at a late date, multiple fetuses outgrow their support system at an early one. In Fig. 5-3, five curves of fetal weights from 1000 to 4000 g are plotted from 28 to 40 gestational weeks. The straight uppermost line is theoretical, representing growth calculated for a uterine environment without limitations. The curve below

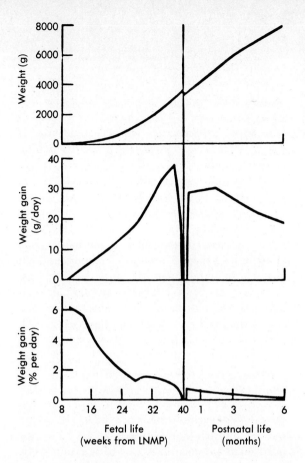

Fig. 5-1. Three intrauterine-postnatal growth curves. *Top:* Steady weight gain becomes linear from 28 to 39 weeks when it is interrupted at birth to resume linear pattern shortly thereafter. *Middle:* Gain in *grams per day* increases with virtual linearity until birth. Postnatal gain resumes but with fewer grams per day. *Bottom: Percent* gain diminishes because of aging placenta and limited uterine size. Interrupted gain at birth is shown again, and postnatal *percent* gain declines steadily. (From Usher, R., and McLean, F. In Davis, J., and Dobbing, J., editors: Scientific foundations of paediatrics, Philadelphia, 1974, W. B. Saunders Co.)

Fig. 5-2. Limitations on growth exerted by uterine size and aging placenta are reflected in earlier diminution in the rate of fetal weight gain as the number of fetuses increases from singleton to quadruplets. Singleton decelerated growth starts at 39 weeks; twins at 30 weeks; triplets at 28 weeks; and quadruplets at 26 weeks. (From McKeown, T., and Record, R.: J. Endocrinol. 8:386, 1952.)

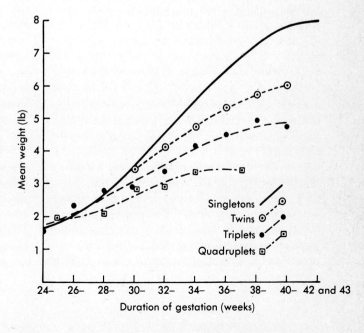

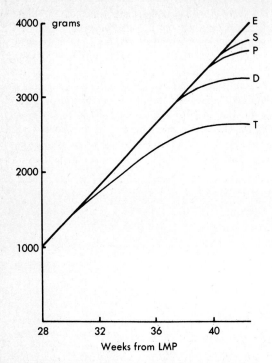

Fig. 5-3. Birth weight curves in different populations indicate the varied times at which growth slows because of limited fetal supply from mother. *E* is calculated growth that would occur if fetal supply line remained adequate throughout gestation. Compare to actual growth rates in Sweden, *S;* Portland, Oregon, *P;* Denver, *D;* and for twins, *T.* (Modified from Gruenwald, P.: Ciba Foundation Symposium 27, Amsterdam, 1974, Elsevier Science Publishers.)

it *(S)* indicates decreased growth velocity at 39 weeks in a Swedish population. Populations in Portland, Oregon *(P)*, and Denver, Colorado *(D)*, revealed a diminished growth rate at 38 and 37 weeks, respectively. The leveling of growth rate in twins *(T)* is seen in Fig. 5-3 at 30 weeks. The normal single fetus gains approximately 100 g during the twenty-eighth week, 240 g in the thirty-fifth week, and significantly less in subsequent weeks, depending on onset of a physiologic decrease in growth rate. Intrauterine limitations impede the growth rate of multiple fetuses when their combined weight is approximately 3000 g

and of singletons at approximately the same weight. The slowed fetal growth rate persists several days postnatally, and it then resumes the pace of unrestricted intrauterine growth that had existed previously.

Head circumference. Head circumference is accurately measured by placing a tape around the cranium at the level of the supraorbital ridges anteriorly and the occipital protuberance posteriorly. Head circumference is generally interpreted to indicate the status of brain growth, but the relationship is not consistently straightforward. However, subnormal measurement is a straightforward indication of inadequate brain size. On the other hand, circumferences that exceed normal rarely indicate supranormal brain size as such, but rather they indicate increased size of the head resulting from other factors such as hydrocephalus. In most instances, head circumference correlates well with brain weight. Growth of the head is linear, beginning with the latter half of pregnancy to about 32 weeks. Beginning at 26 to 28 weeks there is a spurt in head growth that reaches maximum at 32 weeks. At the maximal growth rates between 30 and 32 weeks, head circumference increases by 1.2 mm daily. Daily increments then diminish gradually, and at 40 weeks the rate of growth has subsided to 0.2 mm daily. The findings of ultrasound examinations parallel these data. By ultrasonic visualization the fetal biparietal diameter increases in a linear fashion until approximately 30 weeks. There is some diminution in growth between 30 and 34 weeks, after which growth rate decreases sharply. Postnatally, head circumference grows 1.1 mm daily, which is close to the intrauterine pace that existed before the slowing of growth.

Length. Length increases in the twenty-fifth gestational week by 1.0 cm weekly. Peak lengthening, 1.3 cm weekly, occurs between 31 and 34 weeks. After that, growth velocity diminishes and at 40 weeks the incremental rate is 0.5 cm/week. The postnatal pattern for length growth is similar to weight and head size; growth returns to the rate that existed in utero at 32 gestational weeks.

Growth. The phenomenon of postnatal "catch-up" growth occurs in all three parameters—weight, length, and head circumference. There is a constant addition to fetal dimensions during the second and early parts of the third trimester. Near term, growth continues in all parameters but at notably diminished rates, as if restrained by an outgrown growth support system. Resumption of more rapid rates close to intrauterine maximum then occurs after birth. The pattern of fetal, and then neonatal, growth can be logically attributed to suppression of fetal growth potential followed by postnatal removal of restraints inherent to the outgrown intrauterine support system.

The normal pattern of the fetal-neonatal continuum is an indispensable point of reference in understanding abnormalities discussed later in this chapter. "Normal" is defined and summarized for various populations in growth curves constructed from worldwide data and interpreted over the years. It is possible, therefore, to anticipate normal growth rate and size, identify aberrations, and then seek chemical, structural, and clinical associations that suggest causes. These considerations must also address normal characteristics of diverse geographic and genetic origins. Mean birth weights at term vary considerably among different populations the world over. The difference in mean weights can be as great as 1500 g. The maternal support system, rather than intrinsic growth capacity of the fetus, is considered the principal cause of these population variations. The well-being, nutrition, and socioeconomic environment of mothers are therefore major contributors to effective growth support systems and ultimately to birth weights at term. The father's role is nonexistent; once conception has occurred, the male is a biological redundancy. Thus the course of intrauterine growth is largely determined by maternal factors.

Body composition of the fetus and neonate

The progressive changes in body composition, particularly those involving water and fat content, are pertinent to postnatal therapy of sick babies.

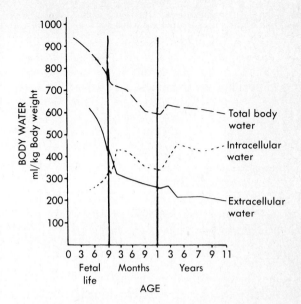

Fig. 5-4. Total body water (ml/kg body weight) diminishes as fetus, infant, and child mature. Commensurate with that diminution, intracellular water increases and extracellular water decreases (in ml/kg body weight). (From Uttley, W., and Habel, A.: Clin. Endocrinol. Metabol. **5:**3, 1976.)

Water. Water contributes the largest proportion of body weight in both fetus and newborn. The smallest embryo ever subjected to analysis weighed less than 1.0 g; water comprised 93% to 95% of total weight. The percentage of water contribution to body weight falls throughout gestation (Fig. 5-4). At 26 weeks it is 85% of body weight; at 30 weeks it is 80%; at 38 weeks water is 74%; and at 40 weeks, 71% of the total body weight. As total body water diminishes, the distribution also changes. Extracellular water diminishes and intracellular water increases as the fetus matures. Expansion of intracellular water occurs with advancing differentiation and cell hypertrophy. Cell size increases and cellular proliferation decreases as intracellular water accumulates. The altered distribution pattern of body water continues past birth. At term, *extracellular* water is 45% of body weight; 2 months later it is 30% of body weight.

These trends in diminished water volume and the changes in distribution are critical considerations in the management of thermal environment for small infants (Chapter 4) and in the maintenance of fluid and electrolyte balance (Chapter 7).

Fat. Fat is indeed sparse during the first 20 gestational weeks, comprising only 1% of total body weight. Subsequently it is deposited at an accelerated pace, mostly late in the last trimester when subcutaneous fat accumulates rapidly. The fetus generates fat from glucose and, to a smaller extent, from transplacentally derived essential fatty acids. Brown fat deposits appear early in the second half of gestation (see Chapter 4). White fat is primarily located in subcutaneous tissue. It stores excess energy for future use if intake becomes suboptimal, as in postmaturity. White fat generates heat as a by-product of metabolic activity, but it differs from brown adipose tissue in that it cannot respond to cold stress. At 26 weeks fat is approximately 3% of body weight; at 35 weeks, 8%; at term, fat is 15% of weight, with 80% of it in the subcutaneous tissue. Body water diminishes as fat accumulates and organ mass increases. Fat accretion, water depletion, and organ differentiation are synchronous phenomena of the maturational process.

Protein. Protein synthesis is from amino acids transferred across the placenta. The fetus generates protein independently; amino acid content of protein molecules is similar to the adult. The only "ready-made" proteins transferred across the placenta in significant quantities are the immunoglobulins, preponderantly immunoglobulin G (gamma globulin).

CLASSIFICATION OF INFANTS BY BIRTH WEIGHT AND GESTATIONAL AGE
Terminology

In 1961 the World Health Organization recommended that babies who weigh less than 2500 g be designated as "low birth weight" (LBW) infants. This definition eliminated all implications of prematurity. It disregards gestational age. Definitions of gestational age correspondingly disregard any consideration of birth weight. A *premature (preterm)* infant is born before the end of the thirty-seventh week. A *term* infant is born between the beginning of the thirty-eighth week and the completion of the forty-first week. A *postmature (postterm)* baby is born at the onset of the forty-second week or anytime thereafter. Gestational weeks are calculated from the first day of the last menstrual period (LMP). These definitions of fetal age have nothing to do with weight, length, head circumference, or other measurements of fetal size. However, the *relationship* of these physical attributes to calculated age is of great importance.

The various types of low birth weight infants (under 2500 g) are as follows:

1. Infants whose rate of intrauterine growth was normal at the moment of birth. They are small only because labor began before the end of 37 weeks. *These premature infants are appropriately grown for gestational age (AGA).*

2. Infants whose rate of intrauterine growth was slowed and who were delivered at or later than term (end of 37 weeks). These term or postterm (postmature) infants are undergrown for gestational age. *They are small for dates or small for gestational age (SGA).*

3. Infants whose in utero growth was retarded and who, in addition, were delivered prematurely. These premature infants are small by virtue of both early delivery and impaired intrauterine growth. *They are small-for-dates, premature infants.*

The corollary of 2500 g for low birth weight is 4000 g for high birth weight. Optimum weight for the lowest perinatal mortality is between 3500 and 4000 g. Above the latter level, mortality begins to increase, and on that basis, the weight of 4000 g serves to delineate high birth weight infants. *Babies are considered large for gestational age (LGA), at any weight, when they fall above the ninetieth or ninety-fifth percentile on the intrauterine growth curves.*

Intrauterine growth curves

The intrauterine growth chart offers a simple and effective way of assessing growth and maturity of newborn infants. It was derived by plotting birth weights of a large neonatal population against the weeks of gestation to show the range of expected weights for each week. The graph lists birth weights vertically and weeks of gestation horizontally. Data from the Colorado intrauterine growth chart are most widely used for this purpose. They plot birth weights from 500 to 5000 g against gestational ages from 24 to 46 weeks or more. Two curves are drawn across the charts, dividing the population into three groups: above the 90th percentile, below the 10th percentile, and between the 10th and 90th percentiles. Weights below the 10th percentile curve are observed in only 10% of the population for any given gestational age. These infants are considered undergrown (SGA). Weights above the 90th percentile curve are higher than the remaining 90% of the population, and these infants are overgrown (LGA). Babies who are categorized between the 10th and 90th percentiles are appropriately grown for their gestational age. All infants below 2500 g, as well as any high-risk baby, regardless of weight, should be evaluated with these or similar graphs soon after admission to the nursery. Consider a neonate you have admitted who weighs 2000 g at 40 weeks. According to the growth chart, this mature infant is well below the 10th percentile, presumably as a consequence of intrauterine growth retardation. There is thus a risk for several disorders that require special measures.

Plotting an infant's weight and gestational age on the chart (Fig. 5-5) demonstrates that growth is appropriate, excessive, or diminished for age and that the baby is either premature, term, or postmature.

The Colorado growth curves categorize infants into percentiles, delineating abnormal growth in the areas on the chart that are above the 90th and below the 10th percentiles. Other systems utilize standard deviations. In these systems the abnor-

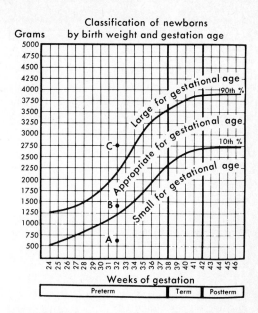

Fig. 5-5. Intrauterine growth status for gestational ages, according to appropriateness of growth. Points *A*, *B*, and *C* (added to original diagram by author) correspond to babies shown in Fig. 5-6. See text for explanation. (From Battaglia, F. C., and Lubchenco, L. O.: J. Pediatr. **71:**159, 1967.)

mal areas are beyond ±2 standard deviations from the mean. These standard deviations correlate with the 97th and 3rd percentiles, respectively. The designation of growth aberrations by standard deviation is more selective for any given population. Infants beyond ±2 standard deviations are more likely to be abnormal. Furthermore, the standard deviations are probably more realistic for infants born at or close to sea level. Colorado data were derived from an infant population that was born at 5000 ft above sea level.

Interpretation of growth curve data

An infant whose weight is appropriate for gestational age (AGA) has presumably grown at a normal rate in utero, whether the birth was premature, term, or postmature. Preterm babies whose weights are between the 10th and 90th percentiles are appropriately grown for gestational age (AGA) but small because normal intrauterine growth was interrupted by early onset of labor. If these same premature infants are below the tenth percentile for birth weight, they are small for gestational age (SGA) as well. Consider, for instance, a 1500 g infant whose gestational age is 36 weeks. According to the intrauterine growth charts, this infant is below the tenth percentile for birth weight at that age and is thus clearly undergrown. Demeanor, appearance, and course in the nursery will differ considerably from those of an appropriately grown infant of the same size who is born at 31 weeks.

An infant who is SGA has presumably grown at a retarded rate in utero, regardless of age at birth. Although this phenomenon may occur at any gestational age, most SGA infants are born at or close to term. Inspection of the intrauterine growth chart reveals that at term most infants who are SGA weigh less than 2500 g. At first glance

these babies may appear prematurely born. At our institution 40% of all low birth weight infants are born at or near term. They are thus mature SGA babies; yet according to the old concept, which interpreted weight and age interchangeably, they would have been considered premature infants. The unique attributes of SGA infants are discussed in more detail later in this chapter.

Infants who are large for gestational age (LGA) have presumably grown at an accelerated rate during intrauterine life. Less is known about them than the SGA. Infants of diabetic mothers are characteristically LGA, but they constitute a minority of all oversized babies. Inaccurately short estimates of gestational age are probably responsible for mistaken classification of many of these infants, although the frequency of these errors has not been documented (p. 119).

Fig. 5-6 shows three infants of different sizes who were born at 32 gestational weeks. From left to right, their birth weights were 600, 1400, and 2750 g, respectively. The largest baby is the infant

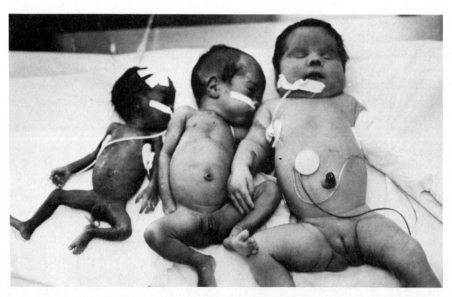

Fig. 5-6. Three babies, same gestational age, weigh 600, 1400, and 2750 g, respectively, from left to right. They are plotted on Fig. 5-5 at points *A*, *B*, and *C*.

of a diabetic mother, and the two small babies are twins delivered of a toxemic mother. On the growth curves in Fig. 5-5, points *A, B,* and *C* represent each of the infants on the 32-week line at their respective weights. At the same age, they are, respectively, small *(A),* appropriate *(B),* and large *(C)* for gestational age. Their clinical problems vary because their intrauterine growth problems were produced by diverse etiologies. The smallest baby is grossly malnourished, probably by virtue of impaired placental circulation. The middle baby is small only because of premature delivery. Growth, which was progressing at a normal rate, was interrupted by birth. The largest baby was growing more rapidly than normal in utero, as is characteristic of most diabetic pregnancies. These problems in management, as well as the mechanisms by which babies of different size emerge at the same gestational age and by which babies of equal size emerge at different gestational ages, are discussed later in this chapter.

PRENATAL ESTIMATION OF GESTATIONAL AGE
History of pregnancy; maternal examinations

Estimation of gestational age has traditionally involved counting the weeks that have elapsed since the first day of the last menstrual period (LMP); in the majority of instances this procedure is still reasonably reliable. Accuracy of historic data is thus totally dependent on the mother's recall. A valid history is best obtained early in pregnancy, when recall of the LMP is more likely to be accurate. The mother's history should not be underestimated; properly taken, it is valid in at least 75% to 85% of patients. For some women, accurate dating of LMP is virtually impossible. Irregular menses in the nonpregnant state frequently complicate the calculations, or the interval between pregnancies is so short that a normal menstrual pattern has yet to be reestablished. In nursing mothers, menstruation may not resume for months after the end of pregnancy. Another

cause of miscalculation is the occurrence of postconceptional bleeding, which is often misinterpreted as a menstrual period, thereby erroneously shortening the calculated gestational age.

The obstetrician uses certain physical milestones in pregnancy to estimate fetal age. The height of the uterine fundus above the symphysis pubis provides some indication of the length of pregnancy. Fundal height varies from 25 cm above the symphysis at 26 gestational weeks to approximately 33 cm in the thirty-eighth week. Fundal height is often misleading; some authors consider it useless for estimating gestational duration. Ultrasound visualization has replaced it. Other useful indications are the first maternal perception of fetal movement at approximately 16 weeks and the perception of fetal heartbeats at approximately 20 weeks.

Prenatal tests for maturity

Estimation of fetal maturity in utero by analysis of amniotic fluid and by other means is important in troubled pregnancies that may require a rapid decision regarding cesarean section. This is particularly true of pregnancies complicated by diabetes and other chronic illnesses. Discussion of prenatal evaluation is presented in Chapter 1. It should be reviewed for a better understanding of the application of prenatal data to the postnatal problems discussed in this chapter.

POSTNATAL ESTIMATION OF GESTATIONAL AGE

In the nursery, examination for certain external characteristics and neuromuscular signs is extremely valuable for assessment of maturity. Once learned, these observations can be made in a few minutes. The neonatal nurse should be familiar with these physical characteristics and neuromuscular responses. The system used in most nurseries was reported by Dubowitz and co-workers in 1970. Their study utilized confirmatory observations by three nurses who had no previous experience with these examinations. Once instructed in the procedure, the nurses' appraisals were reliable, correlating well with those of the principal investigator.

Using this system, an estimate of gestational age is usually accurate within 2 weeks. The accuracy of the method has been confirmed in studies primarily concerned with term infants. Other studies have confirmed accuracy in babies of very low birth weight (less than 1500 g), large for gestational age, and small for gestational age babies,

and even in infants with major neurologic malformations. Measurements can be made any time up to 5 days after birth, but because the information is so important in management of sick infants, the examination is best performed within 24 hours after delivery. The accompanying notes on techniques describe the procedures for evaluating postures and primitive reflexes; Fig. 5-7 illustrates responses elicited and the scores as-

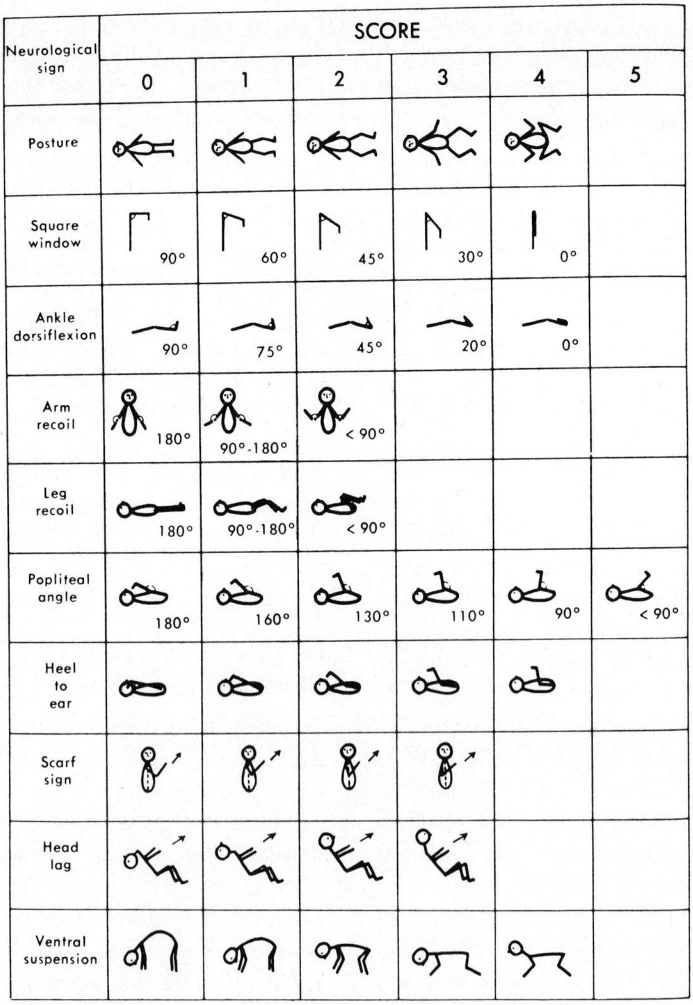

Fig. 5-7. Scoring system of neurologic signs for assessment of gestational age. (From Dubowitz, L. M. S., Dubowitz, V., and Goldberg, C.: J. Pediatr. **77:**1, 1970.)

SOME NOTES ON TECHNIQUES OF ASSESSMENT OF NEUROLOGIC CRITERIA
(for use in conjunction with Fig. 5-7 on p. 120)*

Posture: Observed with infant quiet and in supine position. Score 0: Arms and legs extended; 1: Beginning of flexion of hips and knees, arms extended; 2: Stronger flexion of legs, arms extended; 3: Arms slightly flexed, legs flexed and abducted; 4: Full flexion of arms and legs.

Square window: The hand is flexed on the forearm between the thumb and index finger of the examiner. Enough pressure is applied to get as full a flexion as possible, and the angle between the hypothenar eminence and the ventral aspect of the forearm is measured and graded according to diagrams (Fig. 5-7). (Care is taken not to rotate the infant's wrist while doing this maneuver.)

Ankle dorsiflexion: The foot is dorsiflexed onto the anterior aspect of the leg, with the examiner's thumb on the sole of the foot and other fingers behind the leg. Enough pressure is applied to get as full a flexion as possible, and the angle between the dorsum of the foot and the anterior aspect of the leg is measured.

Arm recoil: With the infant in the supine position the forearms are first flexed for 5 seconds, then fully extended by pulling on the hands, and then released. The sign is fully positive if the arms return briskly to full flexion (Score 2). If the arms return to incomplete flexion or the response is sluggish, it is graded as score 1. If they remain extended or are only followed by random movements, the score is 0.

Leg recoil: With the infant supine, the hips and knees are fully flexed for 5 seconds, then extended by traction on the feet, and released. A maximal response is one of full flexion of the hips and knees (Score 2). A partial flexion scores 1, and minimal or no movement scores 0.

Popliteal angle: With the infant supine and his pelvis flat on the examining couch, the thigh is held in the knee-chest position by the examiner's left index finger and thumb supporting the knee. The leg is then extended by gentle pressure from the examiner's right index finger behind the ankle, and the popliteal angle is measured.

Heel to ear maneuver: With the baby supine, draw the baby's foot as near to the head as it will go without forcing it. Observe the distance between the foot and the head as well as the degree of extension at the knee. Grade according to diagram. Note that the knee is left free and may draw down alongside the abdomen.

Scarf sign: With the baby supine, take the infant's hand and try to put it around the neck and as far posteriorly as possible around the opposite shoulder. Assist this maneuver by lifting the elbow across the body. See how far the elbow will go across and grade according to illustrations. Score 0: Elbow reaches opposite axillary line; 1: Elbow between midline and opposite axillary line; 2: Elbow reaches midline; 3: Elbow will not reach midline.

Head lag: With the baby lying supine, grasp the hands (or the arms if a very small infant) and pull him slowly toward the sitting position. Observe the position of the head in relation to the trunk and grade accordingly. In a small infant the head may initially be supported by one hand. Score 0: Complete lag; 1: Partial head control; 2: Able to maintain head in line with body; 3: Brings head anterior to body.

Ventral suspension: The infant is suspended in the prone position, with examiner's hand under the infant's chest (one hand in a small infant, two in a large infant): Observe the degree of extension of the back and the amount of flexion of the arms and legs. Also note the relation of the head to the trunk. Grade according to diagrams (Fig. 5-7).

If score differs on the two sides, take the mean.

*From Dubowitz, L. M. S., Dubowitz, V., and Goldberg, C.: J. Pediatr. 77:1, 1970.

Table 5-1. Scoring system for external criteria*

External sign	Score†				
	0	**1**	**2**	**3**	**4**
Edema	Obvious edema of hands and feet; pitting over tibia	No obvious edema of hands and feet; pitting over tibia	No edema		
Skin texture	Very thin, gelatinous	Thin and smooth	Smooth; medium thickness; rash or superficial peeling	Slight thickening; superficial cracking and peeling especially of hands and feet	Thick and parchment-like; superficial or deep cracking
Skin color	Dark red	Uniformly pink	Pale pink; variable over body	Pale; only pink over ears, lips, palms, or soles	
Skin opacity (trunk)	Numerous veins and venules clearly seen, especially over abdomen	Veins and tributaries seen	A few large vessels clearly seen over abdomen	A few large vessels seen indistinctly over abdomen	No blood vessels seen
Lanugo (over back)	No lanugo	Abundant; long and thick over whole back	Hair thinning especially over lower back	Small amount of lanugo and bald areas	At least ½ of back devoid of lanugo
Plantar creases	No skin creases	Faint red marks over anterior half of sole	Definite red marks over > anterior ½; indentations over < anterior ⅓	Indentations over > anterior ⅓	Definite deep indentations over > anterior ⅓
Nipple formation	Nipple barely visible; no areola	Nipple well defined; areola smooth and flat, diameter <0.75 cm	Areola stippled, edge not raised, diameter <0.75 cm	Areola stippled, edge raised, diameter >0.75 cm	
Breast size	No breast tissue palpable	Breast tissue on one or both sides, <0.5 cm diameter	Breast tissue both sides; one or both 0.5 to 1.0 cm	Breast tissue both sides; one or both >1 cm	

*From Dubowitz, L. M. S., Dubowitz, V., and Goldberg, C.: J. Pediatr. **77:**1, 1970; modified from Farr, V., et al.: Dev. Med. Child. Neurol. 8:507, 1966.
†If score differs on two sides, take the mean.

Table 5-1. Scoring system for external criteria—cont'd

External sign	Score				
	0	1	2	3	4
Ear form	Pinna flat and shapeless, little or no incurving of edge	Incurving of part of edge of pinna	Partial incurving whole of upper pinna	Well-defined incurving whole of upper pinna	
Ear firmness	Pinna soft, easily folded, no recoil	Pinna soft, easily folded, slow recoil	Cartilage to edge of pinna, but soft in places, ready recoil	Pinna firm, cartilage to edge; instant recoil	
Genitals					
Male	Neither testis in scrotum	At least one testis high in scrotum	At least one testis right down		
Female (with hips ½ abducted)	Labia majora widely separated, labia minora protruding	Labia majora almost cover labia minora	Labia majora completely cover labia minora		

Table 5-2. Dubowitz score/gestational age

Score	Weeks of gestation
0-9	26
10-12	27
13-16	28
17-20	29
21-24	30
25-27	31
28-31	32
32-35	33
36-39	34
40-43	35
44-46	36
47-50	37
51-54	38
55-58	39
59-62	40
63-65	41
66-69	42

signed to each, and Table 5-1 describes external features and their scores. The scores from all the neuromuscular findings and from all the external characteristics compose a maximum total of 70. Gestational age may be read from the corresponding score given in Table 5-2. A score of 50 thus corresponds to 37 gestational weeks, and a score of 20 corresponds to 29 weeks. The gestational age and birth weight may now be plotted on the intrauterine growth chart for the classification of an infant according to growth characteristics and age at birth, as previously described. Proficiency depends on repeated careful performance of this entire procedure. With experience, a nurse can perform it accurately in 5 to 8 minutes.

Having estimated gestational age, the nurse can now plot this information against birth weight on the intrauterine growth chart for assessment of growth as it relates to age.

Several variations and abbreviations of the Dubowitz method have been reported since publication in 1970. In some instances, examination of external signs alone is asserted to be as accurate as the combination of external and neuromuscular findings that are used in the Dubowitz procedure. Thus data from a study of 392 babies in England seem to indicate that observation of four external signs is all that is necessary to provide an accurate assessment. This method assigns scores for various gradations in skin texture, skin color, breast size, and ear firmness. However, difficulties arise in scoring the skin color of Asian and African infants. Furthermore, determination of gestational age of less than 30 weeks is not feasible because the essential observations cannot be scored.

Most recently, a more balanced system (Ballard score) includes six neuromuscular and six external physical signs (Fig. 5-8) in the assessment. This is in contrast to the ten neuromuscular and eleven external signs that compose the Dubowitz method. The most useful items of the Dubowitz meth-

Neuromuscular maturity

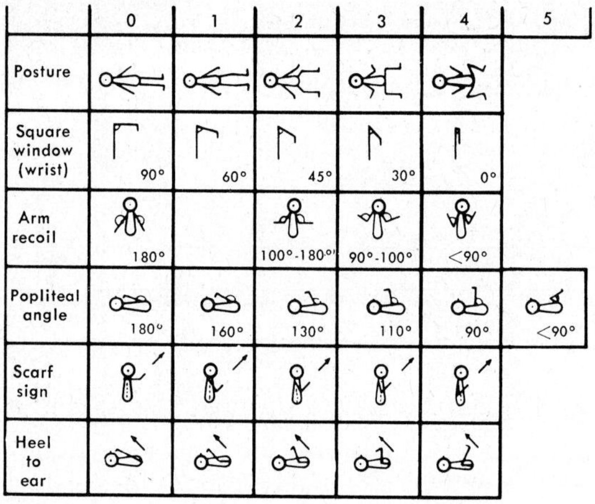

Physical maturity

Skin	Gelatinous red, transparent	Smooth pink, visible veins	Superficial peeling, &/or rash few veins	Cracking pale area rare veins	Parchment deep cracking no vessels	Leathery cracked wrinkled
Lanugo	None	Abundant	Thinning	Bald areas	Mostly bald	
Plantar creases	No crease	Faint red marks	Anterior transverse crease only	Creases ant. 2/3	Creases cover entire sole	
Breast	Barely percept.	Flat areola no bud	Stippled areola 1-2 mm bud	Raised areola 3-4 mm bud	Full areola 5-10 mm bud	
Ear	Pinna flat, stays folded	Sl. curved pinna; soft c slow recoil	Well-curv. pinna; soft but ready recoil	Formed & firm c instant recoil	Thick cartilage ear stiff	
Genitals ♂	Scrotum empty no rugae		Testes descending, few rugae	Testes down good rugae	Testes pendulous deep rugae	
Genitals ♀	Prominent clitoris & labia minora		Majora & minora equally prominent	Majora large minora small	Clitoris & minora completely covered	

Maturity rating

Score	Wks.
5	26
10	28
15	30
20	32
25	34
30	36
35	38
40	40
45	42
50	44

Fig. 5-8. Ballard score (see text). (From Ballard, J. L.: J. Pediatr. **95**:769, 1979.)

od are retained, and these are thought to be valid even in the presence of disease. According to the Ballard score, gestational age is assessable from 26 to 44 weeks. Evaluation can be performed any time up to a postnatal age of 42 hours, but peak reliability is at 30 to 42 hours after birth. In this study, the assessments of both scoring methods (Ballard and Dubowitz) are remarkably close to each other.

Simplification of the Dubowitz examination may be feasible. It is indeed tempting to adapt a shorter, time-saving methodology if a reasonable assurance of accuracy can be shown. A reduction in the number of items would seem to increase the risk of an invalid total score because inaccuracy of a single item then exerts a stronger influence. This is the principal disadvantage of any simplification. In general, the Dubowitz examination has been reliable when properly executed. A variety of abnormal infants have been satisfactorily assessed when compared with estimates of gestational age by maternal dates. These satisfac-

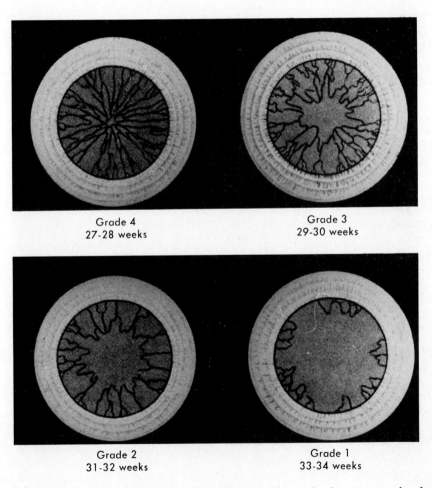

Grade 4
27-28 weeks

Grade 3
29-30 weeks

Grade 2
31-32 weeks

Grade 1
33-34 weeks

Fig. 5-9. Atrophy of fetal vascular network that covers the ocular lens as seen by direct ophthalmoscopy. Disappearance of vascular pattern is correlated with gestational age. (From Hittner, H. M.: J. Pediatr. **91:**455, 1977.)

tory assessments have involved babies who are undergrown or overgrown in utero, ill or well, with or without major neurologic malformations. However, the accuracy of the Dubowitz assessment is not firmly documented for infants below 28 gestational weeks.

An interesting supplementary method for estimating gestational age entails viewing of the cornea with an ordinary (direct) ophthalmoscope. Pupils should be dilated and the ophthalmoscope should be set at +6 to +12 (black numbers), depending on the examiner's needs. The state of the fetal vascular network over the lens can be seen behind the cornea and can be correlated with gestational age. Fig. 5-9 illustrates the four grades of vascular atrophy. At 27 to 28 weeks (Grade 4), the vessels cover the entire surface of the lens (as viewed through the cornea and anterior chamber). At 29 to 30 weeks (Grade 3), the peripheral vessels are less dense, and the central portion of the lens is now cleared of them. At 31 to 32 weeks (Grade 2), peripheral thinning and central clearing of vasculature are more extensive. At 33 to 34 weeks (Grade 1), only a few vessels are visible in the periphery. This examination should be performed during the first 48 hours after birth. The vessels may atrophy and disappear in a few days, even those that were Grade 4 at birth. In babies who are less than 27 weeks, the cornea is cloudy, and visualization of the anterior chamber is thus precluded. After 34 weeks the vascular network has disappeared completely; in some infants, only a few remnant strands are observable.

This superficial ophthalmoscopic examination may be useful in infants who are so severely ill that they cannot be evaluated for several days. The ophthalmoscopic method is obviously not intended to replace the more extensive examinations described in preceding paragraphs.

INTRAUTERINE GROWTH RETARDATION
Terminology

Intrauterine growth retardation is also referred to as dysmaturity, small-for-dates, small for gestational age, pseudoprematurity, and fetal or in-

trauterine malnutrition. We prefer to use the terms *small-for-dates, small for gestational age,* and *intrauterine growth retardation* interchangeably to indicate fetal undergrowth of any etiology. Although the word dysmaturity is used frequently in reference to a small but mature baby, it is not completely accurate; according to its word derivation, it denotes any abnormality of maturity, therefore implying that the baby may be either small or large for his age. The word pseudoprematurity is also unacceptable because it suggests that these small infants appear deceptively premature, which is not the case if they are born at or near term. Fetal, or intrauterine, malnutrition should be reserved for reference to growth retardation caused by a deficient supply of nutrient from the mother to her fetus, thus excluding diminished growth that is caused by intrauterine infections such as rubella or that is associated with other congenital malformations.

Cellular characteristics of growth-retarded infants

Normal cellular growth. Normal cellular growth progresses through three stages that blend into each other. Overall, growth is characterized by the initial production of nuclei by mitosis, followed by the laying down of cytoplasm. Stated differently, nuclei, and therefore DNA, are first produced, and they are responsible for the early growth of any organ. Organ enlargement that results from cell multiplication is called *hyperplasia*. As growth proceeds, each cell enlarges by the addition of cytoplasm. Organ growth caused by cytoplasmic enlargement of existing cells is called *hypertrophy*.

DNA content of any organ can be measured accurately. The amount of DNA in a single nucleus for any given species is uniform. The total number of *cells* in any organ can be calculated by dividing the amount of DNA in a single nucleus into the total DNA determined for that organ. To determine the *average weight per cell*, one need only divide the total weight of the organ by the determined number of cells. The weight/DNA ratio varies from one normal stage of growth to the next, as hyperplasia evolves into hypertrophy. It indicates the amount of cytoplasm relative to DNA for each cell and also varies according to the type of growth retardation.

Data from experiments on rats demonstrate a good correlation between weight/DNA ratios and the normal growth stages. Presumably these same phenomena are applicable to the human growth process. Table 5-3 summarizes the three stages of growth and the role of increments of DNA (new cells) and protein (cytoplasm and cell enlargement) in each.

During the first stage of growth, nuclei proliferate; cytoplasmic mass is minimal, being laid down at approximately the same rate as DNA. During this stage of pure hyperplasia, the weight/DNA ratio is unchanged.

The second stage of growth involves increased production of cytoplasm and decreased proliferation of nuclei (DNA). Existing cells enlarge by addition of cytoplasm, and the rate of cell multiplication declines. Hypertrophy and hyperplasia coexist, but the rate of hypertrophy has increased. Therefore the weight/DNA ratio increases, indicating an increase in cell size.

The third stage of growth involves increasing hypertrophy and even less hyperplasia. Existing cells continue to enlarge, fewer new cells are produced. Weight/DNA ratio now increases further, indicating that cell size is further increased.

In summary, the earliest stages of growth are the result of rapid cell division (mitosis). In the first few weeks of embryonic life, growth occurs entirely by cell division; the most rapid rates occur during the first 25 weeks. After a few weeks of cell division, cellular differentiation is initiated, organs and tissues become recognizable, and each organ is programmed for its unique growth pattern and ultimate contribution to total body weight. Differentiation means cellular enlargement, and as hypertrophy of cells becomes more pervasive, the extent of hyperplasia diminishes. The cells of various organs, on differing schedules, proliferate less as they enlarge more (Fig. 5-7).

Table 5-3. Cellular phases of growth

I   *Hyperplasia* (cell multiplication)
    Increased DNA (nuclei) *maximal*
    Increased protein (cytoplasm) *minimal*
II *Hyperplasia* (cell multiplication)
    Hypertrophy (cell enlargement)
    Increased DNA (nuclei) *moderate*
    Increased protein (cytoplasm) *moderate*
III *Hypertrophy* (cell enlargement)
    Increased protein (cytoplasm) *maximal*
    Increased DNA (nuclei) *minimal*

Differentiation and cellular enlargement are associated with diminished water outside cells and increased water within them. The process that evolves from hyperplasia to hypertrophy and differentiation is a progressive one throughout gestation and after birth as well (Fig. 5-10).

The type of growth impairment suffered by the embryo or the fetus depends on the stage of growth that is disrupted.

Impaired cellular growth. Mention has already been made of two different types of growth retardation, which may occur separately or simultaneously. The hypoplastic type of impairment involves insult to the embryo early in pregnancy, during the initial stage of growth. Because mitosis is impaired, fewer new cells are formed, organs are small, and organ weight is subnormal. The individual cells usually, but not always, have a normal amount of cytoplasm. The initial stage of growth (hyperplasia) is called the *critical period* because it is during this period that susceptibility to congenital malformations and permanent suboptimal growth is greatest. The period of hyperplasia varies in its schedule from one tissue to another. Fig. 5-10 illustrates the varying rates of hyperplasia among four different tissues. Cell multiplication of the brain is shown to virtually cease in infancy, while skeleton and muscle continue their hyperplasia through adolescence. Growth failure that begins later in pregnancy is associated with cellular characteristics that are dif-

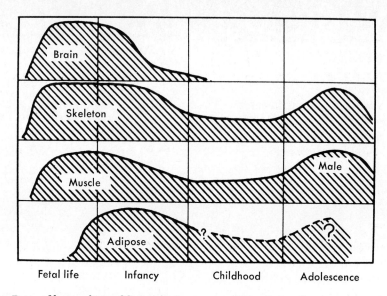

Fig. 5-10. Rates of hyperplasia of four tissues at various ages. New cells cease to appear in the brain during infancy. Note the later hyperplasia of muscle in adolescent males. (From Smith, D. W.: Growth and its disorders, Philadelphia, 1977, W. B. Saunders Co.)

ferent from early disruption. The total number of cells in affected organs is normal or nearly so, but their size is diminished by virtue of reduced amounts of cytoplasm. Abnormally small organ size, in this instance, is thus largely the result of decreased cytoplasmic mass, rather than a diminished number of cells as in hypoplasia. Organ weight/DNA ratios correlate well with these anatomic observations. When the weight of an organ is subnormal only because it contains fewer cells (hypoplasia), the ratio of total organ weight to DNA content is similar to that of normally grown tissue if the number of nuclei and the amount of cytoplasm are diminished approximately to the same extent. On the other hand, if an abnormally small organ contains about the same quantity of nuclei (DNA) as a normally grown one, but the cytoplasmic mass is reduced, the ratio of total organ weight to DNA content is lower than normal. Cytoplasm is decreased, whereas the number of cell nuclei (DNA) is not.

Insult during the first stage of growth (hyper-

plasia) retards the rate of cell division, which results in fewer than normal cells in an organ that is smaller than normal. This type of impairment is not reversible, regardless of attempts to provide optimal nutrition later on. However, if the insult occurs during the hypertrophic stage of growth, individual enlargement of existing cells is impaired. The result is a smaller organ with a normal number of diminutive cells. This impairment is reversible to some extent. With proper nutrition, the cytoplasmic mass may become normal, and the resultant cellular enlargement ultimately imparts normal size to the involved organ.

In animals (rats, monkeys, dogs, pigs), two types of malnutrition have been produced that are correlated with the distribution of organ involvement rather than with their cellular characteristics. Their significance is in the differing effects they exert on the brain. In one type, ligation of placental blood vessels during the latter third of pregnancy produced an asymmetric type of undergrowth. The overall weight of the rats was reduced by 20%; liver weight was reduced by as much as 50%; brain weight was unaffected. Furthermore, liver cells were devoid of glycogen. The ratio of brain weight to liver weight was inordinately large. *This brain-sparing pattern is characteristic of growth retardation that occurs in the third trimester among fetuses of toxemic women.* In them, uteroplacental vascular insufficiency contributes fundamentally to fetal undergrowth. The relationship of a relatively large brain to a small, glycogen-deprived liver is thought to be responsible for the high incidence of hypoglycemia in this type of growth retardation. Glucose demands are greater in the brain than in any other organ; glucose supply is principally from the liver. The demand for glucose by a relatively normal-sized brain on a diminutive liver is probably significant in the pathogenesis of hypoglycemia in babies of toxemic mothers.

A second type of malnutrition was produced in these animals. It entailed maternal protein deprivation throughout pregnancy, rather than interference with uteroplacental blood supply late in pregnancy. The resultant pattern of fetal undergrowth involved all organs to an equal extent. The growth failure was symmetric. Weight and DNA content were both reduced. The liver was not affected any more than any other organ and the brain was not spared.

Two types of fetal undergrowth were thus demonstrated in these animals; the one associated with an insult only during the last third of pregnancy was asymmetric, sparing the brain but profoundly affecting the liver and the rest of the body. The other, associated with insult throughout gestation, was symmetric, affecting all organs similarly, including the brain.

The available data demonstrate heterogeneity in the types of fetal undergrowth. These varying types of undergrowth may be responsible for the different outcomes that have been noted in human infants whose growth was retarded in utero. There seem to be two broad categories of intrauterine growth retardation: intrinsic and extrinsic. The intrinsic variety involves reduction of

growth caused by factors that are operative within the fetus itself, such as severe chromosomal or genetic disorders, intrauterine infection caused by rubella virus or cytomegalovirus, or normal hereditary small stature. The extrinsic variety entails diminution of maternal support to a fetus that otherwise would have been normal. Clinically, diminished maternal support is seen in uteroplacental vascular insufficiency, including toxemia, essential hypertension, severe far-advanced diabetes mellitus, chronic renal disease, multiple pregnancy, recurrent bleeding late in pregnancy from a normally implanted placenta, and probably chronic, severe maternal malnutrition throughout gestation.

Data relating malnutrition to general body growth have stimulated an intense interest in the effects of this phenomenon on growth of the brain. Although the issue is far from resolved, evidence from observations in animals, as described previously, indicates that malnutrition during the period of most rapid brain growth is associated with permanent reduction in the total number of cells. In humans this critical period probably begins at about 15 gestational weeks. Estimates of the time of cessation of hyperplasia vary from 8 to 15 months after term. If this critical period does exist in humans, continuous malnutrition from prenatal into postnatal life may reduce cellular quantity irrevocably and thus permanently impair intellectual capacity. Suggestive evidence in support of this assumption was noted in a severely deprived population of low birth weight infants who died of undernutrition during the first few months of life. There was a 60% reduction in the expected number of brain cells. Among infants who were not of low birth weight, but whose lethal malnutrition was apparently confined to the postnatal period, there was only a 15% to 20% reduction in the number of brain cells. In the first group of infants, the combined effects of prenatal and postnatal deprivation may have resulted in a greater reduction of brain cells than in the second group, which suffered only from postnatal malnutrition. That malnutrition sustained in utero and into early infancy can permanently affect brain structure has indeed been well documented in animals. In humans the similarities are suggestive. The public health and socioeconomic implications of these data are awesome to contemplate if one accepts the hypothesis that malnutrition is a pervasive cause of subnormal mentality on the one hand and that it is socially remediable on the other.

Factors associated with intrauterine growth retardation

Intrauterine growth is associated with a variety of disorders in the mother, fetus, and placenta. Most of these known factors are:

I. Maternal factors
  A. Low socioeconomic status
  B. Toxemia
  C. Hypertensive cardiovascular disease
  D. Chronic renal disease
  E. Diabetes (advanced)
  F. Malnutrition
  G. Cigarette smoking
  H. Heroin addiction
  I. Alcohol
  J. High-altitude residence
II. Fetal factors
  A. Multiple gestation
  B. Congenital malformation
  C. Chromosomal abnormality
  D. Chronic intrauterine infection
    1. Rubella
    2. Cytomegalovirus
III. Placental factors
  A. "Placental insufficiency"
  B. Vascular anastomoses (twin to twin)
  C. Single umbilical artery
  D. Abnormal cord insertion
  E. Separation
  F. Massive infarction
  G. ? Vascular anomalies and tumors
  H. ? Site of implantation
  I. Avascular chorionic villi

Maternal factors

Low socioeconomic status. Infant losses, like low birth weight itself, are profoundly influenced by maternal social class, parity, age, and, in par-

ticular, maternal height. These factors are interrelated and additive when statistical analysis is undertaken. At the happy end of the spectrum is the well-nourished white woman in her twenties, married to a business or a professional man, who is having her second baby. She is more likely than anyone else to have a well-grown, normal infant who weathers labor, delivery, and the immediate neonatal period with no difficulty. At the unhappiest extreme of the spectrum is a malnourished, short, black, adolescent mother who is unmarried, or perhaps a somewhat older woman who is a grand multipara (more than five previous pregnancies) married to an unskilled, often unemployed laborer. Women from these and similar backgrounds are more likely than anyone else to have low birth weight infants who cannot weather the perinatal experience alive or unscathed.

The association of small stature and poor fetal outcome is undoubtedly an indirect one. Aside from genetically determined short stature in any social class, the repeatedly observed association between height and social class suggests that short stature is in part the result of poor nutrition during the growth period in childhood. It thus follows that short stature merely signifies the many unfavorable circumstances that characterize poverty, particularly malnutrition during pregnancy and in the prepregnancy years. Unfavorable socioeconomic status is associated with a heightened incidence of several factors that exert adverse influences on fetal outcome. These biologic fallouts of adverse social status, while high in incidence among the poor, would exert their adverse effects on individuals of any social class. A higher incidence of pregnancy in young teenagers and in women over age 35 has been observed in low economic groups, but this higher incidence obviously is not unique to them. Drug abuse, suboptimal weight gain during pregnancy, cigarette smoking, and lack of prenatal care are more frequent among poor women; and their relationship to abnormal fetal outcome is well established.

Toxemia. Toxemia of pregnancy (pregnancy-induced hypertension) is a maternal disorder that is frequently cited as a cause of fetal growth retardation. Its clinical attributes include hypertension, proteinuria, and edema. The cause of toxemia and the mechanisms by which the fetus is affected are unknown. There is agreement, however, that toxemia is a generalized vascular disorder in which diminution of uterine and placental blood flow impairs the function of the latter organ. Some evidence suggests that maternal malnutrition predisposes to toxemia. Among infants of toxemic mothers, mortality is increased. The principal abnormality in most babies who die is undergrowth for gestational age. Otherwise, a distinctive pattern of morphologic abnormalities has not been identified. Growth retardation is presumably a function of fetal malnutrition in which cellular abnormalities are characterized by diminished cytoplasmic mass in most organs, particularly the liver and adrenals. The brain is usually less affected than are other organs. The gross and microscopic appearance of tissues in these infants closely resembles that of infants who died during the first year of life from postnatally acquired malnutrition.

Hypertension and chronic renal disease. Hypertension and chronic renal disease exert influences on fetal growth that are similar to those of toxemia.

Diabetes (advanced). Most diabetic women (class A or B; see classification in Chapter 11) deliver large-for-dates babies who may nevertheless be born prematurely. However, advanced maternal diabetes involves generalized vascular damage that impairs normal placental blood flow. The woman with advanced (early onset) diabetes is more likely to give birth to a small-for-dates infant rather than a large one, particularly if the diabetes has significantly affected her kidneys.

Malnutrition. The state of maternal nutrition and the course of fetal growth are inextricably entwined. Maternal weight before pregnancy and weight gain during pregnancy exert independent and combined influences on fetal growth. Mothers who are considerably underweight and malnourished are likely to give birth to small babies.

In women who are not obese, weight gain during pregnancy is an important determinant of fetal weight. A gestational weight gain of 25 lb is generally recommended for optimal outcomes. However, in obese women the magnitude of weight gain during pregnancy is not as influential on fetal outcome; they rarely give birth to undergrown infants. Apparently the store of maternal nutrients provides adequate nutrition to the fetus even if maternal weight gain during pregnancy is suboptimal. Except for severely malnourished mothers, nutritional status probably has little effect on growth during the first trimester when demands of the miniscule embryo are easily met. Nutritional demands increase as the fetus enlarges; adequate maternal nutritional status is an absolute requirement for continued normal fetal growth. There is indeed evidence that severe maternal malnutrition affects embryonic growth and differentiation. Affected infants are symmetrically undergrown at birth, and a higher incidence of congenital malformations has been observed.

Two tragic episodes of famine in Europe during World War II, in Holland and in Leningrad, are frequently cited for data that indicate a direct cause and effect relationship between maternal nutrition and fetal outcome. In Holland, maternal malnutrition around the time of conception and during early pregnancy was associated with increased perinatal mortality; the effect of famine during the latter part of pregnancy was not nearly as pronounced. Severely restricted maternal food intake at time of conception was also a major cause of stillbirth and neonatal death during the first postnatal week. The most severe instances of low birth weight occurred when malnutrition existed about the time of conception. It was also noted that the incidence of central nervous system malformations was significantly increased among babies who were conceived during the famine. These associations between famine and fetal outcome gradually disappeared after availability of food was restored. The mean birth weight of infants conceived and born during the famine period was 200 g less than the mean that preceded the food shortage, a difference that often distinguishes developed and underdeveloped populations. A similar famine occurred in Leningrad at about the same time during World War II. The mean birth weight of infants born from that experience had diminished by 500 g.

A positive and healthy effect on fetal outcome has been noted in circumstances of improved nutrition. In Japan, over a period of 20 years following World War II, when widespread severe poverty was replaced by relative affluence, there was an increase of approximately 10% in mean birth weight. The studies from Holland, Leningrad, and Japan indicate the significance of maternal nutrition on fetal growth. The data also relate fetal outcomes to changes in economic conditions, for both better and worse.

That longstanding maternal malnutrition is a dominant cause of fetal undergrowth in low socioeconomic populations has been apparent for some time. Animal experiments indicate a significant role of maternal malnutrition in faulty fetal growth. Maternal undernutrition impairs cellular growth in the human placenta. These placentas are smaller than those of normally nourished women. The growth-limiting effect on the placenta is most profound in the chorionic villi. These anatomic subnormalities apparently exert an adverse effect on function by reducing the total capacity of the placenta to transfer nutrient material to a growing fetus. Epidemiologic data also indicate that the rate of maternal weight gain during pregnancy is related to weight and length at birth. In nutritionally deprived populations, augmented food intake during pregnancy is associated with a significant increase in mean birth weight. The beneficial effects of enhanced food intake during gestation are related to calories, not specifically to a copious quantity of protein. The addition of at least 20,000 consumed calories during gestation begins to increase birth weight significantly.

Cigarette smoking. Among moderate smokers, the incidence of small-for-dates babies is twice that of nonsmokers; among heavy consumers it is three times as great. The end result is related to the number of cigarettes smoked and the duration of the insult. When more than 10 and 15 cigarettes are consumed daily, mean birth weight reductions of 170 g and 300 g, respectively, can be anticipated. Birth weight and body length are reduced. At 7 years of age, children of smoking gravidas are shorter than controls and have a higher incidence of educational retardation, regardless of social class, maternal age, or parity. The statistical association of maternal smoking and the incidence of intrauterine growth is among the most direct and unequivocal of all the maternal factors thus far scrutinized. There is evidence that fetal undergrowth does not occur if the mother ceases smoking at the onset of pregnancy. There is also evidence that consumption of as few as five cigarettes a day may impair fetal growth. The mechanism by which smoking impairs fetal growth has not been unequivocally demonstrated, although several have been suggested. The blood level of carbon monoxide is elevated in affected infants at birth, and therefore carboxyhemoglobin concentration is higher than normal because carbon monoxide has a high affinity for hemoglobin. Less hemoglobin is available for oxygen transport; it is thus possible that affected fetuses are chronically hypoxic. This could account for an impaired rate of intrauterine growth. It has also been suggested that placental vasospasm reduces blood flow, thereby interfering with the transmission of nutrients. The transplacental passage of toxic products of cigarettes has also been proposed as an important consideration. Some authors have concluded that suppression of the smoking mother's appetite exerts the most significant negative influence on fetal growth.

Drug addiction. In some urban hospitals the incidence of addicted babies from maternal addiction is as high as one in fifty deliveries. The threats to survival of the fetus and neonate are multiple, particularly when one considers the daily life most addicts must resort to if their drug need is to be met. Generally, about half the babies born of maternal addicts are low birth weight infants; 40%

of these infants are small for gestational age, and 60% are appropriately grown premature infants. Undergrown offspring of addicted mothers are small by virtue of reduced numbers of organ cells, indicating early growth impairment of the hypoplastic variety. The effect of heroin and morphine is probably independent of the malnutrition that is so frequent among addicts. Intrauterine growth deficiency has been observed among ex-addicts and has been demonstrated in animal experiments. The effect of narcotics therefore seems to persist beyond the period of addiction. The incidence of fetal undergrowth among heroin addicts has been shown to be reduced somewhat by the administration of methadone instead.

Alcohol. Maternal alcohol consumption causes acute effects in the infant immediately after birth; it also causes the chronic effects of fetal undergrowth and malformations (fetal alcohol syndrome). *Acute toxicity* consists of withdrawal symptoms (agitation, hyperactivity, tremors, seizures) up to 72 hours in duration, followed by lethargy for 24 to 48 hours. Subsequently the infant is normal. Alcohol is often detected in the infant's breath soon after birth. Acute symptoms occur in the infant because alcohol freely crosses the placenta. Chronic maternal alcoholism is associated with the *fetal alcohol syndrome*. In addition to fetal wastage, maternal alcoholism causes severe growth deficiency and a constellation of characteristic structural defects. These consist of microcephaly, short palpebral fissures and microphthalmia, epicanthal folds, micrognathia, malformed and immobile joints, dislocation of the hips, cardiac malformations, and malformation of the brain. Severe or mild mental retardation occurs in almost half the infants. Less profound effects have been reported in babies who are apparently only growth retarded. Perinatal mortality is approximately 20%.

Fetal factors

Multiple gestation. Most twins have a subnormal rate of growth late in gestation. This pattern is not unlike the decelerated growth rate in normal singletons, which begins at 36 to 39 weeks and is sustained for several days after birth. This effect is more pronounced in twins, and it begins earlier, at approximately 30 weeks. In either case the slowed rate of growth has been attributed to progressive diminution in the effective transfer of nutrient substances across the placenta, perhaps as a function of placental aging. Tissue abnormalities in twins seem to correlate with the prevalent impression that nutritional deficiency late in pregnancy is responsible for their small size. Subnormal organ weights are primarily a function of diminished cytoplasmic mass. The slowed growth rate of twins has also been ascribed to a lack of intrauterine space for both fetuses. The resultant small placentas can only support small fetuses. In the instance of discordant twins (large discrepancy in birth weight and other body measurements), the smaller twin is nurtured by the smaller placenta. Ordinarily, fetal growth retardation is seen in twins if they are delivered after 30 weeks because, until then, their intrauterine growth parallels that of singletons.

Congenital malformations and chromosomal abnormalities. Anencephalic babies, infants with congenital heart disease, and infants with chromosomal abnormalities are small-for-dates as a result of hypoplasia. This variety of growth retardation originates early in pregnancy, when cell multiplication (hyperplasia) is the predominant factor in the growth process. Mitotic activity is impaired, and the number of cells is reduced. The incidence of a variety of major congenital anomalies is increased severalfold in small-for-dates infants compared with those who are appropriately grown for their age.

Chronic intrauterine infections. Impairment of growth is virtually a hallmark of fetal infections that begin early in pregnancy, particularly during the first trimester. Rubella is the best known example of this phenomenon; infections resulting from cytomegalovirus are similarly implicated. Hypoplastic growth retardation is identical to that described for congenital malformations. The details of these and other infections are discussed in Chapter 13.

Placental factors

General considerations. A great deal of mystery surrounds the role of placental pathology as an original cause of fetal undergrowth. When a placental lesion is identified, the question arises whether it is a manifestation of intrauterine growth retardation or whether it is the original source of fetal difficulty. Vascular anomalies, tumors, infarctions, and abnormal implantation sites have all been observed in association with isolated instances of fetal malnutrition, but apparently they are not responsible for a significant number of growth-retarded babies.

Placental insufficiency. Placental insufficiency is a conceptual term that is frequently invoked to explain the occurrence of fetal malnutrition. It implies impaired exchange between mother and fetus, particularly suboptimal delivery of nutrient material and hormones to the fetus. A number of well-defined pathologic lesions in the placenta seem to be associated with placental insufficiency, but these lesions occur in only a few cases. They include extensive fibrosis, occlusion of fetal vessels in the villi, large hemangiomas, and early separation. Clinical entities such as advanced diabetes and toxemia are apparently associated with insufficiency of placental function. However, in most instances, dysfunction is not associated with morphologic abnormalities, and often there are no apparent maternal disorders. In any case, retarded fetal growth seems to be the end result of placental insufficiency, which is a concept that requires better definition than is presently available.

Intrauterine parabiotic syndrome (twin transfusion). The intrauterine parabiotic syndrome occurs in a small percentage of identical twins. It is a direct result of placental arteriovenous anastomoses that connect the circulations of both fetuses. Blood is transferred from artery to vein (twin to twin) when there is a connection between the arteries of one fetus and veins of the other. The discrepancy in blood volume between the two infants at birth may or may not be associated with weight differences in other body organs, depending on the duration and extent of fetofetal blood transfer. At birth the twin who received the blood (the "venous" twin) is intensely red because of polycythemia, whereas the donor twin (the "arterial" twin) is pale as a consequence of anemia. Increased blood volume in the polycythemic twin may cause congestive heart failure as a result of cardiac overload, and hyperbilirubinemia often occurs because there are more red cells available for breakdown (Chapter 10). The anemic twin may be in shock at birth if blood loss to his sibling was acute. A dramatic discrepancy in birth weight is usually but not always noted. Weight of the recipient twin may exceed that of the donor by as much as 50%, but in many instances a difference in size is less obvious. Polyhydramnios is often present in the recipient baby, whereas oligohydramnios is observed in the donor. The most important initial observation that the nurse can make is the difference in color between the twins. This is sometimes an urgent situation that requires immediate withdrawal of blood from the overloaded baby and a transfusion for shock in the anemic one.

Single umbilical artery. Presence of only one umbilical artery is often associated with a variety of major congenital anomalies, most commonly in the urinary tract. A number of investigators have reported single umbilical artery in 0.2% to 2% of all births. Among such infants, 20% to 65% have congenital anomalies. In the delivery room or in the nursery, the nurse should inspect the cut surface of the umbilical cord to ascertain the presence of two arteries and one vein. Observation of a single artery may lead to the early identification of major congenital malformations.

PHYSICAL FINDINGS OF INTRAUTERINE GROWTH RETARDATION

Most growth-retarded infants simply appear diminutive like AGA premature infants. However, extreme instances of impaired growth are associated with some characteristic physical findings. On first inspection of many small-for-dates infants, several obvious physical characteristics immediately suggest the presence of impaired intrauterine growth. One is struck by the seemingly large head, but head circumference is actually normal or nearly so; it is the chest and abdominal circumferences that are reduced. The head merely appears large for the body. Apparently the brain was spared or less affected by the intrauterine insult, which probably had its inception relatively late in pregnancy. Since the ratio of brain mass to liver mass is large, hypoglycemia is likely to be present in such infants. It was largely the hypertrophic (third) stage of growth that was impaired; one would expect a normal number of cells (nuclei) and diminished cytoplasm in most organs.

The weight/DNA ratio would be smaller than normal. Diminution of subcutaneous fat and loose, dry skin are prominent (Fig. 5-11). Even though the skin appears pale, some of these babies are polycythemic; their venous hematocrit may be greater than 65 vol %. In the extreme, muscle mass over the buttocks, thighs, and cheeks is also wanting. Since body length is not as diminished as subcutaneous fat, these infants often appear thin and long.

Fraternal twins are shown in Fig. 5-12; the longer is minimally undergrown, and the smaller is poorly grown. The paucity of subcutaneous fat in the small baby imparts a relatively long and thin

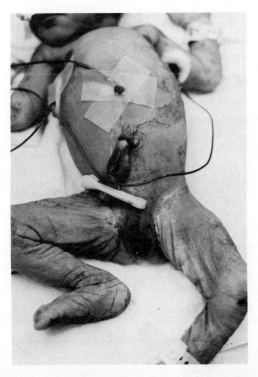

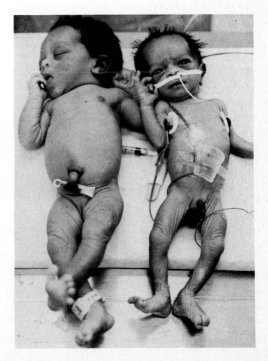

Fig. 5-11. Severe intrauterine malnutrition in a postterm baby. Diminished subcutaneous fat is in dramatic evidence at lower extremities. Cord is stained, thin, and dull. Body is thin and appears long, although length was normal.

Fig. 5-12. Fraternal twins. The smaller infant is typically malnourished. Thin body gives a large appearance to head, longitudinal skin creases in thighs are characteristic of diminished subcutaneous fat, and hair is sparse. Alert appearance is in contrast to sleepy sibling; the wide-eyed look indicates chronic intrauterine hypoxia.

appearance, whereas the head gives the illusion of being large. Longitudinal skin creases in the thighs indicate severe subcutaneous fat depletion, in contrast to the horizontal thigh creases of the larger baby, whose nutritional state is far better. Note the sparse hair of the small twin and the normal hair in the large one. The smaller baby is wide-eyed, presumably as a result of chronic hypoxia in utero. He appears alert compared with his sleepy sibling. The abdomen is sunken (scaphoid), rather than rounded as in the better-nourished baby. At birth the umbilical cord is thin, slightly yellow, dull, and dry in contrast to the normal cord, which is rotund, gray, glistening, and moist. Because all cords wither progressively after birth, their condition after 24 hours of age is of little diagnostic significance. The cords of small-for-dates babies wither more rapidly. Scalp hair is typically sparse; heavy hair growth is exceptional in growth-retarded babies, except in those who are postmature (p. 147). Skull sutures are frequently wide as a result of impaired bone growth. The anterior fontanelle, although large, is soft or sunken, thereby ruling out increased intracranial pressure as a cause of the widened sutures. Ossification centers at the distal femur and proximal tibia are frequently absent in term babies who are undergrown. Most of these infants are more active than expected for their low weight. The vigor of their cry may be particularly impressive. Often, an alert, wide-eyed facial expression is combined with repetitive tongue thrusts that simulate a sucking motion. The apparent vigor is really irritative hyperactivity; the tongue thrusts are probably convulsive equivalents. The overall impression of vigor and well-being is misguided, for these are signs of chronic marginal hypoxia in utero. Many of these babies convulse 6 to 18 hours later, particularly those whose anterior fontanelle is firm as a result of cerebral edema from intrauterine hypoxia. On the other hand, when perinatal asphyxia is severe, the baby is depressed, appearing flaccid and lethargic. Hypoglycemia produces similar symptoms.

Another type of growth retardation is seen in small-for-dates infants whose appearance is different from that just described. These babies, whose insult probably began early and was sustained throughout gestation, do not appear wasted. They are diminutive, but body members are of proportionate size. The head does not appear large for the trunk. The skin is not redundant, but it is thicker (the subcutaneous vascular pattern is obscure or absent) than expected for infants of the same size who are appropriately grown for their gestational age. They are generally vigorous and less likely to be hypoglycemic or polycythemic. These are hypoplastic babies in whom major malformations are present or in whom an early intrauterine infection occurred (rubella or cytomegalic inclusion disease). Their weight/DNA ratio is probably normal, although absolute weight is subnormal.

Table 5-4. Clinical differences of hypoplastic and hypotrophic intrauterine growth retardation

Hypoplastic	Hypotrophic
Universal, proportionate diminution in size and weight; percentiles of head, length, and weight are similar	Selective, disproportionate diminution in size and weight; percentiles of head and length normal, for weight below tenth percentile
Subcutaneous fat appropriate for size; skin taut	Subcutaneous fat diminished for size; skin redundant
Congenital malformation frequent	Congenital malformation infrequent
Intrauterine, nonbacterial infection frequent	Intrauterine, nonbacterial infection rare
Hematocrit usually normal	Hematocrit often elevated
Hypoglycemia, hypoproteinemia uncommon	Hypoglycemia, hypoproteinemia common

Two general types of fetal undergrowth are thus identifiable by body measurement and by reference to intrauterine growth curves (Table 5-4). In one type, the most common one, the insult seems to begin during the last trimester. These babies have a head circumference and body length within the normal percentiles, generally between the twenty-fifth and fiftieth, but their body weight is below the tenth percentile. *These infants are hypotrophic.* Associated maternal factors most frequently include toxemia, chronic hypertension, and chronic renal disease. The second type probably begins early in pregnancy. It is characterized by equally distributed reduction in head circumference, body length, and weight. All these measurements fall below the tenth percentile. *These infants are hypoplastic.* Associated factors include intrauterine virus infection, chromosomal disorders, major congenital malformations, genetically small but otherwise well infants, and probably maternal malnutrition.

PREDISPOSITION TO NEONATAL ILLNESS IN SMALL FOR GESTATIONAL AGE BABIES

Thus far this chapter has been concerned with the fundamental characteristics, classification, and causes of fetal growth retardation. The diagnosis and treatment of certain neonatal illnesses are greatly facilitated by early identification of abnormal growth status. Clinical application of the concepts that have been discussed should reduce neonatal morbidity and mortality. The incidence of undergrowth in premature infants is not known. The illnesses to which SGA infants are vulnerable are discussed in the following paragraphs.

Perinatal asphyxia. Growth-retarded fetuses are often chronically hypoxic for variable periods prior to the onset of labor. Whereas healthy fetuses can withstand the asphyxia of normal birth and are well equipped to compensate for it after delivery, those who are chronically distressed can ill afford the insult; many are undergrown as a result of placental dysfunction. They are thus severely disturbed by normal labor, and at birth recovery is difficult or impossible without proper therapy. Apgar scores at 1 and 5 minutes reflect their depressed state. Hypoxia and acidosis depress brain function and impair myocardial effectiveness. Inadequate cardiac output inexorably accentuates the biochemical abnormalities because perfusion and tissue oxygen deprivation worsen. Even if optimal resuscitative procedure is activated, the damage from asphyxia is sometimes irreversible or only partially remediable. The aftermaths of asphyxia are discussed on p. 59. Appropriate management of these infants in the delivery room is often crucial to their survival. The details of resuscitation at birth are described in Chapter 3. Antepartum evaluation predicts the inability of the fetus to withstand labor. Later, fetal heart monitoring during labor demonstrates the presence of stress. Even if this information is not available, identification of high-risk historic factors are a valuable aid in identifying these infants in advance of their birth. From the maternal history the neonatal nurse can often anticipate the arrival of babies at risk even before the onset of labor. The most common antecedent conditions are toxemia, cigarette smoking, low socioeconomic status, multiple gestation, previously diagnosed infections during pregnancy (such as rubella), and advanced diabetes.

Meconium aspiration. Aspiration of meconium may occur in utero before the onset of labor or during the birth process (see Chapter 8). Small-for-dates infants are more likely to be affected than others because intrauterine hypoxia occurs so frequently among them. The aspiration of meconium is apparently mediated by the fetal response to hypoxia—the release of meconium into amniotic fluid by increased intestinal peristalsis and reflex relaxation of the anal sphincter plus reflex gasping movements that suck the released meconium particles into the bronchial tree. Much of the material in the respiratory tract is aspirated more deeply into terminal bronchioles and alveoli after birth. Respiratory distress thus occurs at birth, and a normal rapid recovery from intrauterine asphyxia is precluded. The extrauterine asphyxial state should be viewed as a continuation of events that have transpired in utero. The meconium aspiration syndrome can be clearly distinguished from hyaline membrane disease by the distinctive radiologic appearance of the lungs in each of these disorders. Diagnosis is also aided by accurate estimation of gestational age; hyaline membrane disease is unlikely to occur in term infants. The prognosis for the baby with syndromes due to aspiration or fluid retention is generally better than for the infant with hyaline membrane disease. These disorders and their complications are discussed in Chapter 8.

Hypoglycemia. The SGA baby is predisposed to hypoglycemia for several reasons. Because intrauterine nutrition is suboptimal, hepatic glycogen stores are scanty and are depleted soon after birth. Glycogen content of hepatic tissue has been shown to be lower in SGA infants than in AGA infants of similar gestational age. The malnourished SGA infant is handicapped by the relationship between an abnormally small liver and a brain of near normal size. Less hepatic glycogen is available per gram of brain tissue, which is the body's largest consumer of glucose.

Vulnerability to hypoglycemia is enhanced by virtue of scanty fat deposits, both subcutaneous and deep. Fatty acids and ketone bodies have their origins in fat deposits which, when scanty, cannot adequately provide the fuels that are alternatives to glucose. Some SGA infants are incapable of a normal level of gluconeogenesis, a process that generates glucose from nonglycogen sources such as fatty acids and proteins. SGA infants do not have adequate supplies of the enzymes that are required to activate gluconeogenesis. The enzymatic deficiency plus a limited supply of fatty acids and protein, which are the substrates of gluconeogenesis, deprive the malnourished neonate of another significant source of glucose. A metabolic energy crunch is thus brought about by meager sources of glucose, and by an increased metabolic rate that requires greater amounts of it. The metabolic hazard is increased by a high incidence of hypoxia, which

depletes already meager glycogen stores. In these metabolic circumstances, hypoglycemia is frequent among SGA babies, whether born at term or before. The incidence may be as high as 40% among the most severely underweight and wasted infants. Babies of toxemic mothers and the smaller of twins are especially at risk when birth weight is below 2000 g. Untreated symptomatic neonates with hypoglycemia are more likely to have neurologic abnormalities and lower mean IQ scores than normal contemporaries. Because of the abnormal sequelae, as well as an endangered survival during the early neonatal period, hypoglycemia must be identified early and treated promptly. SGA infants should be monitored periodically for glucose levels during the first 3 or 4 days of life, and as frequently thereafter as indicated. Most hypoglycemic infants are asymptomatic. The long-term significance of asymptomatic hypoglycemia is unknown. Chemical screening of vulnerable babies is thus essential. Treatment is based on glucose levels, the presence or absence of symptoms notwithstanding.

Hypoglycemia is diagnosed by abnormally low concentrations of plasma glucose in two consecutive samples. During the first 72 hours after birth, infants who are 2500 g or more are considered hypoglycemic when glucose levels are below 35 mg/dl; levels below 45 mg/dl are abnormal thereafter. For infants less than 2500 g at birth, glucose concentrations below 25 mg/dl during the first 72 hours are hypoglycemic; thereafter, levels below 45 mg/dl are abnormal.

Most SGA infants become hypoglycemic at 12 to 24 hours of age, but we have encountered it earlier in severely undernourished premature infants. Although a central laboratory can perform plasma glucose determinations, nurses must screen frequently with Dextrostix. *Optimal management requires that they do so according to their own judgment without physicians' orders.* The details of hypoglycemic syndromes—their pathogenesis, symptoms, and treatment—are discussed in Chapter 11.

Heat loss. SGA infants are ill equipped to conserve body heat because of their disproportionately large surface area and their paucity of subcutaneous fat deposits. However, SGA term infants are more capable of responding to cold stress with increased heat production, compared to equally weighted AGA preterm infants. Brown fat deposits may not be significantly diminished by intrauterine malnutrition. The frequency of asphyxia diminishes the capacity of SGA babies for thermogenesis when cold stressed. Thermogenesis is also depressed during hypoglycemic episodes.

Polycythemia-hyperviscosity. Asphyxiated SGA infants, particularly those who are chronically stressed in utero, are often polycythemic; their blood is hyperviscous. A *venous hematocrit* that exceeds 65% constitutes polycythemia; at this level the viscosity of blood increases significantly. The hematocrit of capillary blood may be used only as a screening device; if it exceeds 70%, a venous hematocrit is indicated.

When blood is hyperviscous, an intrinsic increase in resistance to flow is generated, and "sluggish" movement of blood is the result. A broad spectrum of clinical signs have been attributed to hyperviscosity, but the significance of intrauterine asphyxia is an important consideration. Respiratory distress is common, consisting of tachypnea, retractions, and grunting. These are associated with diminished lung compliance, and they may indeed be attributable to pulmonary hyperperfusion by hyperviscous blood. The occurrence of persistent fetal circulation (PFC syndrome), in which intrauterine pulmonary vasospasm persists after birth, may be caused primarily by perinatal asphyxia. Enlargement of the heart and cardiac failure are likely to be caused by perinatal asphyxia, and perhaps may be exaggerated by polycythemia-hyperviscosity of blood. Central nervous system signs include hypertonia, diminished spontaneous activity, hypotonia, and seizures. These central nervous system abnormalities are also likely to be the result of intrauterine hypoxia. That perinatal asphyxia is the significant cause of brain dysfunction in polycythemic babies is suggested by persistence of abnormalities despite appropriate measures that reduce the hematocrit soon after birth. Hyperbilirubinemia is the result of lysis of excessive erythrocytes. Hypoglycemia is also frequently identified in polycythemic babies. Isolated reports have described pleural effusion, edema of the scrotum, and priapism. Polycythemic SGA infants have an increased risk of necrotizing enterocolitis, presumably because of sludged microcirculation in the intestinal wall. Polycythemia-hyperviscosity is discussed in more detail in Chapter 9.

OUTCOME OF SMALL FOR GESTATIONAL AGE INFANTS

Neonatal mortality is a crude but critical measure of risk imposed by intrauterine growth retardation. The consequences to central nervous system function later in childhood are equally sensitive.

Neonatal mortality. Neonatal mortality for any large population is a function of both birth weight and gestational age. At any given birth weight, mortality increases as gestational age diminishes; at any given gestational age, mortality increases as birth weight diminishes. In general, birth weight probably has a stronger influence on survival. Mortality is lowest in babies who are 3000 to 4000 g at birth. Mortality increases as weights decline from 3000 g to 500 g; it is augmented as weight increases beyond 4000 g.

The differing rates of mortality and their relation to birth weight and gestational age are shown in Table 5-5 and Fig. 5-13. The relationship is clearly demonstrated in Table 5-5 according to five general categories: infants over 2500 g who are above and below 37 gestational weeks, respectively; infants between 1500 and 2500 g who are similarly divided according to gestational age; and a fifth category that includes infants under 1500 g regardless of their age at birth. These groups and the percentage of neonatal mortality for each are from records of single live births in

Table 5-5. Relationship of percentage of neonatal mortality to birth weight and gestational age*

Group	Weight (grams)	Gestational age (weeks)	Weight for age	Percentage of mortality	Increase over group I
I	Over 2500	37 or over	Appropriate term	0.5	—
II	Over 2500	Less than 37	LGA, preterm	1.4	×2.8
II	1501 to 2500	37 or over	SGA, term	3.2	×6.4
IV	1501 to 2500	Less than 37	Appropriate, preterm	10.5	×21.0
V	1500 or less	All	Preterm	70.7	×141.0

*Modified from Yerushalmy, J.: J. Pediatr. **71**:164, 1967.

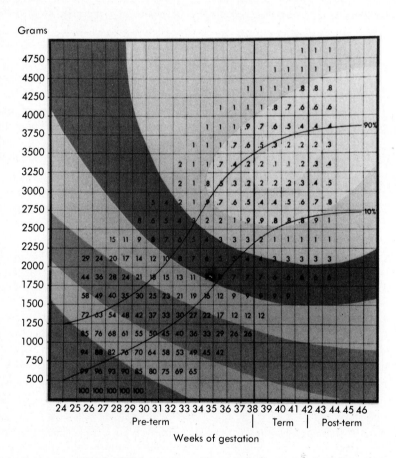

Fig. 5-13. See text, p. 141 for full description. (From Lubchenco, L.: J. Pediatr. **81**:814, 1972.)

New York City over a period of 3 years. The increased risks are indicated in the last column as a multiple of the mortality percentage in group I, which is the lowest-risk category. The column entitled "weight for age" characterizes the majority of infants in each group. Most growth-retarded infants are in group III. In comparison to the appropriately grown term infants in group I, neonatal mortality is increased sevenfold. Additional perspective is gained by comparing the mortality of SGA term babies in group III to premature infants in group IV. Although the outlook for undergrown infants is considerably worse than for those who are normal and at term, it is not as grim as in premature infants of group IV. The gravest prognosis prevails among group V babies who weigh less than 1500 g, over 90% of whom are preterm. Their mortality rate is 141 times greater than that of normal term infants in group I. Little is known about the babies in group II who are large for gestational age, but increased neonatal mortality rates have been noted by a number of investigators. Infants of diabetic mothers, who are at comparatively great risk, usually fall into this category, but they account for only a minority of the babies in group II.

Fig. 5-13 presents a more detailed categorization of mortality by birth weight and gestational age. The statistics are representative of an experience in Denver, and these are superimposed on the Colorado growth curves. Several interesting trends are revealed in the figures on the graph. *Above 36 gestational weeks*, at all birth weights, mortality rates are high among infants below the 10th percentile; they become lower between the 10th and 90th percentiles; and increase again above the 90th percentile. *Below 36 gestational weeks* the pattern differs. Rather than an increase in mortality, a decline occurs above the 90th percentile. The trend becomes more distinct as gestational age diminishes. According to these Colorado growth curves, therefore, increased weight lessens mortality in premature infants, but at term increased weight beyond the 90th percentile enhances mortality. A similar trend is noteworthy using birth weight as the point of reference. At birth weights *below 2500 g*, mortality decreases as gestational age lengthens, even in post-term infants. But mortality does not decrease in post-term infants when their birth weights are *above 2500 g*. Apparently, postmaturity has a more negative effect on the survival of babies who weigh over 2500 g; while it has little effect on low birth weight infants.

Table 5-5 and Fig. 5-13 indicate biologic trends. Since the publication of these data, survival statistics have improved remarkably, particularly among very low birth weight infants. Mortality rates that are related solely to gestational age and birth weight necessarily overlook the multiple factors that actually produce the abnormal gestational ages and weights. These are the factors that are usually directly responsible for mortality. For example, the malformations of congenital rubella are the primary causes of death in babies who happen to be SGA because of impaired fetal growth imposed by rubella. Their deaths are not the result of aberrant growth. Mortality statistics related to birth weight and gestational age are only *associations;* they do not always imply a cause-and-effect relationship. In a substantial number of infants, however, either very short or very long gestational ages and extremely high or low birth weights indeed may be directly implicated in the frequency of neonatal death.

Assessment of neonatal mortality must therefore be considered in finer detail than by means of the statistical associations just described. The variations and disagreements between numbers of published inquiries are no doubt largely a result of the heterogeneous nature of infants who are categorically labeled SGA. Immediate outcomes vary among infants with major malformations, those whose insult began early in pregnancy, and those whose insult began later on; yet in all three categories, the babies are simply labeled SGA. Heterogeneity is even more significant when one attempts to analyze long-term status in regard to stature and central nervous system function.

Postneonatal outcome. Any analysis that seeks to relate fetal growth to stature, weight, and IQ in later childhood must consider the heterogeneity of SGA babies—that is, the magnitude and type of in utero insult, and the time of its inception. Furthermore, the postnatal environmental influences exerted by socioeconomic level must also be assessed in the light of the long-term outcome. Intrauterine growth retardation is most common among poor families, and the socioeconomic factors that influence impaired growth in utero are likely to be operative after birth as well. Thus an abnormal outcome may not be solely caused by intrauterine events. The IQ is a case in point. A study in Scotland has revealed that infants who were undergrown at birth had lower IQ scores at 10 to 12 years of age than those who were appropriately grown at the same gestational age, *but this phenomenon was noted only in poor homes*. On the other hand, in superior homes, IQ scores were virtually identical in both groups. According to these data, fetal malnutrition exerts an influence on intellectual status, but primarily in low socioeconomic families. Apparently the low IQ of children in poor homes cannot be attributed solely to intrauterine growth retardation, unless there exists one type of undergrowth among the poor and yet another among the more favored socioeconomic groups.

There seems little doubt that fetal undergrowth plays a significant role in later subnormal central nervous system function. What remains in doubt are the specific variety or varieties of fetal insult that are implicated and the extent of that implication. It is obvious from years of published studies that not all undergrown neonates fare poorly. Babies who are small by virtue of intrauterine virus infection (rubella, cytomegalovirus) are profoundly affected from direct invasion of the brain by the offending virus, and babies who are SGA by virtue of a chromosomal disorder or some major anomaly are similarly affected. The data are straightforward and uncontested. However, infants who are small for no other reason than that their well-nourished parents are small are not af-

flicted later in life. The data on these infants are also unequivocal. Between these categories is a heterogeneous group of babies whose fetal growth was impeded by an adverse social environment, such as maternal malnutrition, as well as by disorders of pregnancy itself regardless of social class. Any inquiry that does not limit its data and conclusions to specific etiologic categories of fetal undergrowth, insofar as these categories can be determined, will produce equivocal results. This failure to establish specific categories is probably the fundamental reason for the differing literature on this subject. It is furthermore difficult to assess the *severity* of abnormal intrauterine growth. An attempt to evaluate outcome by severity of undergrowth was made in a well-controlled study of approximately 500 babies. It indicated that low birth weight babies (1500 to 2500 g) whose gestational age was at term (40 weeks) were most likely to be smallest in weight and height at 10 years of age compared with babies of similar birth weight but shorter gestational age (34 to 38 weeks). Stated differently, infants of equal weight in whom intrauterine growth was slowest (born after the longest gestations, 40 weeks) were the most deeply insulted group and experienced the worst outcome at 10 years of age. Similar assessment of IQ was not made.

The difficulties that beset a follow-up study of sick infants who are managed in an intensive care facility are clearly exemplified in a report from Toronto. Of 71 SGA infants who were evaluated at 2 years of age, 49% had major developmental handicaps. The authors emphasized that these results bore no direct relationship to the degree of fetal undergrowth. Rather, the *handicaps were strongly associated with central nervous system depression at the time of admission*, which in turn was related to perinatal asphyxia and to postnatal management prior to the transfer of infants to their tertiary care facility. The study infants, all of whom were transferred from other hospitals, were in poor condition on admission. Thus in this report, the evaluation of the long-term effects of intrauterine growth retardation was complicated by a high incidence of perinatal asphyxia (63% were affected) and by transfer from hospitals of birth to the tertiary care unit. Studies that evaluate long-term outcomes of impaired intrauterine growth must therefore also consider a variety of perinatal misadventures that later contribute to subnormality. The issue of inborn versus outborn births is critical in the assessment of outcomes.

It now appears that if one excludes intrauterine infections, chromosomal disorders, and major congenital malformations, SGA *term* infants have a low incidence of severe mental and neurologic handicaps. There is, however, suggestive evidence of a slightly increased risk of cerebral palsy in SGA term infants compared to AGA babies. However, less profound impairments that cause learning difficulties and behavior problems are probably common. From various studies, these impairments include minimal cerebral dysfunction characterized by hyperactivity, short attention span, and poor fine coordination and learning disabilities. Neurologic abnormalities of a mild, diffuse nature are common. Speech defects featuring immature reception and expression are also frequent. The stimulating postnatal environment and optimal nutrition in preschool years that are so essential for all children are probably more urgently required for those who were poorly grown in utero.

School problems among SGA infants born at term are more frequent than in AGA infants. In one study, three times as many SGA infants failed grades as AGA infants, and four times as many required special classes. In another inquiry, even in the presence of average intelligence, half the SGA boys and about one third of the SGA girls performed poorly in school. The same study demonstrated a high incidence of speech and language problems in SGA children; one third of the boys and one fourth of the girls had immature expressive and receptive language capacities. Furthermore, 31% of the boys and 18% of the girls had severe speech defects. Once again, girls fare better than boys. Hearing and visual impairment are not more common in SGA term infants.

The incidence of severe central nervous system handicaps such as mental retardation and cerebral palsy seems to be more clearly a function of gestational age. Premature low birth weight infants have a higher incidence of these unfortunate results, and the more premature the birth, the higher the incidence of abnormality. In terms of central nervous system function, growth impairment in babies born at or near term may result only in some diminution of intellectual capacity, rather than in the severe disabilities that characterize cerebral palsy. Generally the immediate prognosis for survival and the long-term outlook for normal function is better for SGA infants born at or near term than in those who are premature AGA; yet neither group fares as well as the normal-sized term infant.

The SGA premature infant is probably more vulnerable to major handicap than the premature AGA, but the evidence is equivocal. In one study of low birth weight infants, the AGA group was at greater risk for neonatal death; the SGA group was at higher risk for problems in the first year. Another study reported that developmental performance at 9 months through 3 years of age was significantly suboptimal in SGA infants compared to the AGA babies, but the difference was not observed later at 4 to 5 years of age. The authors stressed the importance of long-term follow-up. Another investigation came to a similar conclusion. Initial intelligence tests of SGA prematures were lower than AGA, but the differences disappeared at ages up to 6 years. However, several studies have concluded otherwise. In them, premature SGA infants did not do as well as prematures who were AGA, and the SGA IQ scores were lower.

A classic Scottish study demonstrated that more premature SGA infants had subnormal cognitive capacity, especially when born to parents of low socioeconomic status. The handicaps generally attributed to premature birth, such as hydrocephalus, retrolental fibroplasia, diminished visual acuity, cerebral palsy, and other neurologic deficits, were of relatively high incidence in both

SGA and AGA premature infants. These handicaps may be somewhat more frequent in the SGA group, but the evidence is insufficient for definite conclusions.

The follow-up data on SGA babies, both term and premature, does allow a few clear conclusions:

Socioeconomic status influences the results when follow-up is performed beyond 2 years of age. Lower IQ scores are significantly more prevalent among lower social class SGA infants.

SGA infants whose impaired intrauterine growth was identified before the twenty-sixth week attained significantly lower levels of academic achievement and had a higher incidence of behavior problems. The earlier the insult, the more likelihood of abnormal outcomes.

The combination of intrauterine growth retardation and head circumference below the 10th percentile are well correlated with subsequent neurologic deficit, poor intellectual achievement, and ultimate microcephaly.

Abnormally small head circumference for gestational age may be one of the most important predictors of abnormal neurobehavioral outcome.

The etiologies of growth retardation are diverse, but at least half of all SGA babies are born to mothers who have obstetric complications or chronic vascular disease.

The etiologic diversity of undergrowth in utero causes confusion in the analysis of long-term outcome. Clear conclusions will not be possible until the "lump" called SGA is split into etiologically homogeneous pieces. Accurate prediction of outcomes will be possible only when homogeneous subgroupings are delineated.

PREMATURITY

As discussed at the beginning of this chapter, premature births occur before the end of the thirty-seventh gestational week, regardless of birth weight. The majority of babies who weigh less than 2500 g and almost all infants below 1500 g are born prematurely. Most of them are appropriately grown; some are SGA. On the other

hand, many premature infants of diabetic mothers weigh over 2500 g at birth, LGA.

Prenatal factors

In the past, most studies of the maternal factors associated with prematurity were based on birth weight as the sole criterion of premature birth. Among the so-called premature babies who were studied, a substantial number of low birth weight infants were actually born at term. Despite this difficulty, a number of factors have been shown to be clearly associated with prematurity, although definitive causes are demonstrable in only a minority of affected mothers. The obstetric conditions that play a role in the initiation of premature labor include chronic hypertensive disease, toxemia, placenta previa, abruptio placentae, multiple gestation, and cervical incompetence. Other factors that have been implicated are low socioeconomic status, short maternal stature, absence of prenatal care, malnutrition, and a history of previous premature delivery. The difficulty in evaluating any of the latter group of conditions singly is that they usually occur in some sort of combination with each other. Thus mothers of short stature are often malnourished, do not receive prenatal care, and are the same women who deliver premature infants repeatedly. Furthermore, these particular factors are inseparable from poverty, of which they are the essence. Despite remarkable advances in perinatal medicine, our persistent ignorance of the causes of prematurity remains a major disappointment.

Mortality and morbidity

Mortality rates are highest among premature infants, and these rates increase as birth weight and gestational age decrease. Premature infants are poorly equipped to withstand the stresses of extrauterine life. The lungs may not be ready for air exchange; the digestive tract fails to absorb 20% to 40% of the fat contained in milk feedings. Defenses against infections are relatively ineffective, and an increased rate of heat loss creates serious thermoregulatory problems. The capillar-

Table 5-6. Clinical problems most likely encountered in abnormal birth weight/gestational age categories

Growth/gestational age abnormality	Reference page number

SGA term (<2500 g; >37 weeks)
Perinatal asphyxia
Meconium aspiration
Persistent fetal circulation syndrome (PFC)
Hypoglycemia
Thermal instability
Polycythemia-hyperviscosity
Major congenital malformations
Nonbacterial intrauterine infection
Multiple birth (e.g., twins, triplets)
Intrauterine parabiotic syndrome

AGA premature (<2500 g; ≤37 weeks)
Hyaline membrane disease and immature lung syndrome
Patent ductus arteriosus
Intraventricular-periventricular hemorrhage
Hydrocephaly
Retinopathy of prematurity (retrolental fibroplasia)
Necrotizing enterocolitis
Undernutrition
Thermal instability
Hyperbilirubinemia
Anemia of prematurity
Anemia caused by vitamin E deficiency
Inguinal hernia

LGA term (<4000 g; >37 weeks)
Perinatal asphyxia
Spontaneous pneumothorax, pneumomediastinum
Birth trauma
    Fractured humerus
    Brachial plexus palsy
    Facial palsy
    Depressed skull fracture
Transposition of great vessels

Postmature (any weight; ≥42 weeks)
AGA or SGA
Perinatal asphyxia
Meconium aspiration
Malnutrition; wasting
Thermal instability
Polycythemia-hyperviscosity syndrome

ies are relatively sparse so that perfusion of tissues is at best marginal. Increased capillary fragility predisposes to hemorrhage, especially in the ventricles of the brain.

Premature infants, whether AGA or SGA, are predisposed to the following postnatal disorders: hyaline membrane disease (and immature lung syndrome in the smallest babies), patent ductus arteriosus, intraventricular-periventricular hemorrhage and hydrocephalus, necrotizing enterocolitis, thermal instability, undernutrition, nosocomial bacterial infection, anemia of prematurity, vitamin E deficiency anemia, inguinal hernia, recurrent apnea, and retinopathy of prematurity. Table 5-6 lists the clinical problems that are likely to be associated with various types of abnormal intrauterine growth.

Postneonatal outcome

Premature infants have a relatively high incidence of mental retardation and abnormal neurologic signs. Microcephaly, spastic diplegia, convulsive disorders, and abnormal electroenceph-

alograms are the most frequently encountered signs of brain disorder. The incidence of neurologic abnormality has diminished substantially since the advent of intensive care techniques. Approximately 70% to 90% of very low birth weight infants who survive are neurologically intact. Blindness caused by retrolental fibroplasia was quite common between 1940 and 1955. It was particularly frequent among infants whose birth weights were less than 1500 g. Restriction of oxygen administration resulted in a significantly decreased incidence of the disease, but improved survival rates among the smallest premature infants have been associated with a resurgence that is not clearly attributable to administration of excessive oxygen (see Chapter 8).

Considerable attention has been focused recently on the outcomes of infants who weigh less than 1000 g at birth. Their survival rates have improved astonishingly in the 5 to 6 years preceding this writing. In 1984, 45% of infants below 750 g survived in our nursery; 5 years previously, only 10% survived. Follow-up studies vary in

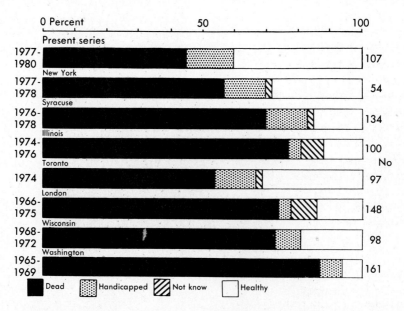

Fig. 5-14. Published outcome studies of babies < 1000 g. The trend is toward lower mortality and a higher percent of healthy survivors. (From Yu, V. Y. H.: Arch. Dis. Child. **57**:823, 1982.)

their findings of handicap and suboptimal outcome. In general the data are encouraging, notwithstanding a persistently high incidence of undesirable outcomes compared to babies who are over 1000 g. During the past several years, improvement in long-term outcome has been observed in virtually every report on the subject. Fig. 5-14 depicts the outcomes from eight published studies. The earliest study data are from babies born between 1965 and 1969 (bottom bar). Results of the most recent study among those depicted are shown in the top bar. A comparison of the top and bottom bars indicates the progress that has occurred during the last two decades. A more recent publication described infants below 750 g who were born between 1975 and 1980. There were 22 long-term survivors among 60 infants; 12 of the 22 (67%) were considered normal. Another report of 69 infants who weighed less than 1000 g at birth, and who were born between 1973 and 1976, describes 36% survival, but only one infant weighed less than 750 g. There was significantly greater morbidity among infants who required assisted ventilation. Overall, 65% of the infants in that study were considered to have had a good outcome, but only 28% of ventilated survivors were normal, while 81% of nonventilated survivors were considered normal. A report from Seattle describes 95 neonates, born from 1977 through 1980, whose birth weights were less than 800 g. Nineteen (20%) survived. Eighty-one percent of these infants were normal when examined at 6 months to 3 years of age. Only one infant was distinctly subnormal. These infants have been observed too soon after birth to allow conclusions, but from this and other studies, the trend toward improved outcome in the smallest infants is clearer with each passing year.

POSTMATURITY

Prolonged gestation is dated from the beginning of the forty-second week; infants born afterward are said to be postmature. By this definition, approximately 12% of all pregnancies are prolonged. Postmature infants may be appro-

priately sized for gestational age; yet often they are SGA by virtue of progressive deterioration of the maternal-placental support system. In such circumstances the infant may be considerably wasted.

Abnormal physical signs of wasting are observed in 4% to 12% of infants who are born in the forty-third week of gestation or later. The incidence of affected infants varies between populations. In the United States, 5% of postmature white infants and 8% of black infants have physical signs of postmature placental dysfunction. In Sweden and Germany, the incidences are 12% and 7%, respectively. There is a higher incidence of Apgar scores below 7 among affected infants, and their hematocrits are more frequently greater than 65%. The physical appearance of a wasted postmature baby differs in several respects from the appearance of his earlier born counterpart of equal size. Changes in the skin, nails, hair, subcutaneous tissue, and body contour are the obvious differences. Vernix caseosa is characteristically absent in postmature babies, except in the deepest skin folds at the axillae and groin, whereas at term the skin of malnourished infants is well covered with this cheeselike material. In postmature babies the skin becomes dry and cracked soon after birth, imparting a parchmentlike texture to it. The nails are often lengthened. Scalp hair is profuse, in contrast to earlier born malnourished infants, whose hair is sparse. Wasting involves depletion of previously deposited subcutaneous tissue; as a consequence, skin is loose, and fat layers are almost nonexistent (Fig. 5-4). The body appears thin and long. Meconium staining occurs frequently, coloring the skin, nails, and cord in shades ranging from green to golden yellow. Release of meconium in response to intrauterine hypoxic stress may occur just before delivery or about 10 to 14 days before. Typically these infants appear alert and wide-eyed, an attractive but misleading feature that is ominous because it may indicate chronic intrauterine hypoxia.

Perinatal mortality is higher in postmature infants than in term infants, particularly in pregnancies that progress into the forty-third week and beyond. In these infants, mortality is two or three times greater than in term babies. Approximately 75% to 85% of all deaths among postmature babies occur during labor. This is not particularly surprising when one considers that fetal oxygenation is marginal or depressed for days prior to the onset of labor. The subsequent stresses of labor are poorly tolerated, and intrauterine demise or severe depression at birth ensues.

Postneonatal outcomes have differed among various studies. In one such study, black infants were no different than their controls in weight, height, neurologic function, and psychologic performance. These parameters were observed on several occasions up to 7 years of age. Weight and height attainment and neurologic and psychologic functions were all normal. Among similarly affected infants in Sweden, IQ score and weight were significantly lower than control infants.

INTRAUTERINE GROWTH ACCELERATION (BABIES LARGE FOR GESTATIONAL AGE; MACROSOMIA)

The highest birth weight recorded in medical literature is 11,350 g (25 lb), a stillborn infant who was delivered in 1916. The *Guinness Book of World Records* (1984) reports the heaviest normal neonate weight at 10,125 g (22 lb, 8 oz); a baby weighing 10,687 g (23 lb, 12 oz) lived less than 24 hours. A stillborn weighing 11,250 g (25 lb) was delivered in 1891. Five percent of infants weigh over 4000 g at birth, and from 0.4% to 0.9% weigh over 4500 g. Whereas low birth weight is delineated below 2500 g for any gestational age, high birth weight is above 4000 g. The same variations in weight for age at birth that were described for small infants are applicable to large ones. An infant who is plotted above the 90th percentile on the intrauterine growth curve (at any week of gestation) is large for gestational age (LGA).

Only a minority of large infants are born of diabetic mothers. Excessive birth weight (over 4000 g) often reflects the genetic predisposition of the fetus. It is proportional to prepregnancy weight and weight gain during pregnancy. Abnormalities of mother and fetus are only rarely accountable for LGA infants. Maternal diabetes is the most notable exception. Large mothers have large babies. These mothers are older, taller, heavier, and they often gain weight excessively during pregnancy. They also have little if any past history of troublesome pregnancy and birth. Large infants are born to multiparous mothers three times as often as to primiparous ones; male infants have long been known to be heavier at birth than females. The small number of infants who have transposition of the great vessels are usually overgrown.

Categorization of babies as large for gestational age has been found, in the majority of instances, to result from miscalculation of dates. The source of error, difficult to avert, appears to be postconceptional bleeding, a spurious menstrual episode after fertilization.

LGA babies are heavier and longer; their heads are larger. The LGA infant of a diabetic mother differs. Excessive birth weight principally is due to the excessive deposition of fat, mostly in the subcutaneous tissue. Fat deposits are enhanced by fetal overproduction of insulin and by augmented transfer of maternal amino acids across the placenta. The volume of extracellular water is diminished in infants of diabetic mothers; it does not contribute significantly to increased birth weight. Length and head size are not greater in infants of diabetic mothers than in normal term babies. The infants of diabetic mothers are macrosomic because of fat deposition. This is documented by measurements of increased skinfold thickness. Inadequate control of maternal diabetes has long been known to be associated with greater fetal deposition of fat and macrosomia at birth. Maternal, and therefore fetal, hyperglycemia stimulates the fetal secretion of insulin, which in turn increases the production of triglycerides followed by excessive deposition of fat.

In diabetic women, birth weight over 4000 g is 4 times more frequent than in nondiabetic women. The discrepancy is of greater magnitude for babies over 4500 g: they are 14 to 28 times more frequent among diabetic women than in the general population.

The mortality rate for large babies born at or near term is higher than for average-sized neonates. The obvious mechanical difficulties posed by delivery of an oversized baby are significant. The need for midforceps and cesarean section is considerably increased. Cesarean section is usually necessary because of cephalopelvic (fetopelvic) disproportion. Shoulder dystocia has been noted in 10% of large babies delivered per vaginam. Fractured clavicle, depressed skull fracture, brachial plexus palsy, and facial paralysis are all increased in frequency, together occurring in 15% of oversized infants. Low Apgar scores occur more frequently in overgrown infants.

Large babies have received relatively scanty attention compared with those who are undergrown. Prenatal identification of overgrown fetuses would seem to be as necessary as the identification of those who are undergrown. Abnormal and traumatic labor and delivery could thus often be averted.

SUMMARY

Expert care of newborn patients requires, among other things, an understanding of the abnormalities of intrauterine growth patterns as they relate to gestational age. An infant's course in the nursery is in large measure determined by these factors, and the illnesses that develop postnatally are often peculiar to a particular type of aberrant intrauterine growth pattern (see Table 5-6). Thus hyaline membrane disease, for all practical purposes, is confined to preterm babies, whereas hypoglycemia is a frequent hazard in SGA infants. With knowledge of maternal factors and with the ability to categorize babies in terms of growth status, the nurse can readily recognize a large number of high-risk infants and plan their management accordingly.

BIBLIOGRAPHY

Allen, M. C.: Developmental outcome and followup of the small for gestational age infant, Sem. Perinatol. 8:123, 1984.

Ballard, J. L., Novak, K. K., and Driver, M.: A simplified score for assessment of fetal maturation of newly born infants, J. Pediatr. 95:769, 1979.

Battaglia, F. C., and Lubchenco, L. O.: A practical classification of newborn infants by weight and gestational age, J. Pediatr. 71:159, 1967.

Beck, G. J., and van den Berg, B. J.: The relationship of the rate of intrauterine growth of low-birth-weight infants to later growth, J. Pediatr. 86:504, 1975.

Bennett, F. C., Robinson, N. M., and Sells, C. J.: Growth and development of infants weighing less than 800 grams at birth, Pediatrics 71:319, 1983.

Campbell, S.: Fetal growth, Clin. Obstet. Gynecol. 1:41, 1974.

Chessex, P., Reichman, B., Verellen, G., et al.: Metabolic consequences of intrauterine growth retardation in very low birth weight infants. Pediatr. Res. 18:709, 1984.

Clifford, S. H.: Postmaturity with placental dysfunction: clinical syndrome and pathologic findings, J. Pediatr. 44:1, 1954.

Commey, J. O. O., and Fitzhardinge, P. M.: Handicap in the preterm small-for-gestational age, J. Pediatr. 94:779, 1979.

Davies, D. P.: Physical growth from fetus to early childhood. In Davis, J. A., and Dobbing, J., editors: Scientific foundations of paediatrics, Baltimore, 1982, University Park Press.

Drillien, C. M.: Prenatal and perinatal factors in etiology and outcome of low birth weight, Clin. Perinatol. 1:197, 1974.

Dubowitz, L. M. S., and Dubowitz, V.: Gestational age of the newborn, Reading, Mass., 1977, Addison-Wesley Publishing Co.

Dubowitz, L. M. S., Dubowitz, V., and Goldberg, C.: Clinical assessment of gestational age in the newborn infant, J. Pediatr. 77:1, 1970.

Escalona, S. K.: Babies at double hazard: Early development of infants at biologic and social risk, Pediatrics 70:670, 1982.

Fitzhardinge, P. M., and Steven, E. M.: The small-for-date infant. II. Neurological and intellectual sequelae, Pediatrics 50:50, 1972.

Freedman, R. M., and Warshaw, J. B.: The low-birth-weight infant: an overview. In Warshaw, J. B., and Hobbins, J. C., editors: Principles and practice of perinatal medicine—maternal-fetal and newborn care, Menlo Park, Calif., 1983, Addison-Wesley Publishing Co.

Gluck, L., Kulovich, M. V., Borer, R. C., Jr., et al.: The diagnosis of the respiratory distress syndrome (RDS) by amniocentesis, Am. J. Obstet. Gynecol. 109:440, 1971.

Gross, S. J., Oehler, J. M., and Eckerman, C. O.: Head growth and developmental outcome in very low-birth-weight infants, Pediatrics 71:70, 1983.

Gruenwald, P.: The fetus in prolonged pregnancy, Am. J. Obstet. Gynecol. 89:503, 1964.

Gruenwald, P.: Growth of the human fetus. I. Normal growth and its variation, Am. J. Obstet. Gynecol. **94**:1112, 1966.

Hirata, T., Epcar, J. T., Walsh, A., et al.: Survival and outcome of infants 501 to 750 gm: a six-year experience, J. Pediatr. **102**:741, 1983.

Hittner, H. M., Hirsch, N. J., and Rudolph, A. J.: Assessment of gestational age by examination of the anterior vascular capsule of the lens, J. Pediatr. **91**:455, 1977.

Horger, E. O., III, Miller, C., III, and Conner, E. D.: Relations of large birthweight to maternal diabetes mellitus, Obstet. Gynecol. **45**:150, 1975.

Iffy, L., Chatterton, R. T., and Jakobovits, A.: The "high weight for dates" fetus, Am. J. Obstet. Gynecol. **115**:238, 1973.

Jones, K. L., and Chernoff, G. F.: Drugs and chemicals associated with intrauterine growth deficiency, J. Repro. Med. **21**:365, 1978.

Kliegman, R. M., and King, K. C.: Intrauterine growth retardation: Determinants of aberrant fetal growth. In Fanaroff, A. A., and Martin, R. J., editors: Behrman's neonatal-perinatal medicine, St. Louis, 1983, The C. V. Mosby Co.

Koenigsberger, M. R.: Judgment of fetal age. I. Neurologic evaluation, Pediatr. Clin. North Am. **13**:823, 1966.

Lubchenco, L. O.: The high risk infant, Philadelphia, 1976, W. B. Saunders Co.

Lubchenco, L. O., Searls, D. T., and Brazie, J. V.: Neonatal mortality rate: relationship to birthweight and gestational age, J. Pediatr. **81**:814, 1972.

Moore, W. M. O.: Prenatal factors influencing intrauterine growth: Clinical implications. In Boyd, R., and Battaglia, F. C., editors: Perinatal medicine, London, 1983, Butterworths International Medical News.

Naeye, R. L.: Human intrauterine parabiotic syndrome and its complications, N. Engl. J. Med. **268**:804, 1963.

Naeye, R. L.: Unsuspected organ abnormalities associated with congenital heart disease, Am. J. Pathol. **47**:905, 1965.

Naeye, R. L.: Abnormalities in infants of mothers with toxemia of pregnancy, Am. J. Obstet. Gynecol. **95**:276, 1966.

Naeye, R. L., Bernirschke, K., Hagstrom, J. W. C., and Marcus, C. C.: Intrauterine growth of twins as estimated from liveborn birth-weight data, Pediatrics **37**:409, 1966.

Orgill, A. A., Astbury, J., Bajuk, B., and Yu, V. Y. H.: Early development of infants 1000 g or less at birth, Arch. Dis. Child. **57**:823, 1982.

Parkin, J. M., Hey, E. N., and Clowes, J. S.: Rapid assessment of gestational age at birth, Arch. Dis. Child. **51**:259, 1976.

Robinson, J. S.: Growth of the fetus, Br. Med. Bull. **35**:137, 1979.

Ross, G., Krauss, A. N., and Auld, P. A. M.: Growth achievement in low-birth-weight premature infants: relationship to neurobehavioral outcome at one year, J. Pediatr. **103**:105, 1983.

Rosso, P., Wasserman, M., Rozovski, S., and Velasco, E.: Effects of maternal undernutrition on placental metabolism and function. In Young, D. S., and Hicks, J. M., editors: The neonate, New York, 1976, John Wiley & Sons.

Rothberg, A. D., Maisels, M. J., Bagnato, S., et al.: Infants weighing 1,000 grams or less at birth: developmental outcome for ventilated and nonventilated infants, Pediatrics **71**:599, 1983.

Shanklin, D. R.: The influence of placental lesions on the newborn infant, Pediatr. Clin. North Am. **17**:25, 1970.

Silverman, W. A.: Dunham's premature infants, New York, 1961, Paul B. Hoeber, Medical Division, Harper & Row, Publishers.

Silverman, W. A., and Sinclair, J. C.: Infants of low birth weight, N. Engl. J. Med. **274**:448, 1966.

Sinclair, J. C.: Temperature regulation and energy metabolism in the newborn, New York, 1978, Grune & Stratton.

Sinclair, J. C., and Tudehope, D. I.: Birth weight, gestational age, and neonatal risk. In Fanaroff, A. A., and Martin, R. J., editors: Behrman's neonatal-perinatal medicine, St. Louis, 1983, The C.V. Mosby Co.

Smith, C. A.: Effects of maternal undernutrition upon the newborn infant in Holland, J. Pediatr. **71**:390, 1967.

Smith, D. W.: Growth and its disorders, Philadelphia, 1977, W.B. Saunders Co.

Starfield, B., Shapiro, S., McCormick, M., and Bross, D.: Mortality and morbidity in infants with intrauterine growth retardation, J. Pediatr. **101**:978, 1982.

Ting, R. Y., Wang, M. H., and Scott, T. F. M.: The dysmature infant, J. Pediatr. **90**:943, 1977.

Vohr, B. R., and Oh, W.: Growth and development in preterm infants small for gestational age, J. Pediatr. **103**:941, 1983.

Widdowson, E. M.: Changes in body composition during growth. In Davis, J. A., and Dobbing, J., editors: Scientific foundations of paediatrics, Baltimore, 1982, University Park Press.

Winick, M.: Cellular growth of human placenta. III. Intrauterine growth failure, J. Pediatr. **71**:390, 1967.

Winick, M.: Cellular growth in intrauterine malnutrition, Pediatr. Clin. North Am. **17**:69, 1970.

Winick, M.: Malnutrition and brain development, New York, 1976, Oxford University Press.

Winick, M., Brasel, J. A., and Velasco, E. G.: Effects of prenatal nutrition upon pregnancy risk, Clin. Obstet. Gynecol. **16**:184, 1973.

Physical examination of the newborn infant

The physical findings associated with birth trauma are described in Chapter 3.

The nurse who learns to evaluate physical signs in the neonate can contribute substantially to his proper management. Contemporary expansion of nursing skills involves many new functions, one of which is the competent performance of a physical examination. Physical findings in the newborn will thus be presented in considerable detail, with emphasis on normal characteristics and their variations, most of which require no therapy. *Some pathologic findings will be described, but they are usually discussed more completely in chapters devoted to the specific diseases in which they occur.*

The initial physical examination should be performed as soon as possible after arrival in the nursery. Its purpose is to identify existing abnormalities and to provide a basis on which future changes can be assessed. After the admission examination a number of observations must be made during the nursery stay. The first passage of stool and the first urination should be noted. Sucking behavior and performance during feedings are extremely important observations. The appearance of jaundice, cyanosis, pallor, excessive salivation, abdominal distention, abnormal stools, respiratory distress, and a number of other events must all be sought in a systematic fashion.

The purpose of the neonatal physical examination is to identify and record evidence of stress, trauma, malformations, and disease during the first days of life. Physical assessment is only one component of the total evaluation. A well-considered chronologic account of antecedent events must be known prior to examination. Laboratory and other procedural data are usually acquired afterward.

SEQUENCE OF EXAMINATION

The sequence in which the various features of the examination are assessed is a matter of per-

151

sonal preference. All examiners eventually develop their own individual approach. Regardless of the system used, it is best to order observations in reference to the amount of disturbance they produce. I prefer to first make assessments that cause the least disturbance, particularly those that require a quiet baby. It seems advisable to then proceed to the more disturbing maneuvers that are not so dependent on the resting state for accurate interpretation.

Inspection without contact. A tremendous amount of information is available by simply looking at a baby, without touching him. The examiner should not, when first confronting an infant, abruptly place a stethoscope on the chest before doing anything else. This maneuver betrays a sad lack of sensitivity to the neonate's reactions and

a total lack of perspective regarding the relative importance of the individual observations that comprise the physical examination.

The infant's overall size and contour are immediately apparent, as is the relative size of the head, extremities, and trunk. Microcephaly or cranial enlargement are obvious. If hydrocephalus is present, the forehead is often prominently protrusive (bossing). The cranial vault is always large in relation to the face (Fig. 6-1). The amount of subcutaneous fat is assessable at a glance. A thin trunk often causes a normal head to appear enlarged. The abdomen is either distended, flat, or sunken (scaphoid), or it may bulge on one side because of a massively enlarged kidney (hydronephrosis, Fig. 6-2).

The baby's *posture* is informative. Normal flex-

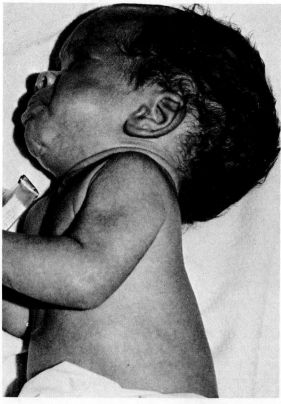

Fig. 6-1. Hydrocephalus. Note the large size of the head in relation to the face. The occiput is prominent, the forehead less prominent than usual. This infant also had severe chorioretinitis. The diagnosis was toxoplasmosis.

ion of the extremities indicates good muscle tone. Lack of flexion is associated with hypotonicity (flaccidity), whereas excessive flexion usually suggests hypertonicity (spasticity). Both these findings are evident in the baby in Fig. 6-3, who had flaccid upper extremities and spastic lower ones. If only one arm is straight instead of flexed, it is probably paralyzed to some extent. This paralysis suggests brachial plexus palsy, which is described on p. 68 and is illustrated in Figs. 2-14 and 2-15. Breech presentations can be identified by the characteristic positions of the lower extremities. These positions are described later in this chapter. The absence of molding plus the position of the lower extremities should suggest a breech delivery. Retraction of the head with relatively normal vertebral posture indicates a face presentation.

A number of features of the *skin* are immediately obvious. If cyanosis is present, its distribution is of great importance because distribution relates to the significance of cyanosis (generalized cyanosis) or lack of it (acrocyanosis). Jaundice, pallor, rash, and evidence of trauma are all there to be discerned by those who will look.

The *face* is informative. Abnormal facies must be appreciated. The alert, wide-eyed baby who appears to be sucking is really agitated as a result of intrauterine hypoxic insult to the brain (Fig. 5-12). Facial paralysis may be evident at rest, or it may not be apparent until the baby cries (p. 70).

Spontaneous movements can be evaluated only if the infant is not disturbed. At rest, sporadic, well-coordinated movements are the rule. If no movement is noted, significant depression is

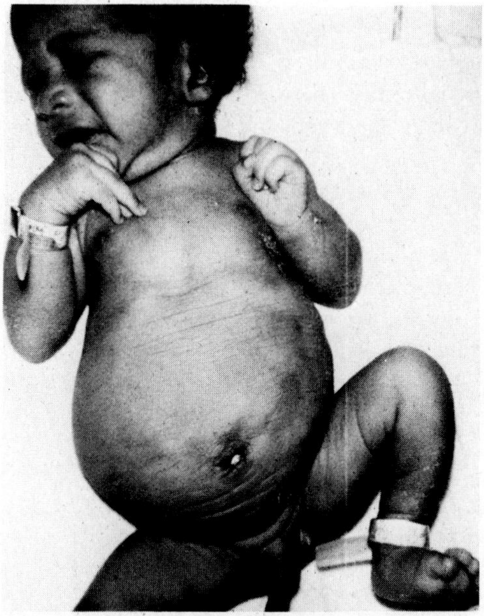

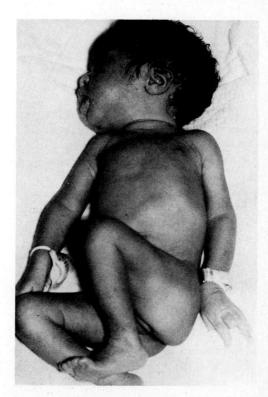

Fig. 6-2. Abdominal distention resulting from unilateral hydronephrosis. Bulging of the right side is immediately apparent.

Fig. 6-3. Upper extremities are flaccid, as seen in the relaxed fingers and elbows. Lower extremities are spastic, and their flexed posture is exaggerated. Note the congenitally amputated finger on the left hand.

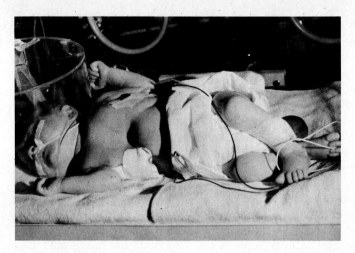

Fig. 6-4. Severe retraction during inspiration. The lower end of the sternum and the subcostal margins are severely indrawn. The upper anterior thorax is expanded. Electrodes to the chest are connected to apnea and heart rate monitors.

probably the cause, whether from hypoxia in utero, maternal anesthesia, hypoglycemia, or any other of a large number of etiologies. The baby who moves little or not at all is usually flaccid as well. Repetitive, rhythmic motions of one or more extremities are convulsive movements. Facial and eyelid twitches are also convulsive phenomena. Absent or diminished movement of one extremity (or two), while the others are used normally, is indicative of paresis or paralysis.

Much information is obtainable for the evaluation of *respiration* by simple inspection. Retractions are obvious (Fig. 6-4); grunting and stridor are audible. Increased anteroposterior diameter of the chest (barrel chest) usually indicates overexpanded lungs (massive aspiration, respiratory distress syndrome type 2). If one side of the chest appears larger than the other, pneumothorax, chylothorax, or diaphragmatic hernia are possible causes. If the left chest is larger, cardiomegaly associated with congenital heart disease is an additional possibility.

Several *scattered observations* by inspection are also of value. The undergrown term or pre-

term infant's hair is sparse (Fig. 5-12), whereas the postmature baby's hair is dense. The cord is thin in mature SGA infants, and it may be the only part of the body that is meconium stained, if meconium release occurs immediately before delivery. Fingernails are long in postmature infants.

These diverse signs are described here to emphasize the value of purposeful inspection without touching. This inspection accomplished, one may then proceed to the more manipulative aspects of the physical examination.

Auscultation, palpation, and other manipulations. With the baby supine, I prefer to palpate the abdomen immediately after the initial inspection. If the infant is disturbed by manipulations beforehand, an adequate evaluation of the abdomen is difficult or temporarily impossible. The fingertips must be gently placed on the abdomen while not exerting any downward pressure. Deep palpation should then proceed gradually. Sudden plunging of the examining hand into the abdomen is thoughtless; it produces discomfort and precludes a successful examination.

The neonate is easily agitated by abrupt manipulations. Auscultation of the anterior chest should follow abdominal palpations. In conjunction with cardiac evaluation, gently palpate the femoral and brachial pulses. Now palpate the extremities by enveloping them with your hand and then move the joints gingerly. This maneuver completed, take the wrists and pull the infant into the sitting position to evaluate head lag. The baby may now be turned to the prone position. Crying caused by the disturbance is of little concern because the resultant deep inspirations and the noise of crying are helpful in auscultation of the lungs. Now move the index finger over the vertebrae down to the sacrum to ascertain the absence of gross anomalies such as agenesis of the sacrum. Separate the buttocks and look at the anus for position and presence. The infant, who is probably crying now, is then returned to the supine position. Manipulate the hip joints to rule out congenital dislocation. The head, neck, and face are next to be examined. With one hand holding a flashlight, gently separate the eyelids with the index finger and thumb. Shine the light tangentially into the eyes to rule out corneal lesions and large cataracts. Now proceed to the neurologic evaluation (p. 173). Examination of the mouth and throat is performed as the last maneuver of the physical evaluation. It is the most agitating. After completing the physical examination, hold the baby in your arms for a few moments. Both of you will feel better.

PHYSICAL FINDINGS
Contour, proportions, and postures

The body of a normal newborn is essentially cylindric; the head circumference slightly exceeds that of the chest. For the term baby, average circumference of the head is 33 to 35 cm (13 to 14 in), whereas for the chest it is 30 to 33 cm (12 to 13 in). Sitting height may be measured from crown to rump, and it is approximately equal to head circumference. These values may vary, but their relationship to each other is normally constant. During the first 24 hours, because of molding, the head may be equal to or slightly smaller than the chest. On the second and third days a normal contour replaces the molded one, and the head circumference increases by 1 or 2 cm as a result. If the head is over 4 cm larger than the chest, and this has been verified by repeated measurements on several successive days, abnormal enlargement resulting from increased intracranial pressure is suspect. In these circumstances, additional signs of increased intracranial pressure are ordinarily detectable. These signs are described later in this chapter.

During the first few days of life, posture is largely the result of position in utero. Placed on the side, the normal infant who was delivered from a vertex presentation tends to keep the head flexed, with the chin close to the chest. The arms are close to the trunk, the elbows are flexed so that the forearms rest on the chest to some degree, and the hands are held in a fisted position. The back is somewhat bent, and the hips are flexed so that the thighs are drawn on the abdomen. Flexion is also maintained at the knees, and the feet are dorsiflexed onto the anterior aspects of the legs. This fetal position is often assumed to some extent by adults and older children while they sleep. During the first days of life, it is the position of comfort for the baby. Frequently the infant may be quieted during crying episodes by taking him up from the crib and gently curling him into this described position.

Other postures are associated with more unusual fetal positions. After a footling breech presentation, the thighs are abducted in the so-called frog-leg position (Fig. 2-8). Some babies born in the frank breech position tend to keep their knees straightened. After a brow or face delivery, the head is extended and the neck appears elongated.

These postures depend on normal muscle tone, which is strikingly diminished in hypoxic babies. Thus affected, they make no attempt to assume previous intrauterine postures but remain in almost any position imposed on them by the examiner. The extremities lie flat on the table surface, and the head turns to one side, depending on the position in which it is placed (Fig. 6-5).

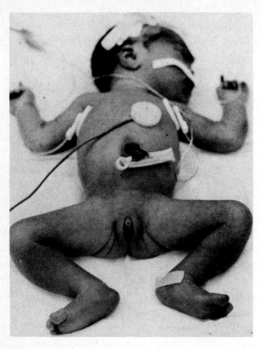

Fig. 6-5. A depressed, flaccid baby delivered in breech position. Extremities lie flat on table, and head remains turned to one side. Note traumatic cyanosis of lower half of body, a result of breech delivery.

Skin and subcutaneous tissue

At birth the skin is covered extensively with *vernix caseosa*, a gray-white substance with a cheeselike consistency. If not removed, it dries and disappears within 24 hours. There is no vernix in premature and postmature babies. For the first day of life the skin is blush red and smooth; toward the second or third days it becomes dry, somewhat flaky, and pink.

In approximately half of all normal newborn infants, *jaundice* is visible during the second or third days of life and disappears between the fifth and seventh days. This is physiologic jaundice; the mechanism of its development is described in Chapter 10. Jaundice in the first 24 hours is abnormal and requires extensive diagnostic evaluation. Icteric skin may be difficult to detect when redness is prominent, but blanching readily demonstrates the underlying yellow discoloration. Jaundice is best demonstrated by blanching the skin over the nasal bridge. Place one thumb on each side of the nose and stretch the skin over the nasal bridge by pressing firmly as each finger is moved a few centimeters laterally. A relatively large area of skin is thereby blanched. Early jaundice is more easily detected on the face than anywhere else.

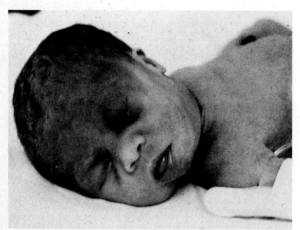

Fig. 6-6. Traumatic cyanosis, with bruising of forehead and scalp. Vertex delivery of a premature infant.

The subcutaneous tissue may be moderately *edematous* for several days. Edema is most noticeable about the eyes, legs, and dorsal aspects of the hands and feet.

Peripheral cyanosis (acrocyanosis) involves the hands, feet, and circumoral area (around the lips). It is evident in most infants at birth and for a short time thereafter. If limited to the extremities in an otherwise normal infant, it is a result of venous stasis and is innocuous. Localized cyanosis may occur in presenting parts, particularly in association with abnormal presentations. In breech presentations, the buttocks or the feet and legs are blue as a result of venous stasis and are edematous (Fig. 2-8); in a transverse lie, a prolapsed arm may be similarly discolored because of obstructed venous return. Occasionally a circular area of edema and cyanosis in the scalp is present at the top of the head as a result of pressure against a dilated cervix (caput succedaneum). Sometimes the forehead and scalp (or even the entire head above the neck) are cyanotic (Fig. 6-6).

Pallor usually accompanies other signs of distress except in anemic babies in whom there has been fetomaternal bleeding across the placenta over a protracted period (chronic hemorrhage in utero; see Chapter 9). Such infants are in no distress even though their pallor may be extreme. Pallor is more commonly a sign of anemia, hypoxia, poor peripheral perfusion due to hypotension (shock), and infection. Subcutaneous edema sometimes imparts a pale appearance, even though blood pressure and hematocrit are normal, because increased water content of subcutaneous tissue impairs transmission of the color of blood. Some postmature infants are pale because they have *parchment skin,* which also transmits less color from blood because it is thicker than normal.

Ecchymoses appear as bruises of varying size anywhere over the body, sometimes involving extensive areas. They most frequently are due to trauma during difficult labor or to brisk handling of the infant during or after delivery. Occasionally they indicate serious infection or a bleeding diathesis. When the extravasated blood in an ecchymosis is broken down, the resultant elevated serum bilirubin levels may occasionally reach dangerous heights. The pathogenesis of hyperbilirubinemia and the role of extraneous blood are discussed in Chapter 10.

Petechiae are pinpoint hemorrhagic areas that occur in a number of disease states involving infection and thrombocytopenia. Occasionally, however, scattered petechiae are noted over the upper trunk or the face as a result of increased intravascular pressure, which causes capillaries to rupture during delivery. These petechiae fade within 24 to 48 hours, and fresh lesions do not appear subsequently. Identification of petechiae may be verified by blanching the skin. Both index fingers are held next to each other, and while maintaining pressure, they are separated to reveal the area in question. Petechiae and ecchymoses do not disappear when the skin is blanched, since blood is fixed in the tissue. Red rashes involving local vascular engorgement disappear completely when the skin is blanched, since blood is emptied from the engorged vessels. The same maneuver reveals underlying jaundice that would otherwise be masked by flushed skin that is suffused with blood.

Mongolian spots are irregular areas of blue-gray pigmentation over the sacrum and buttocks, but they may be so extensive as to cover the back and sometimes the extensor surfaces of the extremities as well. They are common in black infants and in babies of Asian and southern European lineage. These harmless discolorations are caused by pigmented cells in the deep layer of the skin. They disappear by 4 years of age and often much sooner.

Hemangiomas may appear as isolated lesions in otherwise normal infants, or they may be a component of several serious generalized disorders. Microscopically, hemangiomas of the skin are *capillary* or *cavernous*. *Capillary hemangiomas* comprise a mass of dilated capillaries. They are usually found in the superficial skin. *Port wine nevi* (nervus flammeus) are dense concentrations of such dilated capillaries. They may be small and single, or multiple and sparse; they may also involve large areas of skin, even as much as half the body surface. Their color varies from pink to deep purple; in the neonate their surfaces are continuous with that of adjacent normal skin. Edges are clearly delineated. As a rule, they are permanent, but those that are pale may largely disappear. Port wine nevi over the face may indicate Sturge-Weber syndrome (cerebral calcification and glaucoma on the same side as the lesions and hemiparesis on the opposite side) and several other serious generalized disorders as well. *Telangiectatic nevi (stork bites)* are flat, red, localized areas of capillary dilatation seen in almost all neonates. Microscopically the dilated capillaries are considerably less dense than those seen in port wine nevi. They can be eradicated by blanching the skin. They are most commonly situated at the back of the neck, the lower occiput, the upper eyelids, and the nasal bridge. They disappear by 2 years of age, but in many children they often reappear during crying episodes. *Strawberry hemangiomas* are not seen in normal term infants during the nursery stay because they generally appear in the second or third week of life. As a result, they are seen in premature infants who are hospitalized for protracted periods and in term babies after discharge. They are first evident as bright red, flat spots, 1 to 3 mm in diameter, which blanch easily. Subsequently they grow in all directions, protruding prominently from the skin surface. They may not reach their fullest size for 1 to 3 months or more. There is a great temptation to remove these lesions, but it should be resisted because they invariably resolve spontaneously several weeks or months after reaching peak growth. *The cosmetic effect is best when they are allowed to resolve.* Resolution is heralded by a pale purple or gray spot on the surface of the lesion, which grows as the hemangioma shrinks. Appearance of the pale spot indicates spontaneous sclerosis, and thus obliteration, of the capillaries that comprise the lesion. *Cavernous hemangiom-*

as are in the subepidermal layer. They tend to be more diffuse and less sharply demarcated than capillary hemangiomas. Color of the overlying skin may be normal, or bluish as a result of the transmission of color from subjacent blood. Cavernous hemangiomas are usually spongy when touched, but on occasion they are tight cystic masses. Generally these localized lesions have no other significance. They grow at first (like strawberry hemangiomas) and then often resolve spontaneously in a few months or 1 to 2 years. They may be situated so that during their growth they seriously impair the function of an adjacent organ such as the trachea, esophagus, or eye. Cavernous hemangiomas may also be associated with serious thrombocytopenia (Kasabach-Merritt syndrome). *Mixed hemangiomas* are common. They are composed of a superficial strawberry lesion that is continuous with a deeper cavernous one.

Subcutaneous fat necrosis results from trauma. These lesions are sharply demarcated, firm masses of varying size that are located in subcutaneous tissue and are fixed to overlying skin.

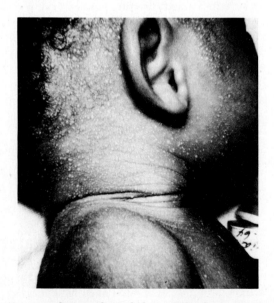

Fig. 6-7. Sudamina (distended sweat glands) appear vesicular. They disappear spontaneously.

Occasionally a pale purple discoloration is in evidence at the surface of these lesions. They occur anywhere over the body, often in the areas to which forceps were applied. Extensive lesions sometimes occur over the anterior thighs and legs and over the back. They disappear spontaneously in days or weeks. During the process of resolution the lesions become soft and fluctuant. Undisturbed, they rarely become infected.

Harlequin color change is a rare, peculiar discrepancy in color between the two longitudinal halves of the body, extending from the forehead to the symphysis pubis. A curiosity of no known pathologic significance, it is elicited by placing the baby on his side for several minutes. The dependent half of the body turns pink while the upper half remains pale. The colors are reversed when the infant is turned onto the opposite side. The same phenomenon may occur in the supine position.

Lanugo is fine hair, sometimes barely visible, that is characteristic of the newborn period. It is more noticeable in premature infants and is most easily seen over the shoulders, back, forehead, and cheeks.

Milia are minute, white papules on the chin, nose, cheeks, and forehead. They represent distended sebaceous glands that disappear spontaneously in several days or weeks. *Sudamina* are tiny vesicles over the face and neck that are formed by distention of sweat glands (Fig. 6-7).

Erythema toxicum is a pink papular rash on which vesicles are often superimposed (Fig. 6-8). The vesicles frequently appear purulent and are sometimes confused with the lesions characteristic of staphylococcal pyoderma. They appear anywhere over the body within 24 to 48 hours after birth and resolve spontaneously after several days. The vesicles contain eosinophils that are demonstrable on a smear prepared with Wright's

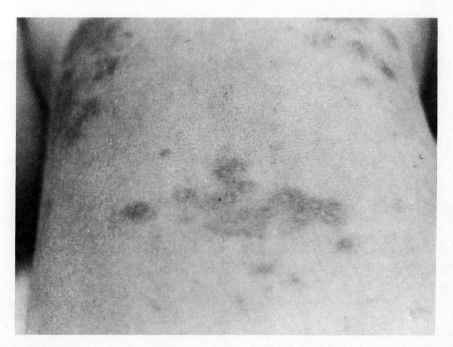

Fig. 6-8. Erythema toxicum. Patches of swollen redness with superimposed vesicles, often mistaken for staphylococcal lesions. Lesions in this instance are distributed over the abdomen and thorax.

stain. The rash is innocuous, and its etiology is unknown.

Sclerema is hardening of the skin and subcutaneous tissue associated with life-threatening disorders such as septicemia, shock, and severe cold stress. As a rule, the cheeks and buttocks are first involved, then the calves and thighs, and eventually perhaps the entire body. The skin is so hard it feels wooden. Sclerema should not be confused with subcutaneous fat necrosis, which is confined to small areas and is usually present in babies who are otherwise well.

Café au lait spots are so named because their color resembles coffee to which milk has been added. In black babies they may be a darker brown color. They are irregularly shaped oval lesions of varying size and distribution, which are not elevated above the skin surface. If six or more of these spots are present, suspicion of neurofibromatosis (an autosomal dominant neurocutaneous syndrome) is appropriate.

Puncture wounds are the result of the attachment of electrodes from fetal monitors. In breech presentations they are incurred on the buttocks or thighs. Rarely, electrodes are accidentally applied to eyelids and other parts of the face. Occasionally, these puncture wounds become infected.

Head

After vaginal deliveries from the vertex position, molding of the head is apparent to some degree in virtually all neonates as a result of pressures exerted during the birth process. The change in shape is more pronounced in first-born infants and in those whose heads are engaged for prolonged periods. Pressure during the usual vertex delivery causes flattening of the forehead with a gradual rise to an apex posteriorly and an abrupt drop at the occiput (Fig. 2-9). In brow presentations the forehead may be unusually prominent, rather than flattened as in vertex deliveries. When the forces of the birth process are not exerted on the cranium, its spherical contour is undisturbed. Thus the head is characteristically

spherical in an infant born from the breech position or delivered by cesarean section. These modes of delivery can be presumed from inspection of the cranial contour. Molding generally disappears by the end of the first or second day of life.

The *cranium* comprises six bones (Fig. 6-9): the frontal, occipital, two parietals, and two temporals. The *frontal bone* runs the width of the cranium at its anterior third. The *occipital bone* occupies the width of the cranium at its posterior third, whereas the two *parietal bones* are situated in the middle third between the frontal and occipital bones. The *temporal bones* are the most lateral and inferior of the cranial bones. They are adjacent to the parietals.

The *sutures* and *fontanelles* of the cranium are extremely important landmarks (Fig. 6-9). They are bands of connective tissue that separate the six major cranial bones. Sutures are palpable as cracks; fontanelles are broader "soft spots" at specific locations. The *coronal suture* runs from one side of the cranium to the other, separating the frontal bone (the forehead) from the two parietal bones posterior to it. In some infants a *metopic suture* bisects the frontal bone into right and left halves. It extends from the frontmost angle of the anterior fontanelle downward toward the nasal bridge. It is usually as wide as the other normal sutures, sometimes wider. The *lambdoid suture*, situated toward the posterior third of the skull, runs from one side to the other, separating the occipital bone from the two parietal bones anterior to it. The *sagittal suture* runs in an anteroposterior direction in the midline, terminating anteriorly at the coronal suture and posteriorly at the lambdoid suture. It separates the two parietal bones. The *squamosal (temporal) sutures* also run in an anteroposterior direction, but they are situated just at the level of the earlobes. They, like the sagittal suture, terminate anteriorly at the coronal suture and posteriorly at the lambdoid suture.

The *fontanelles* are relatively wide, soft areas at the junctions of each of the sutures. The *an-*

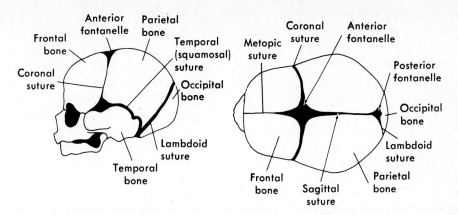

Fig. 6-9. Neonatal cranial bones, sutures, and fontanelles from lateral view and from above. (Modified from Crelin, E.S.: Anatomy of the newborn, an atlas, Philadelphia, 1969, Lea & Febiger.)

terior fontanelle is at the junction of the sagittal and coronal sutures. It is diamond shaped and variable in size. It may be small as a result of molding, but it enlarges as the molding disappears. At its widest point it may measure up to 5 cm. The *posterior fontanelle* is triangular; it measures 1 cm or less in width and is situated at the junction of the sagittal and lambdoid sutures. Four other fontanelles are of less clinical significance. They are at the junctions formed by the squamosal sutures with the coronal and lambdoid sutures.

Appraisal of the head by external examination depends on an appreciation of the contours that are expected as a result of various presentations and on the status of sutures and fontanelles, particularly the anterior fontanelle. At birth and for a day or two afterward, as a result of molding, the edges of the cranial bones may overlap, obliterating the sutures. The lines of overlap seem to be ridges when palpated, and the fontanelles are small (Fig. 6-10). Later, as the shape of the cranium becomes more normal, the bones separate and the sutures can be felt as cracks several millimeters in width. The anterior fontanelle now expands to its full size. In premature infants the overlapping is often easily seen (Fig. 6-10). It may

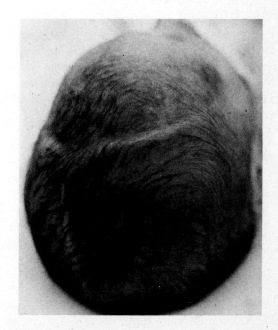

Fig. 6-10. Overlapped cranial bones producing visible ridge in a small premature infant. Easily visible overlapping does not often occur in term infants.

persist for weeks in the smallest infants. In malnourished infants the sutures may be wide at birth, perhaps over 1 cm, because of impaired growth of the cranial bones. The anterior fontanelle is large for the same reason, but it is also flat and soft. Normally arterial pulsations may be seen and bruits heard. Inordinately large, flat, anterior fontanelles and wide sutures also suggest the presence of hypothyroidism, osteogenesis imperfecta, and cleidocranial dysostosis. Unusually *small anterior fontanelles* are the rule in very small premature infants as the result of severe molding during vertex deliveries, in microcephaly of any etiology, and in craniosynostosis. On the other hand, an abnormal increase in intracranial pressure actually separates the cranial bones, expanding suture lines and fontanelles. Rather than being flat and soft, the anterior fontanelle is firm and bulging as a function of high intracranial pressure. These signs, especially those in the anterior fontanelle, are present in babies with hydrocephalus (Fig. 6-1), meningitis, subdural hematoma, and cerebral edema. If there is doubt concerning the firmness and fullness of the anterior fontanelle, the baby should be taken from the crib and held erect in one arm while the fontanelle is palpated. A pathologically bulging fontanelle does not soften and flatten.

Eyes

Eyelids are frequently edematous during the first 2 days after delivery, and the infant rarely opens them. Separation of lids must be accomplished gently because forceful traction easily everts them, thus precluding an adequate view of the eyes.

Instillation of silver nitrate drops into the eyes at birth may cause *chemical conjunctivitis* to appear within an hour or soon thereafter. The resultant purulent discharge disappears without treatment in 1 or 2 days with no residual difficulty.

Purulent conjunctival exudate is also a sign of *conjunctivitis* resulting from infection (Chapter 13). Most commonly, these infections are caused by staphylococci and by a variety of gram-negative rods. Gonorrheal infection, which may also involve the eye itself, occasionally occurs despite application of silver nitrate drops that are ordinarily effective in preventing it.

Subconjunctival hemorrhages are frequent. They result from pressure on the fetal head during delivery, with resultant impairment of venous return and rupture of capillaries in the sclera. They can be seen in the sclerae and are of no pathologic significance, even when the entire sclera is reddened by extravasated blood (Fig. 2-13). *Retinal hemorrhages* are produced by the same mechanism, and they may occur in as many as 10% of normal neonates. They are flame shaped or round and are thought to be harmless. However, extensive hemorrhage over a large segment of the retina usually indicates the presence of a subdural hematoma.

Cataracts, if present, must be identified at the time of the first examination. Cataracts are opacities of the lens that can vary from pinpoint size to involvement of the entire lens. Occasionally they develop several days or weeks after birth. If the entire lens is affected, they are usually seen easily by shining a light into each eye, with the light source held to one side. If the opacity is

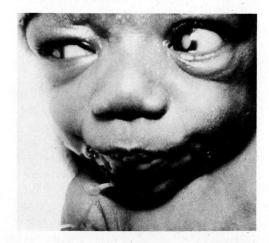

Fig. 6-11. Bilateral cataracts. Note white pupils. Entire lenses were involved. Infant had congenital rubella.

small, it can be identified only with an ophthalmoscope. Bilateral cataracts involving the entire lens are illustrated in Fig. 6-11. In this picture the pupils are white because the opacified lens behind them reflects the light, which is applied close to the eyes from the side of the face. White pupils may also be seen in the presence of lesions deeper in the eye, such as retinoblastoma. Normally the pupils appear black to the bare eye of the examiner when light is directed at them. Cataracts are usually bilateral, but they are sometimes unilateral. They are a major manifestation of intrauterine rubella infection (Chapter 13) and are occasionally seen in cytomegalovirus infection (Chapter 13). They may be hereditary, being transmitted as a dominant trait from an affected parent. In congenital galactosemia, cataracts sometimes appear several weeks after birth.

Corneal opacities are also discerned by directing light to the eyes (Fig. 6-12). They occur after trauma, in association with congenital glaucoma, and as a result of infection such as herpesvirus and congenital rubella. Compare the illustrations

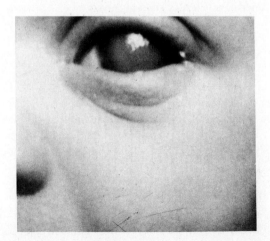

Fig. 6-12. Corneal opacity, unilateral. Cornea is white, its surface rough; overall appearance is that of ground glass. This baby had congenital glaucoma due to intrauterine rubella infection. The cornea is thus abnormally large.

of the cataracts (Fig. 6-11) and the corneal opacity (Fig. 6-12). The two lesions are clearly distinguishable from each other. In the presence of a cataract, the iris can be seen because the affected structure (the lens) is behind it. The cornea is smooth and clear. The corneal opacity involves the eye's outside window (the cornea), and the underlying iris is thus obscure. Furthermore, the surface of the involved cornea is rough, much like ground glass.

Iris coloboma is one of the most common congenital malformations of the eye. The defect varies from a small notch at the inner iris margin to segmental absence, usually at the inferior portion. It is generally limited to the iris and is thus not associated with visual difficulty. Infrequently, the defect involves deeper eye structures such as the retina, macula, and optic nerve, thus impairing normal vision. Rarely, colobomas are associated with serious generalized malformation syndromes.

Nose

Neonates must breathe through the nose; they cannot ordinarily breathe through the mouth. Any obstruction to the nasal passages thus causes some degree of respiratory distress. Partial or complete occlusion may be caused by mucus secretion that has not been removed or by choanal atresia or stenosis. The latter are congenital anomalies of the posterior nares, which may be life threatening (Chapter 8). The nose sometimes is displaced to one side by pressure exerted in utero, particularly in association with oligohydramnios.

Mouth and throat

Complete visualization of the mouth and pharynx is difficult when the tongue is depressed; such attempts are usually met with strong reflex protrusion of the depressed tongue. However, an excellent view is obtained by stimulating a cry before gently depressing the tongue. Examination of the mouth is extremely important for the identification of a cleft palate, which often occurs in the absence of a cleft lip. Cleft palate may involve either the hard or soft palates or both. Occasionally only the uvula is cleft.

Precocious teeth occur infrequently. They are most often situated at the lower central incisor positions (Fig. 6-13). When covered with membranous tissue, they are pink rather than white. If detachment is imminent, they should be removed to prevent aspiration.

Epstein's pearls are small, white papular structures, one on each side of the midline of the hard palate. They are insignificant and usually disappear within a few weeks after birth.

The *frenulum* of the tongue is a sharp, thin ridge of tissue that arises in the midline from the base of the tongue and attaches to its undersurface for varying distances toward the tip. When the attachment extends far forward, a concavity (or a groove) is evident at the tip of the tongue on its upper surface. This condition is referred to as tongue-tie. It rarely if ever interferes with feeding, nor does it produce a speech impediment in childhood. "Clipping of the tongue" by incising the frenulum is therefore rarely indicated, especially since there is some danger of severing a rather large vein in the area of the frenulum. Furthermore, the procedure creates a portal of entry for infection.

Neck

The neonate's neck is characteristically short; abnormalities are infrequent. A *webbed neck* in females is seen in Turner's syndrome. Webbing is characterized by redundancy of skin that extends bilaterally from the posterolateral aspect of the neck, down to the medial portions of the shoulders along the superior margins of the underlying trapezius muscles. *Branchial cleft cysts* may be evident on the lateral aspects of the neck, along the anterior margin of the sternomastoid muscle. They are generally firm, 1 cm or less in diameter, and are covered by normal skin. More commonly, and in the same areas, dimples are evident. These are *branchial cleft sinuses*. Branchial cleft cysts or sinuses are rarely of clinical significance, unless they become infected. They are inherited autosomal dominant traits. *Thyro-*

glossal cysts are superficially evident as subcutaneous structures in the midline of the anterior neck at the level of the larynx above it. They indicate the presence of a *thyroglossal duct,* which is an abnormal remnant of thyroid gland formation during embryogenesis. The duct extends deeply into the neck, often opening at its deep end onto the surface of the tongue at its base (root). The duct may contain thyroid tissue. Later surgical excision is generally indicated. *Goiter* (enlargement of the thyroid gland) is a visible, easily palpated mass in the midline of the anterior neck immediately inferior to, and partially overlying, the larynx. Goiters are generally the result of thyroid medication used in treatment of maternal thyroid disorders. Goiters are not often functional; rarely, however, they are associated with *neonatal hyperthyroidism*.

Thorax

The ribs are flexible; slight sternal retraction is sometimes evident during normal respiration. The *xiphoid cartilage* is at the lower end of the sternum. It may curve anteriorly to produce a prominent pointed protrusion beneath the skin that disappears in several weeks.

Rib fracture may be present in the neonate. Fig. 6-14 depicts the fracture of two ribs that were palpable as rounded, bony masses. They are seen as two opaque, white nodules in the lower left chest that are not present in the lower right chest. Resuscitation was attempted by the ineffective and dangerous method of squeezing the thoracic cage. Vigorous application of this useless procedure resulted in fracture of the anterior portion of the fourth and fifth ribs.

Supernumerary nipples (Fig. 6-15) are occasionally noted inferior and medial to the normal ones, less often they occur superior and lateral to the normal nipples. They are harmless pink or pigmented spots that vary from a few millimeters in diameter to the size of normal nipples, but they do not contain glandular tissue.

Breast enlargement may occur in some infants (Fig. 6-16). It appears on the third day, and toward the end of the first week a milklike substance

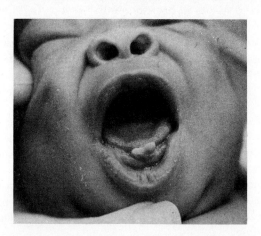

Fig. 6-13. Precocious teeth in the usual location. Teeth were sufficiently loose to threaten spontaneous detachment and aspiration, and they were removed.

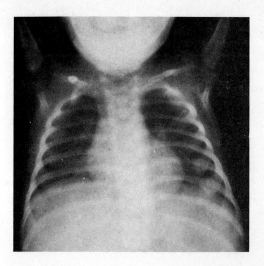

Fig. 6-14. Rib fractures, healing. Round opacities in the ribs to the left of cardiac apex are sites of callus formation during healing process. They were palpated as round, bony masses.

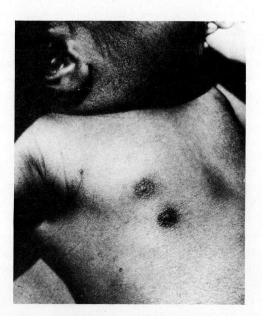

Fig. 6-15. Supernumerary nipple, unusually well developed. The upper nipple is the supernumerary one. Above and lateral to it, near the axilla, is a small spot that is another rudimentary extra nipple.

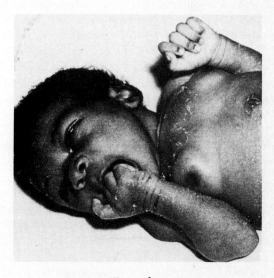

Fig. 6-16. Breast hypertrophy.

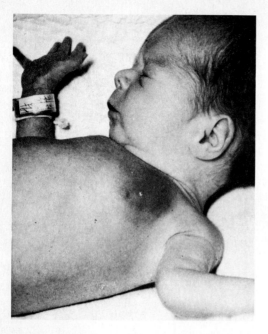

Fig. 6-17. Breast abscess. Note purulent drainage just superior to nipple.

("witch's milk") may be evident. Massaging such breasts with various preparations is a common lay practice that often produces breast abscess. Breast hypertrophy should not be confused with *breast abscess* (Fig. 6-17), which involves asymmetric swelling around the areola and severe erythema of the skin. Pus, which is usually yellow or blood tinged, may exude either from the nipple or through inflamed skin; it should not be confused, therefore, with "witch's milk," which is blank white.

Lungs

Physical examination of the lungs is only a first step, but an indispensable one, in the identification of respiratory disorders. Radiologic and blood gas studies should follow if the suspicion of a respiratory disorder is aroused by positive physical findings. The respiratory pattern should be observed before the infant is disturbed. Normal neonates breathe at rates varying between 40 and 60 respirations per minute. Rapid rates are likely to be present for the first few hours after birth. Fluctuations of respiratory rates are the rule, and for this reason several assessments may be necessary before one can conclude that an abnormality exists. *Periodic breathing*, a frequent normal finding in premature infants that requires no therapy, is characterized by sporadic episodes in which respirations cease for up to 10 seconds. Periodic breathing is not associated with cyanosis or bradycardia, and it is rare during the first 24 hours of life. It should not be confused with apneic episodes, which are of longer duration, often cause generalized cyanosis, and may occur at any time.

In the normal neonate, respiratory movements are predominantly diaphragmatic. The thoracic cage remains relatively immobile while the abdomen rises and falls with inspiration and expiration. Occasionally the immobile chest gives the false appearance of being drawn inward as the abdomen protrudes with each inspiration. This should not be confused with the retractions that characterize abnormal respiration.

Respiratory difficulties can be identified by simply observing the infant. A number of abnormal signs are clearly indicative of distress, generalized cyanosis being the most obvious and serious. A sustained rate in excess of 60 respirations per minute *(tachypnea)* after 3 or 4 hours of age is abnormal, but this condition should be ascertained by obtaining several counts of no less than 30 seconds' duration. Irregular respirations associated with repeated *apneic episodes* are often the result of depressed central nervous system function caused by severe hypoxia or intracranial hemorrhage. *Retractions* indicate obstruction to airflow at any level of the respiratory tract from the nose to the alveoli. They are visible with each inspiration and are characterized by indrawing of the thoracic wall at the sternum, between the ribs, above the clavicles, and below the inferior costal margins (Fig. 6-4). The *respiratory grunt* is an unequivocal sign of difficulty. It is a fascinating compensatory mechanism by which an infant attempts to retain air to increase arterial PO_2 (Chapter 8), to blow air off when trapping occurs, or to hasten transfer of fetal lung fluid across alveolar walls. An audible sigh during each expiration is a variant of the respiratory grunt that serves the same purpose. Air hunger is commonly associated with *flaring of the nostrils* (alae nasi) during each inspiration. As a rule, an infant in respiratory distress has more than one of the abnormal signs just described.

No matter how accurate and well phrased they may be, descriptions of *auscultatory findings* cannot replace experience with the stethoscope. Nevertheless, several introductory remarks may serve to properly orient the examiner. Auscultatory signs in the lungs are of less value in the neonate than in any other pediatric age group. The chest is so small that localization of findings is often impossible. The diminutive lung effectively transmits breath sounds from one region to another. The absence of breath sounds in one part of the lung may not be appreciated because the sounds from the unaffected areas are transmitted from a distance. With experience, diminution of air exchange can be confidently detected, particularly when there is a discrepancy between the two lungs. Diminished breath sounds occur in hyaline membrane disease, atelectasis, emphysema, pneumothorax, and as a function of shallow respirations from any cause. Fine *rales* are produced in terminal bronchioles and alveoli by the rush of air through fluid within them. These rales are classically described as crackling in character. They can be reproduced with some degree of accuracy by rubbing your own hair between two fingers as close to your ear as possible. Rales are heard in some infants with hyaline membrane disease, pneumonia, and pulmonary edema, and occasionally in normal babies immediately after birth. They are sometimes audible only after deep inspiration, which must be induced by stimulating a cry. *Rhonchi* are coarse sounds that resemble snoring. They emanate from large bronchi as air rushes through fluid contained within them.

Rhonchi are most frequently present after aspiration of oral secretions or feedings.

Heart

Inspection occasionally reveals a localized pulsation on the chest wall at about the fifth intercostal space in the midclavicular line, toward the lateral half of the left hemithorax. The pulsations are more evident in small babies with thin chest walls. If pulsations are prominent in the epigastrium, the heart is probably enlarged considerably.

By *palpation*, the normal apical impulse can be identified at the fifth intercostal space. Ascertainment of cardiac position is particularly important in dyspneic infants. Detection of an abnormal position early in the examination is an important initial step in establishing a correct diagnosis. A shift in the mediastinum caused by pneumothorax, for example, moves the apical impulse away from the affected side of the chest (Chapter 8). Pneumothorax in the right chest thus causes a shift of the mediastinum to the left; the apical impulse can be felt farther toward the left lateral chest wall than is normal. On the other hand, if the left chest is affected, the apical beat is palpable closer to the midline of the chest or sometimes to the right of it. Such cardiac displacements also occur in diaphragmatic hernia, which usually affects the left chest (Chapter 8). In the rare occurrence of bilateral pneumothorax, the point of maximal cardiac impulse is displaced downward toward the epigastrium. Abnormal apical location also occurs in dextrocardia, which is a mirror image reversal of cardiac position; the apex is in the right chest. If abdominal organs are also reversed, the anomalous position of the heart may or may not be significant in terms of abnormal cardiovascular function. However, if the abdominal viscera are normally placed and the position of the heart is reversed, cardiac anomalies are more likely. The normal locations of abdominal organs are described on p. 168.

Auscultation is the most informative component of the physical examination of the heart. The ability to perceive abnormalities by evaluating heart sounds depends on continuous, thoughtful practice. The first and second heart sounds are normally clear and well defined. In the neonate they acoustically resemble the syllables toc-tic. The second sound is somewhat higher in pitch and sharper than the first. Heart rates normally fluctuate between 120 and 160 beats/min. In agitated states a rate of 200 beats/min may occur transiently. The heart rate of premature infants is usually between 130 and 170 beats/min, and during occasional episodes of bradycardia it may slow to 70 beats/min or less. *Murmurs* are erroneously considered to be regularly indicative of congenital cardiac malformations, when in fact over 90% of those detected during the neonatal period are not associated with anomalies. Many murmurs are transient. Conversely, murmurs are sometimes absent in seriously malformed hearts. Most murmurs are systolic; they occur after the first sound and end at or before the second sound. Continuous murmurs extend beyond the second sound into diastole. According to their intensity, murmurs are Grade I (softest) to Grade VI (loudest). Murmurs heard soon after birth are likely to indicate cardiac malformations. The appearance of a murmur at any time requires an evaluation of several additional parameters such as the peripheral pulses, blood pressure, the size and consistency of liver, and the size and contour of the heart as revealed by a chest film.

The state of the *peripheral pulses* is important. Brachial, radial, and femoral pulses are the most easily evaluated. Normal pulses are readily discernible, but the examiner's capacity to assess abnormal weakness and fullness depends on careful and experienced observations in normal neonates. Weakness of all pulses is indicative of a diminished cardiac output, peripheral vasoconstriction, or both. This occurs in "hypoplastic left heart syndrome," in the hypoxic myocardium of an asphyxiated baby or in cardiac failure from other causes, and in septic or hemorrhagic shock. Excessively full pulses ("bounding pulses") generally appear several days after birth in premature

infants who have developed a large left-to-right shunt from the aorta to the pulmonary artery through a patent ductus arteriosus (see Chapter 8). Another group of malformations is indicated by a strong right radial pulse and a weak left one. This suggests obstruction to blood flow along the aortic arch resulting from a coarctation that is proximal to (above) the entry of the ductus arteriosus into the aorta. On the other hand, weak femoral pulses and strong radial pulses suggest coarctation distal to (below) the ductus arteriosus. Most aortic coarctations are preductal (proximal to the entry of the ductus). The presence of a murmur also requires assessment of *liver size and consistency*. In babies with right-sided congestive heart failure, the liver enlarges; its inferior edge is palpable 5 to 6 cm below the right costal margin. The enlarged liver is firm because it is tightly distended by blood that has not progressed through the failing heart. Its inferior margin is thus easily palpated. A chest film is indispensable for initial assessment of *cardiac size and contour*. *Blood pressure* is simply and accurately measured with a Doppler apparatus and an ordinary blood pressure cuff. Some types of Doppler equipment provide systolic and diastolic readings; other less expensive types are adequate even though they are limited to systolic readings. The cuff should be no wider than 1 in; in larger babies a 2 in cuff may be essential. Blood pressure readings are usually obtained more easily at the popliteal space with the cuff around the thigh. A loose cuff may result in spuriously high readings; an excessively tight cuff may yield falsely low readings. If the peripheral pulses are weak, the baby may be hypotensive. If the pulse is stronger in one extremity than in another, widely discrepant blood pressures may be demonstrated, and the presence of a coarctation is likely. For intensive care of sick neonates, blood pressures are recorded directly from an aortic catheter.

Abdomen

Inspection. The contour of the abdomen should be noted before it is palpated. It is ordinarily cylindric, sometimes protruding slightly in normal term infants. Several gross abnormalities are apparent on inspection. *Distention* in its most severe form is characterized by tightly drawn skin through which engorged subcutaneous vessels are easily seen. *Localized bulging* at one or both flanks suggests enlarged kidneys, usually hydronephrosis (Fig. 6-2). A grotesque abnormality of contour characterizes the rare malformation known as congenital absence of abdominal musculature ("prune belly" syndrome), in which severe renal anomalies are also present. The anterior aspect of the abdomen is sunken, or perhaps slightly protuberant, whereas the intestines, which are covered only by skin and a thin layer of subcutaneous tissue, bulge pendulously from the flanks (Fig. 6-18).

Palpation. With rare exceptions the edge of the *liver* is normally palpable below the right costal margin, often as far as 3 cm inferior to it. The tip of the spleen can sometimes be felt in normal infants. Examination of the abdomen must include palpation of each *kidney*, and this is most easily accomplished immediately after birth, when the intestines are not yet distended with air. With the infant supine, a finger is placed at the posterior flank (costovertebral angle) to maintain upward pressure while the other hand presses downward toward the posteriorly placed finger. The kidney can be felt as an oval structure between the finger and hand. The lower poles of each kidney are normally situated approximately 1 or 2 cm above the level of the umbilicus. If enlargement is present, they are below this level. By simple palpation the astute examiner can identify approximately 90% of gross renal anomalies. *Bladder distention* should be sought in the suprapubic region. If present, a firm globular mass is palpable. If it persists to any degree after voiding, the bladder is incompletely emptied, and an obstruction may be present at the outlet. *Masses* that are perceptible elsewhere in the abdomen are usually of intestinal origin.

Diastasis recti is an inconsequential longitudinal gap in the abdominal midline between the

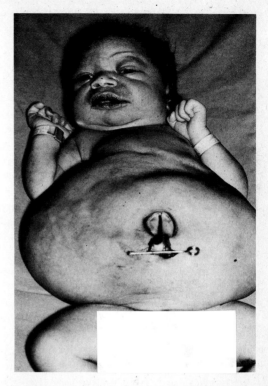

Fig. 6-18. Congenital absence of abdominal muscle ("prune belly" syndrome). Massive bilateral hydronephrosis and hydroureter were present.

two rectus muscles. It can be palpated from the epigastrium to the umbilicus as a linear absence of abdominal wall musculature approximately 1 cm in width. When the infant cries, thereby raising intraabdominal pressure, a bulge is visible through the linear gap in musculature. Diastasis recti disappears within a few weeks.

The normal *umbilical cord* is blue-white and moist at birth. Within 24 hours it begins to dry and becomes dull and yellow-brown. Later it turns black-brown and shrivels considerably. In this gangrenous state it sloughs from its attachment at approximately 1 week of age. After birth, the cut section of the cord reveals three blood vessels (two arteries and one vein). A diagram of the cut surface can be seen on p. 4. The arteries appear to be smaller, round, papular protrusions from the cut surface; the vein is larger and oval. The arterial walls are thick; their lumens are obliterated by vasospasm. In contrast, the venous wall is thin and relaxed; the lumen is thus easily discerned. On the cut surface, the relative positions of the three vessels vary considerably, depending on the level at which the cord is cut, because the vessels pursue a spiral course along the entire length of the cord. A *single umbilical artery* is reason for an assiduous search for congenital malformations of any type. In some reports a significant number of these infants have major congenital anomalies. Other reports assert that there is not a higher incidence of anomalies in surviving infants with a single umbilical artery; the higher incidence of malformations only occurs in babies who do not survive.

If meconium has not been passed by the end of the first day of life, *patency of the anus* should be ascertained by inserting the tip of a thermometer or a plastic feeding tube for a distance not in excess of 1 cm.

Inguinal hernias occur most frequently in males and in a large number of low birth weight babies as well. They are readily discernible when the characteristic swelling is present in the inguinal canal; they are usually unilateral, occasionally bilateral. The swelling in males may extend into the scrotum. Sometimes the hernia is not perceptible until the infant cries. The hernias contain intestine, but in females the ovary and fallopian tubes are also occasionally present. The ovary is palpable as a movable nodular mass in the inguinal canal that is not unlike a swollen lymph node. Surgical correction is required. Infrequently intestinal contents are trapped (incarcerated) in the inguinal canal and cannot be returned (reduced) into the abdomen. Vomiting and progressive abdominal distention appear, and immediate surgical intervention is necessary.

Male genitalia

The *prepuce* covers the entire *glans penis* so that the external meatus is not visible. The pre-

puce is not retractable in the neonate and sometimes cannot be displaced until 4 to 6 months of age. It thus should never be forcibly retracted. This condition is not phimosis, and it is not an indication for circumcision. The trauma of forceful retraction is thought by some to be responsible for phimosis later on. According to a statement by the American Academy of Pediatrics, *"there is no absolute medical indication for routine circumcision of the newborn. It is not an essential component of adequate total health care."* Good penile hygiene accomplishes as much. If the ventral surface of the glans is not covered by preputial tissue, *hypospadias* is present. Hypospadias is characterized by an anomalous position of the urethral meatus on the ventral portion of the glans penis, rather than at its center. It may also be situated on the ventral surface of the penile shaft anywhere along its length.

In term infants the *testes* are in the *scrotum*. In premature infants the testes are in the inguinal canal, or they may not be palpable. The scrotum varies in size in relation to maturity. In premature infants it is small and close to the perineum. In term babies the scrotum is large, hanging loosely at a greater distance from the perineum. The term infant's scrotum is rugated (wrinkled) over its entire surface, back to its perineal attachment. The scrotum of the premature infant is less extensively rugated, becoming smoother toward the perineal attachment. Scrotal rugation is one of the external signs used for the assessment of gestational age (see Chapter 5). A *hydrocele* is frequently observed in the scrotum, particularly in term infants. It is a unilateral (sometimes bilateral) accumulation of fluid that surrounds the testis. When a hydrocele is unilateral, the affected side of the scrotum is larger, appearing tightly cystic. Transillumination of a hydrocele reveals a striking translucency. In an inguinal hernia the scrotal contents comprise intestine or fluid (or both). It is thus opaque to transillumination, or considerably less translucent than the hydrocele. A hydrocele usually disappears spontaneously in a few days or weeks.

Female genitalia

In term babies the *labia minora* are sometimes more prominent than the *labia majora;* in premature infants this is almost the rule. The *clitoris* varies in size. It may be so large as to confound determination of the baby's sex. The diagnosis of adrenogenital syndrome, an endocrine disorder that involves excessive secretions of androgenic and other hormones from the adrenal gland, may then be made. In the affected neonate, life-threatening electrolyte disturbances and dehydration may occur rapidly within a few days after birth.

The *hymenal tag* is a normal redundant segment of the hymen that protrudes from the floor of the vagina and disappears in several weeks. During the first week of life, a milk-white mucoid discharge, which is sometimes blood tinged, may be evident in the vagina. This is a physiologic manifestation of maternal hormonal influences that disappears within 2 weeks.

Extremities

The extremities should be examined for malformations and trauma. Malformations frequently involve the fingers. *Polydactyly* is an excessive number of digits on the hands or feet. In its most common form it consists of a rudimentary digit (digitus postminimus) attached to the lateral aspect of the little finger by a thin pedicle (Fig. 6-19). It is treated by firmly tying a silk suture around the pedicle, close to the surface of the normal finger. Gangrene of the anomalous digit ensues in a few days, and it falls away. Less commonly an extra, fully formed digit is present. *Syndactyly* is the fusion of two digits into one structure (Fig. 6-20), and it most commonly involves the toes.

Fractures have been discussed in Chapter 2. The clavicle, humerus, and femur are respectively involved in descending order of frequency. Fractures should be suspected in any baby who fails to move one extremity as extensively as the others. Malposition and a visible local deformity at the fracture site are often helpful signs.

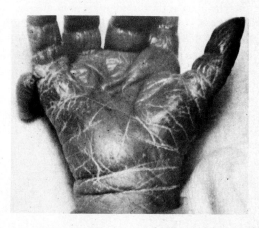

Fig. 6-19. Digitus postminimus (see text). Hypotrophic finger hangs by a thin pedicle from lateral aspect of fifth finger.

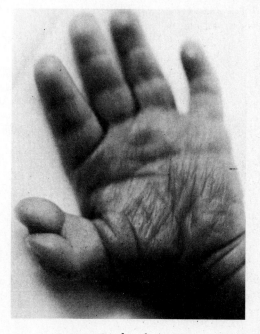

Fig. 6-20. Syndactyly (see text).

Clavicles must be palpated to ascertain their presence as well as to detect fractures. Absence of the clavicles, either total or segmental, is characteristic of *cleidocranial dysostosis* (Fig. 6-21), an inherited disorder of bone formation in the skull, the clavicles, and occasionally the pubic bone. Absence of the clavicles permits innocuous

anterior displacement of the shoulders so that they almost meet in the midline (Fig. 6-21).

Congenital ring constrictions (annular or amniotic bands) are poorly understood malformations that occur infrequently. They affect the extremities, which are thought to become entangled in a local early rupture of the amniotic membrane. Subsequent growth occurs in the presence of constricting amniotic bands. In the extreme, amputation occurs, either of an extremity somewhere along its length or of one or more digits. Milder expressions of this disorder are seen as banded depressions of the skin that are much like a tight rubber band around the extremity (Fig. 6-22). The most common sites of involvement in order of frequency are the fingers, toes, ankle, leg, forearm, and arm. Amniotic bands and the amputations with which they are sometimes associated may involve more than one extremity but are usually unilateral.

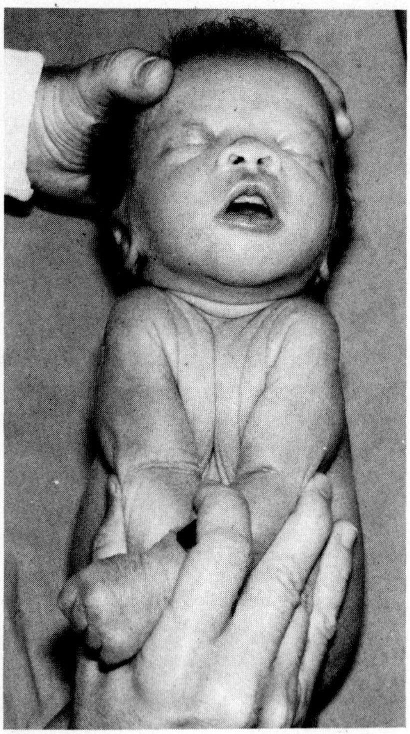

Fig. 6-21. Cleidocranial dysostosis (congenital absence of clavicles). If clavicles were not examined as a routine part of examination, this major syndrome would not have been identified in the neonate, when it should be. Shoulders are drawn anteriorly, and when compressed, they meet in midline.

Fig. 6-22. Congenital amniotic bands above the ankle.

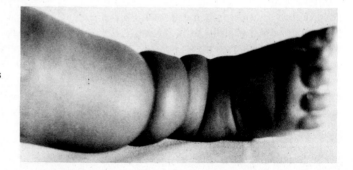

Neurologic evaluation

Abnormal neurologic signs may be transient or persistent. They may disappear by the time the infant is discharged from the nursery, or they may be present throughout the nursery stay. *(Predictions of later brain dysfunction can seldom be made with acceptable accuracy on the basis of neurologic abnormalities during the newborn period.)*

Observations should be made with as little disturbance to the baby as possible. Reflexes that require the greatest degree of disturbance should be elicited toward the end of the examination. Thus *spontaneous movements* should be studied first. Infants who are generally depressed will move little or not at all. They are hypotonic as well. Intrauterine asphyxia, or hypoxia at any time, is the most common cause of this neuromuscular abnormality. Drugs administered to the mother are also frequent causes of depression. These drugs include analgesics (Demerol), hypnotics (barbiturates, magnesium sulfate, alcohol), and local anesthetics (lidocaine). Central nervous system infections, bacterial or nonbacterial, and metabolic disturbances (hypoglycemia, hypothyroidism) also cause depression. Trauma to the central nervous system, most often in the form of cerebral contusion or subdural hematoma, is an additional cause of diminished or absent spontaneous activity.

Spontaneous hyperirritability and exaggerated responses to ordinary tactile or acoustic stimuli are abnormal. These responses may range from severe agitation or jitteriness to frank convulsions. They may thus be manifested as localized twitches, gross rhythmic repetitive jerks of one or more muscle groups (myoclonus), or generalized clonic convulsions. There is little to be gained in attempting to localize central nervous system lesions based on these localized convulsive phenomena, since in the neonate there is generally no such correlation. There is also little use in attempting to differentiate between a severely agitated state characterized by ceaseless movement and a frank convulsion. Usually they are of equal significance. These irritative phenomena are most common during recovery from asphyxia, after a period of depression. They also occur in babies of narcotic-addicted mothers (heroin or morphine withdrawal) and among infants of mothers who are habituated to barbiturates (phenobarbital withdrawal). Hypocalcemia, hypomagnesemia, and hypoglycemia may cause irritative phenomena. Hypocalcemia does not cause convulsive activity (tremors to seizures) during the first 48 to 72 hours after birth. Neonatal hyperthyroidism and pyridoxine dependency are rare causes. Maternal administration of local anesthetics such as lidocaine may produce depression at first, but this is followed by convulsions. Intracranial hemorrhage and, occasionally, central nervous system infection may also produce irritative responses early in their courses.

Asymmetry in movement of the extremities indicates weakness, paralysis, or bone fracture. In brachial plexus palsy, for example, the affected upper extremity is hypoactive or immobile. Failure to move the lower extremities suggests a spinal cord injury. Asymmetry of movement or tone is always abnormal.

Muscle tone is extremely important in the neurologic evaluation of neonates. The normal infant maintains some degree of flexion in all the extremities, and extension by the examiner of any one of them is followed by at least a partial return to the previous position of flexion. Flexion posture is less pronounced in premature infants. Infants who experience intrauterine hypoxia are hypotonic; they may not be flexed at rest. Furthermore, straightening of the extremities is not followed by return to flexion. Poor head control, described later, is additional evidence of abnormally diminished muscle tone.

The elicitation of certain reflex responses is essential for assessment of the infant's neurologic status. The *grasp reflex* is normally strong in term infants. It is elicited by placing a finger across the palm at the base of the fingers. In response, the examiner's finger may be grasped so firmly that, using both hands, the infant can often be raised off the surface of the crib. This response is considerably more feeble in premature babies or in depressed infants. It is asymmetric in some cases of brachial plexus palsy (Klumpke type), being absent or weak on the affected side.

The *rooting reflex* is activated by lightly stroking the angle of the lips. The baby turns his head to the stroked side. Recently fed infants and those who are lethargic or depressed merely purse the lips or do not respond at all. Vigorous infants turn the head briskly and instantly, pursuing the finger as long as contact with the lips is maintained.

The *suck* is evaluated by inserting a sterile nipple into the mouth. In normal infants, particularly those who are hungry, the response is immediate, coordinated, and forceful. Recently fed infants, premature babies, and those who are depressed respond with varying degrees of feebleness.

The *knee jerk* is normally brisk. It is weak in depressed infants, exaggerated to the point of clonus (repetitive jerks) in irritated ones, and asymmetric in babies who have spinal cord lesions, fractures of the femur, or bone and joint infection of the examined extremity.

Ankle clonus is elicited by placing two fingers against the anterior sole of the foot and abruptly, with a short, brisk movement, dorsiflexing it. The response will usually consist of several repetitive jerks (beats) of the foot or none at all. If more than 8 to 10 beats occur, the baby is probably in an irritated state.

Head control in the normal neonate is more effective than is generally realized. With the infant supine the examiner takes the wrists and lifts him slowly to a sitting position. The normal term infant reinforces the maneuver by contracting the shoulder and arm muscles, followed by flexion of the neck. As the sitting position is reached, the infant controls his head by action of neck muscles and thus prevents it from falling forward onto the chest. In many babies the head falls forward but is soon righted to the erect position. Hypotonic infants, such as those with Down's syndrome or those who are hypoxic, have little or no head control, and they do not respond to traction by

activating the muscles of the arms and shoulders. The neck is extremely lax, and the head bobbles in any direction dictated by the combined effects of body position and gravity. There is no attempt to assume an erect posture once the head has fallen to either side or onto the chest.

The *Moro reflex* is demonstrable in all normal neonates (Fig. 6-23). It is often erroneously elicited by slapping the bassinet or jerking it. Some examiners abruptly pull a blanket from under the baby. Others lift him slightly off the crib surface by the wrists and allow him to fall back. The most consistent responses are obtained by holding the baby in a supine position with both hands, one palm beneath the sacrum and buttocks and the other beneath the occiput and upper back. By suddenly slipping the hand down from the occiput onto the back, the head is allowed to fall through an angle of approximately 30 degrees, thus activating the Moro reflex. The normal response is characterized by straightening of the arms and elbows away from the body and by extension of the wrists and fingers. This is followed by return of the upper extremities onto the chest in a position of passive flexion. A cry often accompanies the baby's startled response. Reflex movement of the hips and knees occurs quickly and is of short duration. If an extremity does not respond fully, a localized neurologic defect or fracture is suspect. Suboptimal vigor of the overall response occurs in depressed infants, whereas in premature infants the response is disorganized and incomplete to varying degrees.

Transillumination of the skull is a useful procedure if neurologic disorder is suspected. It is performed with a strong light source from a flashlight fitted with a rubber collar that fits snugly to the skull. In a dark room devoid of light leaks, the examiner must first become dark-adapted. As a rule, dark adaptation is present when the light, placed into the examiner's palm, is transmitted through the hand so that shadows of the distal metacarpal bones are clearly visible as light penetrates the soft tissue between them. The flashlight is then applied to the scalp tightly, and while the snug fit is maintained to avoid light leak, it is moved over the surface of the head. The entire cranium lights up like a red electric bulb in babies who have congenital absence of the cerebral hemispheres (hydranencephaly). In this instance the cranial vault is filled with fluid instead of brain tissue. These infants may behave normally during the newborn period. Severe hydrocephalus produces the same phenomenon. Abnormal light flare is seen locally over subdural hematomas or porencephalic cysts (local absence of cerebral tissue).

A number of conditions cause abnormal light transmission that is not indicative of a brain disorder. Most understandable and common is edema of the scalp, which may occur in infiltration of intravenous fluids being given into a scalp vein or in caput succedaneum. The water-logged scalp transmits more light over a greater area. In the region of the anterior fontanelle, abnormal light transmission is also misleading. The flare of light increases and may extend beyond 2 cm because of the absence of bone. Infants who weighed less

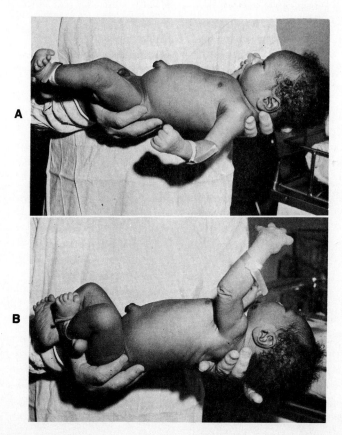

Fig. 6-23. Moro reflex. **A,** The baby is supported beneath the sacrum and upper back, including the occiput. The head is level with the body. **B,** The head is allowed to fall backward. In response, the upper extremities are abruptly thrust upward and outward while the knees and hips are rapidly flexed. Compare changes in position of the head and upper and lower extremities. Compare also this normal response to that in brachial plexus palsy (Fig. 2-15).

than 1250 g at birth, have grown rapidly, and are approximately 1 month of age may often manifest generalized abnormal light transmission. This does not indicate developing hydrocephalus nor cerebral malformation. It is apparently the result of normal enlargement of the subarachnoid space, which seems to occur during this period of rapid growth. Serial measurements of *both head and chest circumferences* will reveal that the apparent rapid growth of the head is actually a component of growth of the entire body. Misinterpretation of this normally increased transillumination, combined with failure to assess head enlargement as a normal component of overall body growth, has resulted in numerous needless pneumoencephalograms, ventriculograms, and other extensive neurologic inquiries.

Final impression of the infant's neurologic status must be formed with great caution. The neurologic examination is not in itself inadequate, but the nature of the neonate's neurologic disorders makes it difficult to localize the disorder or, in marginal situations, to be certain there is any disorder at all. Certainly one cannot take the sum of abnormal findings and arrive at a conclusion in a manner more appropriate for a bookkeeper than a clinician. The incidence of false-positive and false-negative signs is high. Furthermore, repeated observations are absolutely indispensable because abnormal signs are often transient, disappearing in a matter of hours. Extremes are seldom a puzzle; the gross abnormalities and the unequivocal normal state cause little difficulty for the clinician. The in-between phenomena are notoriously troublesome in the total physical examination generally, and in the neurologic evaluation particularly.

BIBLIOGRAPHY

Behrman, R. E., and Kliegman, R. M.: The fetus and the neonatal infant. In Behrman, R. E., and Vaughan, V. C., editors: Nelson's textbook of pediatrics, Philadelphia, 1983, W.B. Saunders Co.

Korones, S. B.: The newborn: perinatal pediatrics. In Hughes, J. G., editor: Synopsis of pediatrics, ed. 6, St. Louis, 1984, The C.V. Mosby Co.

Lucey, J. F.: Examination of the newborn. In Reed, D. E., Ryan, K. J., and Benirschke, K., editors: Principles and management of human reproduction, Philadelphia, 1972, W.B. Saunders Co.

Paine, R. S.: Neurologic examination of infants and children, Pediatr. Clin. North Am. 7:471, 1960.

Phibbs, R. H.: Evaluation of the newborn. In Rudolph, A. M., editor: Pediatrics, New York, 1977, Appleton-Century-Crofts.

CHAPTER 7

Basic principles and clinical significance of acid-base, fluid, and electrolyte disturbances

ACID-BASE BALANCE

In newborn babies almost all serious illnesses eventually involve an acid-base imbalance that in itself may be more hazardous to the baby's survival than the primary disease process. The infant often can be sustained by partial or complete correction of the acid-base disturbance while the primary pathophysiology runs its course. In hyaline membrane disease, for example, there is no effective therapy for eradication of the basic pulmonary pathology (atelectasis), but with spontaneous appearance of adequate quantities of a phospholipid substance known as surfactant, the atelectasis tends to resolve spontaneously in a few days (Chapter 8). In the meantime, if no attempt is made to correct biochemical abnormalities that arise from the primary pulmonary disorder, death is inexorable in severely affected infants. Diarrhea is another case in point. Whether or not antibiotics are ultimately effective in eliminating the etiologic agent (and most often they are not), fluid therapy must be instituted early to rectify the life-threatening acidosis and dehydration that develop so rapidly. Although the diarrhea usually subsides in several days, acid-base balance and optimal hydration must be maintained during its course if the baby is to survive.

An understanding of acid-base disturbances is essential if the nurse is to correlate laboratory data with the clinical course of the disease process and thus assess an infant's progress accurately. Appreciation of the rationale of appropriate therapy is indispensable if the nurse is to participate intelligently in its administration. The discussion that follows will summarize pertinent acid-base factors that are operative in the production of life-threatening illness. Emphasis on terminology is appropriate because understanding of terms and mastery of concepts are inseparable.

pH, acids, and bases

pH. At any given moment acid-base status is determined by the concentration of hydrogen ion (H^+) present in body fluids as a result of the production, neutralization, and elimination of various acids. The higher the concentration of hydrogen ion, the more acid the fluid, and conversely the lower the concentration of hydrogen ion, the more alkaline the fluid. The acidity of a fluid, whether blood, plasma, or urine, is expressed as its *pH*. The mathematic derivation of pH is such that a rise or fall indicates a change of hydrogen

ion concentration in the opposite direction. The pH of a solution is therefore inversely proportional to the concentration of hydrogen ion within it. A pH of 4.0 is more acid than a pH of 5.0, but not simply one-fifth more acid as is superficially apparent from the difference between the two values. Rather, there is a tenfold difference between the two figures because, being negative and logarithmic, each figure represents a multiple of minus 10, or the number of places to the right of a decimal point. Thus a pH of 4.0 represents 0.0001 g of hydrogen ion per liter of solution. This representation is ten times greater than a pH of 5.0, which indicates 0.00001 g of hydrogen ion per liter. Other translations of pH values are listed here to emphasize the large differences in acidity that are indicated by various pH units:

pH 1.0 indicates 0.1 g of hydrogen ion per liter
pH 2.0 indicates 0.01 g of hydrogen ion per liter
pH 3.0 indicates 0.001 g of hydrogen ion per liter
pH 4.0 indicates 0.0001 g of hydrogen ion per liter

A solution with a pH of 1.0 thus contains a hydrogen ion concentration 100 times greater than a solution with a pH of 3.0, or 1000 times greater than at pH 4.0. The reader should again note that the greater the pH value, the less the concentration of hydrogen ion. The accepted normal values for the pH of arterial blood in newborn infants at 24 hours of age is 7.35 to 7.44. The range of pH values compatible with life is 6.8 to 7.8. Most clinically important deviations occur between 7.00 and 7.25. These values represent enormous increases in hydrogen ion concentrations compared with the seemingly small differences between the numbers themselves. Compared with 7.35, a pH of 7.20 represents an increase of 40% in hydrogen ion concentration; pH of 7.10 represents an increase of approximately 80%, and at pH 7.00 the blood is over twice normal acidity (actually an increase of 124%).

Acids. Acids are substances capable of surrendering hydrogen ion (H^+) when in solution. The strength of their acidity depends on the extent to which the hydrogen ion is dissociated from its molecule when in solution, and this varies from one acid to another. Hydrochloric acid (HCl) is powerful because it is dissociated almost completely when in solution, thereby surrendering greater amounts of hydrogen ion than most other acids. The resultant high concentration of hydrogen ion in solution renders a lower pH than other, less-soluble acids in similar concentration. Carbonic acid (H_2CO_3), for example, does not dissociate as readily as hydrochloric acid; it surrenders fewer hydrogen ions in solution and is therefore a considerably weaker acid.

Bases. Bases are alkaline molecules capable of accepting hydrogen ions. When an acid is added to a base in solution, the dissociated hydrogen ion becomes bound to the base, with the resultant formation of a weaker acid. The base thus acts as a buffer by diminishing the potential acidity of a solution. Buffering is indispensable to the continuous maintenance of acid-base balance. In the neonate it is often overwhelmed by pathophysiologic events such as asphyxia, pulmonary dysfunction, or diarrhea. Therapeutic measures to enhance the buffering capacity of blood are therefore applied without delay.

Physiologic maintenance of acid-base equilibrium

Normal metabolism entails a relentless production of acids, principally carbonic acid, which must be neutralized and ultimately eliminated from the body. These acids are categorized as volatile and nonvolatile (or fixed) acids. Carbonic acid (H_2CO_3) is volatile because it is constantly converted to carbon dioxide (CO_2) in the blood and eliminated in the gaseous state through the lungs. The nonvolatile, or fixed, acids are principally lactic, sulfuric, and phosphoric acids. They are buffered in blood and excreted through the kidneys. The three principal mechanisms by which acid products of normal metabolism are neutralized or eliminated are buffering activity in blood, elimination of carbon dioxide (volatile acid) through the lungs, and excretion of fixed acid through the kidneys. The respiratory apparatus directly controls blood levels of carbonic acid; the kidneys directly regulate the concentrations of bicarbonate buffer and hydrogen ion in the blood.

Buffers and buffer pairs. A buffer is a substance that, by its presence in a solution, is capable of minimizing changes in pH caused by the addition of acids or bases. Thus when a strong acid or base is added to a solution that contains a buffer, a weaker acid or base is formed and the change in pH is thus minimized. Buffers exist in pairs that are normally in sufficiently high concentration to stabilize changes in pH. These pairs comprise a weak acid and its salt. The principal buffer pairs in blood are sodium bicarbonate/carbonic acid ($NaHCO_3/H_2CO_3$) and sodium proteinate/acid protein. The protein buffer system resides predominantly in hemoglobin. The first member of each pair is a salt; the second member is a weak acid. The hydrogen ion concentration in blood, and therefore the pH, is determined by a *ratio of the constituents that make up each buffer pair;* the proportion of bicarbonate to carbonic acid (normally 20:1) is the most important determinant. The ratio may be altered by a decrease in bicarbonate or an increase in carbonic acid, thus elevating hydrogen ion concentration and lowering pH.

Buffering of nonvolatile acids. Normally the changes in pH of body fluids caused by the addition of lactic and other nonvolatile acids are minimized and held within physiologic limits principally by the buffering activity of the bicarbonate/carbonic acid system. In this reaction lactic acid is buffered by sodium bicarbonate and converted to sodium lactate plus carbonic acid. Sodium lactate is excreted through the kidneys, and carbonic acid is excreted in the gaseous state (CO_2) through the lungs. These events are represented in the following formulas:

(1) HL (lactic acid) + $NaHCO_3 \rightarrow$
$$Na\ lactate + H_2CO_3$$

(2) $H_2CO_3 \rightarrow H_2O + CO_2$

Other nonvolatile acids also combine with sodium bicarbonate to form salts and carbonic acid.

Buffering of volatile acid (H₂CO₃). Carbonic acid is produced in greater quantity than any other acid during the course of normal tissue metabolism. It is buffered in the erythrocyte by hemoglobin. From tissue fluid it crosses capillary walls to enter the plasma and thence into erythrocytes. By a series of reactions within erythrocytes it is converted to bicarbonate, which is released into plasma as sodium bicarbonate. Thus the carbon dioxide that originates in tissues is largely carried in plasma as sodium bicarbonate. The acid change in pH that would have occurred is held within normal limits by the production of bicarbonate in the red blood cells.

Stabilizing influence of the respiratory apparatus. The concentration of carbonic acid in plasma is determined by the amount of carbon dioxide that is present (Pco_2), which in turn is largely dependent on the capacity of the respiratory apparatus to ventilate normally. In the fetus this process depends on normal placental function. The quantity of carbon dioxide excreted through the lungs increases with the depth and the rate of respiration. The depth and rate of respiration are subject to neural control of the respiratory center in the medulla of the brain, which is exquisitely sensitive to changes in blood pH. The respiratory center directs an increase in rate to eliminate more carbon dioxide when blood pH declines; it directs a decrease in rate to conserve carbon dioxide when the pH is elevated. If the ratio of bicarbonate to carbonic acid falls below normal as a result of an elevated carbonic acid concentration, pH declines. The respiratory rate is then accelerated in response to stimulation of the medullary respiratory center. An increased amount of carbon dioxide is blown off, the ratio of bicarbonate to carbonic acid is restored toward normal, and the pH of blood now rises. On the other hand, if blood pH rises abnormally, as it may when excessive doses of intravenous sodium bicarbonate are administered, the ventilatory rate is slowed. Carbon dioxide is retained, and the level of carbonic acid rises. Although the absolute quantities of carbonic acid and bicarbonate are now increased, their ratio is closer to normal and the pH declines. Ultimately excess bicarbonate is excreted by the kidneys, whereas temporarily retained carbon dioxide is eventually eliminated through the lungs.

Stabilizing influence of the kidneys. Whereas the respiratory apparatus directly regulates the concentration of volatile acid, the kidneys control the blood content of nonvolatile acid. This is primarily accomplished by the excretion of hydrogen ion plus the simultaneous conservation of bicarbonate. In contrast to the rapidly activated compensatory efforts of the lungs, the kidneys respond more slowly, but they tend to carry compensatory mechanisms closer to completion.

Classification of acid-base disturbances

Disturbances in acid-base equilibrium may culminate in a diminished pH (acidosis) or an increased pH (alkalosis). Changes in either of these directions are caused by primary disorders of ventilation (respiratory acidosis and alkalosis) or primary disorders of general metabolism, renal function, or both (metabolic or nonrespiratory acidosis and alkalosis). The distinctions and variations of these disturbances are defined here, having been distilled from a broad literature. When appropriate, the biochemical deviation is described in association with the pathophysiologic event that gives rise to it. Over the years biochemists and physiologists who are concerned with the problems of acid-base balance have been at odds regarding proper definitions of various disturbances. There is frequent mention, in a voluminous literature, of the advantages and pitfalls of a "physiologic language" or a "laboratory language." For us the definitions presented here have facilitated the teaching and clinical applications of the concepts they describe. Table 7-1 summarizes the attributes of the various types of acid-base disturbance and their degrees of compensation.

Uncompensated disturbances. The uncompensated abnormalities defined here are characterized in each instance by the presence of an

Table 7-1. Attributes of acid-base disturbances according to type and degree of compensation

Disturbance	Blood pH	Blood P_{CO_2} (torr)	Blood HCO_3^- (mEq/L)
Normal	7.35 to 7.44	30 to 35	20 to 24
Metabolic acidosis			
Uncompensated	Lowest	Normal	Low
Partially compensated	Low	Low	Low
Fully compensated	Normal	Lowest	Low
Metabolic alkalosis			
Uncompensated	Highest	Normal	High
Partially compensated	High	High	High
Fully compensated	Normal	Highest	High
Respiratory acidosis			
Uncompensated	Lowest	High	Normal
Partially compensated	Low	High	High
Fully compensated	Normal	High	Highest
Respiratory alkalosis			
Uncompensated	Highest	Low	Normal
Partially compensated	High	Low	Low
Fully compensated	Normal	Low	Lowest

abnormal pH. The same underlying abnormalities also exist in compensated forms. They are described later in this chapter.

Acidosis is a condition that causes an inordinate accumulation of acid (nonvolatile or volatile) or loss of base. The net result is an increase in hydrogen ion concentration and thus a diminution of blood pH to levels below normal.

Alkalosis is a condition that causes an excessive accumulation of base or a loss of acid (nonvolatile or volatile). The net result is a decrease in hydrogen ion concentration and thus an increase in blood pH to levels that are above normal.

Metabolic (nonrespiratory) acidosis occurs with an increase in the concentration of nonvolatile acids as a result of (1) deranged metabolism in which there is overproduction of acids, (2) disrupted renal function with impaired excretion of nonvolatile acids, and (3) excessive loss of base through the gastrointestinal tract (diarrhea) and rarely through the kidneys (renal tubular acidosis).

Metabolic (nonrespiratory) alkalosis is characterized by an increased concentration of base (bicarbonate). In the neonate it is most frequently caused by inappropriately large therapeutic doses of sodium bicarbonate. Repeated vomiting resulting from pyloric stenosis is occasionally encountered, causing metabolic alkalosis because a significant quantity of hydrochloric acid is lost in vomited gastric secretions. Rarely metabolic alkalosis results from an excessive renal loss of hydrogen ion or from renal retention of bicarbonate.

Respiratory acidosis follows decreased pulmonary gas exchange with resultant retention of carbon dioxide (increased P_{CO_2}). Perinatal asphyxia and hyaline membrane disease are the most common neonatal clinical entities in which respiratory acidosis occurs.

Respiratory alkalosis, caused by respiratory dysfunction, is characterized by an abnormally low P_{CO_2} resulting from excessive elimination of carbon dioxide during hyperventilation. It is most frequently encountered in therapy with mechanical ventilators that are incorrectly set to deliver respiratory rates and tidal volumes in excess of physiologic needs.

Compensated disturbances. Although definitions in the preceding paragraphs are based on an abnormal pH, acid-base disturbance can also be operative in the presence of a normal or nearly normal pH, provided certain compensatory mechanisms are effective. A description of the data in Table 7-1 is presented in the paragraphs that follow.

Compensation is a physiologic process that occurs in response to an antecedent (primary) derangement of acid-base balance. It tends to restore the ratio of buffer pairs toward normal. If compensation is complete, a normal ratio is reestablished and the pH is normal even though concentrations of the individual members of a buffer pair are abnormal. However, the original source of acid-base disturbance may still exist. The importance of recognizing these compensated disorders cannot be overestimated, since their corrective effects are often only temporary. The underlying disturbance, masked by these compensatory responses, requires cautious therapy.

Compensated metabolic (nonrespiratory) acidosis is characterized chiefly by hyperventilation for the reduction of PCO_2 to levels below normal. Hyperventilation is the compensatory process activated by accumulation of nonvolatile acid that consumes available base (bicarbonate). The excretion of volatile acid (CO_2) through the lungs must be increased to lower carbonic acid concentration to match the lowered level of bicarbonate and thus to restore the sodium bicarbonate/carbonic acid ratio in that buffer pair. In this compensated state the pH is normal or almost normal, but both the PCO_2 and the serum bicarbonate concentrations are low.

Compensated metabolic (nonrespiratory) alkalosis involves hypoventilation that is activated for the purpose of diminishing the elimination of carbon dioxide. Since the primary disturbance is accumulation of bicarbonate, retention of volatile acid (CO_2) tends to restore the ratio between so-dium bicarbonate and carbonic acid. In this compensated state the pH is virtually normal, but the PCO_2 and serum bicarbonate concentrations are elevated.

Compensated respiratory acidosis involves retention of bicarbonate as a result of adjustment in renal function. Since the primary disturbance is accumulation of carbon dioxide, and thus an increase in carbonic acid, the rise in bicarbonate tends to restore the bicarbonate/carbonic acid ratio toward normal. In a fully compensated state the pH is normal, but PCO_2 and serum bicarbonate are increased. Whereas the renal mechanism seeks to restore pH by conserving bicarbonate, the respiratory apparatus attempts to eliminate the accumulated carbon dioxide. The clinically evident result of this activity is tachypnea.

Compensated respiratory alkalosis also involves adjustment of renal function. The primary disturbance is caused by hyperventilation with excessive elimination of carbon dioxide and resultant decline of PCO_2. The kidney thus acts to increase excretion of bicarbonate to restore the bicarbonate/carbonic acid ratio to normal. In the fully compensated state pH is normal, but PCO_2 and serum bicarbonate are individually diminished although in normal ratio.

Mixed disturbances of acid-base balance. Some clinical disorders simultaneously give rise to disturbances of the respiratory and metabolic components of acid-base balance. These are called mixed disturbances, and they are characterized by a concurrence of respiratory and metabolic acidosis or alkalosis. In neonates the most commonly encountered variety is mixed acidosis associated with severe perinatal asphyxia and hyaline membrane disease. In mixed respiratory and metabolic acidosis, the combination of retained carbon dioxide and diminished bicarbonate causes a considerable decrease in pH.

Laboratory procedures for measuring acid-base status

The advent of microtechniques for the direct measurement of blood gases and pH has been a boon to the management of sick neonates. Rational therapy to rectify acid-base disorders is currently based on these procedures. Serial determinations are indispensable during the entire course of an illness because blood gas content and pH may change rapidly and repeatedly. Infants on mechanical respirators, for instance, must be monitored repeatedly and at frequent intervals for blood gas and acid-base status.

The collection of samples should be accomplished with precision and with a minimum quantity of blood. The blood PCO_2, PO_2, and pH can be measured from as little as 0.1 ml. Indwelling umbilical artery catheters are commonly used as a source of arterial blood samples. If this route is unavailable, capillary blood obtained by heel prick may be used for PCO_2 and pH determinations. Capillary blood PO_2 is not accurate. This method of collection requires warming of the heel with a moist pack for a minimum of 5 minutes to dilate capillaries and arterioles. The sample thus obtained is arterialized capillary blood.

An inordinate delay in performing determinations after collection of samples usually causes inaccurate results if the blood is kept at room temperature. The pH drops and the PCO_2 rises because continued glycolysis in the red blood cells produces lactic acid in the sample. The average pH error in normal blood that is analyzed 20 minutes after collection is only minus 0.01 unit. Errors are minimal and clinically insignificant if the blood is stored in ice. Determinations can then be made up to 2 hours later with only a slight fall in pH (less than 0.015 unit). Exposure to room air is another pitfall to be avoided. In these circumstances the PCO_2 falls considerably because it escapes to lower carbon dioxide tensions in the atmosphere, and this causes the pH to rise. When blood is exposed to the atmosphere, PO_2 is also altered, since it tends to equilibrate with the oxygen tension of room air, which is approximately 150 torr.

Heparin is the only acceptable anticoagulant for collection of blood samples. Other anticoagulants, such as citrate, oxalate, and EDTA, have signif-

icant effects on blood pH. Tubes used for capillary samples are commercially prepared with proper amounts of heparin to prevent clotting.

Capillary blood samples are not optimal for PO_2 determinations because they do not correlate with arterial blood levels. Oxygen tension must be monitored from blood taken directly from an artery. This is especially important for premature infants who are given supplemental oxygen; hyperoxia may cause retrolental fibroplasia (Chapter 8). Arterial samples are obtainable from an umbilical artery catheter or from punctures of the radial, brachial. or temporal arteries. Determinations of pH and PCO_2 in capillary blood are valid, however, because they are well correlated with arterial values if the sample is properly collected. However, difficulty arises when the extremities are poorly perfused for any reason. Venous stasis is evident in distressed infants whose extremities are cyanotic. Stasis of capillary blood lowers pH and augments PCO_2; both of these values may thus differ considerably from those of arterial blood, therefore precluding reliable reference to such data for therapy.

All neonatal special care units use blood gas and pH measurements for the characterization of acid-base status. Ideally, personnel and laboratory should be close at hand so that results are available within minutes after they are ordered. The parameters pertinent to acid-base evaluation are as follows:

pH is a measure of hydrogen ion concentration. It expresses the end result of buffer activity and *in itself does not indicate whether an abnormality originates in respiratory or nonrespiratory dysfunction*. Normal values range from pH 7.35 to 7.44.

PCO_2 expresses the partial pressure of carbon dioxide dissolved in plasma. *Deviations from normal are indicative of disorders in the respiratory apparatus*. Normal neonatal values range from 30 to 37 torr.

Plasma bicarbonate measures total bicarbonate concentration. Normal values are between 20 and 25 mEq/L.

Base excess (B.E.) or deficit is a value that is calculated rather than directly measured by the laboratory (see later). It is expressed as a positive or negative value. The negative value is sometimes referred to as a base deficit. Base excess indicates, in milliequivalents per liter, the quantity of blood buffer base remaining after hydrogen ion is buffered. It thus expresses the combined buffering capacity of plasma bicarbonate and hemoglobin. Normal neonatal values range from $+4$ to -4 mEq/L.

Alignment nomogram. Base excess is calculated from the alignment nomogram reproduced in Fig. 7-1. The computation of base excess is

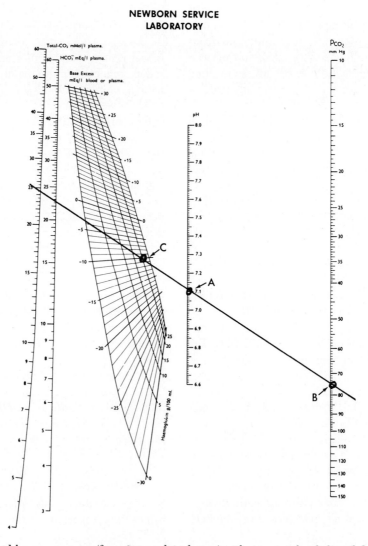

Fig. 7-1. Acid-base nomogram (from Siggaard-Andersen) with an example of plotted data from a sick infant. (See text for explanation.) (Modified from Winters, R. W., Engel, K., and Dell, R. B.: Acid-base physiology in medicine, a self-instruction program, Cleveland, 1967, The London Co.)

possible when hemoglobin concentration and any two of the following parameters are known: blood pH, P_{CO_2} plasma bicarbonate, or total carbon dioxide content of plasma. The variables most commonly used in newborn laboratories are pH and P_{CO_2}.

Assume that an infant in rather severe respiratory distress is admitted to your facility. Blood samples are collected soon after admission, and the following information is forwarded to you:

pH = 7.10 (normal = 7.35 to 7.44)

P_{CO_2} = 75 torr (normal = 30 to 37 torr)

Hemoglobin = 20 g/dl

The values for pH and P_{CO_2} are plotted on their appropriate scales at points *A* and *B*, as shown on the nomogram. A line is drawn through points *A* and *B* across all four scales. The base excess is read at minus 10 mEq/L at point *C*, where the drawn line intersects a grid line representing hemoglobin concentration of 20 g/dl. The plasma bicarbonate concentration can now also be read at 23 mEq/L. If only the pH and bicarbonate are known (as well as the hemoglobin concentration), base excess and P_{CO_2} can be derived by drawing a line through points corresponding to the known values.

Basis of therapy. Intravenous sodium bicarbonate is occasionally used to correct a negative base excess (base deficit). Sodium bicarbonate is available in ampules of a 7.5% solution containing 0.88 mEq/ml. For ease of calculation it is satisfactory in clinical situations to consider the concentration as 1.0 mEq/ml. The dose of sodium bicarbonate is computed from the following formula:

mEq of NaHCO$_3$ to be given = Base deficit ×
    0.3 × Body weight in kilograms

The factor 0.3 represents the approximate portion of body weight composed of extracellular fluid. If the infant whose base deficit was 10 mEq/L weighs 2500 g, calculation of the dose of sodium bicarbonate is as follows:

$$mEq \text{ of } NaHCO_3 = 10 \text{ mEq} \times 0.3 \times 2.5 \text{ kg}$$
$$= 10 \times 0.75$$
$$= 7.5$$

Thus 7.5 ml of the 7.5% solution of sodium bicarbonate will be required. It must always be diluted because the extremely alkaline pH may damage blood vessels near the site of infusion. The required dose should be mixed with at least an equal quantity of water for injection or with 10% glucose water. Generally one fourth to one half of the calculated dose is injected (after dilution) over a period of 2 to 5 minutes, and the remainder is added to intravenous fluid already dripping. In some centers the entire dose is infused, particularly if the infant is profoundly ill.

Summary

Principles of acid-base relationships apply to the management of all neonates admitted to the intensive care nursery. Mechanisms by which these normal relationships are disrupted and restored are operative in every sick baby. Acid-base imbalance is a by-product of the entire spectrum of primary neonatal disorders. It occurs in response to cold stress, during respiratory embarrassment, in gastrointestinal disturbances, as a result of all types of infectious disease, in disorders of the central nervous system, during postoperative periods, and even during the normal birth process. Preoccupation with the obvious symptomatology of these primary disorders often diverts attention from the subtle and perhaps more sinister effects produced by acid-base imbalance. These effects can be identified with certainty only by recourse to laboratory data. It is thus imperative for the neonatal nurse to comprehend the significance of these data.

FLUIDS AND ELECTROLYTES
Changes in quantity and distribution of body water during maturation

As gestational and postnatal ages increase, body water content decreases. Total body water (TBW) diminishes from 67% of body weight in post-neonatal infants to 60% in older children and adults. In the neonate, however, water is 78% of body weight for a term infant, 80% at 32 weeks of gestation, and 95% in a 13- to 14-week fetus. The premature infant has more total body water than the term infant. Postnatal management requires consideration of these and other significant differences.

The distribution of water between the extracellular and intracellular compartments also changes with age. The percent of extracellular fluid (ECF) is greatest in the young. Thus ECF constitutes 20% of body weight in adults and children, 25% in postneonatal infants, 45% in term infants, and 60% in the 5-month fetus. The increased total body water in term and premature infants is largely extracellular.

As the ECF compartment contracts with age, intracellular fluid (ICF) expands from 20% of total weight in a 5-month fetus, to 30% at term, and 40% in adulthood. Total body water, and ECF within it, decreases with age. Conversely, the younger the premature infant, the greater the proportion of ECF. An abrupt change in fluid content occurs regularly in the 3 to 5 days following birth, whether the infant is premature or term. The most premature of infants (very low birth weight) normally lose up to 15% of their body weight, and virtually all of it is ECF. Prevention of this normal fluid loss by intravenous replacement is ill advised. Fig. 7-2 illustrates the declining proportion of total body water with progressing age from fetus to adult. In addition, it further depicts a rising ICF and a falling ECF as total water diminishes.

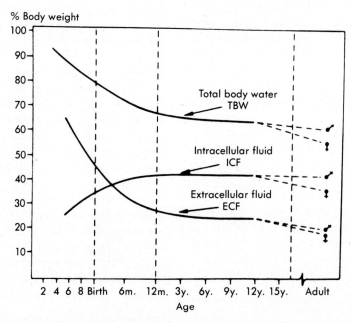

Fig. 7-2. Total body water (as percent of body weight) declines from embryonic period continuously to adulthood as intracellular fluid increases and extracellular fluid decreases. (From Friis-Hansen, B.: In Winters, R. W., editor: The body fluids in pediatrics, Boston, 1973, Little Brown and Co., p. 100.)

Body composition; chemical anatomy

Water and solids. As the fetus grows, solid material increases while water content decreases. The 300 g fetus has a body content of 7% to 8% protein; the term infant has 12.5%. Fat is virtually absent in a fetus of less than 1500 g because it is only deposited toward the end of normal gestation and at an accelerated rate. In term infants, fat comprises 12% to 15% of total body weight.

Distribution of water and solutes: the compartments (ECF and ICF). As traditionally conceived, TBW is divided into extracellular and intracellular compartments (Fig. 7-3). ECF refers to water outside the cells; ICF is water within them. It is useful to think of a different solution in each of two compartments (ECF and ICF), one separated from the other by a continuous semipermeable membrane. The membrane allows free bidirectional movement of water between the compartments. It is semipermeable (rather than freely permeable) because it limits diffusion of electrically charged particles (ions) and blocks passage of large particles that are dissolved in water. Ionic passage occurs normally in certain conditions that require an expenditure of energy by the membrane, such as the sodium pump mechanism, or by the action of hormones, neuromuscular activity, and changes in membrane permeability. Transfer of ions also occurs in disorders that alter the integrity of the membrane to allow abnormal passage of water, particles, or both. Disruption of function is associated with asphyxia, shock, congestive heart failure, severe infections, acid-base imbalance, and dehydration.

Extracellular water and solutes (ECF). Extracellular fluid is distributed between two "spaces": extravascular (interstitial) space and intravascular space. Interstitial fluid surrounds the cells of the body. It constitutes approximately two thirds of the total extracellular fluid volume. Plasma volume comprises one third of extracellular fluid volume. The principal difference between plasma and interstitial fluid is their protein content. Plasma contains a considerable amount of protein; interstitial fluid has virtually none. Plasma proteins are normally present in amounts between 5 and 6 g/dl; 94% to 95% of the plasma is water. The electrolytes are almost entirely dissolved in the water fraction. Capillary membranes are normally impermeable to protein, but electrolytes traverse them freely. The plasma fluid within capillaries, and the interstitial fluid outside them, contain virtually identical concentrations of all the electrolytes that are characteristic of extracellular fluid. The water within red blood cells, while literally "intracellular," is nevertheless considered part of the extracellular compartment, mainly because the red cells are unlike other cells elsewhere. The extracellular fluid is therefore a continuous compartment of water and solutes, even though one portion of it is outside the vascular space and the other is within it.

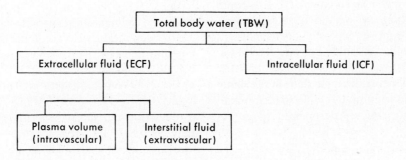

Fig. 7-3. Distribution of body water among principal compartments. (See text.)

The *solutes* of ECF are substances dissolved in its water. Electrolytes, being electrically charged, are dissolved in water as *ions*. The molecules of other substances, such as glucose and urea, are also dissolved in water, but they are not electrically charged and are thus considered *nonionic particles*. *Cations* are ions that have a *positive electrical charge; anions* have a *negative charge*. Normal electrolyte balance requires the total positive charge to equal the total negative charge; the sum of the cations must equal that of anions. This is to say that the total milliequivalent content of each of the two types of ion is equal. The term *milliequivalent* is a quantitative expression of positively or negatively charged particles. This is traditionally expressed as milliequivalents in a liter of fluid (mEq/L). The total of all cations in plasma (and thus also in interstitial fluid) is 155 mEq/L. The total of anions is identical. Sodium (Na^+) is the principal cation of extracellular fluid. Its normal concentration is 142 mEq/L. The other cations are potassium (K^+) at 5 mEq/L, calcium (Ca^{++}) at 5 mEq/L (also often expressed as 10 mg/dl), and magnesium (Mg^{++}) at 3 mEq/L. The major anion of ECF is chloride (Cl^-); the normal concentration of chlorides in plasma is 105 mEq/L. The remaining anions are bicarbonate (HCO_3^-) at 25 mEq/L, sulfate ($SO_4^=$) and phosphate ($PO_4^=$), which together constitute 9 mEq/L, and proteins ($Prot^-$) at 16 mEq/L. When in solution, glucose and urea do not dissociate into ionic particles; their quantity is therefore not expressed as mEq/L, but rather as mg/dl.

Intracellular water and solutes (ICF). Although the intracellular space contains fluid that varies in composition from one type of tissue to another, that compartment can validly be considered as a single one that is composed of "millions of little bags of water, all doing the same thing at the same moment."* In contrast to the *capillary* membrane in the ECF space, the *cellular* membrane in the

---

*From Weil, W. B., and Bailie, M. D.: Fluid and electrolyte metabolism in infants and children, New York, 1977, Grune & Stratton, p. 20.

ICF space does not admit free passage of cations and allows little to anions. When these particles normally traverse cell membranes, they do so by action of transport systems that involve an energy expenditure by the membrane. The energy is derived from chemical reactions within the membrane. As a result of the limited permeability of cell membranes, the ionic separation of ICF and ECF is such that their percent composition differs greatly. Yet, when transfer of ions from one compartment to the other is essential for normal metabolism, the membrane's transport systems accommodate it. The integrity and interdependence of ICF and ECF are thereby preserved.

ICF is more inaccessible to study than ECF; thus less is known about its precise composition. Within an individual cell, fluid of varying constituency is contained in substructures, such as the nucleus and mitochondria. It is nevertheless well established that the major cation of ICF is potassium (K^+); in ECF the major cation is sodium (Na^+). The concentration of ICF potassium is approximately 30 times greater than ECF potassium. Potassium is essentially an intracellular cation. The other intracellular cations are magnesium (Mg^{++}) and sodium (Na^+). Although all these cations are also present in the ECF, their concentrations differ considerably between the two compartments. The intracellular concentration of magnesium (Mg^{++}) is 10 to 15 times greater than the extracellular concentration. Magnesium is therefore considered primarily an intracellular ion. The concentration of sodium (Na^+) in the ICF is only about one fifteenth that of the ECF, and sodium is thus primarily an ECF cation. The concentrations of intracellular anions also differ from that of the extracellular ones. Chloride (Cl^-) is almost nonexistent in the ICF, 2 mEq/L in the cells compared with 105 mEq/L outside them. The reverse relationship exists for phosphate ($PO_4^=$) and sulfate ($SO_4^=$) because together they constitute 126 mEq/L in the ICF and only 9 mEq/L in the ECF. There are 12 mEq/L of intracellular bicarbonate (HCO_3^-) as contrasted with 15 mEq/L of the extracellular anion. ICF protein is 60 mEq/L; ECF protein is only 16 mEq/L. These distinct differences are maintained by the semipermeable cell membranes. The reader has probably already noticed that identical ions are contained in both major fluid compartments; it is their concentrations that vary so considerably. Table 7-2 lists the ionic concentrations of ICF and ECF.

Osmolality and the exchange of water between compartments. A solution exerts osmotic pressure in relation to the number of dissolved particles (solute) within it. The greater the number of particles in a unit of water, the higher the osmotic pressure. These particles may be ionic (Na^+, Cl^-, K^+, and so forth) or nonionic (glucose, urea). Osmotic pressure is not related to the size or weight of particles or to their electrical charge; it is directly determined by the *number* of dissolved particles in a unit of water—the concentration of particles in the solution. Magnesium chloride ($MgCl_2$) dissociates into one magnesium ion and two chloride ions. In solution, the three ionic particles of the $MgCl_2$ molecule exert a greater osmotic pressure in the same volume of water than sodium chloride ($NaCl$), which dissociates into only two ionic particles, one sodium and one chloride ion. Glucose and urea do not dissociate into ions. Theirs are nonionic molecular particles. *Together the ionic and nonionic particles in solution account for the total osmotic activity of the solute*. The term *milliosmole (mOsm)* expresses the unit of osmotic pressure exerted by the solute. *Osmolality* refers to the quantity of milliosmoles per *kilogram* of water (mOsm/kg). *Osmolarity* refers to the number of milliosmoles per *liter* of water (mOsm/L). The values of osmolality and osmolarity approximate each other so closely that both terms can be used interchangeably.

Osmotic pressure of one solution is exerted on that of another when both are separated by a semipermeable membrane. If a difference in osmolality exists, the result is a *net flow* of water into the more concentrated solution until the concentration of particles (milliosmoles) in both solutions

Table 7-2. Ionic concentrations in ECF and ICF

Ions	ECF (mEq/L)	ICF (mEq/L)*
Cations		
Sodium (Na^+)	142	10
Potassium (K^+)	5	150
Calcium (Ca^{++})	5	None
Magnesium (Mg^{++})	3	40
Anions		
Chloride (Cl^-)	105	2
Bicarbonate (HCO_3^-)	25	12
Phosphate ($PO_4^=$) and sulfate ($SO_4^=$)	9	126
Protein ($prot^-$)	16	60

*Concentrations of ICF ions are assumed.

is equal. An exchange of water thus occurs between intravascular fluid (plasma) and interstitial fluid and then between interstitial fluid and intracellular fluid. The transfer of water across a membrane between two solutions is actually a continuous bidirectional one. However a greater volume of water flows into a more concentrated solution, as less is simultaneously transferred in the opposite direction, into the more dilute solution. Thus the *net flow* of water is said to be in the direction of the solution of higher osmolality, and ultimately its osmolality decreases—it becomes more dilute. Constant bidirectional exchange of water occurs across all cell membranes. The difference in osmolality between the two compartments is thus minimized or eliminated, not by exchange of electrolytes across the cell membrane, but by transfer of water in response to discrepant particulate concentrations (osmolality). If sodium (as in $NaHCO_3$, for instance) is infused into the vascular space, it eventually permeates capillary walls (membranes) into the interstitial fluid, but it is slow to cross the cell membrane from the interstitial space. In the meantime the resultant heightened osmolality of interstitial fluid produces a transfer of water from within the cells to the extracellular compartment (interstitial fluid) in an attempt to equalize osmotic pressure. The result is a loss of water from cells. When large quantities of sodium are infused over a short period, the increased intravascular osmolality causes movement of fluid from the interstitial space into blood vessels with a resultant increase in intravascular volume. When this occurs in the fragile capillaries of the premature infant's brain, rupture of capillary walls causes intracranial hemorrhage. This is the basis for caution in the administration of $NaHCO_3$ for metabolic acidosis (Chapter 14).

Physiologic mechanisms for the maintenance of fluid and electrolyte balance

Fluid input and loss. The sole sources of input for the normal term neonate are breast milk or formula. The sick neonate, until he recuperates, receives fluids and electrolytes only by the intravascular route. Consideration of the type and quantity of fluid that is given must be based on a knowledge of how it is lost. Fluid is lost from the body through three routes; evaporative loss from skin and lungs, direct loss from the kidneys, and direct loss from the gastrointestinal tract. Evaporative and renal losses are of primary importance in the neonate. Stool losses, while they occur consistently, are not clinically significant in the sick baby unless diarrhea or loose stools (see Photo-

therapy, Chapter 10) are present. Table 7-3 lists average water losses by the various routes discussed.

Insensible water loss (IWL) and the effects of environmental factors. Evaporative loss occurs visibly in the form of sweat and invisibly in the form of insensible water loss (IWL) from the skin and respiratory tract. Sweating is negligible or absent in babies less than 36 weeks of gestation. IWL constitutes 35% to 45% of total water losses and considerably more in babies below 1000 g at birth. The smaller the baby, the greater the IWL. Approximately 30% of IWL is from the respiratory tract; the remainder is transepidermal water loss (TEWL). The quantity thus lost can be influenced significantly by increasing the humidity of inspired air. If very high levels of humidity are provided, respiratory losses may be reduced by as much as 55%. Cutaneous IWL varies considerably because it is influenced by factors that are operative in the baby and in the environment. The most fundamental of the intrinsic factors is gestational age. The less mature the baby, the greater the evaporative losses in any given environmental circumstances. This occurs for several reasons. The immature baby's surface area per kilogram of body weight is significantly larger than that of the mature infant; the skin is thinner and more copiously vascularized. Water content of the body, and particularly the skin, is higher. The skin is extremely porous, especially in babies who weigh less than 1000 g at birth. The stratum corneum is incompletely developed; keratin is not present in significant quantity for 2 to 3 weeks after birth. Apparently an immature stratum corneum with absence of keratin are the principal factors that promote transepidermal water loss (see p. 91). The immature infant, especially if birth weight is less than 1000 g, is therefore particularly vulnerable to changes in the environment.

Transepidermal water loss (TEWL) is altered significantly by environmental factors. The changes imposed by environmental circumstances, particularly those that entail increased

Table 7-3. Mean water loss (ml/kg/day)

	750-1000 (g)	1001-1250 (g)	1251-1500 (g)
First 2 weeks			
IWL*	62	52	35
Urine	72	72	72
Stool	7	7	7
Second 2 weeks			
IWL*	48	35	30
Urine	80	80	80
Stool	10	10	10

*These values are for babies in incubators. Add 40% to 50% for infants on radiant warmers.

losses, are a critical consideration in calculating proper volumes of fluid input.

Water losses are increased by:
1. High ambient temperature
2. Radiant warmers
3. Phototherapy

Water losses are diminished by:
1. High ambient humidity
2. Heat shields
3. Thermal blankets

High ambient temperature, when above the level required for maintenance of normal body temperature, increases water loss through the skin. Needlessly high environmental temperatures increase the metabolic rate, which is associated with enhanced water loss through the skin. Losses from the respiratory tract are also augmented because the infant's respiratory rate increases in such circumstances.

High ambient humidity diminishes evaporative losses. Heightened humidity principally affects respiratory water loss, which has been shown experimentally to diminish by 55%. Considerably less effect is exerted on cutaneous losses, which in the same experiments were diminished by only 18%.

Radiant warmers enhance TEWL significantly, and this has been a major objection to their protracted use. Studies of this phenomenon have consistently demonstrated greater insensible losses under the warmers than in incubators. These losses vary depending on the type of warmer used, size and gestational age of the infant, and the postnatal age as well. Under radiant warmers, TEWL increases by one half to three times the amount expected in an incubator. Such losses are notably increased in babies whose gestational ages are 30 to 32 weeks or less and whose birth weights are below 1500 g, but especially below 1250 g. They also vary with the type of warmer.

The most important clinical point to be made is that the use of radiant warmers is associated with impressive increments in TEWL, and that these increments can be enormous when gesta-tional age and size are most diminutive. Magnitudes of TEWL have been reported in differing circumstances; even though they vary widely from one study to another, the trends are identical. One report compared babies according to weight (above and below 1500 g) and also according to sources of heat (incubators versus radiant warmers). In incubators, the mean IWL was 17.8 ml/kg/24 h for babies over 1500 g; 37.4 ml/kg/24 h for babies less than 1500 g. Under radiant warmers, these corresponding values were remarkably higher. Mean IWL from babies over 1500 g was as high as 51.6 ml/kg/24 h; under 1500 g the mean was as high as 88.9 ml/kg/24 h. Since that report appeared, others having limited their observations to babies under 1000 g and on radiant warmers, found a TEWL as high as 160 ml/kg/24 h in one baby in a group whose losses ranged from 120 to 160 ml/kg/24 h.

Transepidermal losses are confined to water; electrolytes are not involved. With TEWL of sufficient magnitude, plasma sodium levels become elevated as a function of water loss and renal function (see later in this chapter). Concentration of sodium rises as plasma water declines from TEWL. Serum osmolality thus also becomes elevated (see p. 92). Compared to infants in incubators, higher plasma sodium concentrations have been demonstrated in neonates on radiant warmers when fluid input was not increased.

Variations in gestational age, postnatal age, and size exert a significant influence on these average figures for IWL. Nevertheless, the trend is clear and the data are important; the role of radiant warmers must be considered when monitoring the water balance of sick infants. *A baby who is managed on a radiant warmer will require more fluid than one who is in an incubator if other factors do not differ significantly.*

Heat shields on radiant warmers, if they are the proper type, can significantly reduce IWL imposed by radiant energy. In one study, the use of a cylindric Plexiglas shield (identical to the one shown in Fig. 4-7 on p. 103) was associated with a 25% diminution of evaporative losses. However, the authors did not recommend routine use of these shields because for hypothermic infants the radiant energy of the warmer was less effective in maintaining core temperature. We have measured the quantity of radiant energy delivered to infants beneath this Plexiglas shield, and we have found that 82% of a dose of radiant energy does not pass through the Plexiglas. Body temperature may thus be supported only by the increased heat that is generated within the Plexiglas wall, not the radiant energy delivered to the baby. In contrast, the heat shield shown in Fig. 4-9 on p. 107 utilized a Saran Wrap covering. It reduced the measured quantity of radiance delivered to the body surface by only 18%. Our data also indicate that evaporative losses are reduced by approximately 50% when these particular shields are used (p. 106).

The principal objective of this shield is the reduction of insensible water loss in infants managed on radiant warmers. The material used in its construction should neither impede transmittance of radiant energy significantly nor impair patient visibility and accessibility. Table 7-4 indicates the extent to which the shield diminished the radiant energy requirements for maintenance of normal skin and rectal temperature (by 59%) and diminished IWL by 51%. Fig. 7-4 illustrates the difference in transmission of infrared radiance through different materials when the radiant warmer was at maximal output.

When a Plexiglas heat shield is used in incubators, heat loss and IWL are reduced (p. 106). This study demonstrated a mean decline in IWL of 25%. The infants in that study weighed 695 to 1770 g at birth. Averages from infants whose birth weights vary so widely are often misleading when specific application to an individual infant is required. Although the average decline in IWL for all birth weights was approximately 25%, IWL decreased by as much as 45% among infants who were 1250 g or less. *Plexiglas shields are effective in incubators; their routine use on radiant warmers is ill advised.*

Plastic "bubble blankets" (thermal blankets) were used in one study to minimize water loss in premature infants who were managed in incubators. The plastic blanket, used for commercial packing of fragile merchandise such as china and crystal, is light and transparent. It produced a 70% reduction in IWL. Water loss was 65 ml/kg/24 h without the blanket, 16.2 ml/kg/24 h with it. Similar studies on radiant warmers have not been reported.

Phototherapy exerts a substantial influence on evaporative water loss. Under phototherapy, increased amounts of water are lost through the skin, from the respiratory tract because respiratory rate is increased, and from the gastrointestinal tract because frequent loose stools contain abnormally large quantities of water. Among term infants who receive phototherapy while in an incubator, one can expect a 40% increase in the IWL, and a 160% increase in water loss from stool. These data were derived from term infants, who being otherwise well could compensate for their losses by increasing their oral intake of formula. It is plausible to assume that increased losses incurred on small, seriously ill infants are even more significant, and if neglected, more hazardous. Phototherapy is often used for infants who are under radiant warmers. The addition of phototherapy to babies under 1500 g who are already on radiant warmers increases IWL by almost 50%. *It thus follows that if an infant is transferred from an incubator to a radiant warmer, fluid intake must be increased in anticipation of increased*

Table 7-4. Radiant energy requirements and IWL with and without heat shield

	Radiant energy (mean) mW/cm²/h	IWL (mean) ml/kg/h
With shield	8.7	1.68
Without shield	21.40	3.45
	(p = <0.001)	(p = <0.001)

IWL; if phototherapy is also initiated, fluid intake must be increased still more. Use of an appropriate shield minimizes the increase in fluid requirement.

Role of the kidneys. In normal circumstances renal output of water accounts for 50% to 60% of total water loss. However, this proportion necessarily varies, depending on an infant's maturity and well-being, postnatal age, thermal environment, dosages of fluids and electrolytes, and pharmacologic agents in use. To maintain normal proportions and content of electrolyte and water, the kidney must excrete a given amount of solute (principally sodium, potassium, chloride, bicarbonate, urea, and phosphates) in a given quantity of water. The solute load presented to the kidney cannot be excreted without availability of an appropriate quantity of water. When the largest amount of solute is excreted in the smallest possible quantity of water, the kidney has reached its maximal capacity to concentrate the urine. In the neonate, urine concentration does not usually exceed 600 milliosmoles per liter (mOsm/L), which is equal to a specific gravity of 1.020. The adult can concentrate up to approximately 1400 mOsm/L (specific gravity 1.040). Diluting capacity of the neonatal kidney is also more limited than in older age groups. Maximal dilution is 50 mOsm/L (specific gravity 1.001). Low birth weight infants do have a capacity to respond to a fluid overload by increasing urine volume, but only within restricted limits. Presented with a load of 11.0 ml/kg/h for 2 hours, urine output was shown to increase, but only half the administered fluid could be excreted in a few hours. Concentrating and dilutional limitations of renal function are important considerations in monitoring fluid therapy to avoid dehydration and overhydration.

Development of the fetal kidney is complete at approximately 35 weeks. Before that age, glo-

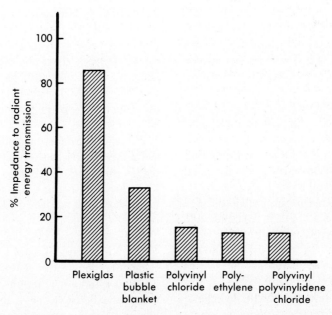

Fig. 7-4. Percent impedance to passage of infrared energy through different substances tested. Plexiglas almost completely blocks transmission of infrared energy. (From Fitch, C. W., and Korones, S. B.: Unpublished data, 1984).

merular filtration rate (GFR) and tubular reabsorptive-secretory capacities are considerably diminished compared to older children and adults. Moreover, using adult function as a reference point, tubular function is even less developed than GFR; a state of glomerular-tubular imbalance is said to exist before 35 gestational weeks. There is therefore a greater capacity for filtration (glomerulus) than for reabsorption (tubule). The functional development of renal tubules in preterm infants after birth is a major determinant of homeostasis and the sodium requirements for maintenance of normal serum levels. Progressive development of renal structure and function is primarily related to conceptional age (gestational plus postnatal ages). An infant born at 30 weeks will proceed in the maturation of renal function at a pace that would have transpired in utero. However, postnatal fluid and solute challenges, plus changes in renal perfusion patterns, seem to accelerate the rate of maturation to some extent. For example, the data for renal excretion of sodium indicate that the most immature babies (less than 30 weeks) ultimately acquire mature function at an earlier postnatal age, but a longer time after birth is required to attain it. Thus, in recent years, deficiencies of sodium homeostasis in premature infants have demonstrated that postnatal persistence of immature renal function is related to conceptional age, and that postnatal maturation is somewhat accelerated. In this context, numerous observations indicate the tendency of premature infants to become hyponatremic early in postnatal life, and in some reports the tendency persists for several weeks thereafter. The observed low serum sodium levels (less than 130 mEq) are largely the result of diminished capacity for tubular reabsorption of the sodium that was excreted into the nephron upstream in the glomerular filtrate. In some studies the excessive rate of sodium excretion continues for 6 weeks after birth. In others, excessive sodium excretion is corrected at a time (conceptional age) corresponding to 33 gestational weeks. The lower the gestational age, the greater the tubular loss of sodium.

The clinical implication of these findings is in the realization that daily sodium requirement is greater than was previously presumed. Severe hyponatremia has been identified repeatedly; it is caused by excessive tubular losses of sodium, and it is enhanced by inadequate daily replacement of sodium.

The role of *aldosterone* in excessive tubular sodium losses has been investigated. Aldosterone is a mineralocorticoid that is released by the adrenal. The kidneys release renin, which stimulates release of angiotensin II, which in turn stimulates adrenal secretion of aldosterone. Aldosterone acts on the distal tubules to promote reabsorption of sodium into the blood stream in exchange for release of potassium into the tubules. A deficiency of aldosterone causes diminished sodium reabsorption and diminished release of potassium; ultimately, hyponatremia and hyperkalemia become manifest. The low serum sodiums and high serum potassiums that have been observed in premature infants could be a result of a maturational deficiency of aldosterone secretion, but high blood and urine contents of aldosterone have been demonstrated in affected infants. Thus aldosterone deficiency does not exist in premature infants. An alternative and plausible explanation for hyponatremia-hyperkalemia is that immature tubules do not respond to aldosterone until 33 to 35 weeks.

These developmental considerations of renal sodium excretion provide rationale for increasing daily sodium requirements to a high of 5 to 7 mEq/kg if the need is apparent. The daily dose of sodium should be increased when serum sodium is below 130 mEq.

Immature renal function (restricted concentrating and dilutional capacity) is also the basis for calculating daily water requirements, but in conjunction with anticipated insensible water losses, which may be immense in the most immature of infants. If inappropriately large amounts of water are lost by IWL, less water is available to the kidney for excretion of solute. At maximal urine concentrations (high urine osmolalities), available water is insufficient for excretion of solute load; solutes are thus retained. Serum sodium is augmented (over 150 mEq/L), and serum osmolality rises abnormally to over 300 mOsm/L. The baby now has hyperosmolar dehydration because a large TEWL was not considered in the calculation of water requirements. If water intake is suboptimal, the kidney excretes less urine to preserve water balance, yet a fixed amount of solute must be excreted if normal electrolyte and acid-base balance is to be maintained. Renal concentration compensates for the relative unavailability of water by using less of it for solute excretion. However, the neonate can concentrate only half as well as the older child; the premature infant concentrates even less. It follows, therefore, that there is less tolerance to insufficient water input and to uncompensated excessive water loss (TEWL). The smaller the baby, the lower the tolerance.

Role of hormones in the maintenance of fluid and electrolyte equilibrium. *Antidiuretic hormone* (ADH) and *aldosterone* play prominent roles in water and electrolyte homeostasis.

ADH produces an antidiuretic effect—it diminishes the volume of water excreted by the kidneys, in the extreme producing severe oliguria, water retention, and overhydration. On the other hand, the absence of ADH increases renal water loss, producing severe polyuria and life-threatening dehydration in the extreme. ADH increases the permeability of renal tubular epithelium to water. Water thus moves from within the renal tubules to the interstitial tissue, and it is retained rather than excreted. In the absence of ADH, renal tubular epithelium is virtually impermeable to water so that an abnormally large volume is excreted. Between the extremes of antidiuresis (severe water retention) and diuresis (abnormally large water loss), varying blood levels of ADH exert appropriate control in response to a fluctuating physiologic need for water retention and excretion. The release of ADH from the posterior pituitary gland may increase or decrease in response to stimuli from osmoreceptors in the hypothalamus, which themselves respond to changes in plasma osmolality. Thus renal water retention occurs if plasma osmolality is high, and diuresis occurs when plasma osmolality is low. A typical sequence of events may be described as follows. When ECF (and thus plasma) is inappropriately concentrated, the hypothalamic osmoreceptors stimulate ADH release. The increased circulating ADH arrives at the renal tubular epithelium to increase its permeability to water. A greater amount of urinary water is now reabsorbed from the tubules, urine volume decreases, and urine osmolality increases. The water thus retained is incorporated into the ECF, and the previously elevated plasma osmolality is reduced. Now reduced plasma osmolality stimulates osmoreceptors to diminish release of ADH, and less water is reabsorbed from the tubules. Urine becomes more dilute, urinary flow is increased, and renal water loss is enhanced. *Renal water excretion varies inversely with the level of circulating ADH.*

The rate of ADH secretion is also influenced by intravascular volume. Receptors that are sensitive to changes in blood pressure (baroreceptors) are situated in the aorta, the carotid arteries, and wall of the atrium. If blood pressure rises, these structures become distended, and the baroreceptors are stretched. In that state they convey impulses to the hypothalamus to diminish the release of ADH. Renal water excretion increases as indicated by a lower urine osmolality. In neonates, hypotension is a more frequent occurrence. The decrease in blood pressure stimulates baroreceptors to signal an increased release of ADH. Renal tubules become more permeable, and water is transferred to renal interstitium. Urinary water loss diminishes, and urine osmolality increases. Retention of water represents an attempt to maintain blood pressure by increasing intravascular fluid volume.

In summary, ADH exerts its powerful influence on the volume of water that is lost from the kidneys by promoting or inhibiting the reabsorption of water from renal tubules. ADH is released in response to a need for retention or excretion of water to compensate for abnormal osmolality of extracellular fluid, and for abnormal intravascular volume.

Aldosterone promotes reabsorption of sodium from the distal renal tubules. This mineralocorticoid causes the reabsorption of sodium into the blood stream primarily in association with an exchange for potassium, which is excreted into the tubules. However, there is actually little, if any, increase in plasma sodium *concentration* because as sodium is reabsorbed from the tubules it carries a commensurate amount of water with it. Overall, there is an increase in extracellular fluid and sodium; concentration therefore remains approximately the same. The effect of aldosterone on plasma potassium concentration is of greater significance clinically. High aldosterone levels can cause serious decreases in plasma potassium concentrations by virtue of the excessive loss from extracellular fluid renal tubules. When plasma potassium concentration diminishes below 50% of normal, muscle paralysis and other signs of hypokalemia become evident. Conversely, if aldosterone is lacking, the urinary excretion of potassium is diminished, potassium is retained, and hyperkalemia results. The renal release of renin, then angiotensin II, and ultimately aldosterone is called the *renin-angiotensin II-aldosterone system*. This normal sequence of hormonal secretion has been identified in neonates, both term and preterm.

Stool loss. The volume of water lost from the gastrointestinal tract is insignificant unless a large number of loose or watery stools are excreted, as in babies with diarrhea. When phototherapy is applied, the water content and volume of stools increase. This does not often cause clinical difficulty.

Disorders of fluid and electrolyte balance

Dehydration. Physiologic equilibrium requires a normal volume of body water, a normal content of solute therein, and a normal distribution of both between the intracellular and extracellular compartments. Dehydration almost always entails a reduced volume of body water in the ICF as well as the ECF. In severe dehydration, blood volume is ultimately reduced because plasma water is so depleted. Dehydration is produced when (1) fluid input is diminished and water loss does not decrease; (2) fluid loss increases and is not matched by an increased input; and (3) increased loss is combined with decreased input. In most instances, dehydration in the neonate occurs when more water is lost than is administered.

Three types of dehydration are clearly identifiable. *Isotonic dehydration* is the result of excessive loss in which water and solute are of the same proportion as in normal body fluids. Serum sodium concentration and osmolality are thus normal because proportional loss of solute and water does not change the concentration of electrolytes in the remaining body fluids. *Hypertonic dehydration* occurs when the volume of lost water is proportionately greater than the quantity of lost solute. Body fluids are thus deprived of greater amounts of water than solute. The result is an abnormal elevation of serum sodium concentration and osmolality. The body fluids that remain are thus hypertonic. *Hypotonic dehydration* is the result of excessive losses that contain more solute than water when compared with normal concentrations in body fluids. The relatively greater loss of solute diminishes serum sodium concentration and serum osmolality. The residual body fluids are hypotonic.

The most frequent cause of dehydration is failure to administer the proper amounts of fluid and electrolytes for physiologic equilibrium, particularly in very small premature infants. Hypotonic dehydration is rare; isotonic dehydration occurs more frequently. *Hypertonic dehydration is the most frequent consequence of inadequate fluid administration.* In this respect, TEWL is probably the most important consideration. Its variations, as influenced by gestational age, size, and use of radiant warmers and phototherapy, are often unappreciated. If TEWL is not approximated by adequate fluid input, dangerous *hypertonic dehydration* occurs because water, not solute, is lost through the skin. Some degree of compensation for the excessive serum sodium concentration can be expected from an increased excretion of sodium by the kidneys. Decreased renal excretion of water partially compensates for the TEWL, but all this renal activity cannot prevent serious water depletion in the face of a protracted inadequacy in fluid administration.

Some *congenital malformations of the kidney* (renal dysplasia and severe hydronephrosis) are characterized by an inability to concentrate urine effectively. The resultant water loss proportionately exceeds the loss of solute, and hypertonic dehydration becomes apparent. *Diarrhea* is not a frequent occurrence in the neonatal intensive care unit, except during outbreaks of infection. Dehydration develops rapidly, particularly in the smallest babies. It is generally isotonic, although hypertonic dehydration is not unusual. The use of *theophylline* for apnea of prematurity has become pervasive. Theophylline causes diuresis, often with a disproportionately large loss of sodium. Either hypotonic or isotonic dehydration may result, depending on the volume of water that accompanies the loss of sodium. Hypertonic dehydration follows *fever* or *high ambient temperature*.

Overhydration. Overhydration refers to an excess of total body water that may be produced by a large input of fluid, a severe diminution in water loss, or a combination of both. Overhydration is usually hypotonic, sometimes isotonic. Hypertonic overhydration is rare, usually occurring postoperatively in the presence of oliguria and injudicious fluid and solute administration.

The clinical signs of overhydration depend on the amount of interstitial fluid that has accumulated (subcutaneous edema) and the extent to which intravascular volume is increased (pulmonary edema, cardiac failure). Edema is the cardinal sign of interstitial fluid accumulation. It usually pits with relatively little pressure, but pitting edema is not present in early overhydration. Furthermore, the neonate is usually supine and un-less the examiner attempts to demonstrate pitting at the flanks and back, its presence will be missed because fluid aggregates in dependent areas. Edema of subcutaneous tissue is itself benign, even though it can be unsightly and it may contribute to pressure ulcers. If, however, plasma volume is expanded, the ultimate result is pulmonary edema and cardiac failure. Overhydration is also characterized by an inordinate weight gain. Whether or not edema is in evidence, inappropriate weight gain indicates overhydration. The most common clinical situations in which overhydration occurs are (1) administration of inappropriately large volumes of fluid and (2) the syndrome of inappropriate ADH (SIADH).

Administration of inappropriately large quantities of fluid is usually the result of an uninformed estimate of the neonate's fluid needs. Ongoing monitoring of fluid balance is indispensable if overhydration is to be avoided. *Acute overhydration from intravascular fluids rapidly leads to pulmonary edema*, particularly in smaller premature infants. In them, the lungs have been likened to a "sump" in which interstitial fluid accumulates rapidly, even in the absence of cardiac failure. *When overhydration develops gradually, it is more likely to produce obvious edema*. Pulmonary edema then appears later if the administration of excessive fluid is not curtailed.

The *syndrome of inappropriate ADH (SIADH)* refers to oversecretion of the antidiuretic hormone. It occurs most often in term infants, although it affects premature infants more frequently than is generally realized. SIADH has been reported at a gestational age as low as 27 weeks. Whether in premature or term infants, virtually all reported instances of SIADH have occurred in association with brain injury resulting from asphyxia, intracranial hemorrhage, and meningitis. Generally, the onset of SIADH in premature infants has been observed at 5 days to 2 weeks of age. In term infants, SIADH occurs most often after perinatal asphyxia. Typically, Apgar scores are low and resuscitation is required in the delivery room. Meconium aspiration is frequently identifiable in these asphyxiated infants. Most of them first convulse at 6 to 12 hours of age. Cerebral edema is indicated by a tight bulging fontanelle and separated sutures. It is in such infants that oversecretion of ADH often occurs. The mechanism by which ADH is copiously released in asphyxiated infants is not understood.

Heightened levels of ADH produce massive reabsorption of water from the renal tubules, considerably exceeding the normal process of compensation for serum hyperosmolality that was described earlier in this chapter. These elevated levels of ADH are initiated in the presence of normal blood volume and serum osmolality. Severe water retention, plus continued renal excretion of sodium, results in severe hyponatremia. Serum sodium may be as low as 110 mEq/L. A unique aspect of SIADH is the high urine osmolality and diminished urine output that occurs and persists even though serum osmolality is low. Abnormally high ADH levels cause massive tubular reabsorption of water; urine osmolalities are thus considerably higher than those of the serum. In contrast to SIADH, overhydration resulting from excessive fluid administration is associated with low (or normal) serum osmolality and low urine osmolality as well. In both instances of overhydration, serum sodium concentration is low because water is retained, not because excessive sodium is lost. This is called *dilutional hyponatremia*. The criteria for the diagnosis of SIADH are hyponatremia and serum hyposmolality, urine hyperosmolality, and normal adrenal and renal function.

SIADH is primarily an inability to excrete water through the kidneys because of massive tubular reabsorption. Fluid input must be severely restricted between 30 and 50 ml/kg/24 h. A daily maintenance requirement of sodium (2 to 3 mEq/kg) should be added to fluid infusions.

Abnormalities of serum sodium concentration. Abnormally low serum sodium concentrations occur below 130 mEq/kg; abnormally high values occur at 150 mEq/kg or more. Disturbances in serum sodium concentrations invariably involve abnormal water content—total body water, maldistribution between ICF and ECF compartments, or both. There is little sodium within cells; it is an extracellular ion. Largely based on the osmolar forces that its concentrations exert, sodium imposes a major influence on the distribution of water between the intracellular and extracellular spaces. Abnormalities of sodium homeostasis are thus inextricably bound to abnormalities of body water content.

Hyponatremia in the neonate is most frequently caused by administration of suboptimal quantities of sodium in the presence of excessive losses from an immature kidney, or from the administration of excessive volumes of water. Less frequently, hyponatremia indicates SIADH (see p. 197). Overhydration attributable to excessive infusion rates generally occurs in small babies for whom glucose requirements necessitate a large amount of fluids. Excessive fluid administration also occurs when insensible water losses are overestimated, particularly in small babies during the second and third weeks of life when TEWL tends to diminish. In essence, these situations entail overhydration; low sodium levels are the result of dilution. Hyponatremia may also occur in the hours immediately after birth, in the presence of maternal overhydration during labor and delivery. Low serum sodium furthermore occurs during the third to sixth week of life when premature infants are maintained by formula feedings. In such instances, urine sodium losses persist by virtue of immature renal function, while the sodium intake provided by formula feedings is below the daily requirement.

Hypernatremia is most often the result of underhydration, which occurs when inadequate quantities of fluids are administered to infants in whom excessive TEWL is not appreciated. Infants on radiant warmers are particularly vulnerable; the addition of phototherapy heightens the hazard. Hypernatremia may also occur in the presence of hyperglycemia. In these circumstances glycosuria causes an osmotic diuresis; inordinate amounts of water are thus excreted in the urine.

Perhaps the most common of circumstances in which hypernatremia occurs are those in which sodium bicarbonate is given repeatedly to correct acidosis, with little attention to the total sodium load thus administered. In the same context, intravenous and umbilical artery flush solutions that contain sodium are frequently overlooked as a significant source of sodium input.

Ongoing assessment of fluid and electrolyte status

The ongoing assessment of fluid and electrolyte status requires several laboratory determinations. Protracted intravascular fluid administration should not be attempted unless such data are available to *personnel who understand their significance*.

The most immediate concern of ongoing assessment is the detection of renal compensatory activity that is called into play by a surfeit or a paucity of infused fluid. At that point imbalance has not yet occurred, and the correction of existing therapy will avoid it. *The earliest recognizable response to inappropriate fluid therapy is the concentration or dilution of urine*. When classically described physical signs of dehydration or overhydration appear, the abnormal process has been long ongoing. It should have been detected earlier by other means. Weight changes are repeatedly emphasized in the literature, and they are indeed useful indicators. However, the state of the "weighing art" in neonatal intensive care units is little better than deplorable. There are too many occasions when accuracy is questionable, and when the "drag" of IV lines and monitor electrodes impair the process. Furthermore, most units still use inappropriately graduated spring scales that were originally designed to weigh meat in supermarkets. In addition, few facilities periodically check the accuracy of these scales with standardized weights. Yet we rely heavily on weights. If normal renal function is present, the process of water depletion or accumulation generally begins with changes in urine osmolality and output. The kidneys concentrate urine to pre-

serve water when input is insufficient to match loss. Conversely, the kidneys dilute urine so that water excretion is increased when input exceeds loss. *This compensatory renal activity is reflected in the urine osmolality or specific gravity, well in advance of abnormalities in serum*. Assuming normal renal function, a urine osmolality between 100 and 300 mOsm (sp. gr. = 1.008 to 1.012) indicates optimal water balance. Furthermore, within these limits, osmolality is associated with a normal urine volume. Osmolalities between 300 and 400 mOsm are acceptable but they suggest that somewhat less than an optimal volume of fluid is being given. Hypertonic urine that is over 400 mOsm indicates a need to increase fluid input until osmolality is 100 to 300 mOsm. If urine osmolality is below 100 mOsm, the quantity of fluid input should be decreased. Specific gravity is a more commonly used procedure for the determination of urine concentration because it is simple and rapid and does not require laboratory personnel. We prefer urine osmolality because it can be better correlated with serum osmolality when assessing the development of serious fluid imbalance. Whether expressed as osmolality or specific gravity, periodic determination of urine concentration is the most valuable screening procedure for careful monitoring.

Monitoring for dehydration. Insufficient fluid input is indicated early by concentrated urine (greater than 400 mOsm). If an inadequate amount of fluid input is allowed to continue, water in the intravascular space diminishes and the increased plasma osmolality is compensated for by movement of water from the interstitial space into the blood vessels. Blood volume and plasma osmolality are thereby temporarily maintained within normal limits (270 to 300 mOsm). Next, body weight decreases to the extent of net water loss, even before the plasma becomes hyperosmolar. Significant weight loss is the first indication of *uncompensated* imbalance. As dehydration progresses, the osmolality of plasma and interstitial fluid rises and serum sodium concentration also becomes abnormally high (over 150 mEq/L). An

Table 7-5. Water imbalance: sequence of events and abnormal values

Dehydration (input < loss)	Overhydration (input > loss)
↓ Urine volume (<1 ml/kg/h)	↑ Urine volume (>3 ml/kg/h)
↑ Urine osmolality (>400 mOsm)	↓ Urine osmolality (<100 mOsm)
↑ Urine sp. gr. (>1.012)	↓ Urine sp. gr. (<1.008)
↓	↓
Weight loss (5% to 15%/24 h)	Weight gain (5% to 15%/24 h)
↓	↓
↑ Serum sodium (>150 mEq/L)	↓ Serum sodium (<130 mEq/L)
↑ Serum osmolality (>300 mOsm)	↓ Serum osmolality (<270 mOsm)
↓	↓
Dry skin, mucous membrane	Subcutaneous edema
↓ Skin turgor	Pulmonary edema
↓	↓
↑ Hematocrit (≥10%)	↓ Hematocrit (≥10%)
↑ Serum protein (>6 g/dl)	↓ Serum protein (<4 g/dl)
↓ Blood volume (variable)	↑ Blood volume (variable)
↓	↓
Shock	Cardiac failure

osmolar discrepancy has now developed between the ECF and ICF, producing movement of fluid from the intracellular space into the interstitial and intravascular spaces. These compensatory activities ultimately become ineffective; plasma volume resulting from net water loss eventually becomes so diminished as to produce an increased hematocrit and plasma protein level hemoconcentration. Diminished blood volume causes shock. Even before shock develops, the skin becomes dry to touch; its turgor is diminished. Mucous membranes lose the sheen that is normally imparted by moisture; they appear dull and dry. The anterior fontanelle is depressed, presumably because the volume of cerebrospinal fluid is diminished. All these abnormal physical signs become apparent late in the process of dehydration. *This entire sequence of events began with the appearance of hyperosmolar urine (over 400 mOsm) when renal compensation was still effective. Dehydration could have been prevented early by increasing the volume of infused fluid.*

Systematic monitoring should also include total fluid input, urine output, urine and serum osmo-

lalities, serum electrolytes, blood urea nitrogen, body weight determination at least every 12 hours, total serum protein and hematocrit, and postoperative fluid losses from surgical repair sites.

Monitoring for overhydration. Fluid input in excess of loss is indicated early by dilute urine (less than 100 mOsm). In these circumstances, plasma fluid increases transiently until excess water diffuses into the interstitial space. At some point fluid volume in both spaces is increased and osmolality of ECF is reduced relative to that of ICF. There ensues a movement of water from the interstitial space into the intracellular space. *Uncompensated* imbalance is first manifested by an inordinate gain in body weight. Serum osmolality is low (less than 270 mOsm), and serum sodium concentration is correspondingly diminished to less than 130 mEq/L. Subcutaneous edema appears if the process of overhydration is gradual; pulmonary edema appears first if the process is rapid. In the extreme, fluid overload leads to congestive heart failure. *This sequence of events began with the appearance of dilute urine (less than 100 mOsm), when compensation could have*

Table 7-6. Maintenance volumes of intravascular fluid by birth weight for the first 2 weeks of life

Birth weight (g)	Days 1-2 (ml/kg/24 h)	Days 3-14 (ml/kg/24 h)
750-1000	100	130-160
1001-1250	90	120-150
1251-1500	90	110-140
1501-2500	80	100-130
2501 and over	70	80-100

been effected by diminishing water input. Table 7-5 lists the sequence of these events and, when applicable, the approximate values that indicate their abnormal nature.

Systematic monitoring must also include total fluid intake and urinary output, blood urea nitrogen, serum electrolytes, total protein, hematocrit, and a recording of weight at least every 12 hours.

Maintenance requirements of fluids and electrolytes

Fluids. Maintenance fluid is administered to replenish the total water loss that occurs from skin, lungs, and kidneys. Water losses are directly related to expended energy as measured in calories. The usual figure given for total water loss in the neonate is 100 ml/100 cal expended. However, in babies who are between 1 and 4 kg, energy expenditure is closely related to body weight. Fluid requirements are therefore accurately expressed as ml/kg of body weight.

Since several factors are known to profoundly influence the loss of water, it is impossible to recommend specific fluid volumes that are applicable in all circumstances. Fluid requirements differ according to the microenvironment provided for infant management such as incubators, radiant warmers, or open bassinets. Requirements vary with weight, gestational and postnatal age, type of illness, humidity during respiratory support, and use of phototherapy or heat shields.

They even differ from one commercial brand of radiant warmer to another. Therefore in providing maintenance fluid, one estimates the standard amount required, alters that quantity according to the presence of influencing factors, and then makes further alterations in response to the available monitoring data.

Intravascular fluid is generally administered within a volume range that is selected according to birth weight and microenvironment. In any given nursery, successful experience generally dictates the quantity of fluids that are customarily administered. Table 7-6 lists intravascular fluid volumes according to birth weight during the first 2 weeks of life. There is little change in these ranges during the ensuing 2 weeks.

Fluid intake should be decreased by 25% of stated quantities during the first 2 days of life. Increases in fluid volume may be required when ambient temperature is higher than usual, with use of radiant warmers and phototherapy, and in the presence of fever, hyperactivity, increased work of respiration (respiratory distress), and fluid drainage from postoperative wounds. The extent to which these conditions impose an increased fluid requirement can only be estimated with the aid of ongoing monitoring data.

Fluid maintenance requirements may diminish if a heat shield is used in an incubator or on a radiant warmer, when a plastic "bubble blanket" is applied to the baby, and when the humidity of inspired air is high. Fluid restriction is necessary in the presence of renal failure from any cause, inappropriate ADH syndrome, congestive heart failure, and patent ductus arteriosus with a significant left-to-right shunt.

Electrolytes. Daily requirements of sodium and potassium are each 2 mEq/kg, and for chloride, 2 to 4 mEq/kg. Infants who are less than 1500 g often require 3 to 4 mEq/kg of sodium daily, often much more because of large renal sodium losses. Normal electrolyte values are listed in Table 7-7 for infants whose birth weights are 1500 to 1750 g. These values are applicable to all premature infants with little clinically significant variation from one birth weight to another.

Table 7-7. Blood chemistry values in premature infants 1500 to 1750 g at birth*

Constituent	Age 1 week Mean	Age 1 week Range	Age 3 weeks Mean	Age 3 weeks Range	Age 5 weeks Mean	Age 5 weeks Range	Age 7 weeks Mean	Age 7 weeks Range
Na (mEq/L)	139.6	133-146	136.3	129-142	136.8	133-148	137.2	133-142
K (mEq/L)	5.6	4.6-6.7	5.8	4.5-7.1	5.5	4.5-6.6	5.7	4.6-7.1
Cl (mEq/L)	108.2	100-117	108.3	102-116	107.0	100-115	107.0	101-115
CO_2 (mEq/L)	20.3	13.8-27.1	18.4	12.4-26.2	20.4	12.5-26.1	20.6	13.7-26.9
Ca (mg/dl)	9.2	6.1-11.6	9.6	8.1-11.0	9.4	8.6-10.5	9.5	8.6-10.8
P (mg/dl)	7.6	5.4-10.9	7.5	6.2-8.7	7.0	5.6-7.9	6.8	4.2-8.2
BUN (mg/dl)	9.3	3.1-25.5	13.3	2.1-31.4	13.3	2.0-26.5	13.4	2.5-30.5
Total protein (g/dl)	5.49	4.40-6.26	5.38	4.28-6.70	4.98	4.14-6.90	4.93	4.02-5.86
Albumin (g/dl)	3.85	3.28-4.50	3.92	3.16-5.26	3.73	3.20-4.34	3.89	3.40-4.60
Globulin (g/dl)	1.58	0.88-2.20	1.44	0.62-2.90	1.17	0.48-1.48	1.12	0.5-2.60
Hb (g/dl)	17.8	11.4-24.8	14.7	9.0-19.4	11.5	7.2-18.6	10.0	7.5-13.9

*Adapted from Thomas, J., and Reichelderfer, T.: Clin. Chem. **14:**272, 1968.

BIBLIOGRAPHY

Al-Dahhan, J., Haycock, G. B., Chantler, C., and Stimmler, L.: Sodium homeostasis in term and preterm neonates. I. Renal aspects, Arch. Dis. Child. **58:**335, 1983.

Al-Dahhan, J., Haycock, G. B., Chantler, C., and Stimmler, L.: Sodium homeostasis in term and preterm neonates. II. Gastrointestinal aspects, Arch. Dis. Child. **58:**343, 1983.

Al-Dahhan, J., Haycock, G. B., Chantler, C., and Stimmler, L.: Sodium homeostasis in term and preterm neonates. III. Effect of salt supplementation, Arch. Dis. Child. **59:**945, 1984.

Bell, E. F., and Oh, W.: Fluid and electrolyte balance in very low birth weight infants, Clin. Perinatol. **6:**139, 1979.

Bell, E. F., Neidich, G. A., Cashore, W. J., and Oh, W.: Combined effect of radiant warmer and phototherapy on insensible water loss in low birth weight infants, J. Pediatr. **94:**810, 1979.

Fanaroff, A. A., Wald, M., Gruber, H. S., and Klaus, M. H.: Insensible water loss in low birth weight infants, Pediatrics **50:**236, 1972.

Finberg, L.: Hypernatremic dehydration. In Finberg, L., Kravath, R. E., and Fleischman, A. R., editors: Water and electrolytes in pediatrics—physiology, pathophysiology and treatment, Philadelphia, 1982, W. B. Saunders Co.

Finberg, L.: Sodium, potassium, and chloride ions: metabolism and regulation. In Finberg, L., Kravath, R. E., and Fleischman, A. R., editors: Water and electrolytes in pediatrics—physiology, pathophysiology and treatment, Philadelphia, 1982, W. B. Saunders Co.

Fitch, C. W., and Korones, S. B.: Heat shield reduces water loss, Arch. Dis. Child. **59:**886, 1984.

Fleischman, A. R.: Special problems of the fetus and neonate. In Finberg, L., Kravath, R. E., and Fleischman, A. R., editors: Water and electrolytes in pediatrics—physiology, pathophysiology and treatment, Philadelphia, 1982, W. B. Saunders Co.

Gennari, F. J.: Serum osmolality—uses and limitations, N. Engl. J. Med. **310:**102, 1984.

Heird, W. C.: Nutrition, body fluids, and acid-base homeostasis. Part III. Provision of water and electrolytes. In Fanaroff, A. A., and Martin, R. J., editors: Behrman's neonatal-perinatal medicine—diseases of the fetus and infant, ed. 3, St. Louis, 1983, The C.V. Mosby Co.

Jones, M. D., Jr., Greshman, E. L., and Battaglia, F. C.: Urinary flow rates and urea excretion rates in newborn infants, Biol. Neonate **21:**321, 1972.

Kildeberg, P.: Clinical acid-base physiology; studies in neonates, infants and young children, Baltimore, 1968, The Williams & Wilkins Co.

Lorenz, J. M., Kleinman, L. I., Kotagal, U. R., and Reller, M. D.: Water balance in very low-birth-weight infants: relationship to water and sodium intake and effect on outcome, J. Pediatr. **101:**423, 1982.

Marks, K. H., Friedman, Z., and Maisels, M. J.: A simple device for reducing insensible water loss in low-birth-weight infants, Pediatrics **60:**223, 1977.

Mendoza, S. A.: Syndrome of inappropriate antidiuretic hormone secretion (SIADH), Pediatr. Clin. North Am. **23:**681, 1976.

Moylan, F. M. B., et al.: Inappropriate antidiuretic hormone secretion in premature infants with cerebral injury, Am. J. Dis. Child. **132:**399, 1978.

Nash, M. A.: The management of fluid and electrolyte disorders in the neonate, Clin. Perinatol. **8:**251, 1981.

Oh, W.: Fluid and electrolyte therapy and parenteral nutrition in low birth weight infants, Clin. Perinatol. **9:**637, 1982.

Oh, W., and Karecki, H.: Phototherapy and insensible water loss in the newborn infant, Am. J. Dis. Child. **124:**230, 1972.

Report of Ad-Hoc Committee on Acid-Base Terminology: Current concepts of acid-base measurements, Ann. N. Y. Acad. Sci. **133:**251, 1966.

Ross, B., Cowett, R. M., and Oh, W.: Renal functions of low birth weight infants during the first two months of life, Pediatr. Res. **11:**1162, 1977.

Roy, R. N., Chance, G. W., Radde, I. C., et al.: Late hyponatremia in very low birthweight infants (<1.3 kilograms), Pediatr. Res. **10:**526, 1976.

Saenger, P.: Disorders of the adrenal gland as causes of electrolyte disturbances: diagnosis and treatment. In Finberg, L., Kravath, R. E., and Fleischman, A. R.: Water and electrolytes in pediatrics—physiology, pathophysiology and treatment, Philadelphia, 1982, W. B. Saunders Co.

Sulyok, E., Varga, F., Györy, E., et al.: Postnatal development of renal sodium handling in premature infants, J. Pediatr. **95:**787, 1979.

Weil, W. B., and Bailie, M. D.: Fluid and electrolyte metabolism in infants and children, New York, 1977, Grune & Stratton.

Williams, P. R., and Oh, W.: Effects of radiant warmer on insensible water loss in newborn infants, Am. J. Dis. Child. **128:**511, 1974.

Winters, R. W.: Terminology of acid-base disorders, Ann. N. Y. Acad. Sci. **133:**211, 1965.

Wu, P. Y. K., and Hodgman, J. E.: Insensible water loss in preterm infants: changes with postnatal development and non-ionizing radiant energy, Pediatrics **54:**704, 1974.

Yeh, T. F., et al.: Reduction of insensible water loss in premature infants under the radiant warmer, J. Pediatr. **94:**651, 1979.

Disorders of the lungs

Although reports on the incidence of pulmonary disorders may vary from one source to another, there is universal agreement that these diseases are the most frequent causes of neonatal morbidity and mortality. Broadly categorized, they result from perinatal misadventures that impair adaptation to extrauterine life, to prenatal and postnatal infections, to congenital anomalies, and to extrapulmonary disorders such as cardiac failure, which secondarily give rise to respiratory dysfunction. This chapter describes the adaptive mechanisms responsible for adjustment to extrauterine respiration and the major clinical entities associated with respiratory distress.

FETAL CARDIOPULMONARY APPARATUS
Pulmonary circulation

The fetal circulation is described in Chapter 1. However, allusion to its pulmonary component is pertinent to the present discussion, particularly in reference to the changes that accompany the first breath (see later). The fetal lung is perfused by only 5% to 7% of cardiac output as a result of the high vascular resistance created by constricted pulmonary arterioles and collapsed alveolar capillaries. Most of the blood emanating from the right ventricle is thus shunted from the main pulmonary artery into the ductus arteriosus, bypassing the lungs. In the mature circulation, all blood from the right ventricle enters the pulmonary circulation directly. Blood supply to the fetal lung is further minimized by diversion of a major portion of inferior vena caval blood into the left atrium by way of the foramen ovale, thus constituting another pulmonary bypass. Establishment of normal extrauterine respiration requires that these fetal pathways be converted to the mature pattern very soon after birth. Further discussion of these changes may be found in Chapter 1.

Development of the fetal lungs

The fetal lung develops in four progressive phases: the embryonic, pseudoglandular, canalicular, and terminal sac periods. During the *embryonic period* (22 to 26 days) the laryngotracheal groove appears. It evaginates to form a midline sac and then divides to form the two lung buds. The bronchial branches develop during the *pseudoglandular period*, which continues to 16 weeks. These bronchial branches are conducting airways. They are small tubules lined by epithelium and embedded in a scantily vascularized mesenchymal mass. The airways divide continuously, forming 15 to 26 generations of branches. The process

of dichotomy is completed by the end of the pseudoglandular period.

The *canalicular period* is the next developmental phase. It continues to 24 weeks. The mesenchyme becomes richly vascular (canalization), and capillaries proliferate as they begin to encroach upon the epithelium that lines the conducting airways. During this phase of development the most distal airways give rise to respiratory bronchioles that extend farther into the periphery. Multiple outpouchings (evaginations) develop along the walls of the respiratory bronchioles to form primitive alveoli. The evaginated bronchioles end in multiple saccules lined by flat epithelium. At about this time (24 to 25 weeks) extrauterine respiration can be mechanically supported in some babies.

The last phase of fetal lung development is the

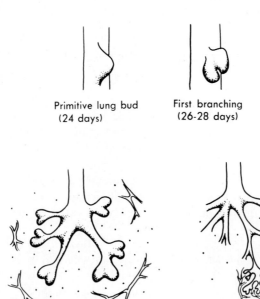

Primitive lung bud
(24 days)

First branching
(26-28 days)

Capillaries differentiate
from mesenchyme;
respiratory bronchioles formed
(20-24 weeks)

Alveolar sacs differentiated;
capillaries contact
alveolar membrane
(24-28 weeks)

Fig. 8-1. Development of primitive lung bud and subsequent branching into surrounding mesenchyme. (Modified from Avery, M. E., and Fletcher, B. D.: The lung and its disorders in the newborn infant, Philadelphia, 1974, W. B. Saunders Co.)

terminal sac period, which continues to term. It is characterized by the appearance of more saccules, which are primitive alveoli. There are approximately 25 million of them, and they are about 8% of the total number of adult alveoli.

At 24 days the *primitive lung bud* appears as a localized pouch from the ventral surface of the *embryonic gut* (endoderm). This segment of gut will ultimately develop into the esophagus; the lung bud will be the trachea (Figs. 8-1 and 8-2). Persistence of a connection between the two structures is the basis for one of several possible types of tracheoesophageal fistulas (p. 278). At 26 to 28 days the lung bud divides into two structures that will become the two major bronchi. Subsequent growth progresses into surrounding mesenchyme (mesoderm), which becomes incorporated into pulmonary structures as differentiation

proceeds; branching of each terminal structure continues as it grows laterally and downward into the pleural space, carrying with it the surrounding mesenchyme. The right and left branches of the original single bud thus give rise to successive generations of bronchi, bronchioles of diminishing size, alveolar ducts, and alveoli as lung development is ultimately fulfilled. The mesenchyme that surrounds these developing airway structures ultimately differentiates into blood vessels, muscle, connective tissue, cartilaginous plates in the bronchi, and the connective tissue that supports and separates alveolar and other structures in the lung.

By 6 weeks the *segmental bronchi* are formed, and at 12 weeks the *major lobes* are delineated. *Respiratory bronchioles* are differentiated at approximately 16 weeks; from them, at about 24

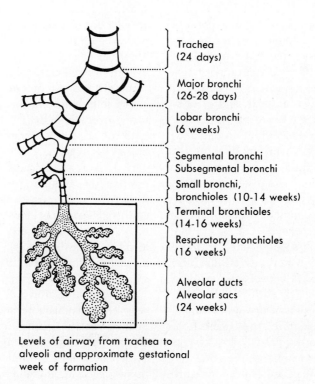

Trachea
(24 days)

Major bronchi
(26-28 days)

Lobar bronchi
(6 weeks)

Segmental bronchi
Subsegmental bronchi

Small bronchi,
bronchioles (10-14 weeks)

Terminal bronchioles
(14-16 weeks)

Respiratory bronchioles
(16 weeks)

Alveolar ducts
Alveolar sacs
(24 weeks)

Levels of airway from trachea to
alveoli and approximate gestational
week of formation

Fig. 8-2. Branching pattern of respiratory tract. The mature structures are indicated, with approximate gestational age of formation.

weeks, alveolar sacs are formed. At birth they are considerably smaller and more shallow than at 1 and 2 months of age. Meanwhile, capillaries have been differentiating from the surrounding mesenchyme since the twentieth week. At 25 to 26 weeks, if live-born, an infant may breathe air successfully if appropriate postnatal support is instituted and if prenatal complications do not preclude survival. At this stage an increased number of capillaries is in direct contact with air spaces that may be functional postnatally. A number of terminal units for air exchange are nevertheless not yet morphologically equipped for extrauterine life. Fewer capillary walls are in contact with potential air spaces, and the remaining mesenchyme (connective tissue) is so abundant that lung compliance will be severely restricted after birth. At 27 to 28 weeks larger numbers of capillaries are in contact with the walls of *alveolar sacs* (alveolar membranes), which themselves have increased in number. The alveolar sacs now comprise most of the cross sectional area of the lung, whereas previously, bronchioles were the most prominent structures. Connective tissue spaces between terminal units are still relatively extensive, however. Lung compliance is low as a result, and in addition, these wide connective tissue spaces may account for the ease with which fluid accumulates within them postnatally. In infants born at this early stage of gestation, the interstitial connective tissue may retain fluid in sponge-like fashion. Furthermore, the relatively large interstitial space in such infants may well account for interstitial emphysema (p. 251) unassociated with an ensuing pneumothorax, which is seen so often in more mature neonates. The wider interstitium also impedes exchange of gases between air sacs and capillaries. At 28 to 29 weeks further differentiation occurs at the distal ends of airways. Terminal saccules are lined with mature type II cells from which surfactant is released. From 30 to 33 weeks new alveolar units appear rapidly. Interstitial tissue is still relatively extensive; alveolar walls are thicker than in the mature infant. At 34 to 36 weeks mature alveolar structures are in evidence.

Most pulmonary growth is attributable to new alveoli. Postnatal ventilation at this gestational age is more affected by perinatal misadventure than by immaturity of structure or function. If unstressed, the neonate at this gestational age can survive by his independent capacity to ventilate and produce surfactant for alveolar stability.

Congenital malformations can be better understood with some knowledge of pulmonary development. Agenesis of the lung and tracheal stenosis are the result of maldevelopment in the earliest differentiation of the primitive lung bud. Tracheoesophageal fistulas of various types probably originate during the earlier branching of the lung bud. Defective deposition of bronchial cartilage from embryonic mesenchyme results in the syndrome of deficient cartilaginous rings. The bronchi collapse during inspiration for lack of supporting tissue. Congenital lung cysts probably result from detachment of respiratory bronchioles, alveolar ducts, and sacs from the proximal airways with which they should normally be continuous. They may enlarge because trapped fluid, secreted by cells in respiratory bronchioles and alveoli, accumulates continuously.

The fetal lungs are metabolically active structures, even though they have no real function until the advent of extrauterine respiration. The blood vessels are narrow, and the alveoli are filled with fluid. Lung fluid differs in origin and composition from amniotic fluid. Lung fluid is derived from cells in the respiratory tract. It is less viscous, and it contains a lower protein concentration than amniotic fluid. Lung liquid must be evacuated soon after birth during the establishment of normal respiration. Its diminished viscosity presumably facilitates postnatal evacuation.

Postnatal lung growth is a vigorous, active process. The chest diameter increases rapidly in early infancy, mostly because of increased number of alveoli and respiratory bronchioles. The term baby is born with 24 million alveoli. At 3 months there are 77 million, and in the adult, 200 to 600 million. The alveolar sacs are considerably more shallow in the neonate, being 50 μm in diameter, compared with 100 to 200 μm in older children and 200 to 300 μm in the adult. The surface area available for gas exchange in the adult is about twenty times greater than in the neonate, which is close to the average increase of adult over neonatal body weight.

Intrauterine fetal breathing movements

It has only been in recent years that human fetal breathing movements have been identified. A considerable amount of investigation in animals preceded the findings in humans. Rhythmical respiratory movements in the human fetus were unequivocally identified when ultrasound techniques became available. These movements are composed of paradoxical excursions of the chest and abdomen. During inspiration the chest is drawn inward and the abdomen protrudes. Contraction pulls the diaphragm down; the abdominal wall is pushed out while the chest wall is drawn in. Excursions are most extensive at the level of the umbilicus, and it is therefore used as a reference point for the assessment of respiratory-type activity.

Fetal breathing movements are episodic. Periods of inactivity have varied from one study to another, most observations having been made during the last 10 weeks of pregnancy. Inactive intervals may last for as long as 2 hours. In fetuses 30 to 31 weeks and 38 to 39 weeks, 24-hour recordings reveal diaphragmatic activity 31% of the time.

Several factors influence breathing movement patterns. At 34 to 35 weeks gestation, prolonged and more frequent periods of activity occur between the hours of 1:00 AM and 7:00 AM during maternal sleep. An increased proportion of time is spent in breathing movements during the 2 and 3 hours that follow maternal meals. Increased fetal activity seems to follow peak levels of maternal glucose, increased movements having been demonstrated after maternal administration of glucose intravenously and orally. Fetal respiratory movements have been observed as early as 18 weeks, but most systematic studies have been conducted during the last trimester.

Maternal cigarette smoking is associated with a decreased incidence of fetal breathing movements. The same response has been noted following the use of chewing gum that contains nicotine, and after maternal ingestion of 1 oz of 80-proof alcohol.

The incidence of respiratory movements is reduced significantly at term, starting from about 3 hours before onset of labor. During labor, episodes of breathing activity are virtually absent.

The potential for clinical usefulness of information on fetal breathing is in the assessment of fetal health and in the evaluation of the role of these movements in normal lung development. Prolonged apnea or apnea with gasping may be associated with poor outcome. In one study fetal compromise was indicated by a reduction in the proportion of time spent in breathing movements. The value of breathing movement data for assessment of well-being seems to be enhanced when combined with heart rate recordings during a nonstress test.

There is some evidence that lung development is influenced by fetal respiratory movements. In animal experiments, a section of the spinal cord between the first and third cervical nerves (high cord section) interferes with diaphragmatic movement, and in these circumstances, weight and DNA content of lungs are significantly reduced. Furthermore, maturation of the lung may be delayed as suggested by immature pressure-volume performance.

FIRST BREATH

Insight into the changes involved in the baby's first breath provides a sound basis for the understanding of pulmonary disturbances of the neonatal period. During intrauterine life, exchange of oxygen and carbon dioxide occurs across the placental membrane from one liquid medium to another. After birth this exchange occurs across the alveolar membrane between a gaseous medium (air in the alveolus) and a liquid one (blood in alveolar capillaries). Among the many changes the infant undergoes at birth, the most abrupt and crucial ones are concerned with adaptation of respiratory function to a gaseous environment. Several requirements must be satisfied before the lungs can assume and maintain these functions:

1. *Respiratory movements must be initiated.*

2. *Entry of air must overcome opposing forces if the lungs are to expand.*

3. *Some air must remain in the alveoli at the end of expiration so that the lungs do not collapse (establishment of functional residual capacity).*

4. *Pulmonary blood flow must be increased, and cardiac output must be redistributed.*

Although these events transpire simultaneously, they lend themselves well to sequential description.

Initiation of respiratory movements

The precise roles of the various stimuli that bombard the infant to initiate his respiratory movements after birth have not been clarified. Their separate effects are difficult to delineate. The identification of intrauterine respiratory movements has given rise to the idea that extrauterine breathing is a continuation of fetal respiratory movements. The neonate may therefore be well practiced by virtue of his fetal experience. If this experience explains the ease with which regular respirations are established after birth, additional explanation is required for the greatly enhanced vigor with which the first extrauterine breaths are executed.

Asphyxia is a significant stimulator of the first breath. Low arterial PO_2, low pH, and high PCO_2 are each known to stimulate respiratory movement under certain conditions. They initiate impulses from the carotid and aortic chemoreceptors that are transmitted to the respiratory control center in the medulla. These asphyxial changes are present to some extent at birth in most normal newborn infants, and they are considered potent stimulators of the first breath. Before the onset of respiration, oxygen saturation of umbilical venous blood (from the placenta to the fetus) varies from 9% to 96%, whereas in umbilical artery blood (returning to the placenta), it ranges from 0% to 67%; yet many of these transiently hypoxemic infants are vigorous. In a substantial number of them, oxygen saturations are below 10%. Some have no measurable oxygen at all, and yet most of them breathe spontaneously within seconds after delivery. The average PCO_2 at birth is elevated to 58 torr, and the mean pH is depressed to 7.28. These asphyxial chemical changes also activate chemoreceptor nerve endings in the carotid arteries and the aortic arch. These short periods of asphyxia are presumably components of the normal birth process. They are characterized by absence of metabolic acidosis (normal buffer base), although respiratory acidosis (high PCO_2 and diminished pH) is present. The first breath may well be a deep inspiratory gasp, stimulated by hypoxia of the central nervous system, that is not unlike the gasps that follow fetal asphyxia. On the other hand, protracted asphyxial episodes are obviously not normal. They are characterized biochemically by metabolic acidosis (diminished buffer base) in addition to respiratory acidosis (hypercapnia) and hypoxemia. Short asphyxial episodes are thought to be powerful stimuli to the first breath; prolonged asphyxial episodes depress it.

Another important stimulus to the onset of respiratory movement is the abrupt drop that occurs in the infant's ambient temperature on arrival in room air. The baby leaves a fluid intrauterine environment of 98.6° F (37° C) and is thrust into a dry ambient temperature of 70° to 75° F (21° to 24° C) in an air-conditioned delivery room. This sudden change in environmental temperature stimulates nerve endings in the skin, with subsequent transmission of impulses to the medullary respiratory control center. This is probably an intense stimulus, and the response is instantaneous. The rapid onset of breathing requires an instantaneous response. At birth, the impact of a cold temperature on the skin (Chapter 4) is probably a further stimulus to breathing. Lambs fail to breathe when delivered into a normal saline bath that is at normal body temperature. The same phenomenon has been noted in human infants. During the first few minutes after delivery, core temperature falls at a rate of approximately 0.2° F (0.1° C) per minute, whereas the decline in skin temperature is three times as great. These temperature changes are apparently within physiologic limits. Purposeful excessive cooling of depressed infants is contraindicated. It causes profound depression due to an abnormal fall in body temperature, which produces the penalties of severe cold stress, including hypoxia (Chapter 4).

The tactile stimulation provided during ordinary handling of infants at birth is probably of only minor significance in the initiation of respiratory movement. Although the traditional slaps to the heels or buttocks may have some influence in stimulating respiratory movement in normal babies, the time so expended on depressed infants is better used for more effective resuscitative measures.

The net result of the initial extrauterine activity of respiratory muscles is the creation of lower pressure within the lungs than in the atmosphere. This negative intrathoracic pressure "invites entry" of air into the lungs. The negative pressure created by expansion of the thorax is largely accomplished by descent of the diaphragm, by contraction of its muscle fibers. The contribution of intercostal muscles to thoracic expansion is relatively minor. The air that is "sucked in" as a result of the normal activity of the diaphragm must now reach the alveoli by overcoming forces that obstruct its free flow.

Entry of air into the lungs and expansion of alveoli

Studies on the initiation of breathing indicate that, normally, respiratory efforts begin from 0.5 to 72 seconds after birth (mean of 18 seconds). Air enters the lungs as soon as intrathoracic pressure falls, but air entry is opposed by surface tension (at air fluid interfaces) and by the viscosity of lung fluid in the respiratory tract. The lungs are aerated almost immediately after birth, and in normal circumstances the rhythmicity of respirations is soon well established. The mechanism of initial breathing is an impressive feat of engineering,

particularly when one considers that the fetal lung is full of fluid. The fluid is not completely absorbed for 12 to 24 hours, but within 2 hours after birth as much as 70% of it may be evacuated. The significance of *unopposed* surface tension forces will become apparent as the functional difficulties of the immature lung are described later in this chapter.

Transpulmonary pressures of 35 to 40 cm H_2O are usually required for the first inspiration, but opening pressures as high as 100 cm H_2O are occasionally necessary. Negative thoracic pressure is almost exclusively created by diaphragmatic descent. The role of chest recoil when the neonate is delivered was formerly thought to be significantly contributory. During transit through the birth canal the squeeze on the chest is considerable, sometimes exerting a pressure as high as 200 cm H_2O. As the baby emerges, release of this constricting pressure causes sudden expansion of the chest. This recoil was previously thought to contribute to air intake as the first breath is activated, but the influence of recoil has been shown to be insignificant. Following the first inspiration, a large positive intrathoracic pressure (mean, 70 cm H_2O) is generated during expiration. This pressure is generated by closure of the glottis, complete or partial, as the baby forcefully pushes air out of the airway. These are the moments in the delivery room when the welcome lusty cry is first heard. The high expiratory pressure thus created serves to distribute air taken in during the first inspiration, while promoting the evacuation of lung fluid across alveolar membranes.

The entry of air into the lungs and the expansion of alveoli require a mechanism for minimizing or eliminating *surface tension forces* and a mechanism for the *evacuation of fetal lung fluid*. These two aspects of the first breath are discussed in the following paragraphs:

Surface tension and surfactant. Surface tension forces are produced by an imbalance in the attraction of one molecule for an adjacent one. Consider a cup of liquid. Below the surface its molecules are attracted to and repelled from each other with equal force from all directions because they are completely surrounded by other molecules. However, the situation is different in the surface layer of molecules because the molecular forces of attraction cannot be equal from all directions. The air above the surface layer exerts little upward pull, and the balance of forces thus favors downward and horizontal directions (Fig. 8-3). The force exerted by this imbalance in intermolecular attraction at the uppermost level of molecules is called surface tension. *It produces a constant tendency for contraction of a surface area.* Now apply this concept of surface area contraction to the spherical inner surface of alveolar walls. In the absence of a counteracting influence (surfactant) and in the presence of an interface with air, surface tension tends to contract alveolar surfaces, thus promoting alveolar collapse.

Alveoli of the lung are similar to a conglomerate of bubbles. Alveolar walls are largely liquid; they envelope air within them. Since an air-liquid interface is present (much like that just described for the uppermost molecular layer of water in a cup), surface-active forces are operative. Intermolecular attraction contracts the surface area of the liquid wall of the bubble (alveolus). Furthermore, in accordance with a law of physics (LaPlace), the smaller the bubble, the stronger the forces of surface tension. Thus the smaller the bubble, the greater its tendency to collapse due to unopposed surface forces. Ultimately the bubble (alveolus) collapses completely (atelectasis).

Pulmonary surfactant is a mixture of approximately ten compounds. It is described as a unique lipoprotein that is predominantly composed of lecithins, and to a lesser extent, of cholesterol, neutral lipids, or other phospholipids. Quantitatively, the major component of surfactant is phosphotidylcholine (PC). It is also the compound that is most active in lowering surface tension forces. Another important component of surfactant is phosphotidylglycerol (PG). The PG fraction of surfactant is far smaller than that of PC, but interest in PG stems from the close correlation of

lung maturity with its first appearance. It may be that PG is the compound of most critical functional significance in maturation of the lung.

Surfactant is synthesized by type II alveolar cells (pneumonocytes). It is stored for a relatively long period prior to its discharge from these cells on the alveolar membrane, where it forms a continuous film on the surface. At this site it functions to diminish the collapsing (atelectatic) effect of surface tension forces on the alveoli.

In the normal lung, surface tension is minimized or eliminated by surfactant, a complex substance principally composed of lipoprotein. It appears in the fetal lung at approximately 22 to 24 weeks of gestation. In terms of body weight, surfactant is present in some fetuses less than 500 g and is demonstrable more regularly as weight increases. Without surfactant, unopposed surface tension forces increase directly with shrinkage of alveoli during expiration, ultimately resulting in alveolar collapse (atelectasis). However, in the presence of surfactant the effects of surface tension forces are eliminated or minimized. As alveoli shrink in the presence of surfactant during normal breathing, surface tension forces diminish rather than increase in magnitude because the surfactant layer, by becoming compressed, is

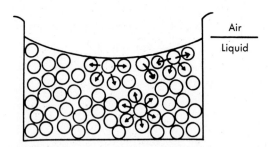

Fig. 8-3. The balance of forces at the air-liquid interface favors displacement downward and horizontally. Away from an air-liquid interface within the water mass, however, there is no displacement because forces are equally exerted in all directions by neighboring molecules. (From Burgess, W.R., and Chernick, V.: Respiratory therapy in newborn infants and children, New York, 1982, Thieme-Stratton.)

made thicker; in this state surfactant counteracts surface forces most effectively by interposing between air and liquid to obliterate the interface. Since there is no air-liquid interface because surfactant molecules have been placed between air and water, there is no significant surface tension. Conversely, the surfactant layer is thinned as alveoli expand during normal inspiration, and in this attenuated state it is less effective in diminishing surface tension. Molecules of surfactant are spread from each other at peak inspiration. Air and liquid now have an interface. Fig. 8-4 clearly depicts this phenomenon. The influence of surfactant is therefore least at peak inspiration, when alveolar expansion is greatest. At this point, recoil of the expanded lung is relatively unopposed, and

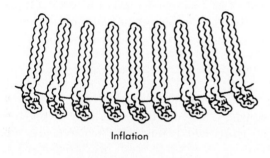

Inflation

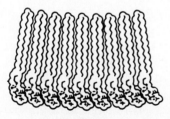

Deflation

Fig. 8-4. At peak inflation when alveolar distention is maximal, molecules of surfactant become separated from each other to expose some air-liquid interface. At end expiration when alveolar deflation is maximal, surfactant is compressed and the molecules obliterate the air-liquid interface. (From Kotas, R. V.: In Thibeault, D. D., and Gregory, G. A., editors: Neonatal pulmonary care, 1979. Reading, Mass., 1979, Addison-Wesley Publishing Co.)

the deflation required for expiration is facilitated. The alveolar lining layer (surfactant) functions principally to maintain alveolar stability (residual expansion at end-expiration) once air has entered the alveolus.

In summary, surfactant is a critical substance. When insufficient in quantity, as in immature lungs, hyaline membrane disease evolves. Surfactant accommodates *initial opening of alveoli* at relatively low pressures. It *prevents alveolar collapse* due to surface tension forces at end expiration, thereby permitting continued gas exchange between respiratory cycles. By providing for alveolar stability, it provides for easy *lung expansion at relatively low pressures* during inspiration. Thus, because it accommodates lung expansion at low pressures, it mediates *increased compliance*. It contributes to the *evacuation of lung fluid* by maintaining alveolar stability. Were the alveoli to collapse at the end of each expiration, fluid from the interstitial tissue would migrate back into the alveolar lumen. Surfactant *promotes optimal capillary circulation* by maintaining maximal alveolar diameter, thereby dilating the precapillary vessels. It forms a *protective film* that covers lining epithelium, thus bestowing some protection against barotrauma.

For over a decade intensive research has sought to characterize the biochemical structure of surfactant and the mechanism of its actions. The goal has been to use a natural or synthetic surfactant for therapeutic instillation into the airway. Clinical trials to determine the therapeutic efficacy of various forms of surfactant are in progress. Surfactant trials are in two categories: preventive therapy that entails insufflation immediately after birth, and "rescue" therapy that involves insufflation when hyaline membrane disease has been diagnosed. Discussion is presented later in this chapter.

Lung fluid. At term the fetal lung is expanded with liquid of intrapulmonary origin. The volume of liquid in the fetal lung is approximately the same as the volume of functional residual capacity (FRC) that is established soon after the onset of extrauterine breathing (30 to 35 ml/kg). The fetal lung is therefore not collapsed, but rather it is distended with fluid that must be replaced by air during the initiation of independent breathing after birth. Fetal lung fluid maintains patency of the developing airway. It begins to appear at some time early in gestation, and as fluid accumulates, periodic expulsion from the fetal lungs delivers it to the posterior pharynx. Some of the fluid is swallowed, but a significant amount makes its way to the amniotic fluid. Since fetal lung fluid contains surfactant, this mechanism is the basis for determinations of surfactant levels in amniotic fluid (L/S ratios). Whereas lung fluid is generated at a steady rate throughout gestation, its formation apparently diminishes considerably in the 48 hours preceding onset of term labor. Fetal pulmonary fluid is thought to be important for normal development of the lungs. In experiments with fetal lambs, protracted drainage of fluid through a tracheal catheter results in pulmonary hypoplasia.

Prior to 1941, lung fluid was thought to have its origin in amniotic fluid. At that time, two stillborn fetuses were described in whom parts of the lung were detached from the airway. There was complete separation from amniotic fluid above, yet the lung contained fluid. In one fetus an anomalous lobe that was not connected to the trachea was nevertheless distended with liquid. In another fetus, complete laryngotracheal obstruction precluded any connection with amniotic fluid in the pharynx. In both fetuses, alveoli were normally developed; the lungs contained liquid. This was a milestone observation, since it indicated the intrapulmonary origin of lung liquid. Subsequent investigations have confirmed these original assumptions.

The volume of fetal lung fluid is approximately 30 to 35 ml/kg, representing the same volume as the functional residual capacity established during extrauterine breathing. Values for pH, bicarbonate, and protein are lower than in amniotic fluid; osmolality, sodium, and chloride concentrations are higher. Protein content of lung fluid is con-

siderably lower than that of plasma; this is a critical factor in the evacuation of lung fluid during the first breaths. The higher concentration of plasma protein imposes an osmotic gradient that favors migration of lung fluid from alveoli into blood capillaries.

Fetal lung fluid is a major force opposing air entry during the first breath. During descent through the birth canal, a strong thoracic squeeze on the fetal chest expels 30 to 35 ml of lung fluid, a third of the total volume in a 3.0 kg neonate. The explusion of lung fluid is often observable during delivery when the head becomes exteriorized while the chest is still compressed by birth canal pressures that may be as high as 200 cm H_2O. Some term infants absorb all lung fluid in the absence of oral drainage, as in those delivered by cesarean section. Most babies delivered by elective cesarean section retain larger volumes of lung fluid, and they cannot evacuate it as rapidly as babies who are delivered vaginally. Thus the incidence of transient tachypnea of the newborn (RDS II) (see later) is considerably more frequent following elective sections. RDS II is thought to be caused by delayed resorption of pulmonary liquid. Most of the fluid (probably two thirds of it) is evacuated across alveolar membranes into capillaries or into interstitial tissue and then to lymphatic vessels. The rate of fluid evacuation by each of these routes has not been defined, but data from animals indicate that half of the absorbed lung fluid is evacuated through the lymphatics, the remainder through blood capillaries. In rabbits, disappearance of lung fluid is considerably more rapid following vaginal delivery (within several hours) than after cesarean section (several days). The mechanical effect of vaginal delivery is apparently important in the evacuation of fluid in humans, but the capillaries and lymphatics are the principal routes of egress.

Several mechanisms seem to be active in promoting the removal of lung fluid during the first few breaths. First, the continuous secretion of fluid diminishes 48 hours before birth. The secreting cells are inactivated by some unknown mechanism. It is clear from conclusive experiments in animals, however, that lung fluid does not accumulate postnatally. Second, the pressure relationship between the airway (alveoli) and interstitial tissue is altered when descent of the diaphragm generates negative pressures up to 80 or 100 cm H_2O. Pressure in the interstitial tissue is therefore considerably lower than in the alveoli, and fluid is forced to flow from alveoli to interstitial space along this pressure gradient. Third, expansion of the lungs has been shown to stretch alveolar walls with resultant enlargement of their pores. In the neonate these pores are six to ten times larger after lung expansion than they were in the fetus. Now, the increased permeability of alveolar membranes and the previously described changes in pressure gradients combine to promote displacement of fluid to the interstitial tissue and to the lymphatics and capillaries. The fourth active mechanism for removal of lung fluid involves the decrease in pulmonary vascular pressure and the increase in pulmonary blood flow that are inherent in the first breath and in adaptation to extrauterine life (see later). With these vascular changes, fluid is displaced into the interstitium, blood vessels, and lymphatics for ultimate evacuation. The fifth mechanism of lung fluid disposition is the osmotic (oncotic) gradient created by the higher concentration of protein in plasma compared to that of pulmonary fluid. Water is thus "pulled" into blood capillaries and lymphatics by osmosis.

In summary, the factors known to promote the evacuation of lung fluid are as follows:

- Reduced fluid production before onset of term labor;
- Vaginal "squeeze" of thorax during birth;
- Pressure gradient; high in room atmosphere, low in blood capillaries;
- Alveolar permeability (pores) during full inflation; and
- Osmotic gradient from plasma to lung fluid.

Aeration of the lungs and evacuation of lung fluid are inseparable requirements of normal postnatal breathing. In essence, the neonate must take the first breaths into a veritable bag of water. Removal of liquid occurs in two stages: displacement from alveolar spaces to interstitial tissue, and from there into lymph and capillary blood vessels. In the normal term infant, displacement to interstitial tissue is rapid, often instantaneous. Complete removal into lymph and blood vessels may take several hours.

Establishment of functional residual capacity (FRC)

If normal respiration is to follow the first breath, some air must remain in the alveoli at the end of expiration to maintain them in a partially expanded state. The volume of this retained air is the lung's *functional residual capacity*. The ability to retain the air is called *alveolar stability*.

In normal term human lungs, the first expansion may require an opening pressure as high as 80 to 100 cm H_2O. At the end of expiration the pressure is again zero, that is, intrathoracic and atmospheric pressure of the room are equal. However, in an effort to keep airways patent and alveoli distended in the presence of relative stiff lungs during the expiratory phase of the first few breaths, a high positive pressure of 20 to 30 cm H_2O is maintained as long as possible by partially closing the glottis. Lung compliance during the first few minutes after birth is only 20% to 30% of its ultimate value in neonates several days of age. Furthermore, during the earliest moments, airway resistance is two to four times greater than later on. Thus, producing a high positive pressure during expiration enhances establishment of functional residual capacity (FRC). At 10 minutes of age FRC is approximately 17 ml/kg of body weight; at 30 minutes it has expanded to 25 to 35 ml/kg, and it remains at that volume until about 4 days of age. More recent studies have also suggested that the neonatal maximum for FRC is attained as early as 3 hours.

If all is well, the lungs retain about 25% of their fully expanded volume after the first few breaths. From a partially expanded state at the end of the first breath, the second or perhaps later breaths

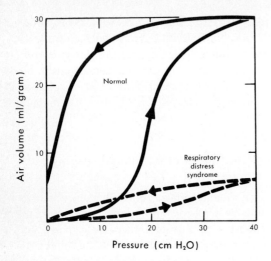

Fig. 8-5. Pressure-volume curves for normal lungs (solid lines) and surfactant-deficient lungs (broken lines). Normal lung expands maximally at 40 cm H_2O. Note that descending limb does not return to 0 level, indicating partial expansion at end expiration (alveolar stability). The hyaline membrane disease curve peaks at a low expansion for 40 cm H_2O because lung compliance is poor. The curve returns to 0, indicating alveolar collapse at end-expiration (no alveolar stability). (From Klaus, M. In Barnett, H., editor: Pediatrics, ed. 15, New York, 1972, Appleton-Century-Crofts, Publishing Division of Prentice-Hall.)

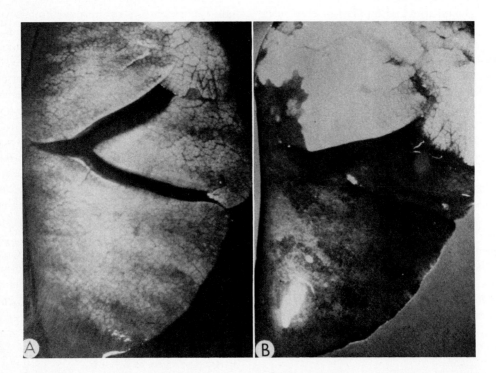

Fig. 8-6. Lung of fetal lamb is inflated in **A**, and deflated in **B**. The upper lobe in **B** contains surfactant and remains partially inflated; the lower lobe does not contain surfactant and it collapses completely. (From Chernick, V.: The first expiration: the role of pulmonary surfactant, Sem. Perinatol. **1:**351, 1977. By permission of the publisher.)

involve considerably less effort. Small pressure changes produce more extensive lung inflation; high opening pressures that were required at first are unnecessary subsequently because alveoli are partially expanded at end expiration and compliance is increased. Alveolar stability and, thus, FRC are not possible in the absence of adequate surfactant activity.

If surfactant quantities are suboptimal, alveolar collapse and failure to retain air are inevitable. Because surfactant activity is deficient, expansion of the immature lung is different from the mature one. At end expiration (zero pressure), alveolar collapse occurs in immature lungs in response to *unopposed* surface tension forces (diminished). The difference between normal and abnormal expansion is clearly depicted in Fig. 8-5. When normal FRC is not established, succeeding inflations require the same high opening pressures as the first one. The work of respiration is vastly increased, continuity of alveolar gas exchange is precluded, and the hypoxic infant becomes fatigued rapidly.

Fig. 8-6 is a different illustration of absent alveolar stability. It depicts the lung of a premature lamb at a point in development when the upper lobe contained surfactant and the lower lobe did not. In Fig. 8-6, *A*, the excised lung has been inflated and appears normal. In Fig. 8-6, *B*, it is deflated; the surfactant-containing upper lobe remains inflated (FRC), but the surfactant-deficient lower lobe is collapsed and airless. Reinflation of the lower lobe requires the high opening pressure similar to that required for the first breath. This failure to establish FRC, as illustrated here in one lobe of the fetal lamb lung, is identical to the phenomenon that occurs throughout both lungs of premature infants with hyaline membrane disease.

Increased pulmonary blood flow and redistribution of cardiac output

Cardiovascular adaptation to extrauterine life proceeds simultaneously with pulmonary adaptation. Five attributes of the fetal circulation must be altered if the mature cardiovascular pattern is to evolve. These fetal characteristics fall into two broad categories:

1. *Pulmonary-systemic pressure relationships*
   High pulmonary artery pressure resulting from increased pulmonary vascular resistance
   Low aortic systemic pressure (placental circuit)
2. *Sites of venous admixture (right-to-left shunts)*
   Foramen ovale
   Ductus arteriosus
   Ductus venosus

The two factors of pivotal significance in initiating the conversion of fetal to neonatal circulation are removal of the placenta and expansion of the lungs with air.

Pulmonary-systemic pressure relationships

Fetal aortic blood pressure lower than pulmonary artery pressure. The placenta receives 40% to 50% of the fetal cardiac output. The fetal placental vessels are apparently not supplied with nerve endings; they are generally relaxed. Therefore they offer little resistance to the flow of blood. The placenta therefore constitutes a low-resistance circuit. The blood that perfuses it comes from the fetal aorta and returns to the fetal inferior vena cava, thus making it a prominent low-resistance component of the *systemic circulation*. Clamping of the cord eliminates the placental vascular bed, thus reducing considerably the total intravascular space in the systemic circuit and also removing the component that offers least resistance to blood flow. As a consequence, at birth the aortic blood pressure is raised. Simultaneously, return flow to the inferior vena cava is reduced by severance of the placenta, and a small drop in pressure occurs in the venous side of the circulation.

Pulmonary artery pressure higher than aortic pressure. This is the result of extremely high pulmonary vascular resistance to blood flow in the fetus. Resistance to blood flow through the lungs is so high as to permit only 5% to 7% of cardiac output to perfuse them, in contrast to the low-resistance placental circuit, which accommodates

40% to 50% of cardiac output. If the lungs expand sufficiently, vasodilatation produces a precipitous fall in pulmonary vascular resistance within the first few minutes after birth. Resistance has been calculated to fall by 80% from fetal levels. A more gradual reduction in resistance transpires over the next 6 to 8 weeks. With the abrupt diminution of resistance comes an equally abrupt increase in pulmonary blood flow. Within minutes pulmonary perfusion has increased approximately five-fold. Relaxation of the pulmonary arterioles is principally in the precapillary segments. An overwhelming stimulus to this vasodilatation is the increase in blood PO_2 that follows the first few breaths. Of secondary significance is the dilatation of capillaries that results from elimination of their compression by alveolar fluid as air enters the alveoli.

High fetal pulmonary arteriolar resistance is not solely a function of constriction. The relative thickness of the muscle layer of these arterioles is considerably greater than it will be later in postnatal life. Thus the gradual diminution of vascular resistance that occurs over the first 6 to 8 weeks is related to thinning out of the muscle layer, rather than to ongoing relaxation of existing muscle. In summary, initial lung expansion and adequate oxygenation diminish blood pressure in the pulmonary circuit by stimulating pulmonary arteriolar relaxation. At the same time, blood pressure in the systemic circuit increases because of greater resistance brought about by severance of the placenta. With this reversal of relative blood pressures in the pulmonary and systemic circuits, the stage is now set for elimination of the fetal sites at which venous admixture occurs (right-to-left shunt).

Fetal sites of venous admixture (right-to-left shunts)

Closure of the foramen ovale. The foramen ovale is an aperture in the interatrial septum. It is covered by a thin flap of tissue that can open like a swinging door in only one direction—into the left atrium. Since, in the fetus, pressure in the right atrium is higher than that in the left

(because pulmonary circuit pressure is high), the flap remains open, permitting most of the well-oxygenated blood from the inferior vena cava to flow from the right atrium into the left atrium. The position of the flap is thus a function of the pressure relationship between both atria. If pressure in the right atrium is *higher* than that in the left, the flap is open and blood flows from the right to left atrium. This is normal for the fetus. When pressure in the right atrium is *lower* than that of the left, the flap closes. This is normal for the neonate. Lung expansion during the first breath causes an abrupt decline in pulmonary vascular resistance and a marked increase in pulmonary blood flow. The amount of blood that flows into the left atrium is therefore increased (pulmonary venous return), causing the left atrial pressure to rise slightly. Left atrial pressure is also augmented by the increase in systemic pressure that follows elimination of the placental circuit. Right atrial pressure falls because of lowered pulmonary vascular resistance. The pressure relationship between the atria is now reversed. When the left atrial pressure increases over that of the right, the swinging flap of tissue abuts against the margins of the foramen ovale. The foramen is now *functionally* closed, and one site of right-to-left shunting is eliminated. The tissue flap does not become immovably adherent to the atrial septum for several months. It is held in the closed position by the higher left atrial pressure. If right atrial pressure again becomes higher than that on the left (the baby is suddenly asphyxiated), the foramen will reopen.

Closure of the ductus arteriosus. The fetal ductus arteriosus is a large vessel, almost equal in diameter to the pulmonary artery. When it constricts, its substantial muscle layer has the capacity of obliterating the lumen. Constriction of the ductus arteriosus occurs in response to the increased blood PO_2 that occurs during the first few breaths. Vasoconstrictive response of the ductus to oxygen is in contrast to the vasodilating response of pulmonary arterioles. If the lungs do not expand normally, failure of PO_2 to rise causes sustained ductus patency. Normally, functional closure (constriction) is complete by 24 to 96 hours after birth in term infants. Anatomic closure (fibrosis) is usually complete by 3 weeks of age. In premature infants the ductus remains patent for much longer and variable periods because the capacity to constrict in reponse to augmented oxygen tension is not yet developed. The reasons for this lack of response have only recently begun to unfold. The ductus remains patent throughout fetal life because of compounds within its tissue that are known as *prostaglandins*. These substances exist in a number of molecular variations. They are synthesized within virtually every tissue in the body. Their functions vary according to the organ (tissue) in which they are synthesized and according to their molecular structure. Arterial oxygen tension and prostaglandins seem to be the principal determinants of ductal constriction. In the presence of prostaglandins, heightened oxygen tension fails to constrict the ductus. The roles played by both these factors are profoundly influenced by gestational age. Early in gestation, as a function of prostaglandin content, there is little constriction of the ductus in response to augmented PaO_2, but as gestational age progresses the vasodilating influence of prostaglandins diminishes and the ductus becomes sensitive to the constricting influence of normal postnatal PaO_2.

Prostaglandins remain in the ductal tissue of premature infants after birth, and it is believed that their presence inhibits the constrictive effect of oxygen after postnatal breathing. The physiologic mechanism by which the vasodilatory effect of prostaglandin E_1 and E_2 is ultimately inhibited has not yet been clarified. The prostaglandins are formed within cells by an enzyme complex known as *prostaglandin synthetase*. The activity of this enzyme can be inhibited pharmacologically by *prostaglandin synthetase inhibitors*. Inhibition impedes formation of prostaglandins, and when this occurs in a patent ductus arteriosus, the vessel proceeds to constrict. Indomethacin is a potent prostaglandin synthetase inhibitor that has been

shown clinically to bring about constriction of the ductus in premature infants. Conversely, in animal experiments, infusion of prostaglandin E_1 or E_2 reversed the constrictive effects of indomethacin. In these experiments, the prostaglandins maintained ductal patency. Discussion of the clinical significance and treatment of patent ductus arteriosus is presented later in this chapter.

Prior to completion of anatomic closure in term or premature babies, the ductus may reopen in response to lowered blood oxygen tension. The older the infant, the less likely is the ductus to reopen. With ductal closure, another fetal right-to-left shunt is eliminated.

Closure of the ductus venosus. The ductus venosus is a channel that, in the fetus, connects the portal (hepatic and intestinal) venous circulation with the inferior vena cava. In the fetus, umbilical vein blood passes through the liver, into the ductus venosus, to the inferior vena cava, and thence to the heart. The mechanism of closure of the ductus venosus is unknown. After birth, very little blood flows through it. Anatomical closure (fibrosis) is completed in 3 to 7 days.

Summary. Changing pressure relationships are responsible for elimination of the fetal sites of right-to-left shunting. With adequate lung expansion, an increase in pulmonary blood flow occurs. This is brought about by the diminished vascular resistance that results from dilatation of pulmonary vessels. Almost all subsequent changes in circulation are a consequence of decreased pulmonary vascular resistance associated with normal lung expansion. Increased blood flow through the lungs leads to a larger flow into the left atrium, thereby raising left atrial pressure above that in the right atrium. When this occurs, the foramen ovale closes, thus eliminating the fetal right-to-left shunt at this site. The ductus arteriosus begins gradual closure by constriction of its wall as a result of a rising arterial Po_2. Earlier, diminished ductus blood flow is a function of changes in pressure relationships between the pulmonary and the systemic circulations. As pulmonary blood pressure declines with lung expansion, pressures in the pulmonary and systemic circuits are almost equalized. Thus there is gradual elimination of the pressure gradient that directed fetal blood from the pulmonary artery through the ductus into the aorta. Constriction of the ductus in response to increased oxygenation when prostaglandin synthesis is inhibited physiologically, plus the change in pressure relationships between the pulmonary and systemic circulations, therefore combine to obliterate another fetal site of right-to-left shunting.

What causes the pulmonary vascular bed to dilate and thus receive a greater flow of blood? Perhaps the most powerful influence is an increase in airway and arterial PO_2. Conversely, hypoxia constricts pulmonary vasculature. Most of this activity occurs in the precapillary arterioles. With the establishment of extrauterine respiration, the increase of arterial PO_2 exerts very different effects on pulmonary arterioles and the ductus arteriosus. The former relax as PO_2 rises; the latter constricts. The alveolar capillaries dilate as the lung expands and alveolar fluid is replaced by air during the first few breaths.

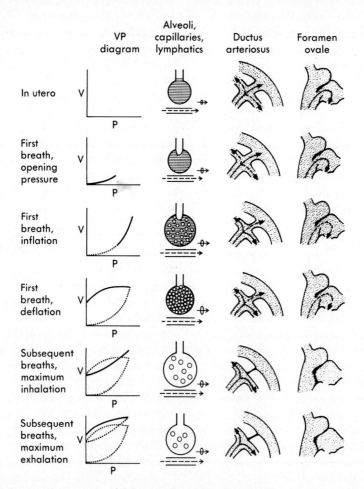

Fig. 8-7. Diagrammatic summary of the first breath. A detailed interpretation is on page 221. (From Scarpelli, E. M.: Pulmonary physiology of the fetus, newborn and child, Philadelphia, 1975, Lea and Febiger).

Diagrammatic summary of the first breath
(Fig. 8-7)

The diagrams in Fig. 8-7 are organized into four vertical columns, representing the progression of events in the initiation of extrauterine respiration. Each horizontal row illustrates the multiple phenomena that transpire at the same times.

In utero (row 1): The alveoli are filled with fluid in which surfactant is suspended (multiple small key-like figures). The capillary beneath the alveolus is constricted and a small amount of fetal blood flow is indicated by a thin, interrupted line in the lumen. The lymphatics are symbolized immediately above the extreme right end of the capillary. Lymphatics in utero are also constricted; very little lymph is within them. The ductus arteriosus is widely patent. The full flow of blood from the pulmonary artery directly through the ductus and thence into the aortic arch is indicated by a solid arrow. The small flow of blood that perfuses fetal lungs is shown in interrupted arrows within the two pulmonary artery branches. Through a patent foramen ovale, blood flow from the right to left atrium is indicated by a solid arrow. Note that the inferior segment of the septum is displaced to the left by the force of blood that streams into the left atrium.

First breath, opening pressure; first breath, inflation (rows 2 and 3): Progression to peak inspiration is indicated in the pressure-volume diagram. Air enters the alveolar duct and alveolus as fluid recedes. Surfactant molecules straddle the newly established air-fluid interface. The capillary and lymphatics dilate, pulmonary vascular resistance diminishes, and blood flow through the pulmonary artery branches increases. The ductus begins to constrict. Ductal flow diminishes, and flow through pulmonary artery branches increases. The lower segment of the septum starts to migrate to the right, closer to the upper segment, as right-sided pressure diminishes because pulmonary vascular resistance has fallen.

First breath, deflation (row 4): At the end of the first deflation, the pressure volume curve shows a functional residual capacity also seen in the alveolus that has retained air at end expira-

tion. Capillary flow is unchanged, but lymph flow increases as more lung fluid is evacuated. There is little change in the ductus arteriosus and foramen ovale.

Subsequent breaths; maximum inhalation (row 5): Alveolar distention is greater than in the previous inflation; liquid is cleared. Surfactant molecules are at the interface of alveolar lining and air. The capillaries are almost completely dilated; they conduct full blood flow. The lymphatics are not as distended as in the previous stage. Ductal constriction is complete; blood flow from pulmonary artery to aorta is eliminated. All blood from the main pulmonary artery flows into its branches and thence to the lungs. The foramen ovale is closed as the lower segment of the septum migrates further right and contacts the inferior edge of the upper segment.

Subsequent breaths; maximum exhalation (row 6): The pressure volume curve and the alveolus show increased FRC. Capillary flow is unchanged, but lymph flow is further diminished. The ductus and the foramen ovale are unchanged. The lungs are expanded and fetal circulatory pathways are converted to mature ones; extrauterine respiration is thus established in a few seconds.

HYALINE MEMBRANE DISEASE (HMD, RESPIRATORY DISTRESS SYNDROME, RDS)

Hyaline membrane disease (HMD) is also known as idiopathic respiratory distress syndrome (IRDS), or simply as respiratory distress syndrome (RDS). It is an acute disorder that is symptomatic at birth or soon thereafter. Primarily characterized by respiratory distress, it occurs almost exclusively in premature infants. Its natural course is 3 to 5 days in duration. In the United States it is estimated that 12,000 infants die of hyaline membrane disease annually.

Incidence and prognosis

Hyaline membrane disease occurs in 1% to 2% of total live births in all races and in all socioeconomic groups. Reports of incidence are variable, but a common trend has been noted in all parts of the world. It is almost exclusively a disease of premature infants, rarely occurring in babies born at term. Furthermore, the incidence varies from one birth-weight group to another. It is most common among infants who weigh between 1000 and 1500 g, next most frequent in those between 1500 and 2000 g, and it is least common between 2000 and 2500 g. In general, 10% to 20% of all premature infants are affected. The incidence of HMD is lower in black babies than in white babies. Severe respiratory distress is even more frequent in babies below 1000 g. In them the clinical picture differs from classic hyaline membrane disease. This disorder occurs in 65% of infants in this lowest birth weight category.

Case fatality rates are too variable to quote precisely, but as one might expect, the lower the birth weight, the less likely is survival. Although recent advances in therapy have diminished the percentage of mortality impressively, it remains high largely as a function of natural and artefactual complications, instead of the inexorable deteriorations that characterized the course of HMD years ago. The overall incidence of hyaline membrane disease has apparently diminished, at least during the last decade. One can only surmise that diminution in its incidence is significantly related to improved obstetric practice. Concurrently, among infants who are affected by the disorder, mortality has also diminished significantly. The consensus is that diminished mortality is a direct result of continuing advances in the intensive care of sick neonates.

Pathophysiology

Comprehension of the pathophysiology of hyaline membrane disease requires familiarity with the events of the first breath. In essence, hyaline membrane disease is a partial persistence of the fetal cardiopulmonary state. Whatever other factors may influence the course of events, the central difficulty seems to be a deficiency in surfactant activity. Hyaline membrane disease is fundamentally a developmental disorder. The maturation of surfactant synthesis has been amply demonstrated

by extensive studies. They have thus far confirmed the validity of L/S ratio measurements, which indicate that, with a few exceptions, the lungs are capable of normal extrauterine function at approximately 35 gestational weeks. The central significance of a developmental concept seems plausible because the disease preponderantly affects premature infants; term infants are rarely affected. A well-defined sequence of biochemical events must transpire in utero before maturation of the lungs is established. If birth occurs prior to completion of this sequence, the neonate with premature lungs is incapable of normally coping with a gaseous environment.

The principal factors that are operative in the evolution of hyaline membrane disease are depicted in Fig. 8-8. The narrative that follows will refer to the numbered squares in the diagram.

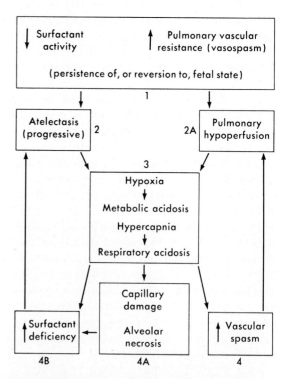

Fig. 8-8. Principal intrapulmonary factors in pathogenesis of hyaline membrane disease. (See text.)

The *persistent fetal state (1)* implies *surfactant deficiency* and increased *pulmonary vascular resistance* as well. The latter would ordinarily disappear in the presence of normal lung expansion, but this disappearance is precluded in the premature lung because of surfactant deficiency. In most instances there is probably enough functional surfactant present at birth to accommodate reasonably effective breathing. Thus, at birth, and for a short time thereafter, some infants breathe with little or moderate difficulty. Soon respiration becomes more labored as surfactant is dissipated. Consequently, normal functional residual capacity (alveolar stability) is not possible. Alveoli that are inflated during inspiration are again collapsed at end expiration. Each breath is like the first; collapsed alveoli require reinflation. The work of respiration is thus relatively tremendous; an effort similar to that expended for the first breath must be mounted for each one that follows. As the infant becomes more feeble, he fails to open more alveoli. *Atelectasis (2)*, already present at birth to some extent, now becomes more widespread. Pulmonary hypoperfusion from vasospasm is present *(2A)*. These two factors *(2, 2A)* produce *hypoxia* and *hypercapnia (3)*. As hypoxia becomes prolonged, anaerobic glycolysis is activated for the production of glucose from glycogen. The by-product of this process is an increased quantity of lactic acid, causing *metabolic acidosis (3)*. Also, carbon dioxide cannot be blown off as a result of atelectasis and the paucity of blood that delivers it to the lungs. The resultant retention of CO_2 (hypercapnia) causes *respiratory acidosis (3)*; blood pH is therefore diminished considerably.

Hypoxia and acidosis accentuate preexisting *vascular spasm (4)*, which in turn increases *pulmonary hypoperfusion (2A)*. Hypoxia and acidosis also inflict *capillary damage* and *alveolar necrosis (4A)*, both of which aggravate *surfactant deficiency (4B)* by impairing its production. As a consequence, *progressive atelectasis (2)* is unabated; unopposed surface tension causes collapse of increasing numbers of alveoli.

Failure of lung expansion and persistence of high vascular resistance result in increased blood pressure in the pulmonary circuit. Venous admixture (right-to-left shunt) through the foramen ovale, as it existed in utero, is maintained after birth. If pressure in the pulmonary circuit is sufficiently high in relation to aortic pressure, a right-to-left shunt (pulmonary artery to aorta) is also present at the ductus arteriosus. The effect of these extrapulmonary shunts is to divert blood from the lungs and thus add to their hypoperfusion. To a variable extent, the fetal cardiopulmonary circulation persists in each patient.

This entire sequence of events can be ascribed to failure of lung expansion and inability to establish alveolar stability as a result of a primary surfactant deficiency. Surfactant deficiency is enhanced by intrauterine asphyxia. Asphyxia causes pulmonary vasoconstriction in utero. The resultant ischemia impairs surfactant production.

The incidence of intrauterine asphyxia in premature infants is indeed higher than in term babies, but the majority of infants who have hyaline membrane disease give no evidence of antecedent stress. Acute asphyxia probably accentuates the maturational inadequacy.

Lung compliance is diminished in hyaline membrane disease. Compliance is a function of the elasticity of lung tissue. It expresses the capacity of the lung to increase in volume in response to a given amount of applied pressure during inspiration. The lungs in hyaline membrane disease require far more pressure than normal lungs for equal amounts of expansion. Pressures of 35 cm H_2O, which usually expand normal lungs, cause little inflation of lungs with hyaline membrane disease. The abnormal lung tissue is thus said to be "stiffer," or less distensible. Compliance is expressed in milliliters (volume change) per centimeter of water (pressure change), or ml/cm H_2O. Compliance of normal newborn lungs is 4 to 6 ml/cm H_2O; in hyaline membrane disease it is one fourth to one fifth as much. The stiffness of affected lungs, and their limited distensibility at end expiration, contributes significantly to the work of breathing in these sick babies. It requires therapy with positive end-expiratory pressure (discussed later).

The role of the hyaline membranes in disruption of pulmonary function has not been delineated. In years past they were believed to arise solely from aspiration of vernix and other particulate matter in amniotic fluid. It has been evident, however, that they are principally the product of cellular necrosis and transudation in alveolar ducts and terminal respiratory bronchioles. Hyaline membranes do not form in alveoli and do not in themselves cause atelectasis. They probably contribute to diminution of compliance.

Predisposing factors

Prematurity is virtually a constant predisposing factor; complications of pregnancy and labor play an additional major role. Maternal bleeding and other causes of fetal asphyxia are associated with the disease but are not identifiable in the majority of babies. Maternal diabetes is an important predisposing factor in itself; it also predisposes to the disease because of the high incidence of prematurity among infants of diabetic mothers (p. 340). The role of cesarean section is still debated. The causes of fetal distress that urgently necessitate cesarean section seem to be the decisive factors. Most studies indicate that elective cesarean (performed in the absence of detectable fetal difficulty) is not associated with an increased incidence of the disease. In other studies, there is impressive evidence for a contributory role by cesarean section itself.

Male infants are twice as likely as females to have hyaline membrane disease. In females, L/S ratios rise toward normal at an earlier gestational age, thus indicating earlier lung maturity. Given a baby with hyaline membrane disease, the risk of its occurrence in subsequently born infants is 90%. The risk of hyaline membrane disease in a second infant is 5% if the first one was unaffected. The second born of twins is considerably more likely to have hyaline membrane disease, probably because of the increased incidence of perinatal asphyxia in the second born.

Morphologic pathology

At autopsy the lungs are purple red, resembling the consistency of liver. They contain little or no air in contrast to normal lungs, which are salmon pink and spongy by virtue of their air content. The microscopic appearance is characterized by widespread atelectasis and hyaline membranes. These membranes are present only in previously aerated portions of the lung, and with usual staining techniques in microscopic sections they may vary in color from pale pink to red (eosinophilic). Generally they have a homogeneous, waxen appearance. They line the surfaces of alveolar ducts and terminal respiratory bronchioles. Epithelial cells are necrotic or absent in areas occupied by membranes and in collapsed alveoli.

Clinical manifestations

Infants with hyaline membrane disease were previously believed to be free of abnormalities for the first few hours of life, but as more careful observations were made, it became obvious that the majority of affected babies had some sort of respiratory difficulty at birth or shortly afterwards. If there is no respiratory distress within 1 to 2 hours after delivery, the diagnosis of hyaline membrane disease is not tenable. In the past, errors were the result of infrequent observation, failure to appreciate the more subtle signs of respiratory difficulty, and failure to perform Apgar scoring at birth.

Increased respiratory rate (over 60 respirations per minute) is the most common sign of abnormal ventilation. Occasionally an expiratory grunt or sigh is the only perceptible sign. The expiratory grunt is a fascinating phenomenon. It is an effort to obstruct exhalation of air temporarily and thus, by increasing "back pressure," to maintain some degree of alveolar expansion to increase functional residual capacity. The epiglottis closes off the glottis. Pressure mounts within the respiratory tract as the outflow of air is obstructed. When the epiglottis is abruptly released, the sudden rush of air over the vocal cords produces a grunt. Infants who grunt can raise their arterial Po_2 by 10 to 20 torr.

Since the exhalation of air must be obstructed by closure of the glottis, passage of an endotracheal tube eliminates the grunt. When infants were intubated during a controlled study, a significant abrupt fall in PaO₂ occurred. However, this should not be interpreted as a contraindication to intubation of severely affected infants who require such therapy.

Retraction of the chest wall during inspiration is a classic sign of respiratory distress or, more specifically, diminished lung compliance. Retractions indicate a failure to fill the lungs with air during efforts exerted by respiratory muscles, especially the diaphragm. They thus indicate inadequate distention of the lungs during inspiration. Retractions are not always a sign of intrinsic lung disease, although this is their most frequent cause. They may also result from obstruction of airflow in the nose, larynx, trachea, or major bronchi. In hyaline membrane disease, airflow is diminished by incomplete expansion of the lungs, which is caused by diminished compliance. The lungs are stiffer than normal, and they fail to inflate fully as the diaphragm descends to enlarge the thorax. Negative pressure persists in the pleural space between the chest wall and the unexpanded lungs, and since the lungs do not expand to fill this space, the flexible chest wall is pulled inward. The net result is retraction of the chest wall.

In addition to *tachypnea, grunting,* and *retractions, flaring of the external nares* is also a frequent sign of respiratory distress. Auscultation of the chest reveals generalized *diminution of breath sounds* and, occasionally, *crepitant rales*. *Apneic episodes* occur in severely affected babies. They are an ominous sign, particularly when observed during the first 24 hours of life. *Cyanosis* in room air is the rule.

Cardiac signs are not ordinarily prominent. The heart rate is usually variable, but it becomes fixed as the disease increases in severity. Bradycardia (less than 100 beats/min) occurs when hypoxemia is severe. Cardiac failure is rare.

Pallor is the result of peripheral vasoconstric-

tion, rather than anemia. *Edema,* which is common in normal premature babies, is more frequent and severe in those with hyaline membrane disease. *Pitting edema* of the hands and feet appears within the first 24 hours and resolves by the end of the fifth day.

Decreased body temperature is frequently observed. In mildly or moderately involved infants it is correctable in an optimal thermal environment, but in severely affected infants it often defies remedial measures. Ambient incubator temperatures of 95° F (35° C) or more may be required to raise the body temperature.

Specific central nervous system signs are few. The muscles are universally *flaccid,* and the infant is *hypoactive* or *motionless*. Severely ill infants assume a frog-leg position, with the mouth open the the head fallen to one side.

Retractions continue for approximately 3 to 5 days and then diminish. Tachypnea often persists for several days afterward. Improvement is signaled by diminution of retractions, increased muscle tone and spontaneous activity, and frequent voiding accompanied by resolution of edema. Death is unlikely after 72 hours except for infants with complications such as intracranial hemorrhage, pneumonia, or pulmonary hemorrhage.

Laboratory data

There are no specific laboratory tests for the clinical diagnosis of hyaline membrane disease. The characteristic biochemical abnormalities (hypoxemia, hypercapnia, and acidosis) are identical to those of perinatal asphyxia and postnatal respiratory failure from any cause. In severely ill infants in room air the arterial Po₂ is below 40 torr (normal lower limit: 50 torr), the arterial Pco₂ is over 65 torr (normal upper limit: 45 torr), and the pH is below 7.15 (normal: 7.35 to 7.45).

Hypoxemia. Inadequate ventilation plus poor perfusion of tissues combine to cause low arterial oxygen tensions. Restoration of normal levels is the primary aim of therapy. Hypoxemia induces metabolic acidosis because lactic acid production increases. It also causes pulmonary arteriolar constriction. Other deleterious effects of hypoxemia include damage to capillary endothelium, impaired metabolic response to cold stress, and ultimately a low systemic blood pressure from diminished cardiac output.

Hypercapnia. Accumulation of carbon dioxide in the bood is a result of inadequate ventilation caused by atelectasis. A rising arterial PCO_2 signifies deterioration of pulmonary function. In the extreme, arterial PCO_2 may exceed 100 torr.

Acidosis. Mixed respiratory and metabolic acidosis is the rule in hyaline membrane disease. Early in the course of the disease respiratory acidosis may predominate, but soon a metabolic component also appears. The arterial pH may approach 6.8. The deleterious effects of acidosis include pulmonary vasoconstriction, irregular heartbeat, depression of myocardial function, further impairment of surfactant activity, and detachment of bilirubin from albumin to cause kernicterus at unexpectedly low serum bilirubin concentrations (Chapter 10).

Other blood chemical values. Serum electrolyte values may remain relatively unaltered, except for potassium, which increases as a result of hypoxic cellular injury in untreated or unsuccessfully treated babies. Lactic acid levels rise in conjunction with hypoxemia. Serum bilirubin levels are generally higher in babies with hyaline membrane disease; this is apparently related to depressed liver function (Chapter 10).

Radiologic findings

The typical x-ray appearance of the lungs is well correlated with the morphologic pathology of the disease. Almost every author who writes about it describes a reticulogranular pattern that is diffuse over both lung fields, occasionally involving one lung more than the other. The general impression one receives on viewing such a film is that the lungs appear clouded or similar to ground glass. White density is particularly prominent and homogeneous at the hilar areas. Close inspection peripheral to the hilar regions reveals tiny, closely

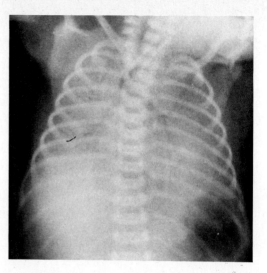

Fig. 8-9. Radiologic appearance of severe hyaline membrane disease. The lungs are dense. The cardiac shadow is barely discernible in left chest. Prominent black streaks emanating from both hilar areas are air bronchograms.

spaced densities that sometimes suggest a heavy snowfall at night. Each of these small densities is an atelectatic area of lung. At the hilar regions, and for some distance peripherally, dark streaks represent air-filled bronchi, which are easily discerned against the white background provided by the collapsed lung. These dark streaks are call *air bronchograms*. Hilar densities, a diffuse reticulogranular pattern, and air bronchograms are thus the cardinal radiologic features of hyaline membrane disease (Fig. 8-9). Table 8-1 summarizes the reported observations from studies on HMD.

Prevention

Hyaline membrane disease is a developmental disorder that centers about the maturation of metabolic pathways to surfactant production. Until prematurity itself can be prevented, the most promising approach seems to lie in attempts to stimulate the elaboration of surfactant in utero. Thus far, trials of corticosteroids (betamethasone and dexamethasone) given to mothers between

Table 8-1. Hyaline membrane disease; categorization of observations*

Established	Probable	Possible
Epidemiology		
Worldwide	Second born twin at greater	Maternal hemorrhage predisposes
Prematurity predisposes	risk	Familial predisposition
Cesarean section without la-	PROM spares	Prenatal corticoids spare
bor predisposes	IUGR spares	Maternal heroin addiction spares
Perinatal asphyxia predisposes	Maternal toxemia spares	Late pulmonary sequelae
Male mortality > female	Maternal diabetes predisposes	
	White > nonwhite race	
Clinical signs		
Onset near the time of birth	Fine inspiratory rales	Pulmonary edema
Retractions and tachypnea	Hypothermia	Persistent patent ductus
Expiratory grunt	Peripheral edema	
Cyanosis		
Systemic hypotension		
Characteristic chest x-ray		
Prominent thymus on first		
day		
Pathophysiology		
Reduced lung compliance	Poor peripheral perfusion	Myocardial malconduction
Reduced FRC	Poor renal perfusion	
Poor lung distensibility		
Poor alveolar stability		
Right-to-left shunts		
Reduced effective pulmonary		
blood flow		
Pathobiochemistry		
Respiratory acidosis	Decreased total serum proteins	Metabolic acidosis
Decreased saturated phospho-	Decreased fibrinolysins	Hyperkalemia
lipids	Low prolactin levels	Pepsinogen in lung
Preceded by low AF L/S ratio	Low thyroxine levels	
Preceded by low AF surfac-		
tant titer		
Pathology		
Atelectasis	Osmiophilic lamellar bodies	Small adrenal glands
Injury to epithelial cells	decreased early, increased	Intracranial hemorrhage
Membrane contains fibrin and	later	
cellular products		
Etiology		
Surfactant deficiency during	Primary surfactant deficiency	Absent corticoid stimulus (in
disease	(in utero)	utero)
		DPL synthesis impaired and/or
		destruction increased
		Autonomic dysfunction
		Primary pulmonary hypoperfusion
		Hypovolemia

*Abbreviations: PROM = prolonged rupture of membrane (>16 hours); IUGR = intrauterine growth retardation; PDA = patent ductus arteriosus; FRC = functional residual capacity; AF = amniotic fluid; L/S = lecithin/sphingomyelin ratio; DPL = dipalmitoyl lecithin.

From Avery, M. E., Fletcher, B. D., and Williams, R. G.: The lung and its disorders in the newborn infant, Philadelphia, 1981, W. B. Saunders Co.

24 hours and 7 days before delivery have yielded promising results. In this group of mothers, if offspring were less than 32 gestational weeks, the incidence of hyaline membrane disease was significantly reduced from that in controls. Mortality from the disease and the incidence of intraventricular hemorrhage were also reduced in babies of the same gestational age. However, even in the group that benefited from betamethasone, hyaline membrane disease occurred in 21%. In addition, betamethasone was ineffective for infants whose gestational age was 32 weeks or more. The betamethasone trial is not in itself a completely successful therapeutic effort, but the results are an encouraging indication that fetal medication is a promising approach to the problem.

Hydrocortisone has been administered postnatally to infants with hyaline membrane disease in a well-controlled trial. A beneficial effect was not demonstrated.

Outcomes

In the 1960s we were frustrated spectators who could only observe hyaline membrane disease as it progressed along a predetermined, irrevocable course. Supportive therapy was meager. Those infants who survived had only minimal or moderate involvement. Many of them were afflicted with permanent brain damage and blindness. The most severely affected could only be offered very limited aid. They tired, with deepening cyanosis, from the struggle to expand their noncompliant ischemic lungs. Today our therapeutic regimens are still no more than supportive, but they are effective because they are directed against specific pathophysiologic mechanisms. It is the advent of newborn intensive care units and their concepts of neonatal care that must be credited with the encouraging results that have been recorded. In that context, continued improvement in outcomes is the result of enhanced expertise in the management of ventilatory support and of expanded understanding of the pathophysiologic requirements for other supportive measures.

Neonatal survival. Compilation of the results from a number of centers indicates impressive improvement in the survival rate. The disease is, of course, still a serious, life-threatening process, but among infants who did not require mechanical support and who were given only constant distending pressure (CPAP), 93% survived. Of those who received only mechanical support, 47% survived. Among infants who were unsuccessfully treated with distending pressure and required subsequent mechanical support, 49% survived. A few years ago, survival for all infants with the disease, regardless of type of treatment, with or without assisted respiration was 61%. More recently, an overall mortality of only 11% was reported for 153 infants who were treated with various modalities of support.

Increased survival of mechanically ventilated babies has been well documented as more effective manipulation of ventilators has evolved. In Britain, for instance, survival of mechanically ventilated infants increased from 11% to 49% in recent years, and this figure represents the most severely affected group of infants. Intraventricular hemorrhage persists as a major problem. It is the most important cause of death among ventilated infants.

Postneonatal outcomes. Long-term developmental assessment is complicated by the possible role of intrauterine misadventure. Results vary from one institution to another, but overall, the majority of infants are developmentally normal. There are specific data to indicate that impaired development is not related to mechanical ventilation, but rather to gestational age, in the infants who were studied. The high degree of variability among neurologic follow-up studies is a result of numerous uncontrollable factors. It is virtually impossible to compare the results from one center with those of another. Differing populations in respect to gestational age are an important consideration for comparison. Probably of even greater importance is the place of birth of the study infants. Outcomes among referred babies (outborn) are far more likely to be abnormal than among inborn infants. Furthermore, at the same birth weight and gestational age, black infants regularly have a higher survival rate than white babies. Follow-up studies have rarely dealt with these racial differences in terms of neurologic sequelae. The age of follow-up also varies among reports, as well as the date of intensive care. Infants who have been treated more recently have survived intact in greater numbers.

The incidence of neurologic defects in reports of ventilated babies has varied from 11% to 29%. These studies have involved babies whose birth weights were below 1500 g to those with mean birth weights as high as 2319 g. Mortality of ventilated babies also differed widely—from 51% in 1974 to 1975 to 79% in 1966 to 1973. The neurologic defects are primarily hydrocephalus or cerebral palsy, presumably as a result of intracranial hemorrhage. Deficits in intellectual function usually accompany these neurologic lesions.

Pulmonary sequelae can be divided mainly into lower respiratory tract infections and bronchopulmonary dysplasia (p. 260). Readmission to the hospital for lung infection increases in frequency when birth weight and gestational age are low. Furthermore, in the absence of bronchopulmonary dysplasia, pulmonary infection after discharge from the nursery does not seem to occur more frequently in babies who were mechanically ventilated.

Sequelae of trauma from the ventilatory process are considerably less frequent than lung infections and bronchopulmonary dysplasia. When nasotracheal intubation is used, ulceration of the nares heals with scar formation and stenosis of the involved nostril or nasal vestibule. Midline clefts of the hard palate have been noted among infants who had orotracheal tubes for a protracted period. The mechanism of cleft formation has not been delineated with certainty, but it is doubtful that the cleft is simply the result of pressure exerted by the endotracheal tube. These tubes are constantly moving about, yet in all the affected infants, the clefts have been located precisely in the midline, suggesting that a disorder of palatine growth has resulted from prolonged intubation.

Damage to vocal cords causes hoarseness and stridor that often disappear or improve but are not uncommonly persistent. Subglottic stenosis occurs rather rarely. It requires tracheostomy because it occludes the airway at the level of the larynx.

APNEA AND PERIODIC BREATHING

Apnea is the cessation of regular breathing. In one form or another, these pauses in respiration compose the most common day-to-day problem encountered in the neonatal intensive care unit. The logical categorization of apneic events is as follows.

Periodic breathing occurs in premature infants whose birth weight is below 1800 g. It is characterized by recurrent failure to breathe for intervals that are no longer than 10 to 15 seconds. The timing is not as important as the absence of associated responses such as bradycardia, cyanosis, limpness, and the infant's capacity to resume regular respirations spontaneously. Periodic breathing generally appears on the second to the fifth day of life. Obviously it cannot be identified in infants who require mechanical ventilatory support for the first few days of life. Periodic breathing has a tendency to disappear by the end of the third week of life, regardless of gestational age.

Apnea is the more serious manifestation of an infant's recurrent failure to breathe. Apneic spells are distinguished from periodic breathing by their longer duration, but more significantly by associated manifestations such as bradycardia (below 100 beats per minute), cyanosis, and limpness. The vast majority of apneic episodes requires some form of stimulation for the resumption of respiration. Thus the mildest spells can be terminated by simple tactile stimulation to the skin, or perhaps more painful stimulation by flicking the fingers on skin. In the extreme, apneic episodes require endotracheal intubation, bagging, and, ultimately, sustained mechanical support. Clinically there are two broad categories of apnea: (1) the apneic spells are secondary to underlying disorders, and (2) the apneic episodes are unassociated with identifiable underlying disease; apnea is a manifestation of incomplete respiratory center development.

Apnea associated with underlying disorders

Apneic spells occur at some time during the course of the clinical disorders listed below. Often they are the first manifestation of an underlying disease.

Impaired oxygenation: anemia, shock, pulmonary edema, patent ductus arteriosus, cardiac failure, hyaline membrane disease, immature lung, and dysfunction of oxygen delivery equipment.
Thermoregulation: hypothermia, hyperthermia, and rapid fluctuations in either direction.
Infection: septicemia, meningitis, and pneumonia.
Brain disorders: perinatal asphyxia, intraventricular-periventricular hemorrhage, seizures, and acute ventricular dilatation secondary to IVH.
Metabolic disorders: hypoglycemia, dehydration and acidosis, hyperammonemia, hypernatremia, and hyponatremia.
Abdominal distention: necrotizing enterocolitis, perforated viscus, and other surgical emergencies such as volvulus and other intestinal obstructions, and gastroesophageal reflux (GER).

The abrupt appearance of serious apneic episodes requires investigation for the possibilities listed above. Identification of underlying disease is particularly urgent in infants who suddenly become apneic after satisfactory progress for days.

Apneic episodes are infrequently caused by primary central nervous system disorders. Apnea as a single manifestation of a convulsive disorder is exceptional. While apneic episodes are frequent accompaniments to convulsions, they are virtually always associated with some other identifiable manifestation of seizure activity, whether subtle or blatant (see seizures, Chapter 14).

Apneic episodes not associated with underlying disease

The majority of apneic episodes cannot be attributed to underlying disorders. They are considered manifestations of incomplete development of the respiratory center in the medulla oblongata. Immaturity of the respiratory center is associated with diminished afferent (input) impulses, and thus a reduction or unpredictable fluctuation of efferent (output) impulses. Morphologically the immature respiratory center is composed of a diminished quantity of synapses, fewer dendritic processes, and minimal central nervous system myelinization.

It is generally believed that hypoxemia precedes apneic episodes, that it depresses function of the immature respiratory center. Several studies have failed to demonstrate an association between antecedent hypoxemia and apneic episodes, but the strong suspicion persists that diminished oxygenation often precedes apnea. There is little known about the pathophysiology of apnea, largely because much investigation remains to be accomplished regarding the nature of normal respiratory control. The clinical problem is nevertheless one of the most commonly encountered in intensive care nurseries. Most units can report that at least half the infants whose birth weights were below 1500 g required treatment for recurrent apnea.

While the data explaining apnea of prematurity has only begun to appear in the last few years, it has become apparent that immaturity of the respiratory center is largely manifested by a diminished response to elevated levels of $PaCO_2$. The term infant increases depth of respiration (greater tidal volume) and alveolar ventilation in response to some elevation of $PaCO_2$. Premature infants with apnea fail to respond to increased $PaCO_2$ levels to the same extent as control infants who are not apneic. Preterm infants with apnea exhibit a diminished inspiratory effort and a blunted response to carbon dioxide. Hypoventilation and hypercapnia ensue. Apnea of prematurity may well be an abnormality in the control of breathing patterns by the respiratory center. The inadequacy of respiratory center function increases as gestational age shortens. Blunted respiratory center response to CO_2 is unusual in infants over 33 weeks gestational age.

In adults, lowered FiO_2 causes a sustained response of increase in ventilation. In preterm infants the response to low FiO_2 is characterized by increased ventilation for approximately 60 seconds followed by a sustained depression of respirations. Some investigators believe that this response to suboptimal oxygenation diminishes the respiratory center's sensitivity to CO_2 levels. The etiologic importance of antecedent hypoxemia has not been precisely defined.

Idiopathic apnea of prematurity is therefore caused by immature dysfunction of respiratory control in the brain stem. Such episodes are composed of cessation of respiratory effort plus undetectable air flow. When air flow is diminished or undetectable but respiratory efforts continue, *obstructive apnea* is said to occur. While apnea in preterm infants is rarely caused solely by obstructive phenomena, such as extreme flexion of the neck, some element of obstructive flow during apneic episodes has in fact been demonstrated.

The treatment of idiopathic apneic spells varies with their severity. Whatever the method, treatment must be instituted as early as possible to forestall continued deterioration during a prolonged apneic episode. Restoration of effective support is more difficult as apnea and cyanosis become more protracted. The mildest spells are easily remedied by tactile or mildly painful stimuli. Recurrent episodes associated with bradycardia and cyanosis require a more aggressive approach. The treatment of choice for sustained prevention or diminution of apnea is theophylline or caffeine. Theophylline is administered intravenously in a loading dose of 5.5 to 6 mg/kg followed by 1 mg/kg every 8 hours. Plasma concentrations must be followed assiduously. Levels between 6 and 13 mg/L are acceptable; a level of approximately 10 mg/L is probably optimal. Caffeine is administered intravenously in a loading dose of 10 mg/kg (20 mg/kg, if caffeine citrate is used), followed by 2.5 mg/kg every 24 hours (caffeine) or 5 mg/kg every 24 hours (caffeine citrate). Monitoring plasma levels of caffeine is critical. Acceptable levels range from 7 to 20 mg/L. Signs of toxicity for theophylline are more often found in cardiovascular function (tachycardia) than central nervous system function (irritated activity, seizures). Gastrointestinal signs occur occasionally (vomiting and abdominal distention). Theophylline is also a known diuretic and natriuretic. Its use in preterm infants requires careful monitoring of urine output and electrolytes. Caffeine toxicity usually involves the central nervous system primarily (irritability and convulsions), but toxic effects are unlikely below plasma levels of 50 mg/L.

However effective the methylxanthines (theophylline, caffeine) may be, the onset of their effectiveness may be too delayed in infants whose apneic episodes require resuscitation repeatedly. When necessary, we institute CPAP for an immediate response, using pressures that range from 2 to 4 cm H_2O. CPAP is then tapered and discontinued as soon as pharmacologic effect of methylxanthines is identifiable (therapeutic plasma levels). The most severe of apneic episodes require mechanical ventilatory support.

MANAGEMENT OF RESPIRATORY INSUFFICIENCY
Use of oxygen

Nothing is more critical to tissue metabolism than an adequate supply of oxygen. The most important aspect of total therapy for respiratory insufficiency is the provision of oxygen. *Once the need for such therapy is apparent for any disorder, its adequacy must be ascertained and its hazards averted by continuous monitoring of arterial oxygen tensions.* In this section, before discussion of practical considerations, it seems fitting to discuss the physiologic principles that underlie rational oxygen therapy, its benefits, and its hazards.

Physiology of oxygen transport: the basis for rational oxygen therapy. The erythrocyte is the vehicle for transport of oxygen. Its basic function is to take up oxygen from the lungs and deliver it to the tissues, carrying sufficient quantities to effect rapid diffusion from capillaries to tissue cells. The performance of this function depends on a number of factors that include an adequate fraction of inspired oxygen (FiO_2) and normal pulmonary function, blood volume, cardiac output, and perfusion. Other aspects are intrinsic to blood. They involve arterial pH and temperature, red hemoglobin cell concentration, and the affinity of hemoglobin for oxygen. Several definitions must be considered before continuing this discussion.

Definitions

Partial pressure of oxygen, or oxygen tension (Po_2). Management of oxygen therapy is based on monitored levels of arterial oxygen tensions (PaO_2), expressed in millimeters of mercury (torr). The partial pressure of a gas is the force it exerts in its tendency to escape from a liquid to a gaseous medium or from one compartment to another, much like the pressure exerted by escaping bubbles in champagne. It is called "partial" when the gas in question is only one of several in a common liquid (or chamber) that exert pressure simultaneously. In arterial (or venous) blood, with the subject breathing room air, partial pressures are measurable for oxygen, carbon dioxide, nitrogen, and water vapor. Total pressure of these gases—that is, their aggregate driving force to escape—is approximately 750 torr. The pressure exerted by oxygen alone, or partial pressure (arterial Po_2), is about 90 torr. The tension attributable to carbon dioxide, the arterial Pco_2, is usually 40 torr. The remaining partial pressures are exerted by nitrogen. The Po_2 is thus the driving force of oxygen, which will move it from one compartment to another—from alveoli to pulmonary capillaries if Po_2 is higher in alveoli than in capillaries, and from capillaries to tissues if partial pressure in the

capillaries is higher than in tissue fluid. The same principle is operative for movement of oxygen from tissue fluid into cells. Movement of CO_2 in the opposite direction, from tissues to blood and thence to alveoli, is governed by a similar pattern of pressure differences. Movement of gas from a higher to a lower partial pressure is movement governed by a *pressure gradient*. If normal arterial blood (Po_2, 90 torr) is exposed to room air (Po_2, 150 torr), oxygen will enter the blood until equilibrium is established, that is, until both have a Po_2 of 150 torr. On the other hand, with arterial Pco_2 of 40 torr and atmospheric Pco_2 of 0 (there is virtually no CO_2 in air), carbon dioxide will ultimately disappear from blood, having moved into room air. The pressure gradient for oxygen movement is from room air to blood; arterial Po_2 rises. For carbon dioxide it is in the opposite direction; arterial Pco_2 declines. This is precisely what occurs when blood collected for blood gas determination is inadvertently exposed to room air. Blood gas determinations in these circumstances are invalid.

Oxygen content (concentration). The oxygen content of whole blood is the total amount in 100 ml. Normal oxygen content is 20.6 ml (vol %). This includes 20 ml bound to hemoglobin and 0.6 ml (approximately 3% of the total) dissolved in plasma.

Oxygen capacity. Oxygen *capacity* must be distinguished from oxygen *content*. Oxygen capacity is the maximal amount that hemoglobin can theoretically hold. Oxygen content is the actual amount held when the determination is made. Most oxygen in blood is bound to hemoglobin. Each gram of hemoglobin has the capacity to bind 1.34 ml of oxygen. If the hemoglobin concentration of whole blood is 15 g/100 ml, the calculated *capacity* at this concentration is 15×1.34, or 20.1 ml of oxygen/100 ml of blood.

Oxygen saturation. Referring only to hemoglobin, oxygen saturation is given as a percentage value that is calculated by dividing the amount of oxygen bound to hemoglobin (content) by the maximal amount that can be bound (oxygen capacity). Normal oxygen saturation is 96% to 98%. Oxygen saturation is governed by the PO_2 and by the affinity of hemoglobin for oxygen.

Affinity of hemoglobin for oxygen. Fetal hemoglobin (Hb F) differs from adult hemoglobin (Hb A). Among its unique attributes is the ability to bind more oxygen at any given PO_2. Therefore, at any given PO_2, oxygen saturation of fetal hemoglobin is higher than the adult's. Fetal hemoglobin thus is said to have a greater affinity for oxygen than adult hemoglobin. The fetal red blood cell therefore takes up more oxygen in the lungs (because Hb F holds more), but this phenomenon is of little overall significance. Of greater potential importance is the fact that increased affinity also causes less oxygen to be released to the tissues because Hb F releases relatively less O_2. Conversely, in the adult, Hb A releases O_2 more readily; more oxygen is unloaded to the tissues at any given PaO_2. Hemoglobin releases bound oxygen in response to a lower tissue oxygen tension (PO_2). In the neonate, the tension must fall farther before fetal hemoglobin releases oxygen, since it is held more avidly than in the adult.

The molecular configuration of fetal hemoglobin differs from that of the adult. This difference, plus the quantity of organic phosphates in the red blood cells, determines the affinity of hemoglobin for oxygen. The principal organic phosphate in the erythrocyte is 2,3-diphosphoglycerate (2,3-DPG). DPG binds to hemoglobin A at specific sites. In so doing it releases oxygen from the hemoglobin A molecule. DPG therefore diminishes the avidity of adult hemoglobin for oxygen, and as a result the adult red cell gives up oxygen to tissue more readily than the fetal (neonatal) red cell. The hemoglobin F molecule has no binding site for DPG. Release of oxygen occurs less readily without DPG binding. Even with DPG in the erythrocyte, hemoglobin F binds oxygen avidly because it has no binding site for DPG. On the other hand, in the absence of DPG, hemoglobin A binds oxygen with the same avidity as hemoglobin F. *The adult level of reduced affinity requires appropriate concentrations of both hemoglobin A and DPG in the same erythrocyte.* Even if DPG is present, the fetal red cell releases less oxygen than the adult red cell. Similarly the adult red cell (hemoglobin A) releases less oxygen if DPG is absent. Red cells give up oxygen readily only if both hemoglobin A and DPG are present.

The affinity of hemoglobin for oxygen in the term infant is greater than that of the adult. The affinity decreases rapidly during the first week of life because a number of neonatal erythrocytes contain hemoglobin A, and DPG accumulates within them. When the term infant is 4 to 6 months of age, oxygen affinity has gradually diminished to approximate adult levels. At this age, hemoglobin A has largely replaced hemoglobin F, and DPG is in properly proportionate concentration in the erythrocyte.

Oxygen-hemoglobin dissociation curve. Normally there is a predictable correlation between oxygen saturation and PO_2. Plotted on a graph in which the percentage of saturation is arranged vertically, and PO_2 horizontally, a typical S-shaped (sigmoid) curve results when the plotted points are joined. Dissociation curves for fetal and adult hemoglobins are shown in Fig. 8-10. The saturation (vertical scale) of fetal hemoglobin is higher than the adult's at all PO_2 levels because there is a greater affinity for oxygen, more is bound to Hb F because there is no competition from DPG. Stated differently, the same percentage of saturation occurs at a lower PO_2 in fetal hemoglobin than in the adult's. This can be clearly discerned by reference to the two shaded vertical bars that indicate zones in which cyanosis is visible, corresponding to fetal and adult values for oxygen saturation of hemoglobin. Cyanosis is apparent when blood is between 75% and 85% saturated with oxygen. These saturations occur at PO_2 levels of 32 to 41 torr in the neonate and 42 to 52 torr in the adult. Fig. 8-10 demonstrates why the newborn is considerably less oxygenated than the adult when cyanosis first becomes discernible. The fetal dissociation curve is said to be shifted to the left of the adult's.

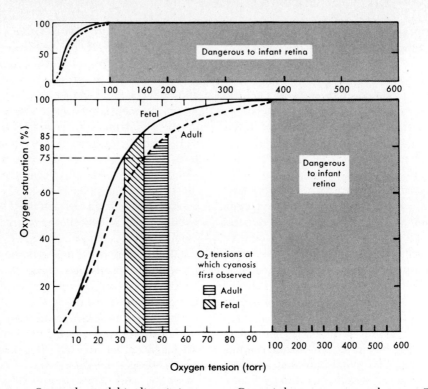

Fig. 8-10. Oxygen-hemoglobin dissociation curves. Cyanosis becomes apparent between 75% and 85% saturation, correlating to lower oxygen tension in neonates than that in adults. Scale at top shows the curves in relation to toxic levels. (From Klaus, M., and Meyer, B. P.: Pediatr. Clin. North Am. **13:**731, 1966.)

The position of the curve (shifted right or left) actually indicates the affinity of hemoglobin for oxygen. When the affinity is decreased, as in the adult, more oxygen is released to tissues at any given oxygen tension. Saturation at any oxygen tension is therefore less than in the neonate. Saturation at any given Po_2 decreases as affinity diminishes. The oxygen-hemoglobin dissociation curve is thus shifted to the right. If affinity is increased, as in the neonate, less oxygen is unloaded to tissues at any given Pao_2. Saturation at any Pao_2 is therefore greater than in the adult. The curve is now said to be shifted to the left.

Two factors intrinsic to blood exert a major influence on affinity of hemoglobin for oxygen. Af-finity diminishes as blood pH decreases and as temperature increases; the curve shifts to the right. Affinity increases as blood pH rises and temperature falls; the curve shifts to the left. The increased affinity caused by lower temperatures explains a common phenomenon. In bitter cold weather, earlobes are bright red because the blood within them is chilled. Affinity for oxygen increases; saturation at any given Pao_2 is thus also increased, and the curve is shifted to the left, as in the neonate. The Po_2 of earlobe tissue may be relatively low, but the increased saturation renders it bright red because hemoglobin retains more oxygen in red blood cells, releasing less to hypoxic tissues as a result of its greater affinity for oxygen.

Practical considerations

Dose and blood level; monitoring FIO_2 and blood gases. Oxygen is like any drug; it must be administered in proper dosage. Unlike many drugs, however, the dose required for optimal and harmless effect varies widely from one infant to another and from time to time in the same infant. Appropriate doses of oxygen can be maintained only by monitoring its ambient concentrations (FIO_2) and measuring the ultimate effect of such concentrations on the infant's arterial oxygen tension PaO_2. The ultimate measure of optimal therapy is the arterial PO_2. Carbon dioxide tension and pH are always determined on the same blood sample. A detailed record of these serial determinations must be kept, particularly in reference to the percentage of inhaled oxygen that is provided. The ambient concentration should always be noted when a blood sample is collected.

By any method of administration, from the simple oxygen hood to the complex mechanical ventilator, oxygen is a medication that requires proper dosage (FIO_2) and repeated blood level determinations (arterial PO_2). PaO_2 over 100 torr is considered hyperoxemic; under 50 torr it is hypoxemic. For sick babies who require supplemental oxygen, there is no correlation whatever between FIO_2 and PaO_2. In most neonatal intensive care units, PaO_2 is maintained between 50 and 70 torr. These levels are achievable at widely varying inspired oxygen concentrations. An infant who is profoundly ill from hyaline membrane disease may require an FIO_2 of 1.00 (100% oxygen) to maintain a PaO_2 of 50 torr. During recovery 5 days later, the same FIO_2 may produce toxic PaO_2 of over 200 torr. Similar radical changes in FIO_2 requirements can occur within an hour or less.

The dose of oxygen is always expressed as its fraction of inspired air (FIO_2). The day has long since passed when oxygen can properly be ordered in liters per minute. This designation merely expresses flow rate of the gas, not its concentration in inspired air. Orders for oxygen administration given as liters per minute betray a sad lack of information.

The dose of oxygen must be monitored continuously. Use of any of several varieties of oxygen analyzers is mandatory for this purpose. At present we prefer an analyzer that is placed in line so that the air mixture is monitored continuously. The FIO_2 should be noted every hour. Prescribed oxygen concentrations are provided through a blender that regulates simultaneous inflow of air and oxygen by adjusting an indicator to the desired level.

The arterial blood level of oxygen should be determined at least every 4 hours for sick babies, often at much shorter intervals (15 minutes) for the most acutely ill infants, and at least every 6 hours for babies who are not acutely ill.

Sites of blood sampling. For blood gas determinations, arterial blood samples are preferred. They are drawn from an umbilical artery catheter, or from the radial arteries by needle puncture. In our laboratory approximately 25% of over 40,000 annual blood gas/pH determinations are drawn by puncture of radial arteries.

Although the great majority of neonatal units use arterial blood for these assessments, a few facilities consider capillary blood samples to be adequate. Blood is collected by heel prick from a foot that has been warmed for 5 minutes. Others prick the lateral aspect of a finger, over one of the digital arteries. Capillary blood values of 35 to 55 torr are said to correspond to arterial tensions of 40 to 65 torr. If capillary PO_2 is above 60 torr, the arterial level may exceed 150 torr. Most centers do not consistently rely on capillary samples for monitoring PO_2, particularly if transcutaneous monitors are available.

Collection of arterial samples through an umbilical artery catheter is widely practiced. Most centers insert the catheter tip to a level between the third and fourth lumbar vertebrae, which is just above the aortic bifurcation and below the origins of the renal arteries. In sick infants who have a right-to-left shunt through the ductus arteriosus, blood taken from the descending aorta is a mixture of oxygenated blood from the left ventricle and deoxygenated blood from the right ventricle that has passed through the ductal shunt. It is a postductal specimen because it came from the descending aorta below (distal to) the ductus opening. If the ductal shunt is substantial, postductal arterial PO_2 is at least 15% lower than preductal blood *when the latter is less than 50 torr*. Arterial blood collected from the right radial artery is preductal. The right subclavian artery (to the right arm) branches from the proximal portion of the aortic arch. Aortic blood from the left ventricle passes the right subclavian artery before it reaches the distal end of the arch where the ductus arteriosus connects to the aorta. It is thus unmixed with right-to-left shunted ductal blood. If a right-to-left shunt is present, ductus arteriosus blood empties into the aorta. This blood is from the right ventricle. It is deoxygenated (venous) blood that has not perfused the lungs. Its presence in postductal aortic blood may lower the PaO_2 substantially. Arterial PO_2 levels in samples from the right radial and brachial arteries, and from either of the temporal arteries (not the recommended sampling sites), are not mixed with postductal blood. These PO_2 levels are thus the same as in blood that perfuses the brain and the eyes. In severe hyaline membrane disease, with a right-to-left ductal shunt, PaO_2 is substantially higher in preductal than in postductal blood. Similarly, if an infant is hypotensive, the relatively higher pressure in the pulmonary circuit produces a significant shunt across the ductus. Postductal PaO_2 in blood from the umbilical artery is therefore substantially lower than in blood from the right radial artery and, in many instances, does not reflect oxygen tension of blood that perfuses the eyes. The PaO_2 in samples from the left radial artery may be similar either to the right radial artery or to postductal aortic samples, since the left subclavian artery (to the left arm) may originate from the aorta at the level of the ductus, slightly above it or slightly below. In the vast majority of infants, PaO_2 in the left arm is similar to that in postductal blood taken from an umbilical artery catheter.

Transcutaneous monitoring of oxygen tension (tcPo₂). The necessity for frequent arterial blood gas samples entails repeated arterial punctures if an umbilical artery is not in place. The need for frequent blood sampling by arterial puncture often taxes the ingenuity of staff and the well-being of babies. Furthermore, resultant values are applicable only to the moment of sampling. We obviously have no idea of oxygen tension during intervals between blood sampling. The need for a noninvasive technique has been met with the use of transcutaneous oxygen monitors, which also provide *continuous* monitoring of PO_2 levels so that minute-to-minute changes are directly in view.

The transcutaneous oxygen apparatus is primarily dependent on a sensor (electrode) attached to the skin. PO_2 values are recorded from warmed skin ($tcPO_2$), and they are generally well correlated with arterial PO_2. $tcPO_2$ is not identical to arterial PO_2. It is not arterial PO_2 that is directly measured. In normal circumstances, PO_2 is zero at the skin surface because skin blood flow is autoregulated to supply only the quantity of oxygen needed for metabolism in the skin. It became apparent during the early days of research on this apparatus that oxygen does, in fact, diffuse through the skin when dermal hyperperfusion is induced. Induction of hyperperfusion and measurement of transcutaneous oxygen diffusion became possible when an appropriate electrode was developed. The electrode contains the same oxygen measuring device used for blood gases in the laboratory. It also houses a coil that provides the heat required for local hyperperfusion. The heat provided by the electrode is automatically regulated by setting the electronic apparatus to which the electrode wire is inserted. A skin temperature sensor relays the level of warmth attained by the heated electrode. More heat is provided if skin temperature falls, and less as it rises, in the same fashion that skin sensors activate heat production for incubators and radiant warmers.

The heated electrode induces local hyperemia

and, as a result, oxygen is delivered to the skin in excess of metabolic needs. The excess oxygen diffuses through the skin and is then measured by the Clark electrode within the heated sensor. The readings obtained are visible by digital display, and also by continuous recording on a strip chart. Resultant values are not identical to arterial PO_2, but they are close enough to be accurate for clinical use. The level of measured transcutaneous oxygen depends on the quantity of oxygen delivered to the skin by hyperperfusion. At skin temperatures between 43° and 44° C, transcutaneous levels closely approximate arterial levels. Any condition that diminishes skin perfusion will cause $tcPO_2$ values to be lower than existing arterial levels. Thus the effect of diminished perfusion is clearly demonstrated by inflating a blood pressure cuff on the arm and measuring $tcPO_2$ distal to the cuff. When the inflated cuff just exceeds systolic pressure, blood flow is obstructed and perfusion distal to the cuff is virtually zero. $tcPO_2$ levels then decline slowly. When the cuff is deflated, obstruction to blood flow is eliminated; $tcPO_2$ values rise quickly.

It must be emphasized that $tcPO_2$ is not a direct measurement of arterial levels. The closeness of arterial and transcutaneous values is a fortunate coincidence that happens to occur at skin temperatures of 43° to 44° C. $tcPO_2$ is vulnerable to changes in numerous clinical circumstances, all of them related to skin perfusion. Increased skin temperature raises $tcPO_2$ above existing arterial levels (hyperperfusion). Hypothermia diminishes skin levels (hypoperfusion). Any condition that impairs blood flow to the skin diminishes $tcPO_2$. Thus in shock from any cause, skin levels are lower than arterial ones.

In alert normal term infants there is considerable minute-to-minute variation of $tcPO_2$. Fluctuations of 20 to 30 torr are physiologic. In deep sleep the $tcPO_2$ remains relatively fixed, but spontaneous crying often produces a precipitous fall of approximately 20 torr, sometimes dipping below 50 torr.

For infants under intensive care, $tcPO_2$ is reliable unless shock or hypothermia is present. $tcPO_2$ is highly variable in babies on ventilators. A significant improvement in respirator care is possible because $tcPO_2$ is visible while the respirator is being manipulated. The alternative is the usual frequent drawing of blood samples, awaiting results from the laboratory. A significant application of skin oxygen monitors is therefore in the rapid adjustment of ventilator settings for relatively rapid optimal oxygenation. The monitors are also helpful in managing infants with chronic lung disease (BPD), but here the interpretation is tricky. In these infants, blood gases are more often spurious than accurate. A crying infant whose pulmonary function is marginal often turns blue. PaO_2 is deceptively low. Furthermore, several studies have demonstrated that $tcPO_2$ lowers significantly in infants who are older than 10 weeks, particularly in the presence of chronic lung disease. Transcutaneous values are probably spuriously low with increased age because the skin is thicker and the skin capillaries are more sparse. Thickness of skin impairs diffusion of oxygen; diminished capillary density precludes the hyperperfusion induced by a heated electrode. Lower $tcPO_2$ readings become more frequent between 8 and 12 weeks of postnatal age, corresponding to 35 to 39 weeks of postmenstrual age.

The hypoxic effect of procedures on transcutaneous readings is impressive. The most extensive hypoxic effects have been demonstrated during the taking of chest x-ray films. Other procedures have produced hypoxia in some infants, but not all. Apparently, any procedure can lower $tcPO_2$. The more disturbing the process, the more consistent the fall in transcutaneous readings. Crying stimulated by manipulation exerts a greater hypoxic effect than spontaneous crying in physiologic circumstances. Although they induce less extensive falls in $tcPO_2$, a number of procedures have been observed to produce some hypoxic effect. These include blood collection from heel prick, chest physiotherapy, weighing, taking of temperature, and heart rate. Even the placement of a $tcPO_2$ electrode itself has been noted to produce transient hypoxia. The trends demonstrated by studies of transcutaneous oxygen levels strongly suggest reevaluation of the routine procedures that comprise intensive care. The need for changing or limiting them, particularly in babies who are most susceptible to hypoxia, is mandatory.

The transcutaneous monitor is not intended to replace blood sampling. In many instances the skin monitor can be the primary source of information on arterial oxygen tensions, but it must be supplemented by periodic blood gas determinations to verify accuracy. In our experience, periodic blood gas sampling, most reliably from an indwelling catheter, is necessary to validate the accuracy of transcutaneous readings. The principal uses of skin monitoring are in the rapidity with which respirator settings can be adjusted for acutely distressed babies, in infants with chronic lung disease whose blood gases are often spurious, and in monitoring the stressful effects of routine procedures used for intensive care.

Hypoxia: detection, prevention, and penalties.
Generally, a PaO_2 less than 50 torr is considered hypoxemic. A number of infants may tolerate lower levels for some time, but it is unsafe to regularly maintain arterial tensions at these lower levels. The acute effects of hypoxemia must be understood; they are often difficult to identify with certainty from clinical manifestations. The clinical recognition of hypoxemia on the basis of *cyanosis* is far from a simple matter. Several factors influence the recognition of cyanosis, including color and thickness of skin, number of capillaries, hemoglobin level, and serum bilirubin. Add to these variables the type and intensity of light, as well as the differences in perception among observers, and one can readily appreciate the complexity of this clinical situation. In the neonate, acrocyanosis (including circumoral involvement) that is present 24 to 48 hours after birth is of no significance insofar as arterial oxygen tensions are concerned.

Cyanosis is not uniformly discernible on all areas of the body, even when oxygen saturations in blood are as low as 70%. Cyanosis of the lips (and perhaps the tongue) is most reliably correlated with hypoxic PaO_2 levels; yet 1 in 10 infants whose lips are not cyanotic may actually be hypoxic. Conversely, 28% of infants whose lips are blue are not hypoxic. They have no need for supplemental oxygen. Hands, nailbeds, and circumoral areas are even less reliable. They frequently appear to be cyanotic despite normal oxygen saturations. The trunk and ears yield a high percentage of false-negative observations; they often appear pink in babies who are actually hypoxemic. *The clinical diagnosis of hypoxia is unreliable. Cyanosis may be absent in hypoxic babies, and it may be present in those who are well oxygenated. Its presence over different parts of the body is variable, and there is little consistency among observers in the ability to recognize it.*

At this point in the discussion, it would be advisable to review the oxygen-hemoglobin dissociation curves (Fig. 8-10). Cyanosis is not visible until saturations fall between 75% and 85%. At these saturations the neonate's PaO_2 is between 32 and 42 torr. Cyanosis in the older child and adult is identifiable at higher PaO_2 levels. The clinical message of the dissociation curve is clear. The pink baby in respiratory distress may be hypoxemic; when cyanosis finally appears, catastrophe may be at hand. The PaO_2 may already be as low as 32 torr. *The ill effects of hypoxemia had transpired while the baby was pink.* The acute responses to hypoxia began as the PaO_2 fell below 50 torr.

Diminished tissue oxygenation causes *metabolic acidosis* resulting from overproduction of lactic acid during anaerobic glycolysis. Peripheral vasoconstriction resulting from acidosis and hypoxemia may cause pallor and a transient rise in blood pressure.

Anaerobic glycolysis also depletes glycogen stores rapidly because more glycogen is required for glucose production. *Hypoglycemia* is therefore another penalty of hypoxia.

The most immediate response to a drop in oxygen tension is *constriction of pulmonary arterioles*, which is greatly accentuated if metabolic acidosis is also present. Hypoxemia worsens because ventilation is impaired by the resultant pulmonary hypoperfusion. Furthermore, surfactant production may diminish as a consequence of alveolar ischemia. One can now see that the fetal cardiopulmonary state is returning: pulmonary artery blood pressure rises, and a shunt is reestablished from the right atrium to the left atrium through the foramen ovale. In the extreme, as in sudden asphyxia from aspiration of a feeding, a right-to-left shunt also appears across the ductus arteriosus.

The thermogenic response to cold stress is reduced or eliminated at PaO_2 levels of 30 to 40 torr. Thus *hypothermia* may develop while the baby is pink. Babies who are marginally hypoxic may become extremely restless. They cry continuously, and their aimless body movements are ceaseless.

The babies who are most often at risk without blood gas determinations are premature, dyspneic, but pink for several hours after birth, though their hyaline membrane disease is progressive. Alveoli collapse continually. They remain hypoxic, but there is no clinical indication of hypoxia. Pulmonary vasoconstriction progresses relentlessly. In this pink baby the meager supply of surfactant that was present at birth is dissipated quickly, and more alveoli collapse as time passes. At 4 to 12 hours they are suddenly apneic, cyanotic, and hypotensive. Therapy should have been instituted while they were pink.

Brain damage from hypoxia may be evident either while the baby is still in the nursery or not until several months later. There is no PaO_2 level that can be regularly correlated with central nervous system damage. Acute and protracted episodes of hypoxia are known to injure brain tissue, but the duration of episodes, the extent to which arterial oxygen tension must decline, and the influence of other variables, such as acidosis and hypoglycemia, have not been defined precisely. There is agreement, however, that these factors produce signs of central nervous system dysfunction immediately after the hypoxic episode or chronically thereafter.

Reducing FIo₂. In the presence of generalized cyanosis, it is advisable to abruptly increase the concentration of inspired oxygen. This is generally understood and widely practiced. However, it is not as generally appreciated that a reduced need for oxygen requires gradual diminution of ambient concentrations. Except for circumstances in which abruptly increased concentrations are maintained for less than 10 minutes, an abrupt change to considerably lower concentrations is contraindicated. "Turning off the oxygen" after administering it in high dosage for some time is a dangerous practice. The longer the duration of therapy, the greater the hazard of abrupt discontinuation; sudden cyanosis and respiratory collapse may follow. This serious reaction is a result of sudden pulmonary vasoconstriction. Called "flip-flop," it is a retrogression that is sometimes more severe than the original disorder. It may persist for several hours or days, or it may be fulminant, leading to death. Infants who have received oxygen for over a week because of intrinsic lung disease may require decrements as small as 3% to 5% every few hours, or even every 24 hours. On the other hand, infants with relatively normal lungs who have received oxygen for less than a few hours and have recovered from perinatal asphyxia may require—and will tolerate—a rapid decrease to avert hyperoxia.

Hyperoxia: oxygen toxicity. The detection of oxygen overdosage is as sensitive as the identification of oxygen deprivation. Here the concern is with the etiologic relationship between retrolental fibroplasia and high arterial oxygen tensions. The absolute upper limit of safety and the length of time oxygen therapy is tolerated have not been documented. At present the consensus is that an arterial PO_2 in excess of 100 torr increases the likelihood of eye injury and is of no value in the treatment of hypoxemia. There are no clinical signs to indicate when this limit has been surpassed.

Methods of oxygen administration. The route of oxygen administration is determined by the infant's needs. If he breathes spontaneously and diminished lung volume (atelectasis) is not a prominent problem, oxygen may simply be given in a head hood. If atelectasis is a major problem, as in hyaline membrane disease, but the baby can breathe spontaneously nevertheless, oxygen is given through a system that maintains some degree of positive pressure throughout the respiratory cycle. CPAP is an example of such a system. If the baby is unable to maintain respiration on his own, if apnea recurs frequently, or if adequate ventilation is not possible while the infant is breathing independently, oxygen must be administered by means of a mechanical ventilator.

Warmth and humidity of oxygen. Oxygen must be warm and humid, regardless of the mechanism that is used to deliver it. This requires equipment that permits regulation of heat in a water reservoir through which oxygen flows before entering the respiratory tract. The infant pays dearly when cold, dry oxygen is thoughtlessly administered.

In an oxygen hood, ambient temperatures about the head and body should be similar. This cannot be accomplished unless oxygen is warmed. Prolonged oxygen therapy by mask is contraindicated, not only because FiO_2 cannot be regulated, but also because cold stress is inflicted on the face. Even if the oxygen is warm, the velocity of flow from the mask results in increased heat loss by convection (Chapter 4). The need for warmth and humidity is often overlooked when oxygen is administered by means of hood or mask. Most caregivers are not familiar with the exquisite thermal sensitivity of nerve endings in the skin of the face and forehead, believing that requirements for thermal environment are met by warming the rest of the body. *If face and forehead are chilled, the infant reacts as though totally cold stressed even when the rest of the body is kept warm.*

In the application of continuous positive airway pressure (CPAP) by either the nasal or endotracheal route, warmth and humidity are indispensable because oxygen is introduced directly over mucosal surfaces. Dry gas increases evaporative fluid loss from the extensive mucosal surfaces, thus augmenting evaporative heat loss. Additionally, mucosal integrity is threatened by the sustained drying effect of unhumidified oxygen. Secretory material, usually copious in small infants, becomes inspissated when humidity is lacking. Resultant obstruction of the respiratory passages, particularly the smaller ones, causes atelectasis.

Incubator and head hood. Concentrations of oxygen in an incubator cannot generally be raised beyond 60% to 70%, sometimes as low as 40% in warm incubators. An imperfectly fitting plastic lid may allow significant escape of oxygen to further limit ambient concentrations. Opening portholes to gain access to the baby also depletes ambient oxygen concentration rapidly.

If environmental oxygen concentration must be raised, a plastic head hood should be used. When a hood is used in an incubator, the portholes may be opened without affecting oxygen concentration in the hood. The head box is obviously essential when infants are treated on an open table supplied with radiant heat from an overhead source. Oxygen delivered to a hood must usually be warmed to 87.8° to 93.2° F (31° to 34° C) and must always be humidified. A constant blast of cold gas to the infant's face produces the responses to cold stress, even though the remainder of the body is in a thermoneutral environment, since thermal sensors of the face are more responsive than the skin sensors in any other part of the body.

Assisted ventilation

Continuous positive airway pressure; CPAP (pressure-assisted spontaneous respiration). Continuous positive airway pressure (CPAP) provides positive pressure at end-expiration for infants who can breathe spontaneously, thus maintaining distention of alveoli in abnormal circumstances where they would otherwise collapse. CPAP has its widest application in hyaline membrane disease, but it is frequently used for a number of other pulmonary disorders. PEEP is positive end expiratory pressure applied during mechanical ventilatory support for infants who cannot breathe for themselves.

Mechanical ventilatory support was introduced in the early 1960s for babies with hyaline membrane disease; its use became widespread in the late 1960s. During these years, results were only fair. Among babies over 2 kg, 65% survived, while below that weight approximately 20% to 30% survived. CPAP was introduced in 1971 for hyaline membrane disease. Among 20 severely affected infants, 16 (80%) survived after 2 to 29 days of therapy. Since that time, end expiratory positive pressure (either CPAP or PEEP) has become pervasive for treatment of hyaline membrane disease and a number of other neonatal lung disorders.

The potential value of CPAP was suggested by a study in Britain that was reported in 1968. The investigators undertook to explain the significance of grunting in babies affected by hyaline membrane disease. They characterized the grunt as forced expiration through a partially closed glottis. Sudden release of glottic closure, and the resultant rush of air, vibrates vocal cords to produce the grunt. When an infant initiates grunting expiration, the glottis is partially closed while the diaphragm expels air forcefully from the lungs. As a result of glottic obstruction to air egress, airway pressure rises until sudden release of the glottis expels the air abruptly. During the time interval that precedes the audible grunt, pressure in the airways rises, lung volume increases, and alveoli are more distended. This is the baby's attempt to maintain distended alveoli. Severely ill infants cannot long compensate by grunting. In that same report, after initially observing the characteristics of grunting, the investigators intubated the study infants. Airway pressure and lung volume failed to increase and the grunt itself was eliminated because the glottis was immobilized by the endotracheal tube. Arterial oxygen tensions were lower when the babies were intubated.

CPAP elevates arterial oxygen tensions, permitting reduction of FiO_2, but the physiologic mechanisms have yet to be elaborated in detail. It is generally postulated that the smaller alveoli (which are most likely to collapse at end expiration) are maintained in a state of partial distention at end expiration by CPAP pressure. The increased number of distended alveoli provides an expanded surface for gas exchange; oxygenation is improved. Respirations, if disorganized beforehand, become regular and deeper a short time after the onset of CPAP. If $PaCO_2$ is high, it may decline slowly, but the major effect of CPAP is rapidly improved oxygenation. The only dependable method for decreasing high $PaCO_2$ is mechanical ventilation. The principal indication for CPAP is hypoxemia resulting from pulmonary insufficiency.

Indications for CPAP vary from one facility to another. All are based on the relationship of PaO_2 to FiO_2. Thus one center may introduce CPAP when a PaO_2 is less than 60 torr at an FiO_2 of 1.0, while at another facility a PaO_2 of less than 50 at an FiO_2 of 0.6 may be the indication. The amount of pressure that is initially applied also varies. Initial pressures of 3 to 6 cm H_2O are recommended. Failure to respond to initial pressures requires progressive increase. The highest recommended levels vary from 10 to 14 cm H_2O. We rarely use pressures higher than 10 cm H_2O at any time, and we usually initiate CPAP at 3.0 to 5.0 cm H_2O.

In the initial report of CPAP, an endotracheal tube was used in most infants; in a few a pressurized head hood was used. Since then the most commonly used modalities are nasal prongs or endotracheal tubes.

CPAP is effective for disorders that require maintenance of alveolar stability. Foremost on the list is hyaline membrane disease. Other disorders include meconium aspiration syndrome, pulmonary edema from any cause (most frequently from patent ductus arteriosus), pulmonary hemorrhage, postoperative thoracotomy, apnea of prematurity, and weaning from mechanical respirators.

CPAP is ineffective when the infant is feeble.

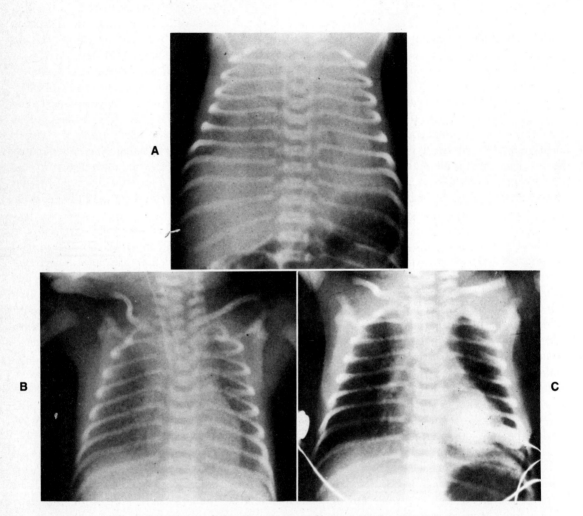

Fig. 8-11. Effect of CPAP on radiologic appearance of lungs. **A,** Before CPAP. Infant had severe hyaline membrane disease. Lungs are dense, with air bronchograms visible. Right cardiac border is obscured. **B,** Twenty minutes after CPAP application. Lungs are not as dense, more air is retained, and the right cardiac border is clearly visible. With better aeration, air bronchograms are not discernible. **C,** One hour after CPAP was applied. Lungs appear normally aerated. Note bulging intercostal spaces indicating some overdistention resulting from CPAP. Cleared x-ray film on CPAP does not indicate disappearance of disease.

It is pressure-assisted support of spontaneous respiration, and it does not directly increase peak inspiratory pressures as in mechanical ventilation. Its effectiveness therefore depends on the infant's capacity to create sufficient negative pressure during descent of the diaphragm, so that tidal volume is adequate. CPAP is inappropriate when respiratory excursions are too shallow to be effective. Ineffectiveness is frequent in infants who weigh less than 1000 g at birth. Their lung compliance is reduced and their musculature scanty. They are thus incapable of expanding lungs adequately because muscle power is insufficient to overcome lung stiffness (poor compliance), thereby minimizing tidal volume. On the other hand, positive pressure mechanical support provides effective tidal volumes by increasing peak inspiratory pressures. CPAP is inappropriate for feeble babies. Obviously CPAP has no place in the support of infants who do not breathe at all when severely depressed by asphyxia, shock, or intraventricular hemorrhage.

CPAP fails in babies with severe hyaline membrane disease. Although respiratory effort may be maximal, lung compliance is so poor that alveolar distention can be accomplished only by the forced (positive pressure) insufflations produced by a mechanical respirator. In these circumstances, inspiratory alveolar expansion requires positive pressure ventilation while alveolar stability is maintained by end expiratory positive pressure (PEEP).

CPAP and PEEP are useless, even hazardous, in infants who have persistent pulmonary hypertension (persistent fetal circulation [PFC] syndrome). Typically the PFC syndrome in its purest form involves little disruption of airways and alveoli (see p. 271). Rather, the primary difficulty is pulmonary vasospasm and hypoperfusion. Lungs are relatively compliant, yet hypoxemia is life-threatening by virtue of pulmonary hypoperfusion. The use of end expiratory positive pressure in infants whose alveolar distention and stability are not significantly diminished, exaggerates hypoperfusion by compressing intrapulmonary vasculature. In the extreme, the end expiratory pressure is transmitted beyond compliant parenchyma; intrathoracic pressure is inordinately elevated throughout the respiratory cycle. Venous return to the heart, from the inferior and superior vena cavae, is diminished (see paragraph to follow).

The principal danger of CPAP (or PEEP) is the use of excessive pressure. When lung compliance is normal or only slightly impaired, end expiratory positive pressure is not tolerated. Even when lung compliance is significantly diminished, excessive pressure creates difficulties; PaO_2 declines and $PaCO_2$ rises. When a lung is stiff, it tends to contain (restrict) applied pressure to the airway and alveoli. When lung compliance is relatively good, applied pressures are transmitted beyond the airway and alveoli to other thoracic organs such as the heart and esophagus. Studies of esophageal pressures in infants whose lungs were poorly compliant revealed that only 20% to 25% of the CPAP pressure was transmitted to the esophagus. In contrast among babies with normal compliance, 90% of the applied pressure was transmitted to the esophagus. If the alveolar walls and the interstitial tissue are sufficiently stiff, and if an appropriate amount of CPAP is applied, very little pressure is transmitted. If pressure is excessive, it is transmitted beyond alveolar walls, compressing pulmonary vessels. As a result, less blood flows through the lungs. As applied pressure is increased, pressure throughout the chest is so high that venous return to the heart from both vena cavae is impeded. Cardiac output is consequently diminished, and the baby becomes acutely hypotensive. Blood pressure is restored to normal almost immediately when end expiratory positive pressure is diminished.

When excessive end expiratory positive pressure is applied during mechanical respiration (PEEP), movement of air in and out of alveoli is diminished. The first indication of excessive PEEP is often an elevated $PaCO_2$; PaO_2 also declines simultaneously in many instances.

In summary, end expiratory positive pressure,

whether CPAP or PEEP, is effective for respiratory support of infants with hyaline membrane disease or any disorder in which alveolar distention at the end of expiration must be maintained. It is also useful in controlling pulmonary edema and pulmonary hemorrhage. While CPAP is effective in the treatment of apnea of prematurity, it has been largely replaced by the use of theophylline or caffeine. CPAP is dangerous if lung compliance is normal. Normally compliant lungs permit transmission of positive pressure to blood vessels in the lung itself and to the large veins that empty into the heart (inferior and superior vena cavae). In these circumstances the transmitted pressure diminishes pulmonary blood flow and impairs venous return to the heart. In the extreme, the heart is small on x-ray examination, and the lungs are overdistended. Cardiac output diminishes, and with less blood in the systemic circulation, there is a measurable fall in systemic blood pressure. On the other hand, when lung compliance is poor ("stiff lungs"), as in hyaline membrane disease or pulmonary edema, positive end expiratory pressure is restricted to the airway; it is not significantly transmissible to other intrathoracic structures.

CPAP produces pneumothorax, but with considerably less frequency than mechanical ventilation. The incidence of pneumothorax with endotracheal CPAP is 5% to 10%; with nasal CPAP it is somewhat lower. Other noteworthy side effects are of an operational nature. The endotracheal tube itself is a source of difficulty. The critical factors in the development of complications from endotracheal tubes include trauma during intubation, impaired mucus transport by ciliary action, duration of intubation, size of the tube, trauma from friction while the tube is in place and while the baby moves or is manipulated frequently, introduction of infection, and occurrence of lobar atelectasis after extubation. The endotracheal tube is obviously irritating to the trachea. It virtually eliminates ciliary activity, and secretions accumulate. It is also a source of respiratory tract infection. It frequently becomes displaced

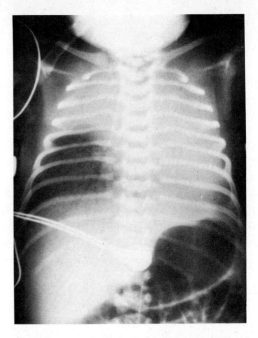

Fig. 8-12. Displacement of endotracheal tube into right main bronchus causes collapse of left lung. In this case, bronchus to right upper lobe is also occluded, causing atelectasis there. Note position of tube deep into right main bronchus.

downward into the right main bronchus, causing atelectasis of the left lung (Fig. 8-12). Tube position must be monitored assiduously. The danger of laryngeal (subglottic) stenosis is small but real. There seems to be little doubt that the development of subglottic stenosis is primarily related to an inappropriately large tube. We use the smallest available tubes (2.5 mm) in babies who weigh below 1300 g and 3 mm tubes for babies between 1500 and 2500 g. If on insertion the operator believes that the fit is too tight, the tube is withdrawn and replacement is made with one of smaller diameter.

Atelectasis after extubation is not an uncommon event. Careful and thorough suction just before withdrawal of the tube has been shown to considerably diminish the incidence of lobar collapse. Nasal CPAP has caused infections of the nose and disfigurement of the external nares, but these complications are rare.

We have been impressed with the discomfort that nasal CPAP causes in a number of infants. The struggle that ensues may predispose them to pneumothorax. Prescribed pressures are sometimes difficult to stabilize. Sedation using chloral hydrate (50 mg/kg of body weight) is usually successful. Nasal CPAP is not usually effective if pressures higher than 10 cm H_2O are required. The infant's open mouth is a natural blowoff valve at this pressure.

At the onset of therapy with CPAP, nasal or endotracheal, we administer the same FIO_2 that failed to oxygenate the baby in a hood (usually 0.60 to 1.00), with a distending pressure of 3 to 5 cm H_2O. In the extreme, pressures are increased to 10 cm H_2O (using tracheal intubation) in an FIO_2 of 1.00. When the PaO_2 is 70 or 80 torr, FIO_2 is diminished by 0.05 to 0.1 periodically, depending on the height of the PaO_2. At an FIO_2 of 0.40, pressure is then gradually decreased. There can be no rigid procedures to raise or lower oxygen or pressure. Decisions must be based on arterial blood gas results.

The nursing skill and close observation required for CPAP are no less demanding than for mechanical ventilation. The nursery that cannot maintain mechanical ventilation, cannot administer CPAP either.

Mechanically assisted ventilation; the use of respirators. In general, the infants who require prolonged ventilatory assistance are severely depressed after perinatal asphyxia. It is indicated in babies with hyaline membrane disease who do not have sufficient vigor to breathe independently or who are repeatedly apneic for prolonged periods and do not respond to CPAP. These babies are hypoxic and they accumulate CO_2, with resultant severe respiratory acidosis. Administration of sodium bicarbonate is contraindicated in severe respiratory acidosis in which PCO_2 exceeds 60 torr. Bicarbonate generates CO_2, which such babies cannot blow off. The result of sodium bicarbonate therapy is a heightened CO_2 and a worsened respiratory acidosis. Mechanical ventilation is the only effective treatment for hypercapnia. Infants whose PCO_2 is over 60 torr are in need of mechanical ventilation.

Respirator therapy is a formidable undertaking that should not be attempted unless proper facilities, equipment, and trained personnel are on hand. The technical problems are numerous; they increase as the baby's size decreases. Scrupulous attention to detail is mandatory, and the major responsibility for these particulars belongs to the neonatal nurse. The endotracheal tube must be maintained in proper position. Once in place, it should not be allowed to slip into the trachea even for a distance of less than 1 cm, since it may then enter the right mainstem bronchus and occlude the left one in bypassing it (Fig. 8-12). The respirator must be observed repeatedly for proper settings. Respiratory difficulties in an infant with hyaline membrane disease are dynamic. Lung compliance may worsen rapidly or improve gradually, requiring adjustments in settings. Bronchial toilet and correct humidification of delivered oxygen must be maintained. Monitoring of blood gases and pH is essential at frequent intervals—so frequent, in fact, that small, simple blood transfusions may be required periodically to replace the sampled blood.

Pressure ventilators are used exclusively in most intensive care units. Their operation is relatively simple and straightforward. Parameters of function, plainly displayed, include oxygen concentration (FIO_2), peak inspiratory pressure (PIP), end expiratory pressure, respiratory rate, inspiratory and expiratory times, and I:E ratio. Most respirators also display alarm limit information that is accompanied by audible warnings when limits are violated.

Peak inspiratory pressure by itself bears no relationship to the tidal volume delivered by a respirator. Tidal volume delivery is determined by the relationship between positive pressure generated by the respirator and resistance to flow imposed by lung compliance. A stiff lung requires higher peak pressures than a compliant lung for delivery of the same tidal volume. Said differently, at the same peak inspiratory pressure a stiff lung receives less tidal volume than a compliant one.

Respiratory rates and *inspiratory-expiratory times* are electrically controlled in most pressure ventilators currently in use. Cycling of respirations is set independently of the pressures. Pressure ventilators in which cycling is regulated electrically are categorized as *pressure-limited, time-cycled respirators*. Within the limits of respiratory rates and inspiratory-expiratory times, peak pressure is influenced by flow rate. The *flow rate* setting is a third independent variable. When high pressure is required during a short inspiratory time, a high flow rate is essential. If the flow rate is insufficient during a given inspiratory time, the desired peak inspiratory pressure will not be attained during the prescribed interval. Failure to reach a prescribed peak pressure means that the desired tidal volume will not be delivered. Flow rate determines the rapidity with which the peak pressure is generated. Peaks are reached more quickly at higher flow rates.

Most clinicians are convinced that pneumothorax, other forms of pulmonary air leak (see p. 249), and bronchopulmonary dysplasia are more likely to occur at high peak inspiratory pressures. However, the influence of the *duration* of high inspiratory pressures is not generally appreciated. *At any given peak pressure, shorter inspiratory times are less likely to produce pulmonary air leak*. High peak pressures may be relatively innocuous if inspiration is sufficiently brief. Unfortunately the severity of illness may preclude short intervals. In general, a safe and effective approach to respirator settings is to apply the lowest pressures and the shortest durations that effectively ventilate the infant. While high pressures are more likely to cause the complications that result from barotrauma, pressures that are too low may result in unacceptably high $PaCO_2$ and low PaO_2. Effective respirator settings require understanding of pathophysiology, knowledge of the capacity and limitations of respirators, and recognition of the significance of blood gas values.

Acid-base balance; fluid therapy

Metabolic acidosis inevitably develops in infants who are moderately or severely ill. Insofar as pulmonary function is concerned, the most direct deleterious effect of acidosis is constriction of pulmonary arterioles. Lung perfusion is thus diminished, and the right-to-left shunt increases. Serial measurements of pH and PCO_2 provide a basis for infusion of intravenous sodium bicarbonate on the rare occasions when this is indicated. Base deficits less than 10 mEq/L do not generally require treatment. The dose of alkali is calculated and administered as described in Chapter 7.

Intravenous fluid is administered from the time of admission. It is given through the umbilical artery catheter and peripheral veins. Umbilical artery catheters should not be used for the primary purpose of fluid administration except in the smallest babies. The umbilical vein is used only in an emergency for short time intervals. Infection, thrombosis, cirrhosis, and portal hypertension later in life are reported from protracted fluid therapy through the umbilical vein. Discussion of fluid and electrolyte therapy is presented in Chapter 7.

Provision of proper thermal environment

The deleterious effects of hypothermia are discussed in Chapter 4. Cold stress increases the need for oxygen in a baby who is already having difficulty with his intake. Furthermore, the increased metabolic rate that occurs in response to cold stress enhances metabolic acidosis in the presence of hypoxia by overproduction of lactic acid. In aggravating hypoxia and enhancing acidosis, and by release of norepinephrine, cold stress causes increased pulmonary vasoconstriction, which probably also impairs the production and activity of surfactant.

Maintenance of blood pressure and hematocrit

Systemic blood pressure is low in many infants with pulmonary disease. Because hypoxemia and acidemia have an early tendency to increase blood pressure, the hypotensive state is sometimes not detectable until they are corrected. Systemic hypotension increases right-to-left shunt through the ductus arteriosus, especially in the presence of inordinately high pulmonary artery pressure. Infants who are hypotensive cannot be oxygenated optimally. The diminished tissue perfusion and hypoxemia associated with shock cause oxygen deprivation of tissues. As a consequence, anaerobic glycolysis occurs, and lactic acid production causes severe metabolic acidosis. Ventilatory support is thus ineffective for optimal oxygenation in the presence of shock. Blood samples persistently demonstrate a low PaO_2 and a high base deficit. Sodium bicarbonate administration has little effect on the metabolic acidosis that accompanies shock.

Hypovolemia is often difficult to identify in the neonate. When blood pressure is low, the issue is straightforward. However, peripheral blood pressure does not decline until circulating blood volume is diminished by 25% to 40% of normal. Thus, many infants are hypovolemic despite normal peripheral blood pressure readings. In these circumstances, hypovolemia may be suggested by a rapid heart rate (over 160 beats/min).

We monitor aortic blood pressure through an umbilical artery catheter. When the umbilical artery catheter is not available, we obtain blood pressures from brachial or posterior tibial arteries with a Doppler ultrasound apparatus. Normal blood pressures are listed below. Blood pressure is generally higher as birth weight increases. The list of blood pressure values (in torr) below contains the range of systolic, diastolic, and pulse pressures (systolic minus diastolic) by various birth weights. There is no significant difference in normal blood pressures for SGA and AGA infants.

750 g:	Systolic	34-54
	Diastolic	14-34
	Pulse	10-29
1000 g:	Systolic	39-59
	Diastolic	16-36
	Pulse	12-30
1500 g:	Systolic	40-61
	Diastolic	19-39
	Pulse	12-31
3000 g:	Systolic	51-72
	Diastolic	27-46
	Pulse	16-34

Having identified hypovolemia by clear-cut blood pressure readings or surmised that it is present because of tachycardia even though blood pressure readings are normal, we immediately administer plasma as a volume expander. Packed red blood cells are ordered from the blood bank at the same time. Plasma is given rapidly in a dose of 10 ml/kg of body weight. Packed red blood cells are given in the same dose as soon as they are delivered to the nursery. If blood pressure remains low after the first dose of plasma, another dose is administered. Blood pressure is monitored frequently.

Hematocrit must also be followed periodically. Most often, it is normal for the first 1 to 3 hours postnatally, even if hypovolemia is present. It falls, however, as the baby attempts to compensate for diminished blood volume by the transfer of tissue fluid into the vascular compartment; hemodilution ensues. We attempt to maintain the hematocrit at 45 to 50 vol%. It is determined at least twice daily during acute illness, and more often if indicated.

Blood sampling for laboratory data is an important and frequent cause of lower hematocrit readings. A record of the amount withdrawn should be kept at the incubator. When 10% of calculated blood volume (85 ml/kg) is withdrawn, a transfusion of packed cells is given.

Umbilical vessel catheterization

Umbilical artery. The risks of umbilical arterial catheterization are well known and very real. In spite of them, most neonatologists do not hesitate to employ these catheters *if the benefits derived significantly outweigh the risks entailed*.

The placement of arterial catheters is a surgical procedure that requires strict aseptic technique. Proper maintenance of the catheter, once it is in place, depends on the skills and knowledge of the nurse.

The safest location for the catheter tip in the aorta is below the origins of the renal arteries. If the tip is between the third and fourth lumbar vertebrae by x-ray films, it is situated below the renal arteries and above the aortic bifurcation. The catheter should have an end hole, rather than side holes, since the dead space at the tip of the latter type of catheter promotes thrombus formation. Furthermore, the catheter should be radiopaque so that its position can be ascertained by x-ray examination immediately after placement. If it is located above the desired level, it can be withdrawn an appropriate distance. If the tip is too low, *the catheter should not be inserted farther after the sterile insertion procedure has been terminated*.

Maintenance requires careful, constant attention to avert infection, to prevent hemorrhage because of loose fittings or accidental withdrawal, and to identify thromboembolic phenomena.

Infection. The incidence of infection varies from one report to another. There is sound basis for applying antibacterial ointment at least once daily to the umbilical stump and to joints in the tubing system. Tubing and stopcock attached to the catheter should be changed daily. After withdrawal of blood from the stopcock, the open portal should be plugged with a sterile insert of some type. We use a syringe. The injection of medication through the stopcock should be meticulous. Care must be exercised to avoid contamination of the syringe tip that is inserted into the stopcock. Inadvertent contact of the syringe tip with contaminated objects (including fingers) prior to its insertion is a common occurrence. The futility of prophylactic antibiotics for infants with umbilical vessel catheters has been well documented.

Hemorrhage. Massive hemorrhage from the umbilical catheter is a real danger if fittings are loosened. Hemorrhage may also occur from the umbilical stump when the catheter is accidentally displaced from its insertion. Aortic blood pressure is high, and considerable blood loss may therefore occur rapidly. This possibility obviously makes constant attention and surveillance by the nurse imperative. Massive hemorrhage into the pelvis has been reported after inadvertent perforation of an artery during the catheterization procedure. We have experienced one such instance.

Thrombosis. Thromboembolic phenomena are the most frequent complications. Varying percentages (as high as 95%) are reported for the incidence of thrombi. In the vast majority of cases they have had no apparent clinical significance; their danger is not negligible, however. Thrombi that encase the catheter or are implanted onto the aortic wall are a potential source of embolization. Emboli are dislodged from these thrombi and released to the lower body, distal to the catheter tip. If they are of substantial size, they obstruct blood flow distal to the vessel they occlude. Necrosis of toes is the most frequent embolic phenomenon. The toes may become progressively cyanotic and ultimately gangrenous. If cyanosis persists for more than 15 minutes, the catheter should be withdrawn. Necrotic ulceration of the skin in the gluteal and perineal regions has been reported in a few infants.

The position of the catheter tip is critical. If the catheter is too high, thrombi may occlude the superior mesenteric artery or, more commonly, the renal arteries, causing infarction of intestines and kidneys, respectively. Hypertension in the neonate has been repeatedly reported as a complication of umbilical artery catheters that may impair renal circulation. The high blood pressure persists for months or years and, if untreated, rapidly leads to cardiac failure. Approximately 80% of cases of neonatal hypertension have been associated with previous umbilical artery catheterization. Opinion differs as to whether thrombi are more likely to occur as the duration of catheterization increases. Thrombosis is more likely in profoundly ill babies.

Vasospasm. The most common manifestation of interrupted blood flow is blanching, which may involve part of a toe, or both lower extremities in their entirety. It is attributed to arterial spasm, and it disappears promptly when the catheter is removed. There is no justification for the past practice of applying moist heat to the uninvolved extremity to relieve spasm of the opposite member.

Infusions. Hypertonic solutions are probably tolerated, if they are infused at a slow rate, because the aorta is large and blood flow through it is rapid. The infused solution is therefore quickly diluted. Sodium bicarbonate should be diluted with equal parts of water or glucose solution and injected at a rate not exceeding 2 ml/min. Rapid injection of any material causes increased turbulence at the catheter tip and predisposes to thrombogenesis. Continuous infusion must be regulated by an automated pump. As a rule, we encounter backflow of aortic blood if the rate of infusion is less than 2 ml/hr.

Umbilical artery catheterization is indicated primarily for sampling in monitoring blood gases and pH. It should never be instituted for the sole purpose of fluid administration.

Umbilical vein. We use umbilical vein catheters only for exchange transfusion or for emergency administration of drugs, fluid, or volume expanders when no other route is immediately available. It is also used to monitor central venous pressure. The incidence of complications from protracted periods of catheterization is unacceptably high. Infection is more common in the vein than in the artery. Hepatic necrosis and thrombosis of the portal vein have also been reported. Portal hypertension at a later age has been attributed to portal vein thrombosis from umbilical vein catheterization during the newborn period.

Complications of assisted ventilation

Extraneous air syndromes (air leak). Extraneous air syndromes are a group of clinically recognizable disorders produced by alveolar rupture and the subsequent escape of air to tissues in which air is not normally present. Table 8-2 lists the sites in which extraneous air has been reported. Although most of these syndromes have long been known to occur spontaneously, their incidence increased as the use of ventilatory support became widespread, particularly since the advent of PEEP. Air leak syndrome now constitutes the most frequent life-threatening complication of ventilatory assistance. The capacity for instant recognition, evaluation, and relief of these disorders is a primary requisite for personnel who assume responsibility for sustained neonatal ventilatory support.

Incidence varies according to type and severity of disease, gestational age, mode of therapy, and

Table 8-2. Extraneous air syndromes

Site of extraneous air	Syndrome
Pulmonary interstitium (perivascular sheaths)	Interstitial emphysema
Alveoli-trabeculae-visceral pleura	Pseudocysts
Pleural space	Pneumothorax
Mediastinum	Pneumomediastinum
Pericardial space	Pneumopericardium
Perivascular sheaths (peripheral vessels)	Perivascular emphysema
Vascular lumens (blood)	Air embolus
Subcutaneous tissue	Subcutaneous emphysema
Retroperitoneal connective tissue	Retroperitoneal emphysema
Peritoneal space	Pneumoperitoneum
Intestinal wall	Pneumatosis intestinalis
Scrotum	Pneumoscrotum

expertise of personnel. Complications are most frequent during treatment for hyaline membrane disease. Interstitial emphysema and pneumothorax, for example, are observed more often in babies with hyaline membrane disease than in infants with other disorders. Frequency is also significantly influenced by the vigor of ventilatory assistance, which itself is usually a reflection of the severity of disease. Interstitial emphysema, pneumothorax, and pneumomediastinum have been reported to occur twice as often with the use of PEEP (39.7%) than without it (20.7%). In babies with hyaline membrane disease, the frequency of pneumothorax increases as therapy becomes more vigorous. Pneumopericardium was described as a "very rare condition" in neonates in 1970; there were descriptions of only seven cases. In 1976 one study described six babies with pneumopericardium in as short a time as 6 months. The authors found 57 cases in their review of the literature. Pneumopericardium, a "very rare condition" in 1970, is now not so rare. Most reports allude to a relationship between the increased frequency of this syndrome and the vigor of ventilatory therapy. A similar course of events has been noted for pneumoperitoneum.

Pathogenesis. All air leaks are caused by high intra-alveolar pressure that results from the inhalation, insufflation, or retention of inordinately large volumes of air. The resultant pressure gradient from affected alveoli to adjacent tissue space may be of sufficient magnitude to rupture alveoli where they overlie capillaries. Air escapes through disruption within the meshes of capillaries. It enters perivascular sheaths and migrates toward the hilum. Pulmonary interstitial emphysema is thus primarily characterized by extraneous air in perivascular sheaths. Often, extrusions of air occur in contiguous connective tissue, and at times in trabeculae through which air migrates to pleura to form blebs. Perivascular sheaths stretch considerably as air accumulates and the enveloped vessels are compressed. The associated circulatory impairment is an important component of interstitial emphysema.

Fig. 8-13 depicts the migration of air from alveolar rupture through lung interstitium into the pleural and pericardial cavities. The chest films in Fig. 8-14 correspond to these diagrams.

Air in perivascular sheaths dissects toward the hilum, invades the mediastinum, and thus causes *pneumomediastinum*. Air bubbles may accumulate at the hilum to form large blebs, which sometimes compress hilar vessels. The blebs are situated where visceral pleura reflects onto parietal pleura. As pressure mounts, rupture of blebs at this location releases air into the pleural space to give rise to *pneumothorax*. Apparently, air also passes from other points in the mediastinal wall to the pleural cavity. The pathway of extension to the *pericardial space* is still conjectural.

Far-flung dispersion of air may occur after alveolar rupture. *Pneumoperitoneum* is thought to result from extension of mediastinal air along the great vessels and esophagus into the peritoneal cavity. We have observed *pneumoscrotum* associated with *pneumoperitoneum*. Presumably migration of air occurred from the peritoneal cavity through the processus vaginalis into the scrotum. *Air embolism* occurs when extremely high pressures are used for ventilatory assistance; air is injected directly into pulmonary capillaries at the time of alveolar rupture. The application of very high peak inspiratory pressure to a lung of low compliance may also lacerate parenchyma, allowing passage of air under a high head of pressure into blood vessels.

The appearance of extraneous air, regardless of its location, always begins with alveolar rupture. Migration of escaped air ensues through tissue planes that offer the least resistance, thus giving rise to a spectrum of clinical syndromes that ranges from interstitial emphysema and pneumothorax to air embolism and pneumoscrotum (Table 8-2).

Clinical aspects. Of the twelve syndromes listed in Table 8-2, pneumothorax and pneumopericardium are the only ones that require instant remedial action lest death or brain damage ensue. On rare occasions, pneumomediastinum requires the same urgency. Interstitial emphysema is a serious manifestation of air leak that is associated with a high rate of mortality. Air embolus is a fatal event, for which there is no effective therapy.

Pulmonary interstitial emphysema (PIE). The migration of air through vascular sheaths regularly precedes the appearance of extraneous air in sites outside the lung. Transient presence of air in the interstitium is most often not evident radiologically. When air accumulates, pulmonary interstitial emphysema is the result. The onset of abnormal clinical signs is relatively gradual. Most infants develop interstitial emphysema during administration of mechanical ventilatory support. Oxygen requirements increase and CO_2 retention may be relentless. Death is eventually caused by failure to adequately ventilate the baby. The extent to which death is attributable to vascular compression, particularly at the hilum, is unknown. The extent to which gas exchange is impaired by the interposition of air between alveoli and blood vessels is also unknown.

Progression of interstitial emphysema to pneumothorax is a frequent event. Approximately 50% of pneumothoraces are associated with interstitial emphysema. A high incidence of interstitial emphysema has been observed during the first 24 hours of life among infants who later developed BPD.

Interstitial emphysema can only be diagnosed radiologically. It is characterized by two basic features: radiolucencies that are linear and those that are cyst-like. The linear radiolucencies vary in width; they are coarse and do not branch. They are seen in the peripheral as well as the medial lung fields. The cyst-like radiolucencies vary from 1 to 4 mm in diameter. In some instances they are oval or lobulated. They may be so numerous that they impart a spongy appearance (Fig. 8-14, *A*). Interstitial emphysema may involve only one lobe, one lung, or more frequently both lungs. It appears within 96 hours after birth in babies who are receiving ventilatory assistance. Attempts should be made to minimize peak inspiratory and distending pressures, but usually the develop-

ment of interstitial emphysema itself imposes a need for more vigorous therapy. High frequency ventilation has recently been reported to be effective in minimizing interstitial emphysema.

Unilateral interstitial emphysema can be treated effectively by selective intubation. Fig. 8-15 demonstrates the sequence of events that follows this type of intubation. The first film (Fig. 8-15, *A*) depicts severe involvement of the right lung and selective intubation of the left lung. We were able to ventilate this infant for 30 hours with an inactivated right lung. Fig. 8-15, *B* shows complete collapse of the previously emphysematous right lung. This occurred within 1 to 2 hours. Fig. 8-15, *C* shows reexpansion of the right lung after the tube was partially withdrawn back to the trachea. Note that the interstitial emphysema cleared completely; it did not recur.

Pneumothorax. Pneumothorax can occur spontaneously (no iatrogenic factors implicated), as a result of ventilatory assistance, or rarely as a complication following certain procedures.

Spontaneous pneumothorax usually occurs during the first few breaths after birth. The vast majority of infants are asymptomatic. Radiologic surveys have demonstrated an incidence of 1% to 2% of all live births, but symptomatic pneumothorax has been noted in only 0.05% to 0.07% of live births. Most investigators have found the highest incidence of spontaneous pneumothorax in term rather than preterm infants. Postmature infants are particularly vulnerable.

Distress is generally evident in the delivery room or soon after arrival in the nursery. Tachypnea (to 130 breaths per minute) is a universal occurrence. A prominent chest bulge on the involved side is characteristic. Grunting, retractions, and cyanosis in room air have been noted in virtually all symptomatic infants. As a rule, they have abnormal chest findings attributable to an underexpanded lung and to displacement of the heart away from the affected hemithorax. Restlessness and irritability are frequent. Spontaneous pneumothorax is sometimes a manifestation of serious lung disease; it has long been reported in

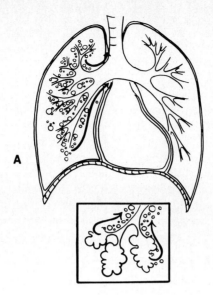

Interstitial emphysema

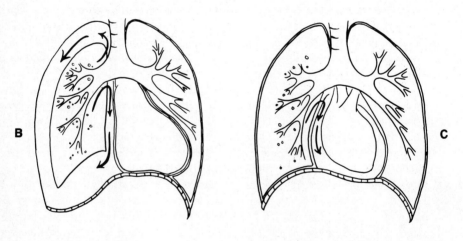

Pneumothorax   Pneumopericardium

Fig. 8-13. A, Air in interstitial lung tissue. Ruptured alveoli are indicated in framed alveoli at bottom. Air dissects from alveoli along vascular sheaths to hilus and thence to pleural space. (See x-ray film in Fig. 8-14, *A*.) **B,** Pneumothorax, indicating origin of air in lung tissue and its pathway to inflate pleural space. Heart shifts to left because of high pressure created in right chest. (See x-ray film in Fig. 8-14, *B*.) **C,** Course of air from lung to pericardial space. Distended pericardial space causes cardiac tamponade, small heart. (See x-ray film in Fig. 8-14, *C*.)

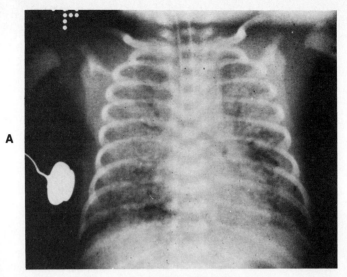

Interstitial emphysema

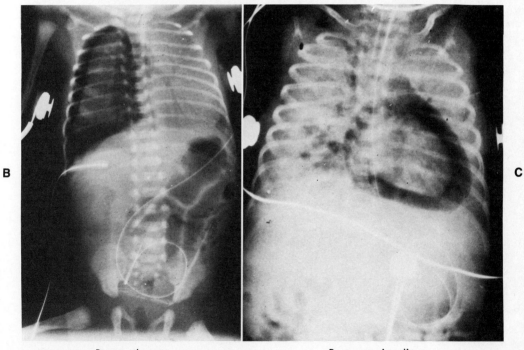

Pneumothorax   Pneumopericardium

Fig. 8-14. A, Interstitial emphysema. Multiple lakes of radiolucency (air), varying in size, impart a spongy appearance to lungs. (See Fig. 8-13, *A*.) **B,** Tension pneumothorax right pleural cavity. The dense right lung is collapsed by pressure in pleural space created by air accumulation. Air-filled pleural cavity is darkest area that envelops right lung. (See Fig. 8-13, *B*.) **C,** Pneumopericardium. Dark halo of air fills pericardial space, outlining the heart itself. Note interstitial emphysema in right lung, indicated by large lakes of air. (See Fig. 8-13, *C*.)

association with meconium aspiration, hyaline membrane disease, pneumonia, pulmonary hypoplasia with renal anomalies, and diaphragmatic hernia. We have also encountered it in infants who had RDS II. Although spontaneous alveolar rupture is sometimes a worrisome portent of serious underlying pulmonary disease, most infants have otherwise normal lungs. Approximately 80% to 90% are mildly ill, requiring no therapy other than an oxygen-rich environment.

Pneumothorax during ventilatory assistance is common. Mild courses are exceptional; tension pneumothorax is the predominant form of the disorder, particularly in babies who are on mechanical ventilators with PEEP. Vigilance by expert nurses is effective for early detection; better yet, a significant number of pneumothoraces are predictable. Short gestational age, hyaline membrane disease, and high ventilatory pressures are the most significant predisposing factors. Their

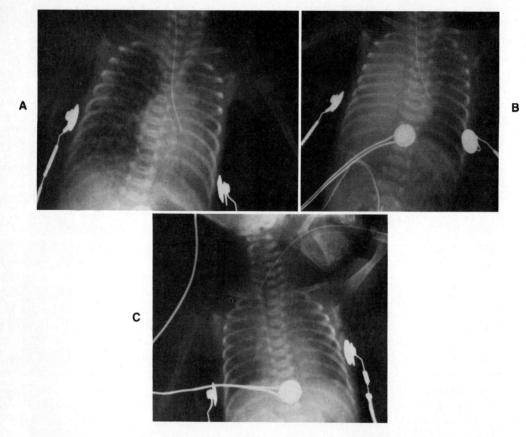

Fig. 8-15. Sequence of films depicting results of treatment of unilateral interstitial emphysema by selective intubation. **A,** Severe involvement of the right lung required intubation of the left main stem bronchus. The baby was successfully maintained only on the left lung for 30 hours. **B,** The desired complete collapse of the right lung was evident approximately 6 hours after intubation of the left lung. **C,** Withdrawal of the endotracheal tube to its usual position in the trachea 30 hours after selective intubation of the left lung reveals complete disappearance of interstitial emphysema on the right.

presence imposes a high risk for air leak. The role of gestational age and hyaline membrane disease can be appreciated from the example of our own experience. In a 12-month period, pneumothorax occurred in 10 of 28 infants (35.7%) whose gestational age was 26 through 28 weeks, yet only 1 out of 12 (8.3%) was involved when gestational age was 35 to 36 weeks. Pneumothorax was 3.5 times more frequent in the presence of hyaline membrane disease than in other abnormalities. The predictive value of these factors is helpful but not specific. Predictions based on chest films are more specific because interstitial emphysema is a frequent precursor, preceding pneumothorax in up to 50% of cases. Pneumothorax follows the appearance of interstitial emphysema within 2 to 72 hours. Pneumomediastinum is another predictor of pneumothorax.

Identification and relief of pneumothorax can be accomplished within a few minutes by detection of abnormal signs. Tension pneumothorax produces abrupt duskiness or cyanosis. There may be significant declines of arterial blood pressure, heart rate, respiratory rate, and pulse pressure before the expected abnormal chest signs. Detection of diminished breath sounds, bulging of affected hemithorax, and mediastinal shift to the unaffected side are nevertheless valuable indications. We use transillumination of the chest. Prior to availability of transillumination, we proceeded to aspirate air from the pleural cavity on the basis of abnormal physical signs. If the infant's status permits, the presence of pneumothorax is first verified radiologically (Fig. 8-14, *B*).

Immediate evacuation of air is urgent. We insert a rubber catheter (no. 12 to no. 14) for attachment to continuous suction. One should be cautioned against the use of a needle for aspiration of air. At autopsy needle tracts have been demonstrated in the myocardium of the left ventricle, presumably as a result of the resumption of normal cardiac position as tension pneumothorax was relieved by the aspiration of air.

The definitive treatment for tension pneumothorax is placement of a chest tube and application of continuous suction (10 cm H_2O), particularly if end expiratory pressure is used for ventilatory assistance. Recurrence of pneumothorax during chest drainage is frequent. In such circumstances the existing tube must be replaced if it is demonstrably occluded; if the tube is not blocked, a second one must be inserted. The most difficult pneumothorax we have ever treated was a bilateral one that ultimately required 28 tube insertions. At 1 year of age this child was normal.

Pneumothorax as a result of certain procedures is a rare occurrence. Several reports describe pneumothorax after birth of babies whose mothers had an amniocentesis shortly before. In one instance, attention was called to the pneumothorax during the baby's bath when a nurse palpated subcutaneous emphysema in the chest wall. Spontaneous resolution was complete 7 days later. These pneumothoraces may result from entry of the amniocentesis needle into the fetal chest. Three infants have been described to have developed pneumothorax following perforation of bronchi by suction catheters.

Of the three etiologic groups of pneumothorax described here (spontaneous, during ventilatory assistance, following certain procedures), the most significant are those that occur during ventilatory assistance. These account for increased incidence, for protracted morbidity, and for most of the mortality attributable to pneumothorax.

Pneumopericardium. Pneumopericardium usually occurs in association with one or more of the other extraneous air syndromes. It is uncommon in the absence of mechanical respiratory support. In most instances very high ventilatory pressures are required for adequate therapy. The first sign of its onset is often a sudden appearance or deepening of cyanosis. Heart sounds are muffled; in the most severe cases, heart sounds are inaudible though reduced voltage cardiac activity is evident on the oscilloscope or ECG. If sufficient air accumulates in the pericardial space, pressure within it rises, and eventually stroke volume diminishes. Arterial blood pressures falls and, in the extreme, peripheral pulses are not palpable.

As hypoxia worsens, bradycardia becomes evident. Metabolic acidosis develops in response to hypoxemia and to the generally diminished tissue perfusion that results from low cardiac output resulting from tamponade. The most distinctive features that suggest the onset of tamponade are the abrupt appearance of cyanosis, hypotension, inaudible heart sounds but with cardiac activity visible on ECG or oscilloscope, and persistent pulsations of fluid in the umbilical artery catheter. Diagnosis by x-ray film is definitive. A broad radiolucent halo completely surrounds the heart, including the diaphragmatic surface (Fig. 8-14, C). In the lateral projection a broad area of radiolucency separates the anterior surface of the heart from the sternum and, to a lesser extent, from the diaphragm as well. We have also identified pneumopericardium by transillumination.

Pneumopericardium varies widely in severity. We have made the diagnosis accidentally on a routine chest film from a baby who had no abnormal cardiac signs. The pericardial air disappeared spontaneously 6 hours later. A review of the literature up to 1976 revealed 63 cases. Approximately 60% survived. Of those infants who were treated with pericardiocentesis, 79% survived. Conservative management (no needle aspiration) was associated with 32% survival. These authors make a case for aggressive management with needle aspiration or catheter insertion. On the other hand, two other reports advocate conservative management. They would not aspirate until cardiac tamponade appears, as indicated by a fall in aortic blood pressure.

Treatment usually consists of multiple pericardial taps as indicated for accumulation of air. The incidence of reaccumulation after initial pericardiocentesis is said to be 53%. Insertion of a no. 14 French Bardex catheter, which remains in place in the pericardial space, is an effective procedure. Pneumopericardium with tamponade should be managed according to the same underlying principles that govern management of tension pneumothorax.

Pneumomediastinum. This is a common isolated disorder when it occurs spontaneously in otherwise healthy infants. It occurs in hyaline membrane disease spontaneously, after resuscitation immediately following birth, and during ventilator therapy. Spontaneous pneumomediastinum has been observed to occur at a rate of 25 per 10,000 live births. As in spontaneous pneumothorax, postmature infants were more vulnerable than others, presumably for the same reason—a higher incidence of meconium aspiration.

Pneumomediastinum, when it occurs in otherwise normal infants at birth, is generally asymptomatic. In other circumstances it produces mild to moderate abnormal clinical signs. Tachypnea, bulging sternum, muffled heart sounds, and cyanosis occur with varying frequencies. The chest film is diagnostic in the lateral projection. Anteroposterior projections often appear spuriously normal. In the lateral view air is seen as a radiolucent area behind the sternum, in the superior portion of the mediastinum if the infant is upright. Occasionally the thymus is visible above the heart. In the anteroposterior view a halo is seen around the heart but not along its diaphragmatic (inferior) border. Sometimes it is quite broad so that it extends toward the lateral reaches of the lungs. The "spinnaker sail sign" is commonly apparent in this projection. It is produced by lifting of the thymus from the heart by the interposed air (Fig. 8-16). Pneumomediastinum resolves spontaneously with rare exceptions. Careful observation is essential; nothing more aggressive is indicated.

Pneumoperitoneum. Free air in the peritoneum usually suggests perforation of an abdominal viscus, requiring immediate surgery. In recent years several reports have shown pneumoperitoneum to be secondary to air leak. Air migrates through the diaphragm to the retroperitoneal space and then to the peritoneal cavity. Fig. 8-17 demonstrates the development of a pneumoperitoneum by extension of air from the posterior mediastinum through the diaphragm and then into the

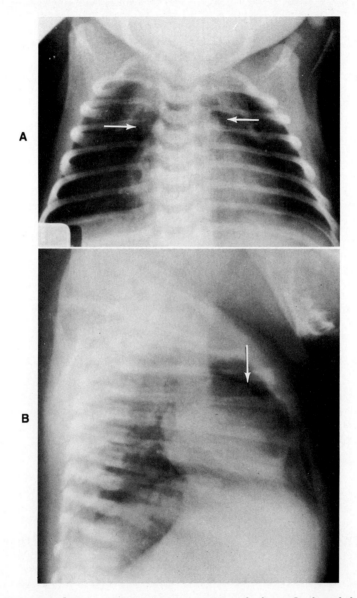

Fig. 8-16. Pneumomediastinum. **A,** Anteroposterior view. The butterfly-shaped shadow of the thymus is above mediastinal air. The air (arrows) separates the thymic shadow and the cardiac shadow beneath it. **B,** Lateral view. Mediastinal air (arrow) is visible in the darkest area immediately beneath the sternum. Since air is situated between the heart and the anterior chest wall, the intensity of heart sounds is substantially diminished.

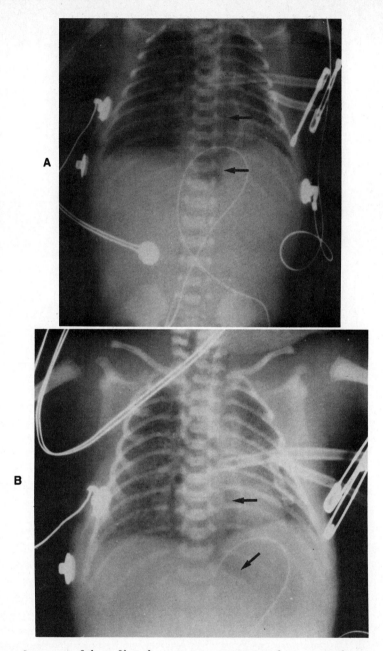

Fig. 8-17. Sequence of three films demonstrating extension of pneumomediastinum through the diaphragm with resultant pneumoperitoneum. The upper arrow in each film indicates collection of air in the posterior mediastinum. The lower arrow of each film indicates the extension of air. Pneumoperitoneum is fully developed in **C.**

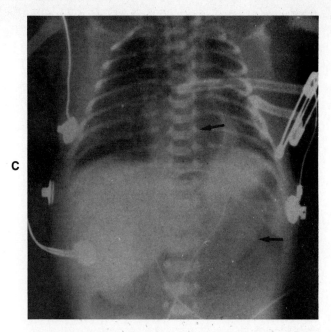

Fig. 8-17, cont'd. For legend see opposite page.

peritoneal space. These films were taken over an interval of 8 hours. The thoracic collection of air on the left side of the vertebral column is in the pulmonary ligament in the midmediastinum, instead of the more common anterior accumulation shown in Fig. 8-16. The principal clinical difficulty in this situation is exclusion of a serious surgical disorder. The simultaneous presence of aberrant air in the chest is good evidence that the situation is nonsurgical. Absence of peritoneal fluid, normal thickness of bowel wall, and absence of air fluid levels in the intestine are additional evidence of the nonsurgical nature of the pneumoperitoneum. Another serious effect of pneumoperitoneum is splinting (immobilization) of the diaphragm that results from massive accumulation of intraperitoneal air. Effective respiratory support can only be restored by continuous drainage of air through a peritoneal catheter in place. Fig. 8-18 demonstrates the curious extension of a pneumoperitoneum through the processus vaginalis into the scrotum.

Air embolus. This rare condition is the most sinister of the extraneous air syndromes. It occurs when extremely high pressures are required to ventilate extremely stiff lungs. As a result, it is thought that parenchymal lacerations occur and that air is injected into the pulmonary vasculature. In most infants with air embolus, inflation pressures up to 55 cm H_2O were necessary to provide satisfactory tidal volume.

The clinical presentation of infants with air embolus is a catastrophic event. Sudden cyanosis and circulatory collapse become evident. The heart slows, but with each beat the air-blood mixture is heard to crackle and pop. Withdrawal of blood from the umbilical artery catheter yields alternating segments of air and blood, similar to what one would expect if a stopcock connection were loose. The x-ray film reveals a bizarre picture of intracardiac and intravascular air. Fig. 8-19 shows air in the portal vessels as well as in the heart. There is no effective treatment for massive intravascular air.

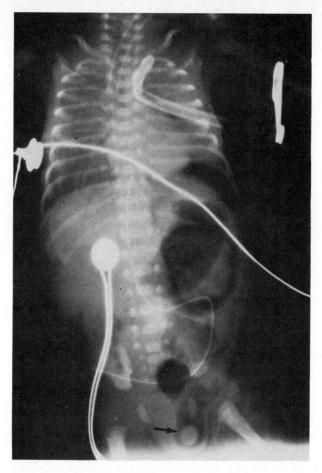

Fig. 8-18. Extension of air in peritoneal space (pneumoperitoneum) through the processus vaginalis and into the scrotum. Arrow at bottom of film indicates the pneumoscrotum.

Bronchopulmonary dysplasia (BPD). When administered in high concentrations, oxygen is injurious to the lungs, but damage is not related to blood oxygen tension. It is a direct result of a high FIO_2 and other factors as well. Histologic damage is characterized by thickening and eventual necrosis of alveolar walls, basement membranes, and bronchiolar epithelial lining layers. Atelectasis and fibrosis are also present. Presumably these changes impair diffusion of oxygen from alveolar lumens to capillaries. Respiratory dysfunc-

tion is thus prolonged, and the resultant abnormal radiologic appearance of the lungs may not resolve for several months.

Bronchopulmonary dysplasia (BPD) is a progressive chronic lung disease that follows protracted periods of mechanical ventilation with high concentrations of oxygen by means of an endotracheal tube. The clinical, pathologic, and radiologic features of the disease were first reported in 1967. In the vast majority of instances, hyaline membrane disease precedes the onset of BPD,

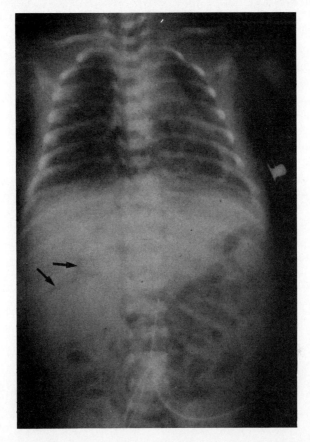

Fig. 8-19. Massive air embolus as a result of high pressures on mechanical ventilator. The heart is filled with air. The arrows indicate air in the portal vasculature.

but other acute pulmonary disorders may play similar roles. Whether preceded by hyaline membrane disease or some other pulmonary disorder, BPD is virtually always associated with administration of high concentrations of oxygen by mechanical ventilation through an endotracheal tube; the relative etiologic significance of each of these factors has yet to be defined satisfactorily.

Radiologic characteristics. The radiologic abnormalities of BPD are well delineated in several reports, but the original descriptions of clearly

demarcated stages imply a steady progression from mild to severe forms. Actually, BPD is not often progressive through the stages that were first described. The descriptions of x-ray appearances are here categorized in terms of severity. *Moderate* disease may not worsen, or radiologic appearance may be equivocal for 3 weeks, at which time *advanced* disease becomes evident.

Moderate BPD is sometimes characterized by diffuse, virtually homogeneous opacification of the lungs, which obscures cardiac margins. This pattern is not always the first indication of moderate BPD. Frequently the first indication is replacement of the early x-ray changes seen in mild disease by coarse, irregularly shaped densities that are often confluent and that occasionally contain very small vacuolar radiolucencies (Fig. 8-20). The areas of density are apparently cast by interstitial and septal edema and by atelectasis due to obstruction of small bronchioles by luminal debris. The small vacuolar radiolucencies represent early foci of emphysema.

In the *severe* form of BPD, the lucent vacuoles have expanded and are now identifiable as air cysts among dense patches, which themselves have become smaller than previously described. The cysts are evidence of progressive multifocal emphysema. The dense patches, compressed by expanding air cysts, are largely indicative of collapsed alveoli, edema and fibrosis of the interstitium, and distention of lymphatics.

In *advanced* BPD the lungs appear bubbly on x-ray films, as air cysts continue to enlarge. Opacities are further reduced in size to strands, streaks, and small patches. Overall, the lungs are extensively hyperinflated; emphysema has progressed considerably (Fig. 8-21). The presence of cardiomegaly usually portends right heart failure.

Clinical course. The incidence of BPD varies from about 10% to 20% among infants with hyaline membrane disease who require mechanical ventilation. In a report of a 12-year experience, advanced BPD was identified in 21% of 299 infants who required at least 24 hours of ventilation with oxygen. The incidence of moderate and advanced BPD has decreased by 50% since the application of distending pressure during ventilatory assistance. End expiratory pressure usually lowers FIO_2 requirements.

About 30% of affected infants are dead by 7 to 8 months of age. In a recent reported experience, a mortality of 38.7% (24 of 62 babies) was noted

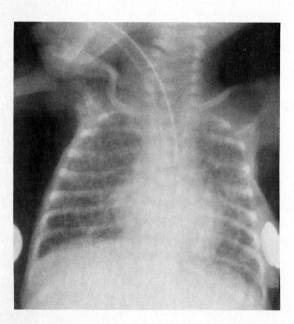

Fig. 8-20. Moderate BPD. Interstitial edema and focal atelectasis produce a diffuse density in both lungs.

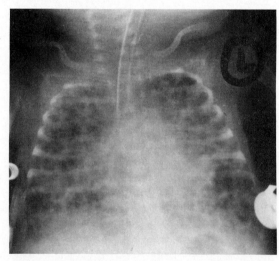

Fig. 8-21. Radiologic appearance of bronchopulmonary dysplasia in advanced stage. White strands are seen throughout both lung fields, representing fibrosis. Multiple areas of regional emphysema impart a cyst-like pattern throughout the lungs.

at all ages. Nineteen of these babies died during their original hospitalization between 1 and 7 months of age. The remaining five died of cardiopulmonary failure after discharge from the initial hospitalization, between 3 months and 3½ years of age.

The onset of BPD may be marked by an increase in oxygen and ventilatory pressure requirements shortly after recovery from hyaline membrane disease has begun, or it may become apparent when there is continued need for such support at a time (between 5 and 10 days of age) when signs of recovery should have developed. Retractions and diminished breath sounds persist, and crepitant rales become audible. This early phase of the clinical course is associated with an x-ray appearance of moderate disease. During the ensuing days or weeks, oxygen concentrations and ventilatory pressures must be increased to maintain satisfactory arterial blood gas levels. As emphysema progresses, barrel-chest becomes obvious; on the x-ray films, the diaphragms are severely flattened and the lungs are increasingly overexpanded (severe and advanced disease). Oxygenation is more difficult and CO_2 retention increases. Respiratory acidosis results; renal conservation of bicarbonate eventually compensates partially for the imbalance. Right heart failure occurs as pathologic changes in pulmonary vasculature progress. In a reported autopsy series, right heart failure was considered the immediate cause of death in 30% of the infants studied. Even in the absence of cardiac failure, right ventricular hypertrophy is almost universal.

In those infants who recover, decrements of inspired oxygen are feasible only at a very slow rate; room air is eventually tolerated after a course of weeks or months. Survival beyond 7 or 8 months of age is associated with normal cardiopulmonary function by 5 to 6 years of age. During this period, recurrent episodes of pulmonary infections and wheezing are characteristic of the disease; some infants experience repeated bouts of acute pulmonary edema as well.

Most of the reported experience concerning the incidence and mortality of BPD is in babies who received oxygen and ventilatory assistance during the years preceding widespread use of continuous distending pressure. Recent observations are more encouraging in that the frequency of BPD seems to have declined by more than half since that time.

Etiologic considerations. In the original description of BPD, high concentrations of inspired oxygen was considered the most likely cause. Affected infants had been given concentrations of 80% or greater for at least 6 days. Although high FIO_2 was considered the primary cause, it was nevertheless speculated that intermittent positive pressure ventilation and endotracheal intubation may have also played a role.

Contemporary consensus holds that advanced BPD is the result of several factors. A prominent and often underemphasized factor is pulmonary immaturity. Developing elastic and connective tissue components of the lung are apparently vulnerable to injuries of any type—those inflicted by oxygen and those caused by ventilator pressures (barotrauma). The severity of the antecedent pulmonary disease, severe hyaline membrane disease for instance, is also an important consideration. Immaturity of lung and severity of insult set the stage for injuries from barotrauma and oxygen, and these injuries are inherent to mechanical ventilation. Whereas originally the etiology of BPD was considered primarily a result of oxygen toxicity, now barotrauma is thought to be more important even though oxygen toxicity is a significant factor. Clinical experience incriminates barotrauma. Rarely, if ever, does an infant develop BPD unless mechanical ventilatory support has been used. Infants who are only in hood oxygen do not develop BPD. A number of other factors have been cited as contributory. There is at least an association between the occurrence of pulmonary interstitial emphysema (PIE) and subsequent development of BPD. That PIE is directly responsible for BPD is unlikely. Rather, it may be that the barotrauma, which produces PIE, is also responsible for BPD. In any event, babies with pulmonary interstitial emphysema are more likely to have BPD later on. Patent ductus arteriosus is also associated with an increased frequency of BPD. A significant left-to-right shunt causes pulmonary edema and thus is thought to initiate the development of bronchopulmonary dysplasia. In the same context, several authors have stated that pulmonary edema from fluid overload may likewise predispose to BPD.

The individual roles of oxygen, intermittent positive pressure ventilation, and endotracheal intubation have yet to be defined precisely despite a bountiful literature on the subject. The contemporary consensus is that all three of these factors are of etiologic significance.

In the years that have passed since BPD was first described, there has been an interesting downward spiral in the oxygen concentration and the duration of therapy that has been considered toxic. As early as 1969, BPD was reported in babies who had received rather low oxygen concentrations for less than 24 hours. In 1975 the appearance of BPD at oxygen concentrations over 40% for over 72 hours was reported. Later on, in the analysis of data from a 12-year experience with BPD, another report concluded that the duration of therapy with over 40% oxygen was the best predictor of BPD but nevertheless, the concentration of inspired oxygen mattered little because if given over a sufficiently long time, BPD will follow. BPD was diagnosed in babies who were exposed to oxygen concentrations as low as 22% to 30%, but for as long as 53 days.

The importance of peak inspiratory pressure during mechanical ventilation has been emphasized. Apparently there is a statistically significant correlation between pressures over 35 cm H_2O and appearance of severe BPD. However, it is our impression that long inspiratory times at almost any high inspiratory pressure are an important cause of lung injury. We make every effort to shorten inspiratory times to the limits that permit acceptable gas exchange (0.3 to 0.5 seconds, depending on rate).

It is thus not surprising that there are no magic numbers. The clinician can only guess the risk for BPD based on a varied reported experience. At best such estimates are as artful as they are scientific. The importance of lung trauma from high pressures during mechanical ventilation and the significance of oxygen concentrations are difficult to separate. The implication of endotracheal intubation is generally agreed on, but the mechanism of involvement is conjectural. Yet another factor to consider is the vulnerability of lungs with hyaline membrane disease to all three of these therapeutic insults. The most seriously ill infants receive high concentrations of oxygen with necessarily high peak pressure by means of an endotracheal tube. If mechanical ventilation must be used, the incidence of BPD will probably be minimized by using the lowest possible FIO_2 and airway pressures and the shortest possible inspiratory times.

Management. The management of an infant with BPD entails the maintenance of effective gas exchange in the presence of damaged lungs, the administration of appropriate fluid volumes and nutrition, and the prevention of widespread pulmonary infection.

Infants whose disease process is mild require oxygen by hood. Severe disease usually requires protracted mechanical ventilation. Ventilator settings should be as low in all parameters as is required to maintain arterial PO_2 at 50 to 70 torr, arterial PCO_2 at 50 torr or slightly higher, and pH in the normal range. Infants whose BPD is advanced have an unalterable tendency to retain CO_2 above desirable values, yet pH gradually becomes normal. Respiratory acidosis is eventually buffered by renal retention of bicarbonate. Therefore in advanced disease, despite the inordinate retention of CO_2, pH is normal because bicarbonate levels are high. Ventilator settings should be at the lowest peak inspiratory pressures that are tolerable. Generally a PEEP level of 2 to 4 cm H_2O is required. Peak inspiratory pressures are gradually lowered to the point of tolerance and respiratory rates are diminished as blood gases indicate effective spontaneous respiration between ventilator insufflations. Mechanical ventilation at slow rates that allow spontaneous respirations between insufflations are called intermittent mandatory ventilation (IMV). This is a common pattern of respiratory support for infants with chronic lung disease.

Edema of the interstitial lung tissue contributes significantly to respiratory insufficiency. Accumulation of fluid in the lung diminishes lung compliance. It also increases airway resistance. The mechanism by which the lung retains excessive water has not been clearly demonstrated. There is good evidence, however, that the administration of furosemide improves lung compliance and diminishes airway resistance. Furosemide is a diuretic. Some studies have demonstrated that the evacuation of lung fluid is associated with the diuretic effect of furosemide; others indicate that furosemide acts directly on the lung. In either event, the administration of furosemide improves lung function within 1 or 2 hours after intravenous administration. The effect persists for approximately 6 hours, perhaps longer. Furosemide is commonly used in the long-term management of BPD. It is generally given two to three times daily, but the schedule of administration varies from one center to another.

Infants with BPD often have acute episodes of bronchospasm, indicated by their wheezing. Some infants wheeze between these acute episodes. Long-term therapy of BPD often includes drugs to promote bronchodilation. Theophylline has been used with some success if infants are less than 30 days of age. Beyond this age fibrosis is extensive, bronchial muscle is replaced by fibrous tissue, and the bronchodilating effect of theophylline is thus precluded. Bronchodilation has also been successfully effected by isoproterenol aerosol therapy. Insufflation of isoproterenol is performed two to four times daily; airway resistance diminishes significantly.

The provision of optimal nutrition is critical. The hope of recovery from BPD is largely based on a capacity to generate new and uninjured alveoli. The process of alveolar formation is impaired if nutrition is suboptimal, and it is obviously impaired by continued use of mechanical ventilation. Adequate caloric intake must be provided either orally or by use of parenteral alimentation. The provision of adequate calories entails considerations that are inseparable from those of fluid administration. The infant with BPD is prone to develop pulmonary edema. Nutrition must be planned utilizing volumes of fluid that are minimal but still compatible with normal water balance. Concentrated formulas containing 24 calories per ounce are advisable. If parenteral alimentation is used, fluid volume must be minimized.

The management of BPD is a protracted challenge to the ingenuity of nursery staff. One must be aggressive in the diminution of mechanical ventilatory support, but inappropriately rapid withdrawal often results in setbacks that prolong the course of illness. Nutritional requirements must be met in the lowest volume of fluids. Infant stimulation and parental support must be actively pursued through the weeks and months of the infant's respiratory incapacity. Infection, particularly pneumonia, is inevitable in infants who must have mechanical respiratory support for weeks. Recurrent acute infections must be identified and treated. Antibiotics must be used judiciously in the interim.

Retinopathy of prematurity (ROP); retrolental fibroplasia (RLF). Retrolental fibroplasia is a disorder of the eyes that, in a few affected infants, ultimately leads to blindness or near-blindness. It was formerly believed to be caused solely by the administration of excessively high oxygen concentrations, which then result in toxic levels of Pao_2. Thus, until recently, retrolental fibroplasia was considered an iatrogenic disease that was largely preventable if caution was exercised in maintaining nontoxic Pao_2 levels. That this is not the case will become apparent as this discussion proceeds. The current consensus holds that toxic Pao_2 levels are indeed an important contributory factor, but that a host of other circumstances, as yet incompletely delineated, are also causative.

Retrolental fibroplasia is no longer considered a completely preventable disorder. Furthermore, some investigators believe that oxygen has no direct effect; that the clinical disorders requiring oxygen therapy are more directly implicated.

Retrolental fibroplasia has long been the accepted name of this ocular disease, which was first described in 1942. However, *retinopathy of prematurity* is now believed to be more appropriate. Literally, retrolental fibroplasia means scar formation behind the lens, which is indeed the culmination of this disorder, but which occurs in only a few affected infants. *Retinopathy of prematurity* is a more inclusive term in that it describes abnormal events in the retina during which a number of stages unfold, beginning with vascular changes, progressing to retinal edema and detachment, and culminating in fibrosis. Progression through all of these stages to scar formation occurs in few infants. In most the process arrests in the early stages of vascular change.

The abnormal events that characterize ROP begin with arteriolar constriction, which may or may not be associated with oxygen administration or with a number of other factors. A month or two later the vessels dilate and proliferate (neovascularization). This new capillary formation may be associated with hemorrhage. New blood vessels leave the surface of the retina to permeate the vitreous. At any time up to this point, the process may come to a halt with no residual visual disturbance, or perhaps only a slight or moderate one. If extensive retinal detachment occurs, varying degrees of scarring ensue. Retinal detachment may be focal or it may involve the entire retina. The stages of development that follow retinal detachment involve scar formation (cicatricial stage) that, in the extreme, comprises a fibrotic retrolental mass invariably associated with total blindness. If scar formation is focal, it may diminish visual acuity insignificantly.

During the decade that followed the first description of the disease in 1942, there occurred what is now referred to as the "first epidemic" of blindness among infants. We are apparently in the midst of a "second epidemic" in which the annual number of blind infants is thought to be comparable to that observed during the first one. In the 1940s and early 1950s, approximately 36 etiologic possibilities were postulated, or were thought to be documented. By the mid 1950s there was widespread acceptance of the concept that excessive oxygen was the only factor directly responsible for the initiation of events in the retina. Acceptance of the role of oxygen overdosage was immediately followed by rigid restriction of therapeutic oxygen; ambient concentrations had to be kept below 40%. During those years, blood gases were not commonly available; there was little reference to PaO_2 levels. These precautions were thus limited to FiO_2 maintenance. A firm conviction prevailed all over the world: If ambient oxygen exceeded 40%, retinal disease was more likely, but if ambient oxygen was held below 40%, retinal disease could be virtually eliminated. Furthermore, prudent use of oxygen required administration for the shortest possible intervals. These rigid events concerned *ambient oxygen concentrations;* PaO_2 was not clinically available.

The rigid recommendations regarding oxygen administration were not without noteworthy basis. Three prospective control studies in the 1950s demonstrated wide discrepancies in the occurrence of retinopathy between groups of babies who received "high" oxygen concentrations and those who received "low" concentrations. Yet in each instance the investigators, and authoritative commentators as well, emphatically cautioned that the data did not justify the assumption that oxygen was the sole cause of ROP. Many insisted that the importance of other causative factors could not be disregarded.

When blood gas determinations became routine in neonatal intensive care, the hazard of retinopathy was said to appear at a PaO_2 greater than 100 torr. There was no experimental basis for this pervasive belief; it was applied because the PaO_2 of infants who were breathing room air seldom exceeded 100 torr. Yet to this date it has been impossible to document a PaO_2 above which retrolental fibroplasia is likely to occur. This a major contention against the predominant role of oxygen toxicity. It has been impossible to establish a fixed level, or even a range of levels, at which eye damage is likely to occur.

Rigid adherence to ambient oxygen concentrations below 40% apparently resulted in a diminished incidence of retinopathy. Some investigators contend that the precipitous drop in incidence was spurious, because in 1958 a significant rise in mortality was reported among infants with hyaline membrane disease who were treated according to the dictum of the day, with restricted oxygen concentrations. The diminished incidence of retinal disease is said to be unreal because a large number of potentially affected infants did not survive. Indeed, in Britain it was estimated that for every infant whose sight was preserved by restricting oxygen, 16 infants did not survive.

The contemporary approach to oxygen therapy is based on PaO_2. Oxygen is administered in any concentration that will effectively maintain PaO_2 between 50 and 80 torr. However, there is still no evidence to define a PaO_2 at which the risk for retinal disease increases significantly.

Current resurgence in the incidence of retinopathy is attributable to an increased survival rate among infants whose birth weight is below 1000 g. In particular, percentage of survival of the smallest infants (between 500 and 750 g) has increased remarkably in just the last few years. A preponderance of the retinopathy now encountered is occurring in the low birth weight babies. We now see a resurgence of ROP despite our capacity for assiduous monitoring of PaO_2 levels with advanced techniques, even with the continuous monitoring provided by transcutaneous oxygen tensions. Most investigators are convinced that the current epidemic results from factors other than oxygen administration, factors that are inherent in the disorders and therapy for survival of these smallest infants. Since the first description of this disease in 1942, it has been clear to one and all that its incidence becomes higher as birth weights decline. The smallest infants are at

greater risk for disease, either self-arresting or blinding. Among infants whose birth weight is less than 1 kg, cicatricial disease occurs in approximately 20% to 40% of survivors, but 5% to 10% of them are actually blinded. Among infants who weigh 1 to 1.5 kg at birth, 2.2% have cicatricial disease; only 0.3% to 1.1% are blinded. The current epidemic is estimated to add approximately 550 newly blinded premature infants to our national population annually.

The exaggerated etiologic importance of oxygen has been recurrently suggested in the literature for years. Now evidence has accumulated and a large number of reports can be analyzed with a perspective that is possible only after accumulated years of experience. At the outset, one must review the data from the three prospective studies conducted in the 1950s. While the important role of oxygen is in fact evident from these investigations, interpretations of the data have tended to overlook the substantial number of infants who developed retrolental fibroplasia despite low ambient oxygen concentrations, and the impressive number of infants who did not develop the disease when exposed to high concentrations. In addition, over 60 full-term infants are known to have developed ROP, and the majority of them did not receive oxygen. It may be that the retinas of these term infants were incompletely developed and were thus vulnerable. Furthermore, the role of oxygen as a sole cause of ROP becomes seriously questionable when one considers that 95 low birth weight infants have developed retinopathy yet never received supplemental oxygen. It is also pertinent to note that the disease has been reported in two infants with cyanotic congenital heart disease, and of even greater interest are 11 affected anencephalic infants of whom 10 were either stillborn or did not survive more than a few days. In those infants a postnatal event is unlikely to be etiologic for ROP.

The issue of causation is also confused by substantial data suggesting that retinal *hypoxia* is a more likely cause of the neovascularization that characterizes the disease. The earliest of vascular changes (spasm) may well be a result of hyperoxia, but it is hypoxia that seems to stimulate the ensuing changes characterized by the formation of new vessels. Early changes of retinopathy have been described in stillborn infants, and at birth in surviving low birth weight infants. It has been suggested that the changes of ROP are associated with those complications of pregnancy that cause retinal hypoxia. Among infants of mothers with complications, retinal changes were found to be over twice as frequent as among control infants. Extreme prematurity (birth weights below 1000 g) is associated with the greatest of vulnerabilities. Retinopathy has recently been cited in approximately 7% of infants whose birth weights are between 1001 and 1500 g; but in survivors who weighed 500 to 750 g at birth, the incidence leaps to 42%. A number of investigators have suggested that the incidence of retinal changes may be as high as 75% among surviving infants whose birth weight was less than 1000 g. This group of the smallest babies is particularly susceptible to intraventricular hemorrhage, recurrent apnea, septicemia, hypoxia, and hypercarbia. They are also most likely to have vitamin E deficiency.

In the late 1940s vitamin E was administered in an effort to prevent the occurrence of retinopathy. The study found an impressive reduction in the incidence of the disease among premature infants who were given vitamin E orally. Subsequent investigations failed to confirm the results of the initial study, and interest in the role of vitamin E waned considerably. In the 1970s, investigations into the mechanism of direct oxidative tissue injury rekindled an interest in vitamin E because it is a known scavenger of the free radicals that result from overoxygenation. In minimizing or eliminating these free radicals, cell membranes are protected from oxidative damage. Furthermore low birth weight infants have been known for years to be at risk for the clinical signs of vitamin E deficiency. More recent trials of vitamin E administration to prevent or ameliorate the effects of retinopathy suggest that the severity of the disease, and therefore the incidence of

blindness, is considerably diminished among treated infants. These studies offer hope, but most investigators believe that more data are necessary to determine the extent of vitamin E toxicity before its widespread use is established.

In summary, the role of oxygen is indeed critical, but its importance has been exaggerated since the original studies of the 1950s. During the early epidemic of blindness, protracted use of oxygen was a major etiologic factor. The current epidemic of blindness involves a different population. We now treat premature infants in whom the excessive use of oxygen does not seem to play the same major role that was described during the experience of the 1950s. The literature appropriately emphasizes that retrolental fibroplasia is not a preventable disease in the low birth weight infant, because in these infants the causes are not known.

PATENCY OF THE DUCTUS ARTERIOSUS (PDA)

In premature infants, persistent patency of the ductus arteriosus gives rise to hyperperfusion and edema of the lungs when a significant left-to-right shunt has developed. The ductus remains patent in 50% to 85% of preterm infants under 1200 g of birth weight; the incidence diminishes as birth weight increases. This discussion is concerned with the syndrome of ductal left-to-right shunting in premature infants, which commonly gives rise to life-threatening pulmonary insufficiency and occasionally to congestive heart failure. It most often appears at 5 to 10 days of age, when ventilatory support for hyaline membrane disease is in the process of gradual withdrawal because of improved lung function. As recovery from hyaline membrane disease progresses, pulmonary vascular pressure decreases hour by hour, until it falls below aortic pressure. The new gradient thus established, blood now flows from aorta to pulmonary artery through the patent ductus arteriosus. The quantity of blood shunted may be as high as 40% of left ventricular output. The result of this redistribution of blood flow is hyperperfusion of lungs with capillary engorgement followed by pulmonary edema. Furthermore, the large amount of aortic blood that is shunted to the pulmonary circuit leads to a correspondingly diminished perfusion of those organs supplied by postductal blood from the aorta. Hypoperfusion of the intestinal tract is thought to be responsible for a higher incidence of necrotizing enterocolitis in babies with significant left-to-right shunts.

It is our experience that an elevation of $PaCO_2$ is the most frequent early sign of significant ductal shunting in premature infants under treatment for hyaline membrane disease. Recurrent apnea (if the infant is not on a ventilator) and need for an increased FIO_2 are also frequent manifestations. These findings are impressive because they appear abruptly when recovery from hyaline membrane disease seems imminent—when FIO_2 requirements and ventilator pressures have been confidently decreased to their lowest levels.

The elevation of $PaCO_2$ usually occurs as end expiratory pressure (CPAP or PEEP) is lowered. With less end expiratory pressure in alveoli to oppose it, transudation of fluid occurs from engorged capillaries; pulmonary edema appears. Decreased compliance of the edematous lung develops and exhalation of CO_2 is therefore impaired. This is very soon reflected as an elevated $PaCO_2$. With few exceptions, the $PaCO_2$ can be lowered by increasing CPAP or PEEP back to its immediately preceding level. This raises alveolar pressure, and fluid transudation is halted. Much of the interstitial fluid probably re-enters the capillaries. Eventually, FIO_2 can be lowered again. In some instances one is confronted with a bizarre situation in which CPAP or PEEP remain indispensable for the control of pulmonary edema, but only room air is needed for normal oxygenation.

In addition to the changes in blood gases and the typical response to elevations of end expiratory pressure, significant ductal shunts are suggested by several physical signs. The murmur that is so often described as characteristic of patent ductus arteriosus is not particularly significant because the presence and intensity of that murmur are poorly correlated to the seriousness of the left-to-right shunt. On the other hand, a heaving precordial impulse (hyperactive precordium) is a certain indication of an overactive, overloaded left ventricle that must supply blood to a significant ductal shunt. Bounding pulses are also a most reliable indication. If pulmonary edema is advanced, and fluid from capillaries has entered the alveoli from interstitial tissue, crepitant rales are audible and are particularly profuse over the baby's back.

The chest film often reveals slight or moderate enlargement of the heart and irregular, fluffy lung densities that characterize pulmonary edema (Fig. 8-22). The lung densities diminish considerably when CPAP or PEEP are increased to minimize the pulmonary edema.

The echocardiogram is considered the most reliable diagnostic modality. It demonstrates left atrial enlargement, which occurs because large quantities of blood return to the left atrium from hyperperfused lungs. On the echocardiogram, measurements are made of the diameters of the left atrium and the aortic root. This is called the LA/AO ratio. If it exceeds 1.0 to 1.2, a significant ductal shunt is considered to be present.

The management of symptomatic patent ductus arteriosus entails general support measures, administration of indomethacin, and surgical ligation. In a number of infants, general support measures seem to suffice. In others, indomethacin must be administered for pharmacologic closure of the ductus. In still others, surgical closure of the ductus is necessary when the two previously mentioned modalities of treatment are ineffective. The indications and timing of treatment with medical support and indomethacin vary from one center to another. The indications for surgical ligation vary even more widely.

General measures are composed of respiratory support that relies principally on end expiratory positive pressure to minimize pulmonary edema. Elimination of lung fluid is even better effected by use of a diuretic such as furosemide (1 to 2 mg/kg in a single intravascular dose). Some cen-

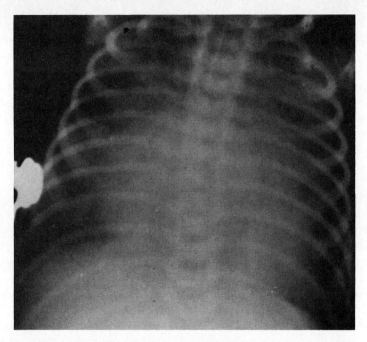

Fig. 8-22. Pulmonary edema and moderate cardiac enlargement are typical radiologic signs of patent ductus arteriosus associated with a significant left-to-right shunt.

ters use digoxin; most are unimpressed with its effectiveness. Furthermore, premature infants require higher doses of digoxin, and the possibility of toxicity is thus more imminent. Support measures also include restriction of fluids to the smallest volume compatible with adequate fluid and electrolyte balance.

The use of indomethacin for pharmacologic closure of the ductus is now pervasive. Successful closure of the ductus has been reported in 50% to 80% of infants to whom it was administered. The drug is usually administered orally, but intravenous preparations would appear to be superior in terms of predictable plasma levels. Generally the dose employed is 0.2 mg/kg of body weight. At some centers, 0.25 mg/kg is administered to babies who are older than 7 or 8 days. The incidence of successful treatment diminishes at 10 to 16 days of age. Three doses are administered at 12-hour intervals. Intravenous admin-

istration of indomethacin results in higher peak plasma concentrations than the orally administered preparation, but the relationship of plasma levels to effectiveness is not established. Contraindications to the use of indomethacin are as follows:

- BUN >30 mg/dl.
- Serum creatinine clearance ≥1.8 mg/dl.
- Total urine output <0.5 ml/kg/h for the preceding 8 to 12 hours.
- Platelet count <60,000/mm³.
- Significantly positive test for blood in stool.
- Identifiable bleeding diathesis.
- Necrotizing enterocolitis.
- Evidence of intracranial hemorrhage within 24 to 48 hours preceding treatment.

Toxic effects of indomethacin have not been troublesome. The drug is widely known to impair platelet adhesiveness and therefore to increase bleeding time. However, significant and hazardous bleeding as a result of indomethacin therapy has not been reported to date. Furthermore, there is no substantial evidence to indicate that the incidence of intracranial hemorrhage is higher as a result of therapy. Transient elevation of serum creatinine concentrations is common after the initial dose of the drug. As a rule, creatinine concentrations do not rise significantly with subsequent doses. Diminution in urine output is almost the rule. Previously normal outputs (1 to 4 ml/kg/h) may decline to 0.5 ml/kg/h. There is no firm evidence to indicate increased incidence of necrotizing enterocolitis among treated infants. The incidence of retinopathy of prematurity (retrolental fibroplasia) may be diminished among treated infants, but evidence is far from conclusive.

In most centers, surgical ligation is the last resort for closure of the ductus. There is a wide difference of opinion regarding an appropriate time for surgical intervention. In some studies, early ligation diminishes morbidity and shortens hospital stay, but has no effect on mortality before discharge from the nursery. There has been no demonstrated difference in mortality between pharmacologic and surgical treatments.

In summary, the efficacy of therapeutic measures for closure of the ductus must be interpreted in a context that also considers complicating conditions such as pulmonary insufficiency, and particularly the incidence of spontaneous closure. In infants whose gestational age is 34 weeks or greater, spontaneous closure is almost the rule. Also, spontaneous closure is not uncommon in the smallest premature infants. General support measures are always necessary for symptomatic babies. Furthermore, a trial of indomethacin is considered appropriate in any baby with a symptomatic (hemodynamically significant) left-to-right shunt. Maximal benefit from indomethacin therapy will only be possible when there is clear evidence for the best appropriate time of therapy, for the most effective dosage schedule, and for reliable early identification of infants who will benefit from therapy. The potential for benefit

probably extends beyond cardiopulmonary considerations. For instance, a large patent ductus arteriosus causes abnormal flow patterns in the cerebral arteries; diastolic flow is retrograde, decreased or absent. The possibility that this constitutes a predisposition to CNS ischemia must be investigated as part of the global approach to assessing the value of early treatment.

PERSISTENT FETAL CIRCULATION (PERSISTENT PULMONARY VASOSPASM; PERSISTENT PULMONARY HYPERTENSION)

Persistent pulmonary hypertension in the immediate postnatal period results from pulmonary arteriolar constriction. This phenomenon is identifiable as a component of a number of clinical entities; it is also a clinical entity in its own right. Pulmonary vasoconstriction causes pulmonary artery pressure to rise above aortic pressure; a right-to-left shunt across the patent ductus arteriosus results. In addition, pressure in the right atrium may be higher than pressure in the left atrium; right-to-left shunting thus occurs at the atrial level as well. Furthermore, vasoconstriction results in pulmonary hypoperfusion, and the total quantity of oxygenated blood leaving the lungs (destined for the left atrium) is regularly diminished. These pulmonary vascular phenomena are components of a variety of clinical entities: hyaline membrane disease, RDS II, pneumonia (especially group B streptococcal), aspiration of milk, diaphragmatic hernia, and cold stress. Vasoconstriction often follows injudicious decrements in FIO_2 in babies receiving oxygen therapy. This is called "flip-flop," and it may be so severe as to be irreversible, even if treated with an FIO_2 of 1.0 on a mechanical ventilator.

Pulmonary vasospasm causes hypoxemia and cyanosis. Depending on the tenaciousness and extent of vasoconstriction, amelioration may be possible with simple hood oxygen, or this failing, with mechanical ventilation. Treatment with tolazoline or with hyperventilation to produce respiratory alkalosis may be urgently required in the most severe cases. Any of these approaches is appropriate when hypoxemia is attributable to pulmonary vasospasm, whether it exists by itself or is a component of one of the clinical entities listed above.

Pulmonary vasospasm in the immediate postnatal period is a response to intrauterine or extrauterine asphyxia. When pulmonary vasospasm is identified in the absence of other disorders, and particularly in the absence of parenchymal lung disease, the diagnosis of *persistent fetal circulation* is justifiable. This form of pulmonary vasospasm occurs in infants who are at or near term. In the vast majority of them, there is a history of perinatal asphyxia. Apgar scores are usually 5 or below at 1 or 5 minutes. The onset of clearly abnormal respiration may be delayed for as long as 12 hours, but in most instances this is discernible within an hour after birth. Tachypnea is the rule; retractions are usually minimal or moderate. Cyanosis occurs soon after delivery. Auscultation of the lungs indicates good air exchange, and there are no blatant signs of cardiac abnormality. Systemic blood pressure is normal. Response to oxygen enrichment may be satisfactory at first, but soon hypoxemia eventuates even in pure oxygen.

The chest film is most often normal. Occasionally, slight cardiomegaly is observed, and not uncommonly, dense streaks emanate from the hilar regions to the peripheral lung fields. Occasionally the lungs are overexpanded.

Arterial oxygen tensions are low. With rare exception, the postductal PaO_2 is at least 15% lower than in the preductal sample. A 15% discrepancy is usually clinically significant if the preductal PaO_2 is less than 50 to 60 torr. The $PaCO_2$ is normal or low. Elevated $PaCO_2$ is a rarity because in this disorder there is no significant parenchymal lung involvement.

Low concentrations of serum calcium and glucose have been described, as well as high hematocrit levels (polycythemia). These have been considered of etiologic significance by some authors. Correction of the calcium and glucose abnormalities is, however, unlikely to relieve pulmonary vasospasm. Correction of a high hematocrit level may occasionally be of some benefit. It is noteworthy that these aberrations have also been described as sequelae of fetal asphyxia in numerous publications; it is more plausible to regard them, and the pulmonary vasospasm itself, as neonatal consequences of fetal asphyxia.

If a response to an FIO_2 of 1.0 in a hood is inadequate, we do not hesitate to administer tolazoline; it has been lifesaving on numerous occasions. Emphasis must be placed on accurate selection of infants in whom pulmonary vasospasm is virtually the sole cause of severe hypoxemia. In our experience, at least 90% of infants so selected respond dramatically to fairly rapid infusion of 2 mg/kg of tolazoline. We add the drug to 10 ml/kg of plasma volume expander. However, we prefer to first try hyperventilation to a $PaCO_2$ of 20 to 25 torr, which usually raises arterial pH to above 7.50.

A note of caution is in order regarding the use of PEEP in babies whose lung parenchyma is not abnormal. In these circumstances, CPAP or PEEP usually worsens the hypoxemia. If mechanical ventilation is used for oxygenation, it should be used without PEEP.

SYNDROMES RESULTING FROM ASPIRATION OR FLUID RETENTION

Among the multiple causes of neonatal respiratory distress, there is a spectrum of abnormalities presumably caused by aspiration of amniotic fluid and its contents into the respiratory tract or by retention of fetal lung fluid. The actual event of aspiration is believed to occur in utero or during delivery—undoubtedly a valid concept. However, in some infants the clinical signs of distress may result from impaired evacuation of fetal lung fluid that would normally be absorbed into the pulmonary circulation during the first few breaths (p. 209). In either case the end result is similar: the flow of air is obstructed in varying degress by the presence of fluid, particulate matter, or both in the respiratory tract.

Most of the clinical signs that characterize these

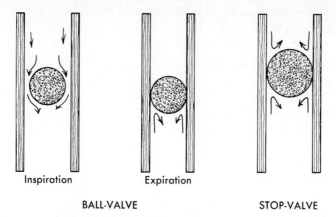

Inspiration   Expiration

BALL-VALVE   **STOP-VALVE**

Fig. 8-23. Mechanisms of airway obstruction. The ball-valve type allows entry of air peripheral to it but blocks air egress, resulting in emphysema. The stop-valve variety allows neither entry nor egress of air, resulting in atelectasis beyond the obstruction. (Modified from Caffey, J.: Pediatric x-ray diagnosis, ed. 5, Chicago, 1967, Year Book Medical Publishers.)

entities can be explained by two simple obstructive phenomena that may occur at any level of the respiratory tract. Fig. 8-23 illustrates both mechanisms: partial obstruction (check-valve, or ball-valve) and complete obstruction (stop-valve). The ball-valve mechanism permits entry of air past the obstruction during inspiration while obstructing its complete egress during expiration. This is possible because the calibers of bronchi and bronchioles become larger during inspiration and smaller during expiration. When bronchioles enlarge, air passes around the obstruction, but when they diminish in caliber during expiration, the lumen becomes completely occluded and air is trapped peripheral to the obstruction. By this mechanism progressive accumulation of trapped air may produce diffuse or regional overexpansion of the lungs (emphysema). On the other hand, a complete obstruction (stop-valve) does not permit entry of any air, and as a result, the portions of lung peripheral to it are collapsed. Both amniotic fluid, with its contents (principally vernix and meconium), and fetal lung fluid are capable of producing either or both of these obstructive phenomena. The spectrum of abnormalities is thus characterized at one end by diffuse emphysema

of both lungs without collapse and at the other end by collapse of large areas of the lungs. The clinical entity in which emphysema predominates has been called *transient tachypnea of the newborn, respiratory distress syndrome type II, or obstructive emphysema of the newborn*. The clinical condition in which occlusion and collapse are more prominent is known as meconium aspiration, or the massive aspiration syndrome.

Respiratory distress syndrome, type II (RDS II; transient tachypnea of the newborn)

Affected infants are at or near term. Respiratory distress begins at birth or shortly thereafter and is characterized by tachypnea, retractions, flaring of the nostrils, "barrel chest," and expiratory grunt. Usually there is little or no difficulty with the onset of breathing. Cyanosis in room air may be noted, but usually clears in relatively small increments of ambient oxygen concentration. Grunting and retractions may resolve within 6 to 24 hours, or they may persist for several days.

The roentgenogram is characterized by generalized overexpansion of the lungs, which is identifiable principally by a flattened contour of the diaphragm, in contrast to the distinctly domed configuration that is seen in normal infants. Dense streaks radiate from the hilar regions. Only occasionally are patches of density evident, representing areas of collapse and/or large fluid accumulations.

The blood pH is moderately depressed, arterial PCO_2 is elevated, and the base deficit is usually 10 mEq/L or less. Alkali therapy is seldom required, since these infants, despite respiratory dysfunction, seem to manage their alveolar gas exchange sufficiently well to maintain normal blood gas tensions. They rarely require assisted ventilation of any type.

The clinical appearance of these babies suggests hyaline membrane disease, but RDS II is a distinctly different abnormality with a far brighter prognosis. As a rule, affected babies recover, and there has thus far been no evidence of chronic lung disease among those who were followed to 5 or 6 months of age.

The grunting that occurs in this syndrome requires comment because it apparently serves a purpose that differs from the expiratory grunt of hyaline membrane disease. Since transient tachypnea involves diffuse emphysema (air trapping), the expiratory grunt probably represents an attempt to eject as much of the trapped alveolar air as possible. In hyaline membrane disease the grunt attempts to retain as much air as possible in an effort to maintain alveolar expansion.

RDS II primarily involves retention of fetal lung fluid. Presumably the infant's lungs are sufficiently mature to function postnatally, save for failure to evacuate this fluid. The syndrome is frequently called "wet lung," but this is an unfortunate designation because fluid is retained in any lung that fails to expand normally after the first few breaths. Thus the immature lungs of an infant at 32 weeks of gestation are also "wet," as are those affected by hyaline membrane disease. RDS II should be designated in infants who are at or near term, whose respiratory distress is predominantly attributable to the presence of retained lung fluid. With clearance, clinical signs disappear.

In our experience, RDS (type II) is protracted among infants in whom perinatal asphyxia has occurred. Some of these infants require hood oxygen for as long as 4 days. A serious hazard in assuming the diagnosis of RDS II is the neglect of group B streptococcal pneumonia. During the first 12 to 24 hours the clinical course of both these disorders may be identical. The real possibility of pneumonia is suggested by an abnormal white blood cell count and differential, hyperglycemia, persistent metabolic acidosis, poor perfusion, and in some instances tachypnea associated with only minimal retractions.

Meconium aspiration (massive aspiration syndrome)

Meconium aspiration is a consequence of fetal asphyxia (Fig. 8-24). It rarely occurs in preterm infants. The asphyxial episode in utero apparently increases intestinal peristalsis and relaxes the anal sphincter to release meconium. It also stimulates fetal gasping. The amount of meconium aspirated in utero is variable. In most instances the major portion is aspirated postnatally during the first few breaths. The airway is thus completely or partially

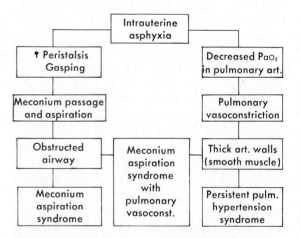

Fig. 8-24. Meconium aspiration in utero and pulmonary vasoconstriction are responses to fetal asphyxia. Meconium aspiration and persistent pulmonary hypertension syndromes may occur singly or in combination.

obstructed at various levels, and alveolar ventilation is either severely decreased in the emphysematous areas or entirely eliminated in the atelectatic areas.

In addition to obstructive phenomena, the airway is also affected by an inflammatory response to meconium—chemical pneumonitis. In animals, inflammation has been demonstrated 48 hours after the instillation of meconium into the trachea. Thickened alveolar walls and interstitial tissue now pose a barrier to the passage of oxygen from alveoli to alveolar capillaries. Thus the diffusion of oxygen is impaired, in addition to the aforementioned obstruction to its inflow.

Pulmonary vasospasm is another important component of the meconium aspiration syndrome. Vasoconstriction of arterioles occurs in response to intrauterine asphyxia and is sustained postnatally in a substantial number of infants. Persistence of pulmonary vasospasm redirects blood through fetal channels (see fetal circulation, Ch. 1), thus maintaining a right-to-left shunt. In such circumstances mechanical ventilation fails to oxygenate the infant with meconium aspiration. In the extreme, uncorrectable hypoxemia results in death. Treatment with *tolazoline*, a powerful vasodilating drug, is often lifesaving. In our experience, it is most effective when there is less airway involvement; it is least successful when parenchymal involvement is extensive. Furthermore, because it dilates blood vessels throughout the body, a moderate, sometimes extreme, fall in blood pressure follows its intravascular administration. Tolazoline must be used with extreme caution in carefully selected babies. The most frequent indication for its use in the presence of pulmonary vasospasm is the failure to oxygenate by mechanical hyperventilation to a $PaCO_2$ of 20 to 25 torr. A significantly higher PaO_2 from the right radial artery (preductal) than from the descending aorta (postductal) is characteristic of clinically significant pulmonary vasospasm. Pulmonary artery pressure is higher than aortic pressure in the presence of pulmonary arteriolar vasoconstriction. Venous blood is shunted from the pulmonary artery across the ductus to the aorta where venous admixture occurs. The PaO_2 in the postductal blood sample, collected from the descending aorta, is thus lower than in the right radial artery where venous admixture is not as extensive. The reader is referred to the description earlier in this chapter of the fetal circulation and the changes that occur in it during the first breath and also to the discussion of persistent pulmonary hypertension on pp. 217 and 271.

Meconium aspiration syndrome is thus a neonatal consequence of fetal asphyxia. Its postnatal manifestations result from obstructed airways and often pulmonary vasospasm as well. Both of these factors are responses to a single antecedent event—fetal asphyxia.

Meconium is passed into amniotic fluid in approximately 10% of all pregnancies; it is a sign of fetal distress. Some fetuses aspirate particles of meconium, which, during the first few breaths, may be inspired more deeply toward the alveoli, if this has not already occurred in utero. In contrast to transient tachypnea, affected infants often have difficulty establishing respiration. In some, respiratory distress may be delayed. It has been shown in puppies that delayed symptoms are associated with gradual progress of small particles toward the more peripheral airways with each breath. Presumably the same process operates in human infants. At least this explanation for the delayed distress observed in these babies is plausible. The signs of respiratory distress are similar to those described for transient tachypnea, except that the rales are often present.

The radiologic appearance of the lungs is characterized by multiple patches of density, interspersed areas of emphysema, and thick streaks that emanate from the hilar regions (Fig. 8-25). The patchy densities represent relatively large areas of atelectasis that are produced by complete obstruction (stop-valve). They are considerably more prominent and extensive than in transient tachypnea. In most instances, overdistention of the lung is predominant, even in the presence of widespread atelectasis. The x-ray film thus also

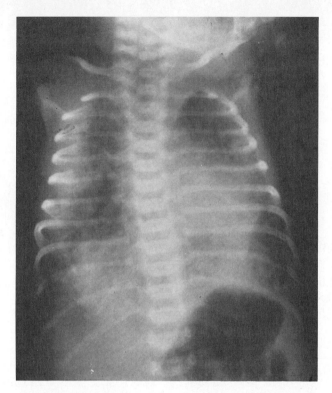

Fig. 8-25. Meconium aspiration is severe in this chest film. Broad areas of density represent atelectasis and interstitial fluid. Regional emphysema is seen in the remaining radiolucent areas. The overall effect of diffuse airway obstruction is overexpansion of the lungs, as indicated by the low position of the diaphragms.

shows flattened diaphragms and bulging intercostal spaces.

Respiratory abnormalities usually subside in a few days, although they may persist longer. Death has been reported in 28% of affected infants. Pneumomediastinum and pneumothorax may complicate the course (see later).

Blood gas and pH determinations indicate varying degrees of mixed respiratory and metabolic acidosis.

The intensity of respiratory and other types of support is often equal to that required for hyaline membrane disease. With rare exception, these infants are born at term; often they are postterm. In most, there is evidence of some sort of intra-uterine distress. Apgar scores at 1 and 5 minutes are usually below 5. Pneumothorax and pneumomediastinum are not infrequent, though they appear in a minority of infants.

Meconium aspiration syndrome is a serious and frequent pulmonary disorder. Recent data demonstrate that *much of the morbidity and virtually all the mortality is avoidable by appropriate management in the delivery room*. Thus, in one inquiry among meconium-stained infants whose tracheas were suctioned immediately, the incidence of respiratory distress was less than half of that in nonsuctioned infants. Death occurred in approximately 1% of the suctioned infants and 28% of the nonsuctioned infants.

In a prospective investigation involving tracheal aspiration of all cases of meconium-stained amniotic fluid, meconium was removed from the trachea in 57% of the babies. Abnormal x-ray films were noted in half of them. Postnatal respiratory distress was noted in every baby who had both an abnormal x-ray film and tracheal meconium. If either of these factors was absent, the infant's subsequent course was uneventful. Other babies, who were admitted from outlying hospitals and had not been suctioned, had an impressively higher morbidity rate. They also required assisted ventilation more often, and the incidence of pneumothorax and pneumomediastinum was higher. In our own experience, 91 babies were admitted with the diagnosis of meconium aspiration syndrome in a recent calendar year. Of the 23 who were referred to us from other hospitals, six died (26%); of the remaining 68 who were inborn, only one baby died (1.5%).

The best management of meconium aspiration syndrome requires aspiration of the trachea in all babies who emerge from stained amniotic fluid *and are in respiratory distress*. At the moment of birth, tracheal aspiration must be performed by application of gentle suction from the masked mouth of the operator, through an endotracheal tube. Use of a catheter is inadequate for this purpose because large particles cannot be evacuated. Mouth suction is maintained while the endotracheal tube is withdrawn so that if larger meconium masses are adherent to the tip of the tube, they are removed. Intubation is repeated until meconium is no longer in evidence. After arrival in the nursery, physical therapy to the chest, followed by suction, is repeated as often as indicated. Oxygen mixtures must be warm and well humidified. Mechanical ventilation (with or without PEEP) is often essential. The use of steroids has been advocated in the past, purportedly to minimize the inflammatory response to meconium. A well-controlled study has demonstrated that hydrocortisone does not diminish the need for assisted ventilation, nor does it reduce mortality. It does, however, prolong morbidity; compared with untreated babies, those who receive hydrocortisone require a significantly longer period to wean to room air.

PNEUMONIA

Infection of the lungs may be acquired in utero (congenital pneumonia) or after birth. The congenital disease is more often lethal. Pneumonia is a common serious perinatal infection. It has a number of attributes that are unique to the neonate and is thus presented in Chapter 12 as a part of the general problem of perinatal infections.

CONGENITAL ANOMALIES

Malformations of the respiratory tract are numerous. A few of the major anomalies are discussed here.

Choanal atresia

The choanae are the posterior nares that open into nasopharynx. Atresia or stenosis is an uncommon malformation that produces dramatic symptoms and requires immediate recognition. Complete or partial obstruction of one or both apertures is caused by a membranous or bony structure covering them. Since the neonate can breathe only through his nose, catastrophic respiratory distress may result from obstruction. The first breath is usually normal because it is taken through the mouth. Cyanosis and severe retractions appear as the infant subsequently attempts to breathe through the nose. Thick mucoid secretions characteristically fill the nose. The anomaly can be demonstrated by failure to pass a catheter or probe through the nose into the nasopharynx. If a membrane covers the choanae, it can be punctured to open the airway. Most often this is not the case. An oral airway should be inserted to accommodate mouth breathing pending ultimate surgical correction of the obstuction. Occasionally respiration is possible only after endotracheal intubation. Choanal obstruction may impede the exhalation of carbon dioxide, and as a consequence, diffuse emphysema and an elevated arterial PCO_2 develop.

Tracheoesophageal fistula

Among the congenital malformations that cause neonatal respiratory distress, tracheoesophageal fistula is the most common. Several variations have been recognized (Fig. 8-26). The most frequent form of this anomaly is atresia of a segment of the esophagus, which is thus divided into an upper blind pouch and a lower separated portion that communicates with the stomach in a normal fashion. A fistula connects this lower esophageal segment with the trachea. This lesion is present in 85% of infants with esophageal atresia. In another variety, which is far less common, esophageal atresia is the only malformation, the tracheobronchial tree being intact. A third type is characterized by a fistulous connection between an otherwise normal trachea and esophagus, the so-called H type of fistula. The other variations are extremely rare.

A distinctive triad of clinical signs is usually recognizable in the most common variety of tracheoesophageal fistula: (1) accumulation of secre-

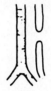

Type A
Esophageal atresia without
tracheoesophageal fistula.
Frequency 8%

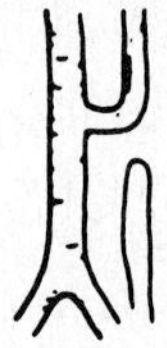

Type B
Esophageal atresia with
proximal tracheoesophageal
fistula.
Frequency 1%

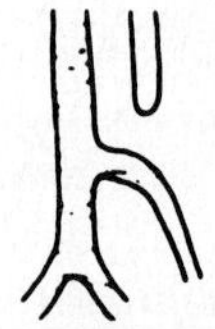

Type C
Esophageal atresia with
distal tracheoesophageal
fistula.
Frequency 86%

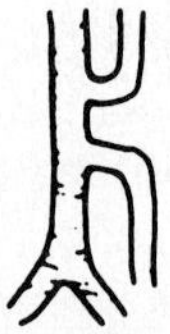

Type D
Esophageal atresia with
both proximal and distal
tracheoesophageal fistulae.
Frequency 1%

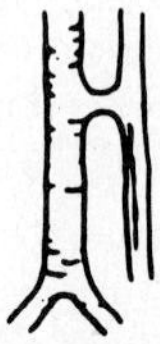

Type E
Tracheoesophageal fistula
without esophageal atresia
(H-type).
Frequency 4%

Fig. 8-26. (From Sunshine, P., et al.: In Fanaroff, A. A., and Martin, R. J.: Behrman's neonatal-perinatal medicine, 1983, St. Louis, 1983, The C. V. Mosby Co.)

tions in the mouth and hypopharynx, often requiring urgent and frequent suction, (2) continuous or sporadic respiratory distress, and (3) repeated regurgitation of feedings. The first two signs should immediately suggest this diagnostic possibility to the nurse. A trial feeding should not be necessary; it could be dangerous because of aspiration. In affected infants, the mouth is full of bubbling saliva, and some degree of respiratory distress is clearly apparent. Often the abdomen is distended because air continually enters the stomach through the fistulous connection between the trachea and the lower esophageal segment. Pneumonia and atelectasis, particularly in the right upper lobe, are also rather frequent signs. The nurse should attempt to pass a catheter into the esophagus of any infant with these signs. The obstruction is not always perceived because the catheter may curl on itself in the esophageal pouch while it seems to pass with ease. One or 2 cc of air should be injected into the catheter while the nurse listens over the stomach for gurgling to indicate that the catheter tip is in the stomach. Listening for gurgling is not consistently reliable.

A chest film usually reveals the blind pouch filled with air. Instillation of dye contrast medium into the pouch, although frequently performed, is not necessary for the diagnosis because the air-filled pouch is plainly visible. If air is also present in the intestinal tract and esophageal atresia has been demonstrated, a tracheoesophageal fistula is undoubtedly present. We use two techniques to demonstrate the pouch by x-ray film. The pouch is dramatically visible if it can be inflated with air at the moment the x-ray film is taken. The nurse uses bag and mask, insufflating five or six times. Then, with the next squeeze of the bag, the x-ray technician takes the film. Even more diagnostic is the passage of an umbilical artery catheter. It is radiopaque, and it loops within the blind pouch. Fig. 8-27 shows three films of a tracheoesophageal fistula. The first is routine chest film in which the air-filled esophageal pouch is visible. Our clinical nurse supervisor suspected pathology from this film. The second is an x-ray film taken while the pouch was inflated by bag and mask. The third demonstrates the position of an umbilical artery catheter within the pouch.

Infants whose only anomaly is esophageal atresia (without a fistulous connection) have pooling of secretions and feeding difficulties. Respiratory symptoms, if they are present, are a consequence of aspirated secretions.

The H type of fistula is well known but rare; it is often suspected but seldom demonstrated early in the course. Respiratory distress is typically at its worst when the baby is fed, since milk enters the lung from the esophagus through the fistula. Tachypnea may persist between feedings, and pneumonia is almost a constant accompaniment. The tract must be demonstrated by feeding contrast medium while the baby is in a prone and somewhat oblique position. Fluoroscopic visualization is usually possible, but repeated attempts are often necessary because the fistula does not always fill with dye.

We diagnosed a case of H type fistula by measuring changes of intragastric oxygen concentration in response to insufflating the lungs alternately with 100% oxygen and room air. After passing a nasogastric tube, the exterior end was attached to an oxygen analyzer to register fluctuations of intragastric oxygen concentrations. An endotracheal tube was passed just below the vocal cords. The tip of the tube was thus above the tracheal aperture of the H fistula. The baby was gently insufflated with 100% oxygen, which crossed the fistula into the stomach and resulted in an increased intragastric oxygen concentration. This was registered on the oxygen analyzer to which the outside end of the nasogastric tube was attached. Oxygen concentration was observed to fall when insufflation was continued, but with room air. The fistula was successfully repaired.

All forms of tracheoesophageal fistula must be repaired surgically. As technical surgical problems have been surmounted, pneumonia, septicemia, and associated anomalies have emerged as the major causes of death. For term infants without other anomalies or pneumonia, a 100% survival rate can be expected. Overall survival of term babies is approximately 70%, and for premature infants, 52%. From available data, it has been surmised that improved management of pneumonia and septicemia would substantially diminish mortality. The later the diagnosis is made, the more hazardous are the procedure and post-operative course. Surgery can be delayed with impunity only if optimal supportive care is available. As a rule, the nurse is the infant's first attendant and thus can best direct initial attention to suspicious signs.

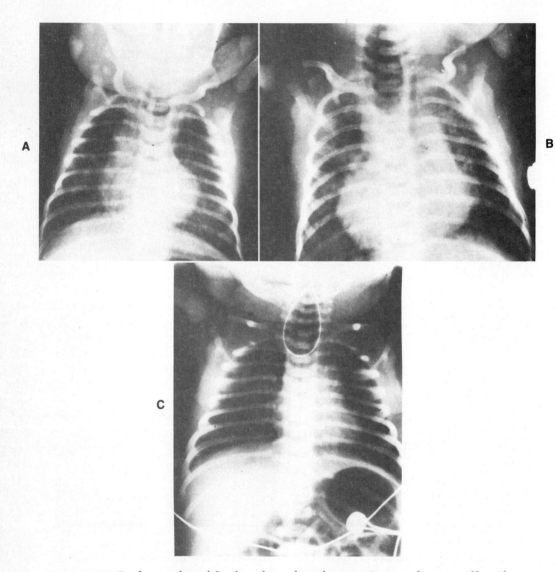

Fig. 8-27. A, Tracheoesophageal fistula with esophageal atresia. Routine chest x-ray film. The radiolucent pocket overlying the vertebrae just superior to the heart is the air-containing esophageal pouch. **B,** Inflated pouch during bagging with mask. **C,** Umbilical artery catheter looped in esophageal pouch.

Diaphragmatic hernia

Incomplete embryonic formation of the diaphragm results in a congenital defect that allows displacement of abdominal organs into the thoracic cavity. Severe respiratory distress occurs at birth or shortly thereafter. The left side is involved five to ten times more frequently than the right side. Herniation occurs through one of several possible defective segments of the diaphragm; the most common is at the posterolateral segment (foramen of Bochdalek). Defects at the anterior portion directly beneath the sternum (foramen of Morgagni) and at the esophageal hiatus are considerably less frequent.

In left-sided involvement the intestine, stomach, and spleen compress the lung. The gastrointestinal tract, distended with air, occupies most of the space preempted from the lung, and the mediastinum is dislocated to the right. In right-sided involvement the liver and/or intestine are the herniated abdominal organs; they displace the mediastinum to the left.

The severity of symptoms is related to the amount of lung compressed by the dislocated abdominal organs. The pattern of respiratory distress is no different from that caused by other neonatal disorders. The most severely affected babies gasp a few times at birth, never establishing respiration. If respiratory distress is not particularly severe at birth, it frequently progresses alarmingly as the intestine in the chest expands with the normal entry of swallowed air (Fig. 8-28).

The diagnosis can sometimes be anticipated before birth if there is a history of polyhydramnios. Polyhydramnios occurs in over half of affected infants because the thoracic location of intestine is obstructive to intrauterine flow of amniotic fluid. The presence of a diaphragmatic hernia is invariably suggested by difficult respiration. Dis-

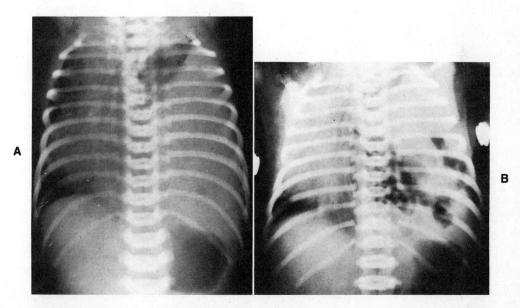

Fig. 8-28. A, Left diaphragmatic hernia immediately after birth. The left chest is opaque, filled with gasless intestine. The heart is displaced to the right chest. **B,** Intestine in left chest has begun to fill with air. The heart is now farther to the right. Fortunately, the infant was bagged with mask for only a short time. Longer periods fill the intestine to produce more tension in left chest, as seen in Fig. 8-29.

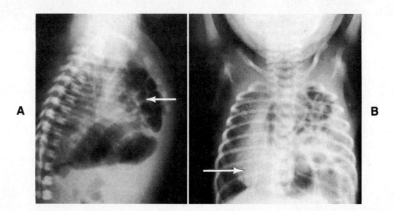

Fig. 8-29. Diaphragmatic hernia. **A,** Lateral view. The cystic appearance in the chest (arrow) is caused by air-filled loops of intestine. **B,** Anteroposterior view. Gas-filled intestinal loops fill the left chest, displacing the heart (arrow) into the right chest. Heart sounds are thus heard in the right chest, and breath sounds in the left chest are virtually absent. (Courtesy Webster Riggs, M. D., LeBonheur Children's Hospital, Memphis, Tenn.)

placement of the cardiac impulse to one side of the chest is the most telling indication of the diagnosis, but pneumothorax can produce the same displacement. If the cardiac impulse is shifted to one side or the other, there should be an immediate realization that one is not dealing solely with the type of perinatal asphyxia in which resuscitative measures would be expected to alleviate much of the difficulty. The abdomen is sometimes sunken (scaphoid), but this condition depends on the displacement of a considerable amount of intestine. More often, the abdominal contour is normal. Diminished breath sounds are the rule in the involved hemithorax.

A chest film confirms the diagnosis. The diaphragmatic margin is absent on the defective side, and the presence of inappropriate thoracic structures is readily discerned. The gas-filled intestines may impart a multicystic appearance to the left chest (Fig. 8-29). If the right side is affected, the liver casts a homogeneous density in the area it occupies. Absence or diminution of the normal liver shadow in the abdomen is another revealing radiologic sign.

The case fatality rate is high, being influenced by the rapidity of diagnosis and surgical correction. Even with optimal management, death is frequent because severe pulmonary hypoplasia precludes effective ventilation. Surgery is the only effective treatment, and it must be done with dispatch. Some infants expire before surgery can be initiated.

RESPIRATORY DISTRESS OF EXTRAPULMONARY ORIGIN

Respiratory distress may be the most prominent sign of a number of disorders of extrapulmonary origin. They fall into four broad categories: (1) congenital heart disease, (2) depression resulting from drugs, (3) metabolic acidosis of nonpulmonary origin, and (4) central nervous system disorders.

Congenital heart disease

In most instances, by the time respiratory difficulty appears in infants with major cardiac anomalies, congestive failure is well developed. In our experience, patent ductus arteriosus in small premature infants is the most common condition associated with congestive failure and pulmonary edema. A high mortality rate during the neonatal period among these infants is well documented. Of the many types of lesions involved in cardiac anomalies, approximately eight of them account for most deaths. Three of these eight anomalies are responsible for almost half the deaths: hypoplastic left heart syndrome (hypoplasia of the left ventricle, aortic atresia, and mitral atresia), coarctation of the aorta, and transposition of the great vessels. The remaining five conditions that are most frequently lethal in the first month of life include hypoplastic right heart syndrome with pulmonary arterial atresia or stenosis, tetralogy of Fallot, truncus arteriosus, endocardial cushion defect, and ventricular septal defect.

Respiratory distress of cardiac origin usually can be identified with the aid of a few simple observations. Breathing is rapid, but not often labored or obstructed. *Cardiovascular pathology is a prominent diagnostic probability in infants who require oxygen and who breathe rapidly with little or no retraction of the chest wall.* Congenital heart disease and septicemia are the most likely probabilities. Occasionally, early pneumonia causes this same pattern of respiration in babies who require oxygen. Heart sounds are loud and rapid. A gallop rhythm is particularly indicative of heart failure. Enlargement of the liver (more than 3 cm below the right costal margin), when present, is also a valuable sign. Enlargement of the heart can be seen on the chest film of almost all infants in congestive heart failure. These signs indicate primary cardiac dysfunction, and with few exceptions the electrocardiogram is abnormal in their presence.

Effects of drugs

Respiratory distress resulting from drugs is characterized by depressed function rather than the rapid, facile breathing associated with heart disease or the rapid, labored breathing so typical of intrinsic lung disorders. Drugs that depress neonates are administered to their mothers during labor; they are usually anesthetics and analgesics. Almost all of these agents are known to cross the placenta. Affected infants usually initiate respiration, but the breathing that follows is shallow and slow. If depression is sufficiently deep, generalized cyanosis may be prominent. Cardiac activity is normal, unless hypoxemic bradycardia occurs as a result of depressed ventilation. The breath sounds are diminished, but only because respiration is shallow, thus reducing air intake. Painful stimuli cause little response in depressed infants, and, at best, the cry is feeble.

Barbiturates are notorious depressive agents. They cross the placenta rapidly. Infants who are born a few hours after maternal barbiturate administration have significant blood levels of the drug for several days after birth. Liberal use of barbiturates during labor and delivery has been curtailed.

Inhalational agents are often used in combination with other drugs during labor, and their individual effects are difficult to evaluate. Anesthetic concentrations of nitrous oxide over 75% generally produce asphyxiated infants. Maternal overdosage with any of these agents will cause depressed respiratory function in the neonate.

Narcotic analgesics are used extensively during the management of labor and delivery. Meperidine is most commonly employed, and its administration in doses that depress the infant is widespread. If it is given intramuscularly between 1 and 3 hours before delivery, some degree of neonatal depression is almost inevitable. If it is administered intramuscularly within an hour of birth in appropriate dosage, significant depression does not usually occur. The effects of meperidine are potentiated if barbiturates are used in combination with it.

Metabolic acidosis of extrapulmonary origin

Rapid respiration is stimulated by an abnormally low pH; if the lungs are normal, increased carbon dioxide excretion occurs and the arterial Pco_2 is reduced. Metabolic acidosis of extrapulmonary origin is most often caused by renal disorders, diarrhea, infection, and a peculiarity of protein metabolism in premature infants called "late metabolic acidosis." The respiratory rate usually subsides after proper alkali therapy for correction of the blood pH.

Central nervous system disorders

Intracranial hemorrhage occurs most frequently in premature infants in whom it is usually of intraventricular or subarachnoid origin. In term infants, subdural and intracerebral hemorrhages are more common. These episodes severely depress respiratory function. Sporadic apnea and irregular breathing are characteristic. Blood gas and pH alterations are identical to those of perinatal asphyxia.

SUMMARY

Respiratory problems are the most frequent cause of neonatal mortality and morbidity. Although most often attributable to intrinsic lung disease, some form of abnormal respiration is inevitable in any type of serious illness; the diagnostic possibilities suggested by breathing difficulties are thus numerous. Several situations require immediate diagnosis and therapy; such optimal management is often lifesaving. No one can better make the first discovery of serious respiratory dysfunction than the nurse, nor is anyone else better equipped to ascertain that therapy is proceeding effectively and without jeopardy to the infant.

REFERENCES

Avery, M. E., Fletcher, B. D., and Williams, R. G.: Hyaline membrane disease. In The lung and its disorders in the newborn infant, Philadelphia, 1981, W. B. Saunders Co.

Avery, M. E., Gatewood, O. B., and Brumley, G.: Transient tachypnea of newborn, Am. J. Dis. Child. **111:**380, 1966.

Avery, M. E., and Said, S.: Surface phenomena in lungs in health and disease, Medicine **44:**503, 1965.

Bancalari, E., and Berlin, J. A.: Meconium aspiration and other asphyxial disorders, Clin. Perinatol. **5:**317, 1978.

Berman, W., Dubynsky, O., Whitman, V., et al.: Digoxin therapy in low-birth-weight infants with patent ductus arteriosus, J. Pediatr. **93:**652, 1978.

Butler, J. N., and Claireaux, A. E.: Congenital diaphragmatic hernia as a cause of perinatal mortality, Lancet **1:**659, 1962.

Chernick, V.: Continuous distending pressure in hyaline membrane disease: of devices, disadvantages, and a daring study, Pediatrics **52:**114, 1973.

Chernick, V.: Onset of breathing at birth, Sem. Perinatol. **1:**343, 1977.

Chernick, V.: Mechanics of the first inspiration, Sem. Perinatol. **1:**347, 1977.

Chernick, V.: The first expiration: role of pulmonary surfactant, Sem. Perinatol. **1:**351, 1977.

Chernick, V., and Reed, M. H.: Pneumothorax and chylothorax in the neonatal period, J. Pediatr. **76:**624, 1970.

Cifuentes, R. F., Olley, P. M., Balfe, J. W., et al.: Indomethacin and renal function in premature infants with persistent patent ductus arteriosus, J. Pediatr. **95:**583, 1979.

Collaborative Group on Antenatal Steroid Therapy: Effects of antenatal dexamethasone administration in the infant: long-term follow-up, J. Pediatr. **104:**259, 1984.

Comroe, J. H., Jr.: Physiology of respiration, ed. 3, Chicago, 1974, Year Book Medical Publishers.

Corazza, M. S., Davis, R. F., Merritt, T. A., et al.: Prolonged bleeding time in preterm infants receiving indomethacin for patent ductus arteriosus, J. Pediatr. **105:**292, 1984.

Corbet, A.: Surfactant secretion and turnover. In Stern, L., editor: Hyaline membrane disease—pathogenesis and pathophysiology, Orlando, 1984, Grune and Stratton.

Corbet, A., and Adams, J.: Current therapy in hyaline membrane disease, Clin. Perinatol. **5:**299, 1978.

Cotton, R. B., Stahlman, M. T., Kova, I., and Catterton, W. Z.: Medical management of small preterm infants with symptomatic patent ductus arteriosus, J. Pediatr. **92:**467, 1978.

Danford, D. A., Miske, S., Headley, J., and Nelson, R. M.: Effects of routine care procedures on transcutaneous oxygen in neonates: a quantitative approach, Arch. Dis. Child. **58:**20, 1983.

Dawes, G. S.: Fetal circulation and breathing, Clin. Obstet. Gynecol. **1:**139, 1974.

Drummond, W. H., Peckham, G. J., and Fox, W. W.: The clinical profile of the newborn with persistent pulmonary hypertension: observations in 19 affected neonates, Clin. Pediatr. **16:**335, 1977.

Duc, G.: Assessment of hypoxia in the newborn, suggestions for a practical approach, Pediatrics **48:**469, 1971.

Ellison, R. C., Peckham, G. J., Lang, P., et al.: Evaluation of the preterm infant for patent ductus arteriosus, Pediatrics **71:**364, 1983.

Fanaroff, A. A., and Martin, R. J.: The respiratory system: other pulmonary problems—meconium aspiration syndromes. In Behrman's neonatal-perinatal medicine, St. Louis, 1983, The C. V. Mosby Co.

Fenner, R., Muller, H. G., Busse, M., et al.: Transcutaneous determination of arterial oxygen tension, Pediatrics **55:**224, 1975.

Fitzhardinge, P. M.: Follow-up studies in infants treated by mechanical ventilation, Clin. Perinatol. **5**:451, 1978.

Fletcher, B. D.: The radiology of respiratory distress syndrome and its sequelae. In Stern, L., editor: Hyaline membrane disease—pathogenesis and pathophysiology, Orlando, 1984, Grune and Stratton.

Fox, W. W., et al.: Pulmonary hypertension and the perinatal aspiration syndromes, Pediatrics **59**:205, 1977.

Fox, W. W., Gutsche, B. B., and DeVore, J. S.: A delivery room approach to the meconium aspiration syndrome (MAS), Clin. Pediatr. **16**:325, 1977.

Friedman, W. F., Heymann, M. A., and Rudolph, A. M.: Commentary: new thoughts on an old problem—patent ductus arteriosus in the premature infant, J. Pediatr. **90**:338, 1977.

Friedman, W. F., Fitzpatrick, K. M., Merritt, T. A., and Feldman, B. H.: The patent ductus arteriosus, Clin. Perinatol. **5**:411, 1978.

Gerhardt, T., and Bancalari, E.: Apnea of prematurity. I. Lung function and regulation of breathing, Pediatrics **74**:58, 1984.

Gerhardt, T., and Bancalari, E.: Apnea of prematurity. II. Respiratory reflexes, Pediatrics **74**:63, 1984.

Gersony, W. M., Peckham, G. J., Ellison, R. C., et al.: Effects of indomethacin in premature infants with patent ductus arteriosus: results of a national collaborative study, J. Pediatr. **102**:895, 1983.

Goldman, H. I., Maralit, A., Sun, S., and Lanzkowsky, P.: Neonatal cyanosis and arterial oxygen saturation, J. Pediatr. **82**:319, 1973.

Gregory, G. A., Gooding, C. A., Phibbs, R. H., and Tooley, W. H.: Meconium aspiration in infants: a prospective study, J. Pediatr. **85**:848, 1974.

Gregory, G. A., et al.: Treatment of the idiopathic respiratory distress syndrome with continuous positive airway pressure, N. Engl. J. Med. **284**:1333, 1971.

Hall, R. T., and Rhodes, P. R.: Pneumothorax and pneumomediastinum in infants with idiopathic respiratory distress syndrome receiving continuous positive airway pressure, Pediatrics **55**:493, 1975.

Hallman, M., Merritt, T. A., and Ardinger, R.: The development and functional significance of lung surfactant. In Stern, L., editor: Hyaline membrane disease—pathogenesis and pathophysiology, Orlando, 1984, Grune and Stratton.

Harding, R.: Fetal breathing. In Beard, R. W., and Nathanielsz, P. W., editors: Fetal physiology and medicine—the basis of perinatology, New York, 1984, Marcel Dekker.

Harned, H. S., Jr., and Ferreiro, J.: Initiation of breathing by cold stimulation: effects of change in ambient temperature on respiratory activity of the full-term fetal lamb, J. Pediatr. **83**:663, 1973.

Harrison, V. C., Heese, H. de V., and Klein, M. B.: The significance of grunting in hyaline membrane disease, Pediatrics **41**:549, 1968.

Hart, S. M., McNair, M., Gamsu, H. R., and Price, J. F.: Pulmonary interstitial emphysema in very low birthweight infants, Arch. Dis. Child. **58**:612, 1983.

Hartmann, A. F., Jr., Klint, R., Hernandez, A., and Goldring, D.: Measurement of blood pressure in the brachial and posterior tibial arteries using the Doppler method, J. Pediatr. **82**:498, 1973.

Hislop, A., and Reid, L.: Growth and development of the respiratory system: anatomical development. In Davis, J. A., and Dobbing, J., editors: Scientific foundations of paediatrics, Baltimore, 1982, University Park Press.

Hittner, H. M., Godio, L. B., Rudolph, A. J., et al.: Retrolental fibroplasia: efficacy of vitamin E in a double-blind clinical study of preterm infants, N. Engl. J. Med. **305**:1365, 1981.

Hittner, H. M., Godio, L. B., Speer, M. E., et al.: Retrolental fibroplasia: further clinical evidence and ultrastructural support for efficacy of vitamin E in the preterm infant, Pediatrics **71**:423, 1983.

Huch, A., and Huch, R.: Transcutaneous, noninvasive monitoring of PO_2 Hosp. Prac. **11**:43, 1976.

Jobe, A.: Respiratory distress syndrome—new therapeutic approaches to a complex pathophysiology. In Barness, L. A., editor: Advances in pediatrics, vol. 30, Chicago, 1984, Year Book Medical Publishers.

Johnson, J. D., Malachowski, N. C., Grobsein, R., et al.: Prognosis of children surviving with the aid of mechanical ventilation in the newborn period, J. Pediatr. **84**:272, 1974.

Kao, L. C., Warburton, D., Platzker, A. C. G., and Keens, T. G.: Effect of isoproterenol inhalation on airway resistance in chronic bronchopulmonary dysplasia, Pediatrics **73**:509, 1984.

Kao, L. C., Warburton, D., Sargent, C. W., Platzker, A. C. G., and Keens, T. G.: Furosemide acutely decreases airways resistance in chronic broncho-pulmonary dysplasia, J. Pediatr. **103**:624, 1983.

Karlberg, P.: The first breaths of life. In Gluck, L., editor: Modern perinatal medicine, Chicago, 1974, Year Book Medical Publishers.

Kattwinkel, J., Fleming, D., Cha, C. C., et al.: A device for administration of continuous positive airway pressure by the nasal route, Pediatrics **52**:131, 1973.

Klaus, M. H.: Cleansing the neonatal trachea, J. Pediatr. **85**:853, 1974.

Koop, C. E., Schnaufer, L., and Broennie, A. M.: Esophageal atresia and tracheoesophageal fistula: supportive measures that affect survival, Pediatrics **54**:558, 1974.

Korones, S. B., and Eyal, F. G.: Successful treatment of persistent fetal circulation with tolazoline (abstract), Pediatr. Res. **9**:367, 1975.

Kotas, R. V.: Surface tension forces and liquid balance in the lung. In Thibeault, D. W., and Gregory, G. A., editors: Neonatal pulmonary care, Reading, Mass. 1979, Addison-Wesley Publishing Co.

Krauss, D. R., and Marshall, R. E.: Severe neck ulceration from CPAP head box, J. Pediatr. **86:**286, 1975.

Kuhns, L. R., Bednarek, F. J., and Wyman, M. L.: Diagnosis of pneumothorax or pneumomediastinum in the neonate by transillumination, Pediatrics **56:**355, 1975.

Langston, C., and Thurlbeck, W. M.: Lung growth and development in late gestation and early postnatal life. In Rosenberg, H. S., and Berstein, J., editors: Perspectives in pediatric pathology, New York, 1982, Masson Publishing USA.

Levy, R. J.: Persistent pulmonary hypertension in a newborn with congenital diaphragmatic hernia: successful management with tolazoline, Pediatrics **60:**740, 1977.

Liggins, G. C.: The prevention of RDS by maternal steroid therapy. In Gluck, L., editor: Modern perinatal medicine, Chicago, 1974, Year Book Medical Publishers.

Lucey, J. F.: A reexamination of the role of oxygen in retrolental fibroplasia, Pediatrics **73:**82, 1984.

Marriage, K. J., and Davies, P. A.: Neurological sequelae in children surviving mechanical ventilation in the neonatal period, Arch. Dis. Child. **52:**176, 1977.

Martin, C. G., Snider, A. R., Katz, S. M., et al.: Abnormal cerebral blood flow patterns in preterm infants with a large patent ductus arteriosus, J. Pediatr. **101:**587, 1982.

Merenstein, G. B., Dougherty, K., and Lewis, A.: Early detection of pneumothorax by oscilloscope monitor in the newborn infant, J. Pediatr. **80:**98, 1972.

Merritt, T. A., DiSessa, T. G., Feldman, B. H., et al.: Closure of the patent ductus arteriosus with ligation and indomethacin: a consecutive experience, J. Pediatr. **93:**639, 1978.

Milner, A. D., and Vyas, H.: Lung expansion at birth, J. Pediatr. **101:**879, 1982.

Morrow, G., III, Hope, J. W., and Boggs, R., Jr.: Pneumomediastinum: a silent lesion in the newborn, J. Pediatr. **70:**554, 1967.

Najak, Z. D., Harris, E. M., Lazzara, A., and Pruitt, A. W.: Pulmonary effects of furosemide in preterm infants with lung disease, J. Pediatr. **102:**758, 1983.

Neal, W. A., and Mullett, M. D.: Patent ductus arteriosus in premature infants: a review of current management, Pediatr. Cardiol. **3:**59, 1982.

Northway, W. J., Jr., Rosan, R. C., and Porter, D. Y.: Pulmonary disease following respirator therapy of hyaline-membrane disease: bronchopulmonary dysplasia, N. Engl. J. Med. **276:**357, 1967.

Oski, F. A., and Delivoria-Papadopoulos, M.: The red cell, 2,3-diphosphoglycerate, and tissue oxygen release, J. Pediatr. **77:**941, 1970.

Owens, W. C., and Owens, E. U.: Retrolental fibroplasia in premature infants, Am. J. Ophthalmol. **32:**1631, 1949.

Patrick, J.: Fetal breathing and body movements. In Creasey, R. K., and Resnik, R., editors: Maternal-fetal medicine—principles and practice, Philadelphia, 1984, W. B. Saunders Co.

Patrick, J.: Fetal breathing movements, Sem. Perinatol. **4:**249, 1980.

Peckham, G. J., Miettinen, O. S., Ellison, R. C., et al.: Clinical course to 1 year of age in premature infants with patent ductus arteriosus: results of a multicenter randomized trial of indomethacin, J. Pediatr. **105:**285, 1984.

Perelman, R. H., and Farrell, P. M.: Analysis of causes of neonatal death in the United States with specific emphasis on fatal hyaline membrane disease, Pediatrics **70:**570, 1982.

Phelps, D. L.: Retinopathy of prematurity: an estimate of vision loss in the United States—1979, Pediatrics **67:**924, 1981.

Phelps, D. L., and Rosenbaum, A. L.: Effects of marginal hypoxemia on recovery from oxygen-induced retinopathy in the kitten model, Pediatrics **73:**1, 1984.

Phelps, D. L.: Vitamin E and retrolental fibroplasia in 1982, Pediatrics **70:**420, 1982.

Philip, A. G. S.: Oxygen plus pressure plus time: the etiology of bronchopulmonary dysplasia, Pediatrics **55:**44, 1975.

Primhak, R. A.: Factors associated with pulmonary air leak in premature infants receiving mechanical ventilation, J. Pediatr. **102:**764, 1983.

Rhodes, P. G., Graves, G. R., Patel, D. M., et al.: Minimizing pneumothorax and bronchopulmonary dysplasia in ventilated infants with hyaline membrane disease, J. Pediatr. **103:**634, 1983.

Robert, M. F., Neff, R. K., Hubbell, J. B., et al.: Maternal diabetes and the respiratory distress syndrome, N. Engl. J. Med. **294:**357, 1976.

Rome, E. S., Stork, E. K., Carlo, W. A., and Martin, R. J.: Limitations of transcutaneous PO_2 and PCO_2 monitoring in infants with bronchopulmonary dysplasia, Pediatrics **74:**217, 1984.

Rooth, G.: Transcutaneous oxygen tension measurements in newborn infants, Pediatrics **55:**232, 1975.

Rowe, R. D.: Abnormal pulmonary vasoconstriction in the newborn, Pediatrics **59:**318, 1977.

Rudolph, A. M.: Congenital diseases of the heart, Chicago, 1974, Year Book Medical Publishers.

Scarpelli, E. M., and Moss, I. R.: Transition from fetal to neonatal breathing. In Gootman, N., and Gootman, P. M., editors: Perinatal cardiovascular function, New York, 1983, Marcel Dekker.

Silverman, W. A.: Retinopathy of prematurity: oxygen dogma challenged, Arch. Dis. Child. **57:**731, 1982.

Spitzer, A. R., and Fox, W. W.: The use and abuse of mechanical ventilation. In Stern, L., editor: Hyaline membrane disease—pathogenesis and pathophysiology, Orlando, 1984, Grune and Stratton.

Stahlman, M.: Recovery from the respiratory distress syndrome, Pediatrics **52:**280, 1973.

Stahlman, M. T.: The history of hyaline membrane disease and the development of its concepts. In Stern, L., editor:

Hyaline membrane disease—Pathogenesis and pathophysiology, Orlando, 1984, Grune and Stratton.

Stahlman, M., Hedvall, G., Dolanski, E., et al.: A six-year follow-up of clinical hyaline membrane disease, Pediatr. Clin. North Am. **20**:433, 1973.

Stern, L.: The use and misuse of oxygen in the newborn infant, Pediatr. Clin. North Am. **20**:447, 1973.

Stevenson, D. K., et al.: Refractory hypoxemia associated with neonatal pulmonary disease: the use and limitations of tolazoline, J. Pediatr. **95**:595, 1979.

Strang, L. B.: Onset of breathing and its control in the neonatal period. In Neonatal respiration: physiological and clinical studies, Philadelphia, 1977, Blackwell Scientific Publications.

Strong, R. M., and Passey, V.: Endotracheal intubation, Arch. Otolaryngol. **103**:329, 1977.

Sundell, H., et al.: Studies on infants with type II respiratory distress syndrome, J. Pediatr. **78**:754, 1971.

Thibeault, D. W., Lachman, R. S., Laul, V. R., and Kwong, M. S.: Pulmonary interstitial emphysema, pneumomediastinum, and pneumothorax, Am. J. Dis. Child. **126**:611, 1973.

Ting, P., and Brady, J.: Tracheal suction in meconium aspiration, Pediatr. Res. **7**:398, 1973.

Tyler, D. C., Murphy, J., and Cheney, F. W.: Mechanical and chemical damage to lung tissue caused by meconium aspiration, Pediatrics **62**:454, 1978.

Versmold, H. T., Kitterman, J. A., Phibbs, R. H., et al.: Aortic blood pressure during the first 12 hours of life in infants with birth weight 610 to 4,220 grams, Pediatrics **67**:607, 1981.

Vidyasagar, D.: Clinical features of respiratory distress syndrome. In Stern, L.: Hyaline membrane disease—pathogenesis and pathophysiology, Orlando, 1984, Grune and Stratton.

Walsh, S. Z., Meyer, W. W., and Lind, J.: The human fetal and neonatal circulation, Springfield, Ill. 1974, Charles C Thomas, Publisher.

Wigglesworth, J. S.: The respiratory system. In Bennington, J. L., editor: Perinatal pathology, Philadelphia, 1984, W. B. Saunders Co.

Workshop on bronchopulmonary dysplasia, J. Pediatr. **95**:815-920, 1979.

Yao, A. C.: Cardiovascular changes during the transition from fetal to neonatal life. In Gootman, N., and Gootman, P. M.: Perinatal cardiovascular function, New York, 1983, Marcel Dekker.

Yeh, T. F., Vidyasagar, D., and Pildes, R. S.: Neonatal pneumopericardium, Pediatrics **54**:429, 1974.

Yeh, T. F., Srinivasan, G., Harris, V., and Pildes, R. S.: Hydrocortisone therapy in meconium aspiration syndrome: a controlled study, J. Pediatr. **90**:140, 1977.

Yu, V. Y. H., Liew, S. W., and Roberton, N. R. C.: Pneumothorax in the newborn: changing pattern, Arch. Dis. Child. **50**:449, 1975.

Hematologic disorders

Perplexing hematologic problems are more frequent during the neonatal period than at any other time in childhood. The most common manifestations of neonatal blood disorders are anemia, hemorrhage into tissues, hyperbilirubinemia, and polycythemia. Anemia may be the end result of hemolysis, blood loss, or impaired red cell production. Hemorrhage into tissues is produced by disorders of the clotting mechanism. Hyperbilirubinemia follows intravascular hemolysis or the degradation of extravasated blood. Polycythemia is the result of an oversupply of blood to the fetus.

HEMOGLOBIN CONCENTRATIONS IN NORMAL NEONATAL BLOOD

The normal neonate's blood volume at birth is influenced by the quantity of blood allowed to flow from the placenta before the cord is clamped. The placental circulation contains approximately 75 to 125 ml at term, comprising one fourth to one third of total fetal blood volume. The infant's blood volume may be increased significantly by allowing the placenta to empty. At birth, infants held at levels below the placenta tend to acquire blood, and those held above it may lose some. In normal circumstances approximately 25% of the placental blood is transfused into the infant within 15 seconds after birth; at the end of 1 minute 50% of blood is transferred. If a term infant is held below the level of the placenta and clamping of the cord is delayed several minutes, blood volume can be increased by 40% to 60%. The increase is proportionately greater in a premature infant because the same quantity of blood is transferred from the placenta to the smaller intravascular volume of the premature infant. Placental blood content changes little during the last trimester so that potential volume of placental transfusions will not differ as gestational age advances.

Whether this added volume has a salutary effect on the baby's subsequent course has not been well defined. Thus some studies indicate a lower incidence of respiratory distress if cord clamping is delayed, whereas others do not demonstrate such an association. In any event, during the first few days of life, hemoglobin concentrations are higher in babies whose cords are clamped late, but there is no evidence that the additional hemoglobin is of any particular benefit.

Hemoglobin and hematocrit determinations may vary according to sampling site. At birth and for several days thereafter, hemoglobin concentration is higher in capillary than in venous blood. Normal hemoglobin concentration in cord blood ranges from 16 to 19 g/100 ml (mean, 16.8 g/100 ml), whereas capillary values may be 2 to 8 g/100 ml higher. Even higher capillary levels may result from peripheral circulatory stasis, in which slowed blood flow causes stasis of the red blood cells, thereby increasing their concentration.

Normally, hemoglobin concentrations rise up to 6 g/100 ml during the first few hours of life, particularly if the cord is clamped late. This rise is a result of shifts of fluid that result in decreased plasma volume. After 24 hours they decline slightly, and by the end of the first week hemoglobin levels are at least equal to or greater than that of cord blood. In normal term infants, there is ordinarily no significant decrease in hemoglobin during the first week of life. A drop during this period usually indicates blood loss or hemolysis. Venous values below 13 g/100 ml or capillary hemoglobin less than 14.5 g/100 ml are indicative of anemia. A normal decrease continues after the first week. At birth the reticulocyte count is 4% to 5% at term, but by the end of the first week it is 1% or less. In premature infants on the first day, reticulocytes range from 10% to 12% at 26 gestational weeks, down to approximately 4% at 36 weeks.

ANEMIA RESULTING FROM HEMOLYSIS

An abnormally rapid rate of red cell breakdown causes anemia and hyperbilirubinemia. Ordinarily, erythropoiesis increases in response to hemolysis, thus augmenting the number of reticulocytes and nucleated red cells in circulating blood. The hallmarks of hemolysis are anemia, hyperbilirubinemia, reticulocytosis, and increased numbers of nucleated red cells. The most common causes of fetal and neonatal hemolysis are isoimmunization (maternofetal blood incompatibility) and infection. Less frequently, hemolytic anemia results from toxic drug effects, erythrocyte enzyme defects, or abnormal red cell morphology.

Isoimmunization: Rh incompatibility (erythroblastosis fetalis)

Erythroblastosis fetalis is also known as *hemolytic disease of the newborn*. Before the widespread use of anti-Rh gamma globulin (Rhogam) to prevent fetal disease, approximately one third of all cases of isoimmunization involved Rh incompatibility; this form of the disease is often serious. In the U.S., Rh disease is now infrequent because of Rhogam immunization.

Most cases of isoimmunization now result from ABO incompatibility, which is generally mild, occasionally severe.

Antigens and blood group factors. The terms *blood group antigens* and *blood group factors* are used interchangeably. There are a number of blood group systems, of which the Rh and ABO systems are the most significant. Other antigenic systems are only rarely involved in maternofetal blood incompatibilities. An antigen is a substance that stimulates the production of antibodies. Thousands of discrete patches of red cell antigens are situated on or in the covering cell membrane. The Rh system is composed of six factors: C,c, D,d, and E,e. Although the terms *Rh positive* and *Rh negative* strictly indicate the presence or absence of any Rh factor, in common usage these terms refer to the D factor, which is involved in 95% of Rh incompatibilities.

Pathogenesis. In the pathogenesis of Rh disease, fetal red cells pass across the placenta to an Rh-negative mother, who produces antibodies to Rh antigen on fetal red cell surfaces. These antibodies are transmitted across the placenta to the fetus; they become attached to fetal red cells, and hemolysis follows. This course of events requires maternal antibody production, which can occur only in the presence of incompatibility between mother and fetus (Rh-negative mother, Rh-positive fetus). *The mother produces antibodies to fetal antigens only if her own cells lack these antigens.* This is the basis of Rh incompatibility. Thus an Rh-negative mother (whose cells lack D factor) is the recipient of erythrocytes from her Rh-positive fetus. She responds by generating anti-D antibodies, which pass across the placenta and become attached to the D antigen on fetal red cells, causing their eventual dissolution.

During normal pregnancy, small quantities of fetal blood (0.1 to 0.2 ml) may cross the placenta into the maternal circulation, whereas larger amounts are transferred during placental separation. During a first pregnancy, initial sensitization to D antigens does not occur prior to the onset of labor because at least 0.5 to 1 ml is required for a sensitizing maternal immune response. Thus the minute leakage of fetal blood before labor is insufficient to sensitize a primigravida, but the larger amount of blood transferred during placental separation is sufficient to cause sensitization. During the second pregnancy with an Rh-positive fetus, the usual small amount of fetal blood leakage now acts as a booster dose because the mother has been previously sensitized, and her antibody production increases remarkably. Offspring of this and all subsequent pregnancies may thus be affected. Firstborn babies may be erythroblastotic if maternal sensitization has occurred after past transfusion of Rh-positive blood or if there was previous abortion of an Rh-positive fetus, but these events are not common.

The incidence of Rh (D) disease in a given population varies inversely with the extent of *immunization by Rh immunoglobulin (Rhogam)*. For over 20 years we have had the capacity to eliminate the disorder worldwide, not unlike the contemporary elimination of smallpox throughout the world. The prevalence of Rh disease also varies considerably by *race*. Thus the highest incidence is among Caucasians, 15% of whom are Rh negative. In contrast, the incidence of Rh negativity among Asians is zero. Among blacks (American) the incidence is between 5% and 6%.

The incidence of maternal sensitization to Rh (D) factor among Rh-negative women is estimated at approximately 20% after the second pregnancy. Thus there are several variables that ultimately affect the appearance of fetal disease. *The maternal capacity to react* to Rh (D) antigen is one, because the response to Rh antigenic stimuli is not universal among Rh-negative women. Multiple injections of Rh-positive red cells into Rh-negative individuals causes Rh (D) antibodies in only half the injected subjects. *ABO incompatibility* is another variable that affects sensitization. It can diminish the response to Rh antigen in women who would otherwise react to it. The protective effect of ABO incompatibility is a result of destruction of type A or B Rh-positive red cells by anti-A or anti-B antibody. Anti-A or anti-B destruction occurs before the cells can stimulate maternal production of anti-Rh (D) antibodies. This early destruction of ABO-incompatible erythrocytes is not a universal phenomenon. There are many exceptions. Fetal Rh disease does in fact occur in the presence of an associated ABO incompatibility, but Rh sensitization may be reduced significantly.

The *volume of fetal blood transferred* to a mother across the placenta is especially important. The greater the volume of transplacental fetomaternal hemorrhage, the more likely the occurrence of Rh sensitization. The importance of obstetric factors is preeminent. The clinical entities associated with larger volumes of transplacental hemorrhage are as follows:

- Toxemia;
- Cesarean section;
- Breech delivery;
- Transverse lie;
- Twin pregnancy;
- Placenta previa;
- Abruptio placentae;
- Manual removal of placenta;
- External cephalic version;
- Amniocentesis complicated by placental hemorrhage; and
- Abortion (particularly therapeutic).

Clinical manifestations. The disease begins in utero, at which time its severity can be estimated by analysis of amniotic fluid (Chapter 1). In response to hemolysis, the rate of erythropoiesis is accelerated, and immature red cells (erythroblasts) appear in the fetal circulation. Red cell destruction releases hemoglobin, thus increasing the formation of bilirubin, which is largely, although not entirely, excreted across the placenta into the maternal circulation. At birth most affected infants have slightly elevated bilirubin levels, but jaundice is rarely evident. Anemia is present in proportion to the severity of hemolysis.

If amniocentesis has not been performed, the first visible indication of the severity of the disease may be the color of amniotic fluid at the time of membrane rupture. Straw-colored fluid is usually associated with mild or absent fetal disease; deep yellow fluid indicates a severely involved fetus. Intrauterine death may be associated with green- or brown-tinted fluid.

Most mildly affected infants appear to be normal at birth, although the liver and spleen may be somewhat enlarged. If the fetus is profoundly affected, pallor is obvious because of anemia.

Jaundice. The hemolytic process that originated in utero continues after birth. Bilirubin production increases as a function of hemolysis, and now it accumulates in the infant because placental excretion is precluded. Although jaundice is usually not apparent at birth, it may appear 30 minutes later in the most severely affected babies. As a rule, it is evident within 24 to 36 hours.

Anemia. Anemia may be progressive and severe, or it may be minimal. Most infants are mildly anemic. Much depends on the infant's capacity to replace erythrocytes by active erythropoiesis. In severe disease, neither fetus nor neonate can compensate for the anemia that follows erythrocyte destruction. Most red blood cell destruction occurs in the spleen, but rarely in profoundly affected infants hemolysis may be intravascular. In either case, red cell volume diminishes, plasma volume increases, and total blood volume is unchanged. Intravascular hemolysis releases hemoglobin into plasma and results in hemoglobinuria. If anemia is sufficiently severe, oxygen content of blood is lowered to cause significant tissue hypoxia and then metabolic acidosis.

Hepatosplenomegaly. Hepatosplenomegaly occurs in virtually all affected infants. Most of the enlargement results from an extensive extramedullary hematopoiesis that is clearly visible by light microscopy. Splenomegaly is also caused by massive erythrocyte destruction. The enlarged spleen is fragile, and it may rupture as the infant is manipulated during delivery, resuscitation, abdominal palpation, or during the exchange transfusion.

Bleeding. Bleeding occurs in severely affected babies. It is always associated with thrombocytopenia, and sometimes with coagulation defects as well. Ecchymoses and petechiae in the skin are common signs; hemorrhages into lungs and brain also occur.

Hypoglycemia. Hypoglycemia is a result of hyperplasia of beta cells in the islets of Langerhans, thereby increasing plasma insulin levels. Symptomatic hypoglycemia (see Chapter 11) is frequent in Rh disease; it occurs most often in babies whose cord blood hemoglobin is less than 10 g/dl. The more severe the hemolysis, the more likely is hypoglycemia. Signs of low blood glucose may appear before, during, or after exchange transfusion. Posttransfusion hypoglycemia may have no relation to hyperinsulinemia. After transfusion, hypoglycemia is a response to the transient elevations of blood sugar that often occur during the procedure. At that time, insulin production is stimulated. When the transfusion is terminated, the source of increased glucose (ACD or CPD donor blood) is removed, but circulating insulin is still copious and hypoglycemia follows. This reaction is not different from the hypoglycemia caused by the cessation of glucose input when an IV infiltrates. The posttransfusion response is exaggerated in babies whose severe Rh disease is associated with beta cell hyperplasia.

Hydrops fetalis. Hydrops fetalis is the most severe expression of Rh disease. Progressive anemia due to intense hemolysis leads to fetal hypoxia, cardiac failure, generalized edema, and effusion of fluid into the pleural, pericardial, and peritoneal spaces. Hypoproteinemia largely resulting from diminished plasma albumin is common. Some authors attribute the universal edema to low albumin levels. Others consider heart failure to be most contributory. Hydrops is a frequent cause of intrauterine death among infants with Rh disease. It generally appears between the thirty-fourth and fortieth gestational weeks. Intrauterine transfusion apparently supports some of these infants until an exchange transfusion can be performed after delivery. At birth, the most striking findings of hydrops fetalis include universal edema (anasarca) and alarming pallor. The edema may

be so extensive that the infant is almost twice the expected birth weight for gestational age. Respiratory distress is sometimes severe. Jaundice is usually not apparent until later. Immediate exchange transfusion is urgent, but hydropic infants seldom survive.

Laboratory diagnosis. Fetal diagnosis of the disease and an accurate estimate of its severity are accomplished by analysis of amniotic fluid for bilirubin (Chapter 1). Repeated amniocentesis is usually essential to monitor the extent of fetal involvement. Erythroblastosis can also be anticipated by demonstrating a rising titer of anti-D antibodies in maternal serum during pregnancy, but this is not as reliable as amniotic fluid studies. These antibodies are produced by the mother in response to D factor on fetal cells that leaked through the placenta into her circulation. In the infant the diagnosis is made postnatally by demonstrating these same antibodies on the surface of red blood cells. These maternal antibodies crossed the placenta to enter the fetal circulation. The diagnosis is accomplished by the direct Coombs' test. If anti-D antibody has become attached to D antigen on the infant's erythrocytes, the addition of Coombs' reagent causes visible agglutination of the cells, thus establishing the diagnosis of erythroblastosis. The diagnosis can be excluded if the Coombs' test is negative; but in a few instances of mild hemolysis in which very little antibody coats the infant's red cells, the Coombs' test may also be negative.

The hematologic abnormalities in affected infants are not specific for Rh or other disorders of blood incompatibility, but are rather characteristic of any process of blood loss; hemogloblin concentration decreases, reticulocytes and nucleated red blood cells increase. Strictly interpreted, high reticulocyte counts in Rh disease clearly indicate vigorous erythropoiesis, which in turn suggests an attempt to compensate for loss of hemoglobin. The associated hyperbilirubinemia indicates that loss of hemoglobin results from hemolysis. Hyperbilirubinemia is generally of greater magnitude when anemia is profound. On the other hand, severe hyperbilirubinemia may occur without any significant anemia if erythropoiesis produces sufficient numbers of red cells to replace those that are hemolyzed. In these circumstances, newly generated red cells are a source of additional hemolysis, thus prolonging or exaggerating hyperbilirubinemia. In Rh disease, reticulocyte counts are generally greater than 8%, and nucleated red cells may exceed 10 or 12 per 100 white cells. Severe Rh disease also produces thrombocytopenia; exchange transfusion itself may do likewise.

Treatment: exchange transfusion. The most effective treatment is exchange transfusion. Details of this procedure are well described in monographs devoted to erythroblastosis. Although the indications for exchange transfusions can be complex and equivocal, they are generally performed when bilirubin concentrations reach 20 mg/100 ml in term infants, 15 mg/100 ml in larger premature infants, and lower levels in smaller ones.

The primary purpose of an exchange transfusion is removal of "target organs," namely, the Rh-positive erythrocytes. The exchange removes bilirubin and Rh (D) antibody as well, but these soon reappear in circulating blood because they are distributed between the intravascular and extravascular spaces. Thus they migrate into the blood from interstitial tissue as blood concentrations are reduced during and after the exchange transfusions. The goal of treatment is to prevent the most sinister complication of the disease, kernicterus (p. 327), and to eliminate the possibility of progressively severe anemia. A "two-volume" exchange is used. This term refers to the exchange of an amount of donor blood that is twice the infant's blood volume. Donor blood is thus given at 170 ml//kg of body weight. This volume replaces 85% of the infant's blood. Fresh Rh-negative blood is used, either type O or the infant's own type. The transfusion is given through a catheter in the umbilical vein by removing 4 to 5 ml/kg of body weight and infusing like amounts of donor blood. The procedure is usually completed in 60 to 90 minutes. Each exchange of

blood should take 2 minutes to complete. Careful attention to thermal balance is essential. The procedure thus should be performed under a source of radiant heat. In experienced hands the mortality rate from the complications of exchange transfusion is less than 1%.

Electronic cardiorespiratory monitoring is essential during the procedure. Blood pressure should be taken periodically, or it should be known by continuous electronic display.

Banked blood for exchange transfusion is available in several anticoagulant preservatives, acid-citrate-dextrose (ACD), citrate-dextrose-phosphate (CPD), CPD-adenine (CPD-A), and heparin. CPD-A is currently the preferred anticoagulant preservative. Heparinized blood is not generally recommended because (1) heparin increases lipolysis to elevate levels of free fatty acid, which compete with bilirubin for albumin binding, thus raising concentrations of unbound bilirubin (see Chapter 10); (2) the relatively low blood glucose of heparinized blood may cause hypoglycemia; (3) the anticoagulant effect of heparin may be exaggerated to cause bleeding in sick infants; (4) heparinized blood must be administered within a few hours after collection.

The use of "fresh blood" for exchange transfusion has been universally advocated, but until recently "fresh blood" was defined as banked blood that is no older than 4 or 5 days. However, alarmingly high potassium levels have been noted in blood stored for less than 2 days. In a telling study, 28 separate units of whole blood were sampled for potassium content. None was over 4 days of age, and all were stored in a CPD anticoagulant. Approximately 20% of the units contained potassium in excess of 11 mEq/L. Thirty percent contained more than 9 mEq/L. Normal serum potassium (4.5 mEq) was identified in only 10% of the samples tested. The authors believed that the concentration of preservative was sufficiently hypertonic to damage red cell membranes and cause seepage of potassium from within red cells into the plasma. They found that in some blood units no older than 24 hours, potassium levels were already unacceptably high. This particular study was stimulated by the occurrence of fatal hyperkalemia after exchange transfusion of a sick premature infant with CPD blood that was less than 2 days old. The potassium content of that unit was 13 mEq/L. Thus whenever feasible, blood should not be over 1 or 2 days old. Furthermore, plasma potassium concentration should be determined on whole blood to be used for exchange transfusion, and should be discarded if potassium levels exceed 10 mEq/L. The blood preparation of choice is composed of frozen red cells that are washed and reconstituted with fresh frozen plasma immediately before exchange transfusion.

Although there is considerable hazard of hyperkalemia in whole blood used for *exchange transfusion,* packed red cells used for *simple transfusion* are safe even when potassium levels are considerably elevated. In one study the mean potassium concentration of packed cells on the second day of storage was 16.2 mEq (range, 10.1 to 25.6 mEq). From the fourth through the seventh days of storage, potassium levels rose continuously; the highest level was 30.3 mEq/L in blood that had been stored for 7 days. Despite these high levels, transfusion of these packed red blood cells in volumes of 10 ml/kg did not affect serum potassium concentrations of recipient newborns. In fast, their mean serum potassium levels fell from 5.1 mEq/L to 4.9 mEq/L within an hour after transfusion.

Hazards of exchange transfusion. Complications due to faulty technique are as follows:

Thrombosis is most often associated with difficult and traumatic catheter insertion into the umbilical vein. Thrombi form in the portal vein to later cause portal hypertension during the first 2 years of life. Portal hypertension causes splenomegaly as well as esophageal varices that eventually rupture and bleed dangerously. Uneventful catheter insertion is not usually associated with thrombus formation.

Hepatic necrosis may occur if the catheter rests in the liver where clots may form.

Air embolization follows insertion of a catheter that is open at its distal end. A syringe must be attached to the distal end of the catheter, and both syringe and catheter should be filled with saline prior to insertion.

Septicemia is virtually inevitable if the catheter is inserted through an infected cord or periumbilical area, or from careless contaminating technique.

Cardiac arrhythmia or arrest may follow placement of the catheter tip within the heart when the catheter has been too deeply inserted.

Hypervolemia or hypovolemia follows imbalances between input and output during the exchange transfusion.

Hypothermia has been attributed to the use of cold blood or a cool ambient temperature. Donor blood should be passed through an apparatus made of plastic tubing no less than 6 ft in length and immersed in a 37° C waterbath. The transfusion should be performed on a servocontrolled radiant warmer, taking care to place the skin probe so that it is not covered by drapes.

Biochemical abnormalities caused by exchange transfusion are as follows:

Hyperglycemia during the procedure results from high concentrations of glucose in preservative anticoagulants, heparin excepted.

Hypoglycemia during the procedure occurs as a result of the low glucose concentration of heparinized blood. *Hypoglycemia after the procedure* is a rebound phenomenon caused by the antecedent insulin response to hyperglycemia during the exchange with ACD or CPD donor blood.

Hypocalcemia and hypomagnesemia are decreased in their ionized fractions because the ions combine with citrate in ACD or CPD preservatives. To prevent low calcium, many clinicians infuse 1 ml of 10% calcium gluconate after exchange of 100 ml of blood. Although ionized calcium does in fact decline during the procedure, symptoms are nevertheless rarely evident, and normal levels return spontaneously in a relatively short time. Thus at some centers calcium is not infused periodically during the transfusion. Hypomagnesemia has been observed but its significance and incidence are questionable. Cardiac monitoring must be ongoing during the transfusion to detect electrocardiographic changes associated with hypocalcemia (prolonged Q-T interval).

Following are *blood pressure changes* that occur during the procedure.

Vacillations in arterial pressure are intrinsic to a single pass (withdrawal and infusion). Undulations are often of greater magnitude when a pass is completed rapidly, in less than 1 minute, compared to a pass of longer duration. A decline in blood pressure during slow withdrawal is usually restored during the following infusion, but restoration is incomplete if withdrawal is too rapid.

Undulation of intracranial pressure parallels the changes in arterial pressure. Both diminish during withdrawal and increase during infusion. The undulations are of lesser magnitude when exchange cycles are performed slowly. The implication of these findings is that increased blood flow in the cerebral circulation during infusion may cause intraventricular-periventricular hemorrhage, particularly in sick premature infants.

Following are *other effects of exchange transfusion*.

Neutropenia occurs during the exchange and persists for varying periods thereafter. The return to normal is slower in premature than in term infants. Decreased neutrophils are apparently the result of replacement with donor blood that is virtually free of white cells. Multiple exchange transfusions may be associated with neutrophil counts as low as 242/mm^3.

Thrombocytopenia is also brought about by exchange transfusion. A rebound to higher platelet counts usually occurs within 24 hours.

The *effect on drug levels* is surprisingly minimal in most instances. Table 9-1 lists a number of commonly used pharmacologic agents and their calculated percent loss in blood levels when either a one-volume or two-volume exchange transfusion is performed. Antibiotic therapy is not impaired unless multiple exchanges are performed. Replacement of antibiotics is probably indicated in these circumstances. Determination of antibiotic blood levels before and after multiple transfusions may sometimes be necessary for adjustment of dosages. *Anticonvulsant drugs* (phenobarbital, phenytoin) are minimally decreased by exchanged transfusions; replacement of these drugs is not necessary. However, recurrent transfusions at close intervals require determination of blood levels. The *loss of theophylline* is significant. Thus, if possible, the exchange transfusion should be initiated at the end of a dosing interval, and concentrations should be determined before and after the transfusion. *Furosemide* need not be replaced if given more than 1 hour before exchange, because onset of its pharmacologic effect is rapid. *Digoxin* removal by exchange transfusion is minimal, thus additional dosing is unnecessary.

Table 9-1. Hypothetical drug loss by exchange transfusion

Drug	Percent loss	
	One volume	Two volume
Amikacin	7.1	13.8
Ampicillin	7.7	14.7
Carbamazepine	3.7	7.2
Carbenicillin	5.6	10.9
Colistin	18.7	33.9
Diazepam	2.3	4.5
Digoxin*	1.2	2.4
Furosemide	4.9	9.5
Gentamicin	5.2	10.1
Kanamycin	5.6	10.9
Methicillin	10.1	19.1
Oxacillin	19.6	35.4
Penicillin G (crystalline)	6.0	11.6
Penicillin G (procaine)	2.4	4.8
Phenobarbital	6.4	12.3
Phenytoin	3.1	6.2
Theophylline*	17.8	32.4
Tobramycin	10.3	19.6
Vancomycin	5.7	11.0

*Whole blood volume used in calculation.
From: Lackner, T. E.: Drug replacement following exchange transfusion, J. Pediatr. **100:**813, 1982.

Intestinal perforation resulting from necrotizing enterocolitis usually involves the colon or ileum when it is a complication of exchange transfusion. The signs include abdominal distention, bloody stools, retention of gastric secretion that is often bilious, respiratory distress, hypotension, pallor, and cyanosis. Abdominal distention appears initially, usually within 48 hours of the last exchange. X-ray examination reveals free air in the peritoneal space in most instances of intestinal perforation. Surgery is mandatory when perforation has occurred. Intestinal perforation after exchange transfusion is probably the result of ischemia of the gut. Blood flow in the portal system may be profoundly disrupted during the procedure. Venous pressure in the portal system is elevated during infusions and diminished during withdrawals. When inserted, the catheter should pass from the umbilical vein through the ductus venosus into the inferior vena cava, but it sometimes lodges in the portal vein instead. Blood is thus exchanged directly in and out of this vessel. Since the portal vein drains blood from the intestine, disruption of normal vascular pressure during exchange cycles impairs normal intestinal blood flow to cause ischemia and necrosis of the gut wall. Perforation of the wall follows.

Phototherapy. If one is to use phototherapy as the initial form of treatment for the hyperbilirubinemia of hemolytic disease, several distinct limitations must be borne in mind. First, severe hemolysis causes rapid accumulation of bilirubin at a rate that exceeds the capacity of phototherapy to break down bilirubin in the skin. Second, even if phototherapy effectively controls bilirubin levels by its activity in the skin, hemolysis is ongoing, and severe anemia may ensue. Phototherapy is often successful as initial treatment (in preference to exchange transfusion) for ABO incompatibility because bilirubin does not usually accumulate so rapidly, and severe anemia does not often develop. The same may be said for mild Rh disease in which phototherapy is used in hope of avoiding an exchange transfusion. A number of studies have demonstrated reduction in the rate of bilirubin accumulation within the first 2 days of life and a reduced need for repeated exchange transfusion, but these outcomes were observed principally in babies whose hemolytic process was mild. Using phototherapy before the first exchange, with standard equipment that provided a preponderance of blue light, we noted progressive anemia even though bilirubin levels were controlled. Multiple simple transfusions were essential later, and we were impressed with the resultant prolongation of hospital stay. Thus we withhold phototherapy and perform an exchange transfusion when indications are imminent. Phototherapy is applied after the exchange. By using exchange transfusion as the initial form of therapy, red cells destined for hemolysis are removed, and the principal source of excess bilirubin is eliminated. Subsequent accumulation of serum bilirubin is primarily a consequence of its migration from the extravascular space into the blood, and secondarily the result of sustained hemolysis of new red cells that are generated by the baby.

Prevention. Erythroblastosis is a preventable disease. Maternal sensitization can be prevented by the administration of anti-D gamma globulin (RhIg) to unsensitized mothers. Vaccination of mothers provides passive immunization, which supplies antibodies that temporarily suppress the maternal response to antigen on Rh-positive red cells. The vaccine's mechanism of action is controversial; the following possibilities have been considered: (1) administered anti-D antibody destroys fetal Rh-positive red cells in the maternal circulation before they can immunize the mother against the D antigen; (2) the administered antibody becomes attached to antigen on the surface of cells and blocks its immunogenic capacity; (3) the antibody suppresses reaction to antigen at the central locations where the immune response primarily occurs (spleen and lymph nodes). Whichever the mechanism, the administration of Rh immunoglobulin (RhIg) is universally accepted as an effective modality by which Rh disease in babies has been reduced dramatically.

While the reduction has been dramatic, it has nevertheless been incomplete. It is estimated that approximately 20% of Rh-negative women in the United States do not receive postpartum prophylaxis. This has been referred to as the utilization "gap." It is not entirely a result of failure to administer RhIg after delivery. Rather, it is estimated that failure to administer vaccine occurs in only approximately 5% of deliveries throughout the country. The remainder are newly sensitized women who emerge from a number of other circumstances. Thus vaccine is not given to approximately 15% of women who have spontaneous or induced abortions, and they constitute a major source of de novo sensitization. Another source of new sensitizations is the previously unrecognized sensitization that occurs during pregnancy because of unusually large volumes of fetomaternal hemorrhage that is large enough to sensitize the mother during gestation. Recognition that maternal sensitization occurs in a substantial number of women during the third trimester has led to administration of RhIg between 28 and 32 weeks of pregnancy followed by another dose of vaccine within 48 hours after delivery. Antenatal vaccine creates no hazard to the fetus. Theoretically, it is conceivable that immunoglobulin (IgG) given during pregnancy may cross the placenta. In the fetus, vaccine antibody could hemolyze fetal red cells just as maternal antibodies do in Rh disease. Fetal safety is apparently assured by the small dose of RhIg (vaccine). It has been estimated that approximately 50 such maternal injections would have to be given in a 2-day period to create hazard to the fetus. It is further estimated that five doses of RhIg given during pregnancy would be harmless. There is insufficient Rh antibody in these doses to harm an Rh-positive fetus.

A preponderance of women who fail to react to postpartum vaccine have already been sensitized during the last trimester of pregnancy by large volumes of blood from their fetus. Sensitization before delivery is preventable in most cases by antepartum vaccination with RhIg. Whereas 2% to 3% of Rh-negative primigravidas are sensitized before delivery, administration of RhIg during the third trimester reduces the incidence to 0.3%, provided a postpartum dose is also given.

Isoimmunization: ABO incompatibility

The disorder produced by incompatibility in the ABO groups is usually considerably milder than Rh disease. Group A or B infants of group O mothers are most commonly involved; group B infants of group A mothers are only occasionally affected. Group O infants are never affected, regardless of the mother's blood type.

ABO incompatibility differs from Rh disease in several respects. Preexistent natural anti-A and anti-B antibodies from group O mothers pass to the fetus without previous sensitization by leakage of fetal blood. As a result, firstborn infants are frequently involved, and there is no relationship between the appearance or severity of disease and repeated sensitization from one pregnancy to the next. Stillbirth and hydrops fetalis are rare. Jaundice is common; hepatosplenomegaly occurs inconsistently. Reticulocytosis indicates a hemolytic process, but significant anemia during the neonatal period and later is rare. The direct Coombs' test on the infant's cells is usually positive; the indirect Coombs' test using infant's serum on adult red cells may be strongly positive. Infants whose direct Coombs' test is positive are more likely to be jaundiced, with bilirubin in excess of 10 mg/dl. An affected group A infant has demonstrable anti-A antibody in his serum. A blood smear reveals increased numbers of spherical, mature erythrocytes called *spherocytes*. These cells are thicker and smaller in diameter than normal red cells. They are not observed in abnormally increased number on smears from infants with Rh disease. The usual indication for exchange transfusion for ABO incompatibility is progressive elevation of serum bilirubin concentration to 20 mg/dl in term infants and 12 to 15 mg/dl in premature infants. The donor blood must be group O; it should never be the infant's own type.

Hemolysis resulting from infection

Infectious diseases, bacterial and nonbacterial, are associated with hemolytic anemia. Hyperbilirubinemia, and to a lesser extent anemia, are often prominent signs of septicemia and neonatal renal infection. The nonbacterial infections that cause hemolysis are of intrauterine origin. They include cytomegalic inclusion disease, toxoplasmosis, rubella, herpes-virus, and coxsackievirus infections. Congenital syphilis also causes hemolysis. Hyperbilirubinemia during infections is a result of hepatocellular damage as well as hemolysis. Infections are discussed in Chapter 12.

Other causes of hemolysis

A number of enzymatic deficiencies in red cells are known to cause hemolytic anemia. *Glucose-6-phosphate dehydrogenase (G-6-PD) deficiency* is the most common. It occurs primarily among blacks, Filipinos, Sephardic (not Ashkenazic) Jews, Sardinians, Greeks, and Arabs. It is genetically transmitted, occurring predominantly in males, rarely in females. The disorder is manifest during the newborn period in only a fraction of affected individuals. Jaundice and anemia are the presenting signs. A large number of drugs have been reported to cause hemolysis in G-6-PD–deficient patients. Most of these substances are rarely, if ever, used in the newborn infant.

Large doses of water-soluble vitamin K analogue (Synkavite, Hykinone) have produced hemolysis and jaundice in the past. Vitamin K_1 is generally used rather than the water-soluble analogue because it is safe in respect to hemolysis. Vitamin E deficiency causes hemolytic anemia in premature infants. Virtually all neonates, term and preterm, are born deficient in vitamin E (tocopherol) by adult standards. The smallest infants are most deficient. Tocopherol stores in a 3500 g infant are estimated at 20 mg; at a birth weight of 1000 the stores are 3 mg. Although plasma vitamin E levels are related to maternal levels, vitamin E levels at birth do not exceed 0.6 mg/dl. The risk for vitamin E–deficient hemolytic anemia is restricted to premature infants whose birth weight is less than 1500 g. In larger or older neonates, erythrocyte survival is apparently diminished by suboptimal vitamin E levels, but without detectable anemia. The risk for vitamin E–deficient anemia is related to several factors: maternal nutrition and blood levels of tocopherol, birth weight and gestational age, ability of the infant to absorb orally administered vitamin E, ratio of vitamin E to polyunsaturated fatty acid (PUFA) in milk feeds, and amount of dietary iron. The absorption of vitamin E (and other fat-soluble vitamins) depends on the capacity to absorb dietary fat. Premature infants absorb fat less effectively than term infants, but efficiency of fat absorption increases during the first few weeks of life. Unsaturated fatty acids are absorbed more efficiently than the saturated ones.

The toxic biochemical event is called *lipid peroxidation*, which affects polyunsaturated fatty acids (PUFA), which are important constituents of red cell membranes. Lipid peroxidation damages the membranes, red blood cells are lysed, and hemolytic anemia ensues. Peroxidation occurs when there is an excess of PUFA in relation to the quantity of available vitamin E. In the presence of a relative excess of PUFA, vitamin E is incapable of counteracting lipid peroxidation. In addition, elemental iron enhances the peroxidation reaction. There is thus a three-cornered relationship between vitamin E, PUFA, and elemental iron.

In years past, vitamin E–deficient hemolytic anemia was more common than today. At that time commercial formulas contained excessive quantities of PUFA, principally linoleic acid. The incidence of anemia has diminished considerably, since the quantity of linoleic acid has been reduced in commercial formulas.

Vitamin E–deficiency anemia was first reported in 1967. It occurs among infants whose birth weight is less than 1500 g and is usually first recognized 4 to 6 weeks after birth. Hemoglobin values vary from 6 to 8 g/dl; reticulocyte counts exceed 7%. Platelet counts are elevated beyond 600,000/mm³. In a few infants edema of the lower extremities and the lower trunk is obvious. Serum protein concentrations are normal. Vitamin E concentration blood is less than 0.5 mg/dl.

Treatment entails administration of tocopherol orally in amounts of 100 to 200 units daily for approximately 2 weeks. The response is characterized by diminished reticulocyte and platelet counts, associated with a gradual rise in hemoglobin concentration. The hemolytic anemia can usually be prevented by daily oral administration of 15 to 25 mg of tocopherol. In many nurseries vitamin E supplements are fed to infants whose birth weights are less than 1500 g.

Abnormal morphology of erythrocytes occurs in several varieties; they are uncommon causes of hemolytic anemia. *Hereditary spherocytosis* is the most frequent of these conditions. The red cells are abnormally fragile and thus are predisposed to premature breakdown. The life span of these cells is therefore abnormally short. They are remarkably susceptible to deposition and dissolution in spleen. The responsible molecular abnormality has not been identified. A substantial number of affected individuals have hemolytic anemia in the newborn period. Jaundice and pallor resulting from anemia are the outstanding signs of the disease. The blood smear reveals a preponderance of spherocytes. They are small and round, and they stain densely as a result of their spherical configuration. These cells are similar in appearance to those observed in ABO incompatibility. Treatment during the newborn period includes exchange transfusion for high bilirubin levels or simple transfusion if anemia is the only difficulty.

Hemolytic anemia has also been described in the rare entity known as *hereditary elliptocytosis*. Most of the red cells in affected infants are a bizarre elliptical shape, and those of one of the parents have a similar appearance. Treatment during the newborn period is the same as that for hereditary spherocytic anemia.

ANEMIA RESULTING FROM LOSS OF BLOOD

Causes of fetal and neonatal blood loss

I. Cord
  A. Rupture of varices or aneurysms
  B. Traumatic rupture of normal cord
  C. Torn vessels with velamentous insertion
II. Placenta
  A. Incision into fetal side during cesarean section
  B. Placenta previa
  C. Abruptio placentae
  D. Multilobed placenta with interlobar vessels
III. Fetal blood loss
  A. Fetomaternal (acute or chronic blood loss)
  B. Fetofetal (into twin, acute or chronic blood loss)
IV. Enclosed hemorrhage
  A. Intracranial
  B. Ruptured liver
  C. Ruptured spleen
  D. Adrenal hemorrhage
  E. Retroperitoneal
  F. Subaponeurotic (scalp)
  G. Cephalhematoma
  H. Pulmonary (massive)

Prenatal blood loss

The fetus may lose blood before or during parturition. In utero bleeding may occur into the mother's circulation, directly into the vessels of a twin, or as a result of mishap during the birth process. The latter is usually a result of some factor in the placenta or cord that predisposes to ruptured vessels or to operative complication during cesarean section.

Fetomaternal transfusion is a common phenomenon, but resultant abnormal signs of blood loss in the neonate are infrequent. Fetomaternal transfusion more frequently contributes to Rh disease by stimulating maternal antibody formation (see p. 290). Loss of fetal blood presumably occurs at the intervillous spaces. The precise site of placental leak has not been demonstrated. Fetal blood cells in maternal circulation have been detected in as many as 50% of pregnancies; yet in only 1% of them is blood loss sufficient to cause neonatal anemia. Fetal red cells are easily detected in maternal circulation by the acid elution technique. They do not disappear completely for several weeks after delivery.

Fetofetal (twin-to-twin) transfusion occurs in identical monochorionic (identical) twins through arteriovenous anastomoses in the common placenta. This condition is also known as the *intrauterine parabiotic syndrome*.

Twin placentas are of four structural varieties:
- Separated (2 amnions, 2 chorions)
- Fused (2 amnions, 2 chorions)
- Fused (2 amnions, 1 chorion)
- Fused (1 amnion, 1 chorion)

Of all identical (monozygous) twins, approximately 70% have single chorion placentas (monochorionic). Vascular anastomoses occur, to some extent, between every pair of monochorionic placentas. These anastomoses may be vein-to-vein, artery-to-artery, or artery-to-vein. Fetofetal transfusion occurs in artery-to-vein anastomoses. The effect of blood loss on the donor twin depends on the size of the transfusion and its duration. Clinical signs of acute or chronic blood loss may therefore occur (see later). In general the fetofetal transfusions of longest duration are associated with greater discrepancies in body weight and length. Thus only a chronic process results in impressive weight discrepancy. If the smaller twin weighs at least 20% less than the larger one, the process is surely chronic and the donor is the smaller baby. If the weight discrepancy is smaller, there is little relationship between growth status and the identity of donor or recipient infants. In the extreme, death occurs in utero early in pregnancy. In approximately 15% of monochorionic twins, or perhaps more, significant anemia occurs in the donor; and polycythemia in the recipient. Hemoglobin in the donor has been reported as low as 5 g/dl. Signs of acute or chronic hemorrhage are observed. The *donor twin* is often considerably smaller than the recipient and may be severely undergrown for dates. All the physical attributes of in utero undergrowth are in evidence. Oligohydramnios and hypotension are also common. Postnatal hypoglycemia occurs as a result of intrauterine malnutrition. Pallor is impressive, proportional to the anemia. The *recipient twin* is polycythemic, with a significantly increased blood volume. Hemoglobin concentration may be 20 to 30 g/dl volume. A deep red complexion contrasts dramatically with the pallor of the donor sibling. Polyhydramnios and hypertension are common. The recipient sibling may be strikingly larger than his twin, often appearing overnourished by comparison. *The size of twins differs little if the transfusion occurs late in pregnancy*. Thus, gross differences may exist in blood volume and other hematologic attributes in the absence of other discrepancies of size and development. The cardiovascular, pulmonary, and central nervous system signs of polycythemia (see later) are noted in the recipient baby.

Obstetric misadventure may cause life-threatening fetal blood loss. In all instances the signs of acute hemorrhage are in evidence. Placenta previa and abruptio placentae are often associated with fetal as well as maternal hemorrhage. Anomalous vessels at the insertion of the cord (velamentous) are vulnerable to disruption and hemorrhage. Even the normal cord can be torn if it is inordinately short or regardless of length during unattended delivery. Severe acute hemorrhage may complicate cesarean section if the placenta is inadvertently incised during the procedure. In multilobular placentas, the vascular connections between lobes rupture easily, which may result in severe fetal hemorrhage. During cesarean section, delayed clamping of the cord causes anemia *if the baby is above the level of the placenta*. The infant is usually placed on the mother's abdomen, or is held at approximately that level, when the cord is clamped and cut. A significant amount of blood thus passes from fetus to placenta by virtue of gravity if clamping is delayed. Furthermore, unlike the situation in vaginal deliveries, the uterus is not contracted; it is atonic. This enhances backflow of blood to the placenta because low vascular resistance persists. The result is reduction in blood volume, red blood cell volume, and plasma volume. These values are significantly higher, however, if delayed clamping occurs *while the infant is below the level of the placenta*. In this position the fetus receives transfusion from the placenta.

Acute versus chronic fetal blood loss

Acute hemorrhage may result from any of the conditions listed previously; fetomaternal and fetofetal transfusions are most often chronic. The signs of acute hemorrhage are those of hypovolemia (shock) and anemia. They are generally present at birth and include pallor, cyanosis, tachycardia, feeble or absent pulses, gasping, tachypnea, and retractions. The cry is weak, spontaneous activity is absent or diminished, and flaccidity is severe. Superficially these infants appear to be asphyxiated, but three differentiating clinical signs are helpful. First, babies who are in shock from acute blood loss have a rapid heart rate (over 160 beats/min) until they become hypoxic; infants who are only asphyxiated usually have bradycardia as a result of profound hypoxemia. Second, infants in shock remain cyanotic despite oxygen therapy; asphyxiated babies respond to it. Third, infants who are in shock usually breathe rapidly; asphyxiated infants breathe slowly. Acute blood loss should be suspected in the presence of these differentiating signs. Suspicion is the initial step; without it the baby is lost. The diagnosis is more assured if there is knowledge of an obstetric accident. Low hemoglobin and hematocrit values are diagnostic, but in acute hemorrhage they are misleadingly normal at birth. The hematocrit may remain normal immediately after acute blood loss because 2 to 4 hours must pass before hemodilution occurs from the influx of interstitial fluid into the circulation in attempt to maintain blood volume. Hemoglobin values in capillary blood are a source of error; they can be spuriously high, especially in sick neonates because of severe stasis of peripheral circulation. Venous blood samples are required. Immediate transfusion is lifesaving.

Chronic hemorrhage is associated with slowly developing anemia and compensatory adjustment of blood volume. At birth, affected infants are pale and anemic, but misleadingly vigorous. Several reports have described pale babies, otherwise apparently well, whose hemoglobin concentrations were as low as 5 g/100 ml. After chronic intrauterine blood loss, hemoglobin at birth may range from 5 to 12 g/dl. The temptation to immediately transfuse a chronically anemic baby is often irresistible. If signs attributable to severe anemia (tachycardia, hypoxia) are evident, a packed-cell transfusion is indeed indicated. There is no need to rapidly restore hematocrit or hemoglobin values to normal levels, certainly not to levels higher than 35 vol % or 12 g/dl, respectively. Packed cells should be given as a partial exchange transfusion. The red cell mass required to increase the hematocrit to 35 vol % is calculated, and the packed cells are given in exchange for equal volumes of the infant's blood. This technique avoids volume overload while simultaneously increasing red cell mass. Two characteristics of chronic intrauterine blood loss must be kept in mind for their critical therapeutic implications. Most important is that generally there is no diminution in blood volume in chronic loss that can compare with that of acute loss. Rapid, overzealous transfusion is thus dangerous; it may overload the vascular space and cause failure of a heart that already functions marginally because of severe anemia. Second, chronic blood loss involves iron deficiency. Therefore many of these babies do not require transfusion at all; they need only elemental iron, 5 to 10 mg/kg of body weight daily. The iron therapy should be maintained for a year.

Postnatal blood loss

Postnatal hemorrhage most often occurs into enclosed spaces (see list on p. 299). Defects of the clotting mechanism, also responsible for serious postnatal blood loss, are discussed later. Enclosed hemorrhage is a common cause of anemia during the first 3 days of life. *Intracranial hemorrhage* (subarachnoid, subdural, and intraventricular) may be sufficiently severe to cause a significant drop in hemoglobin, although signs of central nervous system dysfunction are predominant. *Hemorrhage into the scalp* may be extensive, resulting in massive blood loss and a hemoglobin concentration as low as 3 g/dl. The scalp is boggy and thick, obscuring the sutures and fontanelles of the skull, and extending over the forehead to impart a blue suffusion to the skin. Deficiency of vitamin K–dependent and other clotting factors is often present in affected infants. We have encountered severe scalp hemorrhage in an infant with hemophilia. In addition, a high incidence of difficult labor and delivery has been noted. Scalp hemorrhage is first apparent from 30 minutes to 4 hours after birth. Pallor increases as blood continues to accumulate in the scalp, and if hemorrhage is severe, shock ensues. Transfusion is urgent, and intravenous sodium bicarbonate is also necessary because of severe metabolic acidosis. Vitamin K_1 or any other coagulation factor shown to be deficient should be given intravenously.

After traumatic labor, especially in breech deliveries, hemorrhage may occur into the liver, spleen, adrenals, and kidneys. Hemorrhage into the liver is particularly pernicious. It may also follow vigorous external cardiac massage. Blood accumulates beneath the liver capsule for a day or two while the infant appears well, although perhaps pale. When the capsule ruptures and pressure is released, bleeding from the liver becomes copious, and sudden shock ensues. Liver enlargement is easily palpated, and the upper abdomen appears distended, particularly after rupture of the capsule. Rupture of the spleen may occur during traumatic delivery, from severe enlargement in erythroblastosis fetalis, or during exchange transfusion.

Enclosed hemorrhage, in addition to causing shock, often gives rise to hyperbilirubinemia from degradation of the extravasated blood. Treatment first consists of simple transfusion for blood loss, and then if the bilirubin rises phototherapy is indicated (p. 330). Exchange transfusion is necessary if bilirubin continues to accumulate beyond serum levels of 20 mg/dl and at lower levels in preterm infants.

DISORDERS OF COAGULATION

Hemorrhage may result from inherited disorders of the clotting mechanism, from clotting defects created by other disease processes, or from exaggerations of physiologic neonatal clotting deficiencies. Platelet abnormalities are also an important cause of hemorrhage. When trauma is superimposed on coagulation defects, serious hemorrhage may result, as exemplified by massive bleeding into the scalp.

The normal clotting mechanism

The defect caused by injury to a blood vessel gives rise to a series of biochemical events that culminate in the formation of a firm mass of fibrin and platelets—the clot. Fig. 9-1 depicts the scheme of normal clot formation. When vascular endothelium is damaged, subendothelial structures are exposed to blood, while vasoconstriction restricts flow to the injured site. The exposed subendothelial structures, primarily collagen, attract platelets that adhere, aggregate, and accumulate. It is on the surface of this platelet mass that thrombin is formed to induce the appearance of fibrin, which becomes sufficiently firm to form an effective clot. In the best of circumstances, hemorrhage ceases, followed by slow repair of damaged vascular structures and resolution of the clot.

The normal clot evolves in response to injury only in the presence of (1) platelets of normal function and quantity, (2) biochemical conversion of several blood factors that are sequentially activated to generate thrombin from prothrombin, and (3) release of tissue factor from the vessel wall to trigger another sequence of events that also culminates in the conversion of prothrombin to thrombin (Fig. 9-1).

The role of platelets; formation of the platelet plug. The platelet is a small anuclear cell that has broken from a megacaryocyte in bone marrow and is in reality a cell fragment. Its full life in the circulation has been estimated at 10 days. Platelets adhere to exposed subendothelial structures when a vessel is damaged, and a multicellular aggregation (platelet plug) is formed. During this process the platelet generates thromboxane A$_2$, which stimulates local vasospasm and continued aggregation of platelets. Platelets also secrete adenosine diphosphate (ADP), which maintains continued aggregation. At its surface the platelet plug accelerates a "cascade" of reactions that involves several plasma factors called *procoagulants*. Procoagulants lead to the generation of thrombin from prothrombin and then fibrin from fibrinogen. As thrombin is generated, it further enhances platelet aggregation. For major hemorrhagic episodes, the platelet plug temporarily slows bleeding, but in minor episodes the plug is sufficient to halt the bleeding. Three fundamental reactions of platelets contribute to clot forma-

tion—adhesion to vessel wall, release of thromboxane A$_2$ and ADP, and aggregation. Subsequent formation of the fibrin clot depends on the evolving "cascade" of plasma procoagulant reactions and upon the release of tissue factors; both pathways contribute to formation of fibrin strains that enmesh the platelets in the preliminary plug to ultimately form a firm clot.

The preliminary platelet plug halts small blood loss completely. When injury and bleeding are greater, hardening of the plug is required to stop the bleeding. The preliminary platelet plug is important for control of minute ruptures in vessel walls that occur frequently, particularly in the skin. In the presence of thrombocytopenia, formation of preliminary platelet plugs is impaired,

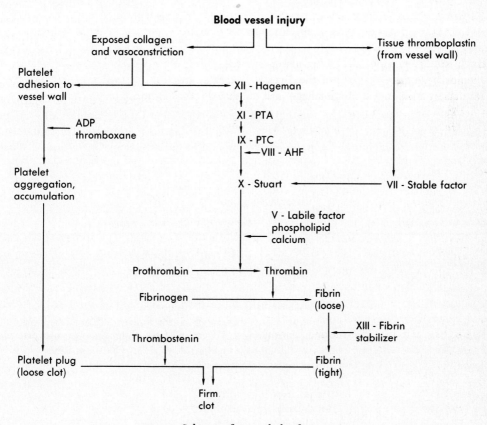

Fig. 9-1. Scheme of normal clot formation.

blood escapes through the unoccluded vessel rupture, and now petechiae are visible.

Formation of thrombin. Thrombin is formed from prothrombin by the coordinated activities of factor X, factor V, phospholipid, and calcium. Prothrombin is a plasma protein (alpha$_2$-globulin) in normal plasma. It is generated continuously in the liver; vitamin K is essential to the process.

Formation of thrombin from prothrombin is directly dependent on activated factor X, factor V, phospholipid, and calcium. Factor X is activated by reactions from two separate sequences, the *intrinsic* and the *extrinsic pathways*. Prothrombin is converted to thrombin only in the presence of sufficient factor X.

The *intrinsic pathway* is a series of reactions among substances known as the *blood coagulation factors* (procoagulants). They are labeled by Roman numerals and are sometimes identified by synonymous names, all of which are listed in Table 9-2. The coagulation factors circulate as inactive substances until they are converted to activity by a sequence of reactions in which each inactive form is converted to activity by its predecessor. This is the coagulation cascade. The cascade is initiated by activation of factor XII after blood has been exposed to the collagen and the basement membrane of injured blood vessels. Inactive factor XII binds to these exposed endothelial structures and is transposed into the active form, which then itself activates the next factor—factor XI. Active factor XI triggers the conversion of factor IX, which now converts factor X to its active configuration. Factor IX activates its successor only in the presence of factor VIII, calcium, and phospholipid. Factor VIII is indispensable for rapid activation of factor X. It is the antihemophilic factor (AHF) that is congenitally absent in hemophilia.

The *extrinsic pathway* is triggered by exposure of blood to tissue factor. Tissue factor is a component of the surfaces of smooth muscle cells and fibroblasts in vascular subendothelial layers. It is particularly copious in placenta, lung, and brain, inducing a configurational change in factor VII, which subsequently contributes to the activation of factor X. In the presence of active factor X, rapid conversion of prothrombin to thrombin proceeds.

The *common pathway* involves conversion of prothrombin to thrombin, and then fibrinogen to fibrin. It is called the common pathway because both the intrinsic and extrinsic sequences culminate in its activation. Once formed, thrombin

Table 9-2. Commonly used names of clotting factors and their synonyms

Commonly used terms	Less frequently used synonyms
Fibrinogen	Factor I
Prothrombin	Factor II
Tissue thromboplastin	Factor III
Calcium	Factor IV
Factor V	Proaccelerin; labile factor; Ac-globulin; Ac-G
Factor VII	Serum prothrombin conversion accelerator; SPCA; stable factor
Factor VIII	Antihemophilic factor; AHF; antihemophilic globulin; AHG
Factor IX	Plasma thromboplastin component; PTC; Christmas factor
Factor X	Stuart factor; Stuart-Prower factor
Factor XI	Plasma thromboplastin antecedent; PTA
Factor XII	Hageman factor
Factor XIII	Fibrin stabilizing factor

Modified from Guyton, A. C.: Textbook of medical physiology, Philadelphia, 1981, W. B. Saunders Co.

cleaves fibrinogen into three separate molecular strands, one species of which links with its identical counterparts to form a polymer of insoluble fibrin. This requires factor XIII (fibrin stabilizing factor). In the presence of factor XIII, polymerized fibrin becomes "tight" fibrin. It is deposited in the form of strands that enmesh the platelets that have aggregated during formation of the preliminary plug. The result is a firm clot.

Calcium is essential for all the reactions of the intrinsic and extrinsic pathways, except those concerning factors XII and XI. Calcium deficiencies do not impair coagulation because the low levels required to impair clotting would first be lethal. However, absence of calcium does prevent in vitro clot formation. This is the basis of the anticoagulant effect of citrate-containing preservatives that are used for banked blood. Calcium is complexed to citrate in the preservative to preclude coagulation.

Containment of the coagulation process

The potential for coagulation is ever present, merely awaiting an appropriate trigger mechanism to become activated. In healthy individuals, there are over 30 substances related to coagulation (procoagulants) and to its inhibition (anticoagulants). The balance between these two groups of substances determines whether coagulation will proceed. Anticoagulants must localize the coagulation process to the affected regions that require it. Otherwise, once initiated, the coagulation process would theoretically extend to all parts of the body regardless of need. The balance between activators and inhibitors is thus constant during normal physiologic states. When an imbalance favors activation of coagulation, the process must still be restricted to the area in need; it must be terminated when the clot is formed, and repair must restore the injured area to its precoagulation state. In the absence of these limiting mechanisms, the slightest endothelial damage would precipitate ongoing generalized thrombosis.

Several controlling mechanisms prevent a tidal extension of the coagulation process. Thus rapid blood flow carries activated components to unaffected parts of the body where they are ineffective. Enzymes of the intrinsic pathway are cleared by the liver. Progress of the cascade requires a disrupted blood vessel surface and a primary platelet plug, which normally localizes the process to an area of injury.

Several distinct plasma proteins are important for the inhibition of various stages of coagulation. These are antithrombin III, antiplasmin, and alpha$_2$-macroglobulin. They are critical modulators of coagulation. The principal inhibiting substance is antithrombin III (ATIII), which modulates the conversion of fibrinogen to fibrin by inhibiting thrombin activity. During the coagulation process, approximately 90% of the generated thrombin is attracted to existing fibrin threads that have developed around and within the evolving clot. This in itself prevents the spread of thrombin to other parts of the body. The other portion of thrombin that is generated during the coagulation process would thus be left to circulate throughout the body were it not combined with an antithrombin-heparin complex that inactivates the thrombin that it binds. *Heparin* is present constantly in small amounts. It is a well-known powerful anticoagulant. It is normally deposited in the cytoplasm of numerous species of cells, and is produced in particularly large volumes by *mast cells* in pericapillary connective tissue throughout the body. Mast cells secrete heparin continuously. *Basophils* in the blood also produce minute quantities of heparin. The anticoagulant effect of heparin depends on its combination with the antithrombin-heparin cofactor. When excessive quantities of heparin are present, the removal of thrombin from circulating blood is instantaneous. Heparin plus antithrombin-heparin cofactor also inactivates factors XII, XI, IX, and X, thereby slowing the progress of the coagulation cascade. *Alpha$_2$-macroglobulin* exerts its anticoagulant influence by binding coagulation factors until they are destroyed. The action of alpha$_2$-macroglobulin is unrelated to heparin.

Blood clots must be dissolved after serving their purpose. Appropriate lysis of blood clots is effected by *plasmin* (or fibrinolysin). Plasmin is formed from plasminogen. Plasmin dissolves fibrin threads and other substances within the clot.

Clot formation includes formation of plasminogen, which is normally converted to plasmin for clot dissolution within several days after clot formation. The lysis of blood clots is relatively slow. It occurs in small vessels and in blood that has

Table 9-3. Hemostatic laboratory values

Hemostatic factor or component	Premature infant	Full-term infant	Age adult level is attained
Vascular and platelet function			
Vasoconstriction	Present	Present	At birth
Capillary fragility	Increased	Normal	At birth
Bleeding time	Normal	Normal	At birth
Platelet count	Normal	Normal	At birth
Platelet function	↓ ↓ Aggregative ability	↓ Aggregative ability ↓ Clot retraction ↓ Platelet factor 3 availability	Not established
Coagulation			
Whole blood clotting time	Decreased	↓ Or normal	At birth
Partial thromboplastin time (PTT)	70-145 seconds	45-70 seconds	2-9 months (35-45 seconds)
Prothrombin time (PT)	12-21 seconds	13-20 seconds	3-4 days (12-14 seconds)
Thrombin time (TT)	11-17 seconds	10-16 seconds	Few days (8-10 seconds)
Thrombotest (II, VII, IX, X)	30%-50%	40%-68%	2-12 months
XII (Hageman factor)	10%-50%	25%-60%	9-14 days
IX (PTA)	5%-20%	15%-70%	1-2 months
IX (PTC)	10%-25%	20%-60%	3-9 months
VIII (AHF)	20%-80%	70%-150%	At birth
VII (proconvertin)	20%-45%	20%-60%	2-12 months
X (Stuart-Prower factor)	10%-45%	20%-55%	2-12 months
V (proaccelerin)	50%-85%	80%-200%	At birth
II (prothrombin)	20%-80%	26%-65%	2-12 months
I (fibrinogen) (g/dl)	150%-300%	150%-300%	2-4 days
XIII (fibrin-stabilizing factor)	100%	100%	At birth
Fibrin splint products (μg/ml)	0-10	0-7	
Antithrombin III	48%	55%	

Modified from Beyer, W. A., Hakami, N., and Shepard, T. H.: J. Pediatr. **79**:838, 1971.

coagulated within extravascular tissue. In large vessels, clots are not usually dissolved by this process.

Normal values and global tests for coagulation status

The tests usually used for the assessment of coagulation status are global ones. That is, they suggest inadequacy within a given group of the coagulation reactions. Tests for specific factors are available and are used when the coagulopathy is thought to be primary rather than secondary to a serious underlying disease such as infection.

The most frequently used global tests are the bleeding time, the activated partial thromboplastin time, prothrombin time, and thrombin time.

Bleeding time. The bleeding time entails a small standard incision in the skin and tests for the time consumed before bleeding stops. The usual normal time interval is 3 to 7 minutes. The test is abnormal if platelet function or number is diminished, or if the structural integrity of vessel walls is abnormal.

Activated partial thromboplastin time (PTT). The PTT tests for abnormalities of the intrinsic system (factors XII, XI, IX, and VIII). It also demonstrates abnormalities of the common pathway.

Prothrombin time. Abnormally long prothrombin times suggest deficiencies of factor VII and the common pathway.

Thrombin time. Thrombin time is a test for the conversion of fibrinogen to fibrin. It indicates suboptimal levels of fibrinogen in plasma or dysfunctional fibrinogen. It also demonstrates the presence of excessive heparin.

Normal values for these tests are presented in Table 9-3. As a rule, prothrombin times greater than 50% of adult values or partial thromboplastin times more than double adult values are indicative of abnormal clotting. Normal thrombin times in the neonate are usually 1 to 3 seconds longer than in the adult.

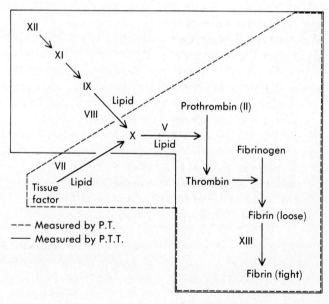

Fig. 9-2. Intrinsic and extrinsic clotting pathways correlated with PT and PTT clotting screens. (From Gross, S. J., and Stuart, M. J.: Hemostasis in the premature infant, Clin. Perinatol. 4:263, 1977.)

Fig. 9-2 depicts the intrinsic, extrinsic, and common pathways accompanied by graphic indication of their applicability to PT and PTT testing.

Platelets. Platelet counts are an indispensable part of the investigation of bleeding infants. Normal values for premature infants (of whatever size and gestational age) and full-term infants are similar. While reported studies indicate that *mean* normal counts *at birth* range from 200,000 to 300,000/mm^3, a platelet count between 100,000 and 150,000/mm^3 merits repeat and further investigation. A count below 100,000/mm^3 is definitely abnormal. Disorders of platelets are discussed later in this chapter.

Hemostasis in the neonate versus the adult

The neonate, especially the premature infant, is vulnerable to hemorrhage on the one hand and thrombosis on the other. Although they are considered physiologic, there are deficiencies of procoagulant factors, anticoagulants, and platelet function in the neonate that are not present in the adult. When a balance is maintained between factors that seem to be counterproductive in their relationship to each other, normal hemostasis is maintained. In the plasma, these factors promote (procoagulants) or impede (anticoagulants) fibrin formation. Furthermore, vascular structure must be intact, and platelets that are functional should be normal in number.

The vitamin K–dependent factors (II, VII, IX, X) are present at lower concentrations at term, and even lower in the premature, compared to the adult. In neonates, factor V is in the adult range of values. Factor VIII is present in the same concentration in the premature as in the adult and is often significantly higher in the term infant. Factors XII and IX are diminished in prematures and term infants; normally, factor XIII is probably diminished.

Plasma fibrinogen concentration is comparable to adult levels at 32 gestational weeks; higher values have been reported in babies who are less than 32 weeks.

The global coagulation tests generally demonstrate longer times in neonates than in adults. The lower values of various factors described above are apparently responsible for protracted prothrombin times and partial thromboplastin times in both premature and term infants. Prolonged PT is attributable to physiologic diminution of factors VII, X, and II. Prolonged PTT is caused by decreases of early contact factor in the intrinsic pathway (XII, IX) as well as lower levels of factors IX and II.

Fibrinolytic activity (lysis of clots) is diminished in neonates. In fact, hypercoagulability of the neonate's blood as evidenced by diminished whole blood clotting time has been postulated. The shorter time to clotting that has been demonstrated in neonates may well result from diminished content of plasminogen, antithrombin III, and inhibitors of factors X and XI. Thus the apparent tendency to bleed more freely, as reflected in diminished levels of various coagulants, is apparently more than counteracted by a greater incapacity to inhibit coagulation. On balance, hypercoagulability best describes hemostasis in the neonate.

Hemorrhagic disease of the newborn: vitamin K deficiency

Hemorrhagic disease of the newborn is a bleeding disorder during the first few days of life that is caused by a deficiency of vitamin K, which is in turn responsible for a deficiency of prothrombin and other coagulation factors (factors II, VII, IX, and X). These factors are generated in the liver, and their production is also dependent on normal hepatic function.

Vitamin K–dependent factors are substantially reduced from adult values at birth. In normal infants, particularly those fed cow's milk early, these levels are gradually restored. Hemorrhagic disease is rare in infants who receive cow's milk on the first day of life. Hemorrhage is most common in breast-fed infants. In a few babies (less than 0.5%), hemorrhage occurs as a result of sustained low levels. The babies of mothers who have taken phenobarbital and diphenylhydantoin (Dilantin) are especially at risk for vitamin K deficiency with severe hemorrhagic complications. They should not be treated in a routine fashion with vitamin K but rather should be treated as though actively bleeding; 1 to 2 mg of the vitamin are thus administered intravenously immediately after birth. Coagulation studies are obtained prior to treatment and should be repeated subsequently. As a rule, the hemorrhagic manifestations become apparent on the second or third day. Bloody or black stools (melena), hematuria, and oozing from the umbilicus are the most frequent signs. Hemorrhage from the nose, from the circumcision site, and into the scalp and skin (ecchymosis) is also visible. The most characteristic laboratory feature of the disease is an extremely prolonged prothrombin time, less prolongation of the partial thromboplastin time (PTT), and lengthened clotting time.

Prophylactic administration of vitamin K at birth prevents deficiencies of the involved clotting factors. Vitamin K_1 is the preferred preparation. The recommended intramuscular dose is 0.5 to 1 mg. Larger doses do not exert an increased prophylactic effect. Cow's milk contains approximately 6 μg of vitamin K per deciliter, and breast milk contains only one fourth as much. The consumption of 10 oz of cow's milk formula during the first 48 hours thus tends to restore the prothrombin time toward normal. In premature infants the response to vitamin K administration and to early feedings is less pronounced, presumably because of immature liver function.

Vitamin K is effective in the treatment, as well as the prevention, of hemorrhagic disease. Intravenous administration of 1 to 2 mg is preferred to intramuscular injection in bleeding infants because the latter route results in large hematomas. This precaution applies to any bleeding diathesis. The coagulation defect is ordinarily corrected within 2 to 4 hours after vitamin K administration. Bleeding may be sufficiently pronounced to require blood transfusion for correction of diminished blood volume, or fresh-frozen plasma to supply the deficient coagulation factors.

Disseminated intravascular coagulation (DIC)

Intravascular coagulation is produced by a diversity of factors that themselves are associated with a multiplicity of disease states. It is therefore the symptom complex that results from a number of serious disorders. It is characterized by inappropriate activation of the clotting process. Inordinately rapid consumption of clotting factors and platelets occurs during intravascular coagulation, and DIC is thus also referred to as *consumption coagulopathy*. The resultant depletion of these factors leads to a paradoxic hemorrhagic diathesis, which constitutes the most serious threat of this syndrome.

The overproduction of thrombin is stimulated by several factors. In these circumstances, plasma fibrinogen is converted to fibrin at a far more rapid rate than normal, and as this accelerated process proceeds, coagulation factors (II, V, VIII, XIII, fibrinogen, and platelets) are significantly depleted. For this reason DIC has been called "consumption coagulopathy." Fibrinolysis is also exaggerated, thereby accentuating the bleeding tendency. Thus plasmin generation increases and the small fibrin clots, formed throughout the body by hypercoagulation, are degraded to produce a copious quantity of fibrin degradation products (FDP). DIC is a bilateral disruption of the normal balance between coagulation and fibrinolysis, giving rise to the severe end results of both processes—thrombosis and hemorrhage.

Any disorder that introduces a stimulus to clotting into the bloodstream can cause DIC (see boxed material on p. 310). In the neonate, infections of bacterial and viral origin are the most common sources of such stimuli. Bacterial septicemia resulting from gram-negative rods, disseminated herpesvirus, and rubella are particularly noteworthy. It has been noted in association with abruptio placentae, presumably in response to the entry of amniotic fluid into the fetal circulation. Severe antigen-antibody reactions, as in Rh disease, also seem to be responsible for triggering this process.

ETIOLOGIES OF DIC CORRELATED WITH MECHANISMS OF COAGULOPATHY

Injury to endothelial cell → activation of intrinsic system through activation of factor XII

Gram-negative sepsis

Gram-positive sepsis

Virus infections: disseminated herpes simplex, cytomegalovirus, rubella

Fungal infections: disseminated *Candida albicans*
Protozoa: toxoplasmosis
Prolonged hypotension (any cause)
Severe acidosis
Hypoxemia
Hypothermia
Polycythemia-hyperviscosity
Intrauterine growth retardation
Breech delivery with severe birth asphyxia
Fetal distress during delivery
Vascular catheters
Cavernous hemangiomas

Tissue injury with libration of tissue factor, which complexes with factor VII and activates the extrinsic system

Abruptio placentae
Preeclampsia
Eclampsia
Dead twin fetus
Amniotic fluid embolism

Brain injury
Surgical procedures

Fetal neoplasms: acute leukemia, solid tumors
    (neonatal neuroblastoma)

Chorioangioma of the placenta

Necrotizing enterocolitis

*Red blood cell or platelet injury →
release of phospholipids, which accelerate
blood coagulation*

Intravascular hemolysis: severe erythroblastosis
    fetalis, incompatible RBC transfusions

Antigen-antibody reactions
Polycythemia (?)

*Reticuloendothelial system injury
with decreased clearance of activated
coagulation factors*

Severe hepatic disease

Modified from Gross, S. J., and Stuart, M. J.: Clin. Perinatol. 4:259, 1977.

Clinical signs are variable and widespread because bleeding may occur anywhere in the body. Bleeding from venipunctures is a common initial sign, even from the punctures inflicted 24 hours previously. Life-threatening hemorrhage into vital organs is cause for considerable anxiety when coagulation factors and platelets are extremely depressed.

The diagnosis can be made by demonstrating prolonged prothrombin time (PT) and partial thromboplastin time (PTT), thrombocytopenia ($<150,000/mm^3$), decreased fibrinogen level (<150 mg/dl), and increased fibrin degradation products (FDP). Factors V and VIII, which should be normal in unaffected premature and term infants, are often diminished in DIC. Thrombin time (TT) is usually prolonged beyond 30 seconds. Strong evidence for the diagnosis is the presence of fragmentation of red cells on a routine blood smear. Their architecture is disrupted as they pass through the smallest vessels in which fibrin thrombi have formed as a result of intravascular coagulation. The red cells are sheared by the microthrombi.

Therapy of DIC is largely unsatisfactory. Mortality seems to be related more to the underlying disease process than to the coagulation defects themselves. The universal recommendation is to treat the underlying disease, but the problem posed by DIC is often immediately life-threatening, and treatment of the underlying disease is often necessarily slow. Obviously in the presence of bacterial septicemia, antibiotics are appropriate. However, the infant may die from coagulopathy before the antibiotics can produce beneficial results. Serious underlying clinical entities involve several dysfunctions that themselves give rise to DIC; some of them are more amenable to relatively prompt control. Thus severe acidosis, electrolyte imbalance, hypoxemia, hypothermia, polycythemia, and hypotension are amenable to more rapid correction than septicemia. When the abnormalities that are produced by underlying diseases are controlled with relative rapidity, intravascular coagulation ceases.

Studies that have addressed direct treatment of the clotting abnormalities of DIC have been inadequately controlled or have failed to clearly demonstrate a superior approach. Fresh frozen plasma and platelets every 12 hours (for replacement of depleted clotting factors and diminished platelets) is used most frequently. Some investigators criticize this therapy because theoretically it provides additional substrate (platelets and coagulation factors) for continuation of accelerated intravascular clotting. Proverbially, the treatment adds fuel to the fire. Exchange transfusion is also widely recommended. Frozen red cells added to fresh frozen plasma is the preparation of choice. The exchange transfusion avoids the fluid overload that is inherent in repeated plasma and platelet transfusions. It may also remove abnormal noxious elements such as fibrin degradation products. Exchanges must be repeated every 12 hours if coagulopathy persists.

Heparin therapy would appear to be the treatment of choice, but it has too often failed. In the presence of cofactor antithrombin III, heparin inhibits activated factors of the coagulation cascade, especially factor X. Heparin also inhibits thrombin formation from prothrombin. It is a powerful anticoagulant that should halt the coagulative tornado that characterizes DIC, but numerous variables, unique to the neonate, preclude its success. Furthermore, monitoring heparin therapy in profoundly ill neonates is an awesome task. Appropriate dosage is difficult to calculate because clearance of heparin is decreased. Results of tests for the toxicity and effectiveness of heparin are often spurious. Most centers do not use it preferentially. Perhaps the clearest indication for its use is evidence that formation of large thrombi, rather than hemorrhage, is the predominant threat to life.

THROMBOCYTOPENIA

Platelets are the smallest cells in the blood. They do not possess nuclei and are normally visible on a routine blood smear in small aggregations. Formed from megakaryocytes in the bone marrow, platelets are indispensable to effective coagulation. They function in the earliest stages of hemostasis by aggregating at points of vascular injury, where they literally act as a plug. They also release substances that are essential for coagulation in its later stages (see normal coagulation, this chapter).

Clinical manifestations of platelet deficiency

Petechiae and ecchymoses are the characteristic lesions produced by platelet deficiencies. They are present at birth, or they appear any time thereafter. Typically, new lesions continue to form in crops if the deficiency persists. Central nervous system hemorrhage is always a potential hazard in the presence of platelet deficiency, but fortunately it occurs infrequently. Although bleeding can sometimes be massive, it is usually insufficient to cause a significant decline in hemoglobin concentration. However, the breakdown of extravasated blood sometimes results in serious hyperbilirubinemia. The principal disorders that produce thrombocytopenia are infectious, pharmacologic, or immunologic in nature.

Thrombocytopenia resulting from infection

Thrombocytopenia is a frequent accompaniment of perinatal infection. Among the bacterial infections, septicemia is by far the most prominent. Congenital syphilis also produces platelet deficiency. Thrombocytopenia, petechiae, and ecchymoses are major clinical signs of congenital rubella, toxoplasmosis, cytomegalovirus infection, and herpesvirus infection (Chapter 12). These bacterial and nonbacterial infections may produce a constellation of signs comprising hepatosplenomegaly, jaundice, anemia, and thrombocytopenia.

Thrombocytopenia induced by drugs

A number of drugs taken by the mother during pregnancy may destroy her platelets and the platelets of her fetus as well. The sulfonamides and quinine are of significance because of their widespread use in the past. These and other drugs stimulate the production of maternal antibodies, which destroy maternal platelets and cross the placenta to exert identical effects in the fetus.

Thrombocytopenia may rarely be produced by the thiazides, a group of diuretics used for the treatment of preeclamptic edema. In these circumstances, platelet antibodies are not produced in the mother; her own platelets remain intact, but those of the fetus are destroyed by toxic effects of the drug. Thrombocytopenia may persist for as long as 3 months after birth. In a few babies, hemorrhage may be extensive, primarily involving the gastrointestinal tract, brain, and lungs.

Thrombocytopenia induced by immune mechanisms

Fetal platelets may be destroyed by placental passage of antibody from the mother. This destruction is rare, and it is produced by two distinct mechanisms. In one type, antiplatelet antibodies are the result of maternal disease. They destroy her platelets and cross the placenta to destroy those of her fetus. This mechanism is operative in maternal *idiopathic thrombocytopenic purpura and systemic lupus erythematosus*.

In another type of immune mechanism, the mother's platelets are unaffected. This pattern is similar to that described for erythroblastosis fetalis. Platelets are serologically distinct because of the different antigens they possess. When fetal platelets enter the maternal circulation, the mother produces antibodies to them that cross the placenta to destroy fetal platelets. The resultant disease is known as *isoimmune neonatal thrombocytopenic purpura*. It varies widely in severity. Intracranial hemorrhage is apparently more common in this type of thrombocytopenia than in most others. Firstborn infants are frequently affected. The clinical signs are otherwise similar to any other type of platelet deficiency.

Thrombocytopenia and giant hemangioma

Congenital hemangiomas, usually large ones, may reduce the number of circulating platelets considerably. These vascular tumors trap and destroy tremendous numbers of platelets, thereby creating thrombocytopenia, which causes generalized bleeding. The platelet count of blood within the hemangioma is higher than in blood taken from other sites. Generalized hemorrhage is usually preceded by abrupt swelling and tenseness of the hemangioma. Treatment consists of irradiation of the hemangioma, which usually shrinks in several days. Removal of the tumor may be urgent if it compresses the trachea when situated in the neck. Irradiation should be given first, surgical excision may follow a few days later.

POLYCYTHEMIA-HYPERVISCOSITY ("THICK BLOOD SYNDROME")

Increased blood volume and hematocrit values may arise from four possible sources: (1) prolonged emptying of placental blood into the infant after birth, (2) continuous transfer of maternal blood to the fetus (maternofetal transfusion), (3) transfusion from a donor twin in utero (fetofetal transfusion), and (4) increased red cell production.

The first three groups are examples of passive acquisition of excessive red blood cells. The last category includes infants who generate excessive erythrocytes in response to intrauterine difficulties, congenital abnormalities, or chromosomal disorders. Table 9-4 lists the etiologies of polycythemia. In the last category are small-for-dates babies, infants who experienced intrauterine hypoxia, and babies with certain chromosomal abnormalities.

Polycythemia is said to occur when *venous* (not capillary) hematocrit is 65% or greater. An increased incidence has been noted in infants who are either large or small for gestational age, also in those who are born at high altitudes. The incidence in Denver (altitude 5000 feet) is reported at 5% of all births; at sea level the incidence is 2.5% or less. It is also reported in approximately 40% of the infants of diabetic mothers. Fetal hyperinsulinemia is often associated with enhanced levels of plasma erythropoietin, which is the primary stimulator of erythropoiesis. Active polycythemia is rare at gestational ages below 34 weeks.

Although hyperviscosity and polycythemia are not synonymous, there is a predictable relationship between the two. Viscosity of blood is largely determined by hematocrit, but also by the rigidity of red blood cells and the viscosity of plasma. By far the most significant factor is hematocrit. At hematocrits of 65% or greater, the blood of almost all infants is hyperviscous, hence the name "thick blood syndrome."

Table 9-4. Etiology of neonatal polycythemia

Active (increased intrauterine erythropoiesis)	Passive (secondary to erythrocyte transfusions)
Intrauterine hypoxia	Delayed cord clamping
Placental insufficiency	Intentional
Small for gestational age infants	Unassisted delivery
Post maturity	Maternal-fetal transfusion
Toxemia of pregnancy	Twin-to-twin transfusion
Drugs (propranolol)	
Severe maternal heart disease	
Maternal smoking (?)	
Maternal diabetes	
Neonatal thyrotoxicosis	
Congenital adrenal hyperplasia	
Chromosome abnormalities	
Trisomy 13	
Trisomy 18	
Trisomy 21 (Down's syndrome)	
Hyperplastic visceromegaly (Beckwith syndrome)	
Decreased fetal erythrocyte deformability	

From Oski, F. A., and Naiman, J. L.: Hematologic problems in the newborn, Philadelphia, 1982, W. B. Saunders Co.

The most frequent cause of polycythemia-hyperviscosity in otherwise normal term infants is delayed cord clamping. Red cells may also be acquired via maternofetal or fetofetal transfusions. These are the passive forms of polycythemia, and they are almost regularly associated with normal reticulocyte counts. In contrast, increased reticulocyte counts are regularly observed during the first few days after birth if polycythemia is a result of augmented fetal erythropoiesis.

The clinical signs of polycythemia-hyperviscosity include a broad spectrum of organ involvement. Presumably, abnormal signs are the result of diminished perfusion rates associated with "thick blood." However, the abnormalities commonly attributed to hyperviscosity are often a result of the underlying disorders that caused polycythemia, particularly fetal asphyxia, which itself produces central nervous system dysfunction. There is some evidence to suggest that sluggish blood flow is in fact a direct cause of central nervous system dysfunction. Thus, in symptomatic hyperviscosity, abnormalities of cerebral blood flow have been demonstrated by the Doppler technique, and these have been shown to become normal following thinning of blood by partial exchange transfusion. Similarly, abnormal renal glomerular blood flow has been rectified by partial plasma exchange.

Infants affected by central nervous system signs are hypotonic and difficult to arouse. Some are easily startled, irritable, and tremulous. In the extreme, some infants convulse. Other signs include enlargement of the liver, jaundice, deep red plethoric skin, and cyanosis during activity. Respiratory distress may be a result of diminished lung compliance. Congestive heart failure has also been observed. Priapism, acute renal failure, necrotizing enterocolitis, and peripheral gangrene have all been reported to be associated with thick blood.

Laboratory findings include occasional instances of thrombocytopenia, reticulocytosis (in infants who actively generated excessive erythrocytes), hypoglycemia, hyperbilirubinemia, and hypocalcemia. Chest films often reveal hyperaerated lungs associated with obvious vascular engorgement; occasionally alveolar infiltrates are discernible. Cardiomegaly is often observed on chest radiographs.

Glomerular filtration and urine sodium excretion are reduced. Glucose disappearance rates are increased, apparently because of enhanced cerebral utilization of glucose or perhaps reduced glucose production in sluggishly perfused liver.

Partial exchange transfusion, using fresh-frozen plasma to replace calculated volumes of blood, is the definitive treatment for polycythemia. The appropriate replacement volume is determined by subtracting the hematocrit desired from the abnormal one existing and then multiplying the result by the infant's blood volume. Finally, this value is divided by the existing abnormal hematocrit, and the volume of blood to be exchanged has been calculated.

Several reports have indicated that an increased incidence of residual abnormal central nervous system signs can be expected beyond the neonatal period in untreated polycythemic babies. Some investigators disagree. Those who are convinced of abnormal outcomes have advocated early partial plasma exchange transfusions when hematocrits exceed 65%. Others prefer to identify polycythemic infants, await the appearance of abnormal signs, and then perform the plasma exchange transfusion.

BIBLIOGRAPHY

Allen, F. H., Jr.: Historical perspective. In Frigoletto, F. D., Jr., Jewett, J. F., and Konugres, A. A., editors: Rh hemolytic disease: new strategy for eradication, Boston, 1982, G. K. Hall Medical Publishers.

Allen, F. H., and Diamond, L. K.: Erythroblastosis fetalis, Boston, 1958, Little, Brown & Co.

Bada, H. S., Chua, C., Salmon, J. H., and Hajjar, W.: Changes in intracranial pressure during exchange transfusion, J. Pediatr. **94:**129-132, 1979.

Bada, H. S., Korones, S. B., and Fitch, C. W.: Reversal of altered cerebral hemodynamics by plasma exchange transfusion in polycythemia, Clin. Res. **29**(5):894A, 1981 (abstract).

Barrow, E., and Peters, R. L.: Exsanguinating hemorrhage into scalp in newborn infants, S. Afr. Med. J. **42**:265, 1968.

Batton, D. G., Maisels, M. H., and Shulman, G.: Serum potassium changes following packed red cell transfusions in newborn infants, Transfusion **23**:163-164, 1983.

Biery, J. G., Corash, L., and Hubbard, V. S.: Medical uses of vitamin E, N. Engl. J. Med. **308**:1063-1071, 1983.

Blanchette, V. S., Gray, E., Hardie, M. J., et al.: Hyperkalemia after neonatal exchange transfusion: risk eliminated by washing red cell concentrates, J. Pediatr. **105**:321-324, 1984.

Bleyer, W. A., Hakami, N., and Shepard, T. H.: The development of hemostasis in the human fetus and newborn infant, J. Pediatr. **79**:838, 1971.

Bowman, J. M.: Efficacy of antenatal Rh prophylaxis. In Frigoletto, F. D., Jr., Jewett, J. F., and Konugres, A. A., editors: Rh hemolytic disease: new strategy for eradication, Boston, 1982, G. K. Hall Medical Publishers.

Clarke, C.: Rhesus haemolytic disease of the newborn and its prevention, Brit. J. Haematol. **52**:525-535, 1982.

Danks, D. M., and Stevens, L. H.: Neonatal respiratory distress associated with a high hematocrit reading, Lancet **2**:499, 1964.

Ehrenkranz, R. A.: Vitamin E and the neonate, Am. J. Dis. Child. **134**:1157-1166, 1980.

Gatti, R. A., et al.: Neonatal polycythemia with transient cyanosis and cardiorespiratory abnormalities, J. Pediatr. **69**:1063, 1966.

Gershanik, J. J., Levkoff, A. H., and Duncan, R.: Serum ionized calcium values in relation to exchange transfusion, J. Pediatr. **82**:847, 1973.

Gill, F. M.: Thrombocytopenia in the newborn, Sem. Perinatol. **7**:201-212, 1983.

Gorman, J. G.: New applications of Rh immune globulin: effect on protocols. In Frigoletto, F. D., Jr., Jewett, J. F., and Konugres, A. A., editors: Rh hemolytic disease: new strategy for eradication, Boston, 1982, G. K. Hall Medical Publishers.

Gorman, J. G.: Rh immunoglobulin in prevention of hemolytic disease of newborn child, N.Y. State J. Med. **83**:42-49, 1983.

Gross, G. P., Hathaway, W. E., and McGaughey, H. R.: Hyperviscosity in the neonate, J. Pediatr. **82**:1004, 1973.

Gross, S., and Melhorn, D. K.: Exchange transfusion with citrated whole blood for disseminated intravascular coagulation, J. Pediatr. **78**:415, 1971.

Gross, S., and Melhorn, D. K.: Vitamin E, red cell lipids and red cell stability in prematurity, Ann. N.Y. Acad. Sci. **203**:141, 1972.

Gross, S., Shurin, S. B., and Gordon, E. M.: The blood and hematopoietic system. In Fanaroff, A. A., and Martin, R. J., editors: Behrman's neonatal-perinatal medicine, ed. 3, St. Louis, 1983, The C. V. Mosby Co.

Gross, S. J., and Stuart, M. J.: Hemostasis in the premature infant, Clin. Perinatol. **4**:259-304, 1977.

Guyton, A. C.: Textbook of medical physiology, ed. 6, Philadelphia, 1981, W. B. Saunders Co., pp. 92-102.

Handin, R. I.: Physiology of coagulation: the platelet. In Nathan, D. G., and Oski, F. A., editors: Hematology of infancy and childhood, ed. 2, Philadelphia, 1981, W. B. Saunders Co.

Hathaway, W. E., and Bonnar, J.: Perinatal coagulation, New York, 1978, Grune and Stratton.

Hathaway, W. E., Mull, M. M., and Pechet, G. S.: Disseminated intravascular coagulation in the newborn, Pediatrics **43**:233, 1969.

Lackner, T. E.: Drug replacement following exchange transfusion, J. Pediatr. **100**:811-814, 1982.

Maisels, M. J., Li, T., Piechocki, J. T., and Werthman, M. W.: The effect of exchange transfusion on serum ionized calcium, Pediatrics **53**:683, 1974.

McDonald, M. M., and Hathaway, W. E.: Neonatal hemorrhage and thrombosis, Sem. Perinatol. **7**:213-225, 1983.

Michael, A. F., and Mauer, A. M.: Maternal-fetal transfusion as a cause of plethora in the neonatal period, Pediatrics **28**:458, 1961.

Naeye, R.: Human intrauterine parabiotic syndrome and its complications, N. Engl. J. Med. **268**:804, 1963.

Orzalesi, M.: ABO system incompatibility: relationship between direct Coombs' test positivity and neonatal jaundice, Pediatrics **51**:288, 1973.

Oski, F. A.: Nutritional anemias. In Walker, W. A., and Watkins, J. B., editors: Nutrition in pediatrics: basic science and clinical application, Boston, 1985, Little, Brown & Co.

Oski, F. A.: Nutritional anemias, Sem. Perinatol. **3**:381-395, 1979.

Oski, F. A., and Naiman, J. L.: Hematologic problems in the newborn, ed. 3, Philadelphia, 1982, W. B. Saunders Co.

Pearson, H. A.: Posthemorrhagic anemia in the newborn, Pediatr. Rev. **4**:40-43, 1982.

Pollack, W., Gorman, J. G., and Freda, V. J.: Rh immune suppression: past, present, and future. In Frigoletto, F. D., Jr., Jewett, J. F., and Konugres, A. A., editors: In Rh hemolytic disease: new strategy for eradication, Boston, 1982, G. K. Hall Medical Publishers.

Rosenberg, R. D.: Physiology of coagulation: the fluid phase. In Nathan, D. G., and Oski, F. A.: Hematology of infancy and childhood, ed. 2, Philadelphia, 1981, W. B. Saunders Co.

Sacks, M. O.: Occurrence of anemia and polycythemia in pheno-typically dissimilar single-ovum human twins, Pediatrics **24**:604, 1959.

Saigal, S., O'Neill, A., Surainder, Y., et al.: Placental transfusion and hyperbilirubinemia in the premature, Pediatrics **49:**406, 1972.

Scanlon, J. W., and Krakaur, R.: Hyperkalemia following exchange transfusion, J. Pediatr. **96:**108-110, 1980.

Setzer, E. S., Ahmed, F., Goldberg, R. N., et al.: Exchange transfusion using washed red blood cells reconstituted with fresh-frozen plasma for treatment of severe hyperkalemia in the neonate, J. Pediatr. **104:**443-446, 1984.

Sisson, T. R. C., Knutson, S., and Kendall, N.: The blood volume of infants. IV. Infants born by cesarean section, Am. J. Obstet. Gynecol. **117:**351, 1973.

Touloukian, R. J., Kadar, A., and Spencer, R. P.: The gastrointestinal complications of neonatal umbilical venous exchange transfusion: a clinical and experimental study, Pediatrics **51:**36. 1973.

Usher, R., and Lind, J.: Blood volume of the newborn premature infant, Acta Paediatr. Scand. **54:**419, 1965.

Neonatal jaundice

According to adult standards, all neonates have hyperbilirubinemia; their serum bilirubin levels exceed 1 mg/100 ml at some time during the first few days of life. These elevations of serum bilirubin levels produce visible jaundice in only half of all newborn infants, and for the majority of these babies the icterus is a normal event; in others it may indicate a number of disorders of diverse etiology (see outline, p. 322).

BILIRUBIN IN THE NORMAL NEONATE
The physiologic itinerary of bilirubin
(Fig. 10-1)

Bilirubin serves no known useful purpose. It is an end product of the breakdown of several substances, primarily hemoglobin. One may thus envision a physiologic "itinerary" that is designed to rid the body of bilirubin at a rate that approximates its formation. Ultimately, bilirubin is delivered to the intestinal lumen where it is excreted in feces. The "itinerary" can be outlined as follows: (1) Bilirubin is formed (mostly from hemoglobin) in reticuloendothelial cells and enters the bloodstream. (2) It is transported in circulating blood bound to albumin molecules. (3) It is extracted from the bloodstream by cells of the liver parenchyma (hepatocytes), involving the following steps: (a) disengagement from albumin binding by the hepatocyte cell membrane, which has a stronger affinity for bilirubin than albumin; (b)

317

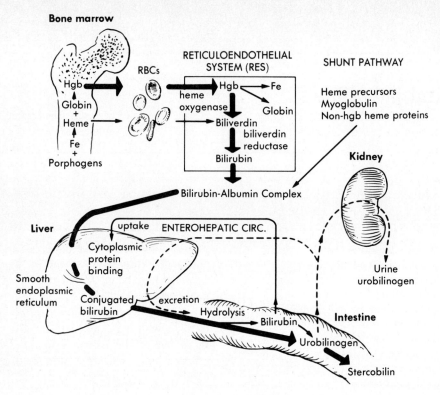

Fig. 10-1. The "bilirubin itinerary": synthesis, transport, metabolism, and excretion. (By Gartner, L. M. In Assali, N. S.: Pathophysiology of gestation, New York, 1972, Academic Press.)

transformation to a water-soluble form (bilirubin glucuronide) within the hepatocyte; (c) secretion of water-soluble bilirubin glucuronide into the canaliculus structurally associated with the hepatocyte; (d) progression from the canaliculus into the bile ducts that comprise the biliary tree; (e) further progress into the extrahepatic biliary tract, including ultimately the common bile duct, which empties into the intestinal lumen.

Description of the steps outlined above first requires an understanding of the characteristics of conjugated and unconjugated bilirubin. Pathologic states entail failure to excrete unconjugated bilirubin alone or both forms together. Failure to maintain an equilibrium between production and excretion (with resultant retention) is a result of

excessive production, which overloads an otherwise normally operating mechanism for excretion, normal production in the face of an *impaired processing mechanism,* or both.

Types of bilirubin (conjugated; unconjugated)

The existence of direct- and indirect-reacting bilirubin has been known for over 50 years, but the chemical differences that characterize them were first demonstrated in the 1950s. Direct-reacting bilirubin is bilirubin glucuronide, which is also referred to as conjugated bilirubin because the free bilirubin molecule undergoes conjugation with a glucuronide radical in the liver. Because the resultant complex is water soluble, it is normally excreted through the biliary tree and also through the kidneys if serum levels are abnormally high. Indirect-reacting bilirubin is unconjugated bilirubin because it has not been converted to the glucuronide form in the liver. Since it is fat soluble and not water soluble, it cannot be excreted in bile or through the kidneys. Because it is fat soluble, unconjugated bilirubin has a high affinity for extravascular tissue, particularly fatty tissue and brain. In plasma it is complexed to albumin. A laboratory report of total bilirubin includes the direct and indirect fractions and does not distinguish between them unless the direct fraction is specifically determined.

Formation of bilirubin

The fetus excretes bilirubin across the placenta into the maternal circulation. Only unconjugated (indirect) bilirubin is discarded by the placental route; conjugated (direct) bilirubin is not. The fetal liver is severely limited in its capacity to conjugate bilirubin. In exceptional circumstances, however, substantial quantities of direct bilirubin are demonstrable at birth. This has been observed in severe Rh disease that is managed by intrauterine transfusions, severe congenital rubella, toxoplasmosis, cytomegalovirus infection, and other severe infections.

Approximately 80% of the body's bilirubin is formed from the breakdown of erythrocytes. The life span of a normal neonatal red cell is estimated at 80 to 100 days by different investigators (adult life span is 120 days); its fragility increases as the cell ages, and it is then sequestered from the blood. Hemoglobin is then split into two fragments, heme and globin. The globin fraction is a protein, and it is utilized as such by the body. Unconjugated bilirubin is formed from heme in reticuloendothelial cells that are primarily located in the spleen and liver. One gram of hemoglobin yields 35 mg of unconjugated bilirubin. The normal neonate produces bilirubin at a rate of 6 to 8 mg/kg/24 hours. The remaining 20% of the body's bilirubin is produced by destruction of early red cell forms soon after their release from bone marrow or within the marrow itself, from nonhemoglobin sources that are predominantly in the liver, and from myoglobin.

Bilirubin transport in plasma (albumin binding)

Once formed, bilirubin is transported in plasma to the liver, where it is conjugated with glucuronide (see later). In plasma, unconjugated bilirubin is bound to albumin; 1 g of albumin binds between 8.5 and 17 mg of bilirubin. The albumin molecule has two binding sites for bilirubin. One of them binds bilirubin tightly, the other more loosely. These loosely bound bilirubin molecules tend to migrate to plasma as free (unbound) bilirubin. After complete saturation of "tight" binding sites, there is a relatively abrupt rise in loosely bound or free bilirubin. The level of bilirubin at which saturation occurs is extremely variable. Bilirubin that is complexed to albumin cannot leave the vascular space. In the liver, however, the hepatocyte membrane apparently has a higher affinity for bilirubin than does plasma. The bilirubin molecule is thus disengaged from its albumin binding site to enter the hepatocyte. A minute amount of the pigment is unbound, in which state it is free to leave the blood and permeate tissues. It is in the unbound state that bilirubin also diffuses into liver cells, where conjugation with glucuronide takes place. When not bound to albumin, bilirubin permeates other extravascular tissues, including the brain. The quantity of unbound bilirubin is increased if albumin binding capacity is reduced or if the affinity of bilirubin for albumin is diminished. This may occur in several circumstances. Thus unconjugated bilirubin may accumulate to levels that surpass albumin binding capacity. This accumulation occurs at varying serum bilirubin levels that cannot be predicted with any degree of consistency. Much depends on maturity and illness of the baby. Furthermore, at any serum level, bilirubin is displaceable from albumin binding sites by several substances having a greater affinity for these sites. These substances include metabolites such as free fatty acids, or drugs such as sulfonamides, salicylates, and sodium benzoate. Albumin binding capacity is reduced in the presence of an acid blood pH. Hypoalbuminemia causes low binding capacity, whereas binding capacity can be increased by giving albumin intravenously. Neonatal serum albumin does not bind bilirubin as effectively as adult serum albumin. Thus, gram for gram, "fetal albumin" has a lower binding capacity than that of the adult. Binding capacity increases with age to approximately adult levels by 5 months. The binding capacity of purified human serum albumin, administered at the time of exchange transfusion to augment bilirubin removal, is half that of circulating serum albumin in adults. Neonatal serum albumin falls between the two.

Bilirubin in the liver cell (hepatocyte); conjugation and excretion (Fig. 10-1)

The cell membranes of hepatocytes disengage unconjugated bilirubin from albumin binding sites in circulating blood. Once within the cell the bilirubin is bound to and transferred by a substance called *ligandin* and also, though less effectively, by "Z protein." These proteins are intracellular carriers of bilirubin and other substances. Within the hepatocyte, ligandin transports bilirubin to the smooth endoplasmic reticulum where the conjugation of bilirubin with a glucuronide radical takes place through a series of reactions culminating in the transfer of glucuronic acid from *uridine diphosphate glucuronic acid* (UDPGA) to bilirubin. This last reaction is catalyzed by the transfer enzyme, *glucuronyl transferase*. The steps that precede the formation of UDPGA require oxygen and glucose. Oxygen deprivation and hypoglycemia may therefore impair UDPGA production and contribute to hyperbilirubinemia. Bilirubin glucuronide is passed from the liver cell into the biliary tree and then into the gastrointestinal tract where it is converted to urobilinogen and then to stercobilin. Some urobilinogen is reabsorbed into the circulation from the intestine to be excreted through the kidneys.

The fetal and neonatal small intestinal mucosa contains a considerable amount of the enzyme *beta-glucuronidase*. This substance can convert the bilirubin glucuronide that has entered the intestine back to unconjugated bilirubin by splitting off the glucuronide. Bilirubin is now fat soluble once again and is absorbed across the intestinal wall into the *portal (enterohepatic) circulation*. Meconium contains 0.5 to 1 mg of bilirubin per gram. Delayed meconium passage thus increases the amount of bilirubin reabsorbed across intestinal mucosa because more bilirubin glucuronide is converted to the unconjugated reabsorbable form. This "enterohepatic shunt" contributes significantly to physiologic jaundice: it may explain the high incidence of hyperbilirubinemia in some cases of upper intestinal obstruction. It is the mechanism by which late feeding, because it promotes intestinal stasis, results in higher mean serum bilirubin levels than early feeding. The old practice of withholding feedings for 48 hours has long been discontinued for this and several other good reasons as well. During the first few days of life the neonate's capacity to excrete bilirubin is only 1% or 2% that of the adult's. This is apparently related to deficient activity of glucuronyl transferase, which increases gradually after a few days, probably attaining adult levels at 2 to 4 weeks of age.

Physiologic jaundice

Although a deficiency of glucuronyl transferase has been said to be the major cause of physiologic jaundice, the diminution in activity of this enzyme is not as profound as previously believed. Glucuronyl transferase deficiency is not the sole cause of physiologic jaundice; a number of other immature functional difficulties are accountable. First, *an excessive amount of bilirubin is delivered to the liver* because synthesis is increased and because there is significant reabsorption of the pigment from the intestine via the enterohepatic shunt (see previous discussion). For several reasons, the neonate generates three times more bilirubin per kilogram of body weight than the adult. The number of red cells per kilogram of weight is greater, and these cells have shorter survival times (70 to 90 days versus 120 days in adults). Therefore senescent red cells are sequestered and dismembered in greater numbers during shorter time intervals to yield a higher rate of bilirubin production. Second, *there is a diminished capacity of the liver to excrete the excessive bilirubin delivered to it* because (1) uptake by hepatic cells is inhibited and (2) there is diminished conjugation of pigment in the liver cell. The inhibited uptake of bilirubin may be attributable to deficient ligandin in the hepatic cell. Hyperbilirubinemia is therefore a regular occurrence in all neonates, but jaundice occurs in only half of them because serum bilirubin levels must exceed 4 to 6 mg/dl before it is visible as pigment in the skin. In term infants a peak unconjugated bilirubin level is reached on the third or fourth day of life; in premature infants it is attained on the fifth or sixth day. This is physiologic jaundice. Physiologic jaundice is a useful clinical concept because it implies a normal state that does not require therapy. As a rule, physiologic jaundice fulfills the following specific criteria: (1) the infant is otherwise well; (2) in term infants, jaundice first appears *after 24 hours* and disappears by the end of the seventh day; (3) in premature infants, jaundice is first evident after 48 hours and disappears by the ninth or tenth day; (4) serum unconjugated bilirubin concentration does not exceed 12 mg/dl, either in term or preterm infants; (5) hyperbilirubinemia is almost exclusively of the unconjugated variety, and conjugated (direct) bilirubin should not exceed 1 to 1.5 mg/dl; (6) daily increments of bilirubin concentration should not surpass 5 mg/dl. Bilirubin levels in excess of 12 mg/dl may indicate either an exaggeration of the physiologic handicap (as in perinatal asphyxia) or the presence of disease. *At any serum bilirubin level, the appearance of jaundice during the first day of life or persistence beyond the ages previously delineated usually indicates a pathologic process.*

CAUSES OF NEONATAL JAUNDICE

The boxed material on p. 322 presents most of the disorders associated with neonatal jaundice, categorized by the mechanisms involved and type of hyperbilirubinemia.

Table 10-1 presents the most important clinical and laboratory data that suggest the causes of abnormal jaundice. It is important to understand that jaundice is probably the most common *potentially* abnormal sign in the immediate postnatal period but that only a fraction of affected infants require detailed investigation. Diagnostic assessment is necessary for babies in whom:

1. Jaundice appears within the first 24 hours after birth.
2. Serum bilirubin is over 12 mg/dl if term, 15 mg/dl if premature.
3. Serum bilirubin rises more than 5 mg/dl in 24 hours.
4. Conjugated (direct) bilirubin is more than 2 mg/dl.
5. Phototherapy is considered necessary.
6. Jaundice persists beyond 7 days if term and beyond 10 to 14 days if premature.

Intrinsic blood disorders

Isoimmune hemolytic disease of the newborn (p. 289). Maternofetal blood group incompatibility (Rh, ABO) is the most frequent cause of pathologic jaundice. Hemolysis is intravascular by virtue of an antigen-antibody reaction on the surface of the red cells.

Polycythemia (p. 313). An increased quantity of erythrocytes results in sequestration of greater numbers of aged cells, which, when broken down, yield excessive amounts of bilirubin. The accumulation of pigment is occasionally sufficiently pronounced to necessitate an exchange transfusion. Hyperbilirubinemia occurs in the absence of maternal blood group incompatibility or any other disorder that accelerates hemolysis.

Structural and enzyme defects of red cells. Enzymatic deficiencies, the most prominent of

CAUSES OF PATHOLOGIC NEONATAL JAUNDICE

Overproduction

Intravascular blood disorders (unconjugated hyperbilirubinemia)
  Maternal-fetal incompatibilities (isoimmunization)
    Rh, ABO, other blood groups
  Structural and enzyme defects of red cells
    Hereditary spherocytosis
    Hereditary elliptocytosis
    Pyknocytosis
    G-6-PD deficiency
    Pyruvate kinase deficiency
  Polycythemia-hyperviscosity syndrome
  Drug-induced hemolysis
Extravascular hemolysis; enclosed hemorrhage (unconjugated hyperbilirubinemia)
  Neonatal swallowed blood syndrome
  Intraventricular-periventricular hemorrhage
  Petechiae, ecchymoses (bruising)
  Hematomas (cephalhematoma)
  Swallowed blood syndrome

Impaired excretion pathway

Hepatic dysfunction due to enzyme, hormone disorders (unconjugated hyperbilirubinemia)
  Glucuronyl transferase deficiencies (types I and II)
  Transient familial neonatal hyperbilirubinemia
  Galactosemia
  Breast-feeding jaundice
Obstructed biliary tree (unconjugated plus conjugated hyperbilirubinemia)
  Biliary atresia
  Choledochal cyst
  Cystic fibrosis
  Cholestasis due to parenteral alimentation

Increased enterohepatic absorption (unconjugated hyperbilirubinemia)
  Swallowed blood syndrome
  High intestinal atresia; stenosis
  Lower intestinal atresia, stenosis
  Annular pancreas
  Meconium ileus (cystic fibrosis)
  Hirschsprung's disease

Mixed (overproduction plus impaired excretion)

Bacterial infection (unconjugated plus conjugated hyperbilirubinemia)
  Septicemia
  Necrotizing enterocolitis
  Pneumonia
  Kidney infection ($\pm$conjugated hyperbilirubinemia)
  Congenital syphilis
Nonbacterial infection (unconjugated plus conjugated hyperbilirubinemia)
  Cytomegalic inclusion disease
  Rubella
  Toxoplasmosis
  Herpes simplex
  Coxsackie virus
  Echovirus
  Hepatitis B

Mechanisms unknown (unconjugated hyperbilirubinemia)

Infants of diabetic mothers
Hypothyroidism

Table 10-1. Significance of clinical data in diagnosis of neonatal jaundice*

Information	Significance
Clinical data	
Family history	
Parent or sibling with history of jaundice or anemia	Suggests hereditary hemolytic anemia, such as hereditary spherocytosis
Previous sibling with neonatal jaundice	Suggests hemolytic disease from ABO or Rh isoimmunization
History of liver disease in siblings or disorders such as cystic fibrosis, galactosemia, tyrosinemia, hypermethioninemia, Crigler-Najjar syndrome, or alpha$_1$-antitrypsin deficiency	All associated with neonatal hyperbilirubinemia
Maternal history	
Unexplained illness during pregnancy	Consider congenital infections such as rubella, cytomegalovirus, toxoplasmosis, herpes, syphilis, or hepatitis
Diabetes mellitus	Increased incidence of jaundice among infants of diabetic mothers
Drug ingestion during pregnancy	Ingestion of sulfonamides, nitrofurantoins, or antimalarials may initiate hemolysis in G-6-PD–deficient infant
History of labor and delivery	
Vacuum extraction	Increased incidence of cephalhematoma and jaundice
Oxytocin-induced labor	Increased incidence of hyperbilirubinemia
Delayed cord clamping	Increased incidence of hyperbilirubinemia among polycythemic infants
Apgar score	Increased incidence of jaundice in asphyxiated infants
Infant's history	
Delayed passage of meconium or infrequent stools	Increased enterohepatic circulation of bilirubin. Consider intestinal atresia, annular pancreas, Hirschsprung's disease, meconium plug, drug-induced ileus (hexamethonium)
Caloric intake	Inadequate caloric intake results in delay in bilirubin conjugation
Vomiting	Suspect sepsis, galactosemia, or pyloric stenosis; all associated with hyperbilirubinemia
Infant's physical examination	
Small for gestational age	Infants frequently polycythemic and jaundiced
Head size	Microcephaly seen with intrauterine infections associated with jaundice
Cephalhematoma	Entrapped hemorrhage associated with hyperbilirubinemia
Pallor	Suspect hemolytic anemia
Petechiae	Suspect congenital infection, overwhelming sepsis, or severe hemolytic disease as cause of jaundice

*Modified from McMillan, J. A., Nieburg, P. I., and Oski, F. A.: The newborn. In The whole pediatrician catalog, Philadelphia, 1977, W. B. Saunders Co.

Continued.

Table 10-1. Significance of clinical data in diagnosis of neonatal jaundice—cont'd

Information	Significance
Clinical data—cont'd	
Infant's physical examination—cont'd	
Appearance of umbilical stump	Omphalitis and sepsis may produce jaundice
Hepatosplenomegaly	Suspect hemolytic anemia or congenital infection
Optic fundi	Chorioretinitis suggests congenital infection as cause of jaundice
Umbilical hernia	Consider hypothyroidism
Congenital anomalies	Jaundice occurs with increased frequency among infants with trisomic condition
Laboratory data	
Maternal	
Blood group and indirect Coombs' test	Necessary for evaluation of possible ABO or Rh incompatibility
Serology	Rule out congenital syphilis
Infant	
Hemoglobin	Anemia suggests hemolytic disease or large entrapped hemorrhage; hemoglobin above 22 g/dl associated with increased incidence of jaundice
Reticulocyte count	Elevation suggests hemolytic disease
Red cell morphology	Spherocytes suggest ABO incompatibility or hereditary spherocytosis; red cell fragmentation seen in disseminated intravascular coagulation
Platelet count	Thrombocytopenia suggests infection
White cell count	Total white cell count less than 5000/mm^3 or increase in band forms to greater than 2000/mm^3 suggests infection
Sedimentation rate	Values in excess of 5 during the first 48 hours indicate infection or ABO incompatibility
Direct bilirubin	Elevation suggests infection or severe Rh incompatibility
Immunoglobulin M	Elevation indicates infection
Blood group and direct and indirect Coombs' test	Required to rule out hemolytic disease as a result of isoimmunization
Carboxyhemoglobin	Elevated in infants with hemolytic disease or entrapped hemorrhage
Urinalysis	Presence of reducing substance suggests diagnosis of galactosemia

which is G-6-PD deficiency (p. 298), are responsible for hemolysis and jaundice because of disrupted erythrocyte metabolism; that is particularly noteworthy in premature black infants.

Abnormal contours of erythrocytes also render them vulnerable to early dissolution and the occasional production of jaundice. Hereditary spherocytosis is the most common disorder in this category. Rare abnormalities of red cell morphology that may also cause icterus are hereditary elliptocytosis (p. 299) and pyknocytosis. In pyknocytosis the red cells are small and stain rather deeply; the cell borders are irregular. Their life span is abnormally short, thereby increasing the rate of hemolysis.

Drug toxicity (chemical hemolysins). Excessive doses of vitamin K_3 have produced hyperbilirubinemia in premature infants. Hemolysis is more severe and more likely to occur in the presence of G-6-PD deficiency. Hyperbilirubinemia has also been reported in infants whose mothers received large doses of vitamin K_3 to protect the infant from hemorrhagic disease of the newborn. Vitamin K should be administered to the infant in the form of K_1, only in an intramuscular dose of 0.5 to 1 mg. Ingestion or inhalation of naphthalene is a rare but fascinating example of drug-induced icterus. It has been reported in G-6-PD–deficient infants whose mothers ingested or inhaled fumes from mothballs.

Extravascular hemolysis (enclosed hemorrhage; unconjugated hyperbilirubinemia)

Degradation of blood in enclosed spaces is relatively rapid. Perhaps the most graphic example is the hyperbilirubinemia that follows the formation of *petechiae* in the skin from any cause. One gram of hemoglobin is transformed into 35 mg of bilirubin; the added pigment from rapid hemolysis of a small amount of blood thus overtaxes the neonate's limited capacity to conjugate bilirubin. Extensive *ecchymosis* from traumatic delivery is not uncommon in small premature infants; an inordinately high level of serum bilirubin often follows. Large *cephalhematomas* produce the same effect, particularly if they are bilateral. Infrequently, *intraventricular-periventricular hemorrhage* is associated with protracted hyperbilirubinemia. If no other cause for protracted jaundice can be identified, a lumbar puncture should be done to demonstrate dark brown blood. This is old blood from an intraventricular hemorrhage, and it is sometimes associated with little or no symptomatology. *Swallowed blood syndrome* occurs when the baby has swallowed maternal blood during delivery. Hemolysis in the intestinal lumen is followed by absorption through the enterohepatic circulation. The overproduced bilirubin exceeds hepatic capacity to metabolize it.

Impaired hepatic function

Deficient glucuronyl transferase activity. Two rare entities that involve glucuronyl transferase deficiency are worthy of mention. *Familial nonhemolytic jaundice* (Crigler-Najjar syndrome) is a heritable, permanent deficiency of glucuronyl transferase that does not involve hemolysis. Unconjugated hyperbilirubinemia persists throughout life because of an inability to form bilirubin glucuronide. The syndrome occurs in a serious, often lethal form (type I) and in a milder form that is apparently a partial deficiency of glucuronyl transferase type II. Type I bilirubinemia ranges upward from 20 to 25 mg/dl. Numerous exchange transfusions are often required in the neonatal period. In contrast to type II, it resists phenobarbital therapy. Kernicterus and death are common. Serum bilirubin in type II disease is generally under 20 to 25 mg/dl, and small amounts of bilirubin glucuronide are in bile. Response to phenobarbital is usually satisfactory. Kernicterus is less likely to occur in the milder expression of the syndrome. Most survivors suffer severe brain damage as a result of bilirubin toxicity. Occasionally kernicterus develops later in childhood.

Transient familial neonatal hyperbilirubinemia (Lucey-Driscoll syndrome) affects all the offspring of one mother. Severe unconjugated hyperbilirubinemia appears during the first few days and subsides during the second or third week. An unidentified factor in the sera of affected mothers and in their infants has been shown to impair glucuronyl transferase activity in vitro.

Infection. Bacterial and nonbacterial infections are often associated with jaundice. Some degree of conjugated (direct) hyperbilirubinemia is frequent, indicating impaired liver function and of-

ten actual destruction of hepatic tissue. Septicemia and renal infection produce hemolysis as well.
The nonbacterial infections and syphilis do likewise; structural liver damage occurs more frequently in them than in the bacterial diseases.

Metabolic factors

Infants of diabetic mothers. The basis for increased incidence of hyperbilirubinemia in infants
of diabetic mothers is unknown. The frequency
of prematurity and respiratory distress among
these babies is probably the most important factor. Depression by asphyxia of hepatic function
that is already immature seems plausible. Furthermore, severe illness diminishes intestinal mobility, thereby enhancing reabsorption of bilirubin from the small intestine.

Galactosemia. Protracted bilirubinemia, with
either moderately or severely elevated levels,
may occur in galactosemia as the only clinical
manifestation. Jaundice may persist over 10 days.
The bilirubin is unconjugated at first, but later,
as liver damage begins, conjugated bilirubin is
retained in the blood.

Breast milk jaundice. This syndrome of unconjugated hyperbilirubinemia occurs in 1% to 5%
of breast-fed term infants. Two substances in
breast milk, a pregnanediol and a free fatty acid,
have been suggested as causes of this syndrome.
Both are believed to inhibit the activity of glucuronyl transferase in the neonatal liver. Unless
the mother has had a previously involved baby,
the syndrome cannot be anticipated during the
first 3 to 4 days of life because only the normal
pattern of physiologic jaundice is discernible.
Breast milk does not augment bilirubin levels during the first 3 days of life. If there has been a
previous infant with breast milk jaundice, there
is a 70% possibility of recurrence in subsequently
born siblings. On the fourth or fifth day of life,
when physiologic hyperbilirubinemia is expected
to subside, bilirubin levels continue to climb until
they reach peak concentrations of 10 to 27 mg/dl
between 10 and 15 days of age. If breast feeding
is not interrupted, bilirubin levels gradually decline from peak to normal levels sometime between 3 and 12 weeks of age. If breast feeding is
discontinued for 48 to 72 hours, a prompt decline
in bilirubin occurs. Resumption of breast feeding
is followed by a rise in bilirubin of only 2 or 3
mg/dl and a subsequent decline. We prefer to
interrupt breast feeding to establish the diagnosis
of this benign syndrome and to allay the maternal
apprehensions that are inevitable in the presence
of protracted jaundice. Affected infants are otherwise well. They feed and gain weight normally,
and their bowel movements are unaffected.

Hypothyroidism. Persistent low-grade hyperbilirubinemia may be, as in galactosemia, the only
sign of hypothyroidism in the first 2 to 4 weeks
of life. Only unconjugated bilirubin is involved.

Biliary obstruction (biliary atresia)

Obliteration of the biliary tree is not common.
It has been noted in congenital rubella infection,
but other causes, still unknown, are operative as
well. Jaundice appears during the first week or
later; half the affected infants are not icteric until
the second week. Conjugated hyperbilirubinemia
always develops eventually, although some degree of unconjugated bilirubin accumulation also
occurs, particularly at the onset of jaundice. The
conjugated hyperbilirubinemia progresses relentlessly in the months or few years left of life.
Biliary cirrhosis eventually becomes so extensive
as to virtually eliminate most of the liver functions.

Currently, biliary atresia is not considered to
be a congenital anomaly but a progressive obliteration of the biliary tract of unknown etiology
that, in only a few instances, may eventually clear
spontaneously. Infection of some sort, as yet un-
demonstrated, is a favored explanation by many.
Obliteration of the bile duct system occurs at any
level—from the microscopic canaliculi in liver parenchyma down to the common bile duct. Thus
intrahepatic obstruction is the sole manifestation
in a minority of infants, extrahepatic obstruction
being far more common. Occasionally, both areas

are involved. The obliterative process may begin in utero or in the immediate postnatal period; the disease progresses postnatally. It has not been found in stillborn fetuses, probably indicating that it is not a completely evolved congenital anomaly.

Biliary atresia is preponderantly a disorder of term infants, affecting females twice as often as males. These otherwise well infants become jaundiced in the second week of life or later; the liver, and eventually the spleen, become massively enlarged. Hyperbilirubinemia, at first unconjugated, soon becomes largely conjugated. Stools are clay colored and putty-like in consistency. For several months these infants appear well, except for the jaundice. Later, as hepatic dysfunction progresses, nutrition and severe growth impairment supervene. Ultimately a bleeding diathesis appears. Surgery may help a minority of infants.

KERNICTERUS (BILIRUBIN ENCEPHALOPATHY)

Kernicterus, the most serious complication of neonatal hyperbilirubinemia, is probably caused by deposition of unconjugated, unbound bilirubin in brain cells. The signs of so-called "classic" kernicterus were described at the turn of this century. They first appear between the second and tenth days of life in infants who are deeply jaundiced. These signs are identifiable in full-term babies; they are rare in kernicteric premature infants. Depression appears at the onset, characterized by coma, lethargy, diminished activity and Moro reflex, hypotonia, and absent sucking and rooting reflexes. Signs of excitation follow the depression, including twitching, generalized seizures, opisthotonos, hypertonia, and a high-pitched cry. Approximately half of affected infants do not survive. Those who do are affected by choreoathetoid cerebral palsy and often by high-frequency hearing impairment. A few are intellectually impaired. Neurologic deficits in later infancy and childhood have been noted when little or no neurologic disturbance has been identified in jaundiced infants during the neonatal period.

The *pathogenesis* of kernicterus is unknown. Though much has been written, little has been elucidated. According to current concepts, damage occurs when unconjugated bilirubin enters neurons. The entry is facilitated by (1) diminished albumin binding of bilirubin so that the free form permeates neuronal cell membranes, and (2) by disruption of the blood-brain barrier, allowing migration of bilirubin into brain parenchyma. In normal circumstances, structure and function of the blood-brain barrier preclude the entry of bilirubin into brain substance. Free bilirubin becomes available for egress from the circulation when (1) accumulation of the pigment exceeds the capacity of albumin to bind it, (2) when the binding capacity of albumin is impaired, or (3) when bilirubin is displaced from its binding sites on albumin by substances such as sulfa drugs and numerous other pharmacologic agents. Albumin binding capacity is diminished in the presence of acidosis. Furthermore, bilirubin may be dispossessed from its binding site by the heme pigment that is produced during severe hemolysis. Similar displacement occurs when free fatty acids accumulate in plasma as a result of hypoglycemia and hypothermia.

Morphologic changes in affected brain cells suggest that kernicteric damage impairs learning, memory, and adaptive behavior among survivors. The most commonly affected regions of the brain, however, are not the cerebral cortex, but rather the basal ganglia, the subthalamic nuclei, and the hippocampal cortex. Kernicterus is identifiable at autopsy by grossly visible yellow discoloration of involved brain tissue. Microscopically, there is also necrosis of neurons in the yellowed regions of brain. It is doubtful that kernicteric damage has occurred unless neuronal damage is also evident microscopically.

The major clinical question, incompletely answered for years, concerns the relationship between bilirubin levels in plasma and the occurrence of kernicterus. The relationship between bilirubin levels and kernicterus was first suggested in the late 1940s and then documented in 1952, but only in term babies who had erythroblastosis. In that study the association between kernicteric brain damage and hyperbilirubinemia was shown by an increasing incidence of encephalopathy as bilirubin levels became more elevated; by jaundice that always preceded the onset of brain damage; and by the diminished incidence of encephalopathy with control of bilirubin levels by exchange transfusion. Ramifications of these initial observations are still unsettled today. Do high bilirubin concentrations cause kernicterus in *nonhemolytic* term infants? There is no evidence for that contention. Do asymptomatic babies whose bilirubin concentrations exceed 20 mg/dl have developmental handicaps in later childhood? Today we can only say "perhaps." Other unanswered questions concern serum bilirubin levels at various gestational ages; their relationship to immediate brain damage and to later developmental impairment is unknown. For example, in premature infants there is no established level of bilirubin that predicts increased likelihood of kernicterus; nor do we know if innocent bilirubin levels at any given gestational age are damaging at lower gestational ages.

There are no generally accepted criteria for treatment and for prediction of outcomes. There is only reluctant consensus. This much seems to be rigidly accepted in practice if not in belief: serum bilirubin concentrations in excess of 20 mg/dl in term infants are an indication for exchange transfusion, *whether or not blood incompatibility (ABO or Rh) is present*. Yet this rigid rule is only based on the 1952 report on *Rh disease in term babies*. Similarly, 15 mg/dl is accepted in larger preterm babies, and 10 to 12 mg/dl is regarded as an indication for exchange transfusion in the smallest premature infants. There is no sound basis for these categorical recommendations. Kernicterus has been reported at considerably lower levels than those recommended, presumably because of a high concentration of unbound (free) bilirubin. Finally, one should also realize that for premature infants we cannot delineate a serum

bilirubin concentration below which kernicterus is unlikely to occur; it has been reported at a level of 3.3 mg/dl!

"Classic" kernicterus is no longer seen in our nurseries. We now recognize kernicterus in small premature babies, but only at autopsy. The early descriptions dwelled upon term or near-term infants who were untreated. Percent survival of very small premature infants was considerably lower than it is today. With the inception of exchange transfusion, there were fewer infants with "classic" kernicterus. When phototherapy appeared on the scene, the rare instance of kernicterus became rarer. Today the use of anti-Rh immunoglobulin (see p. 296), plus anticipatory management of fetal erythroblastosis during pregnancy, has virtually eliminated kernicterus. Bilirubin encephalopathy is still a problem, but only in small preterm babies whose birth weights are less than 1500 grams. Their clinical signs are not at all sim-

Table 10-2. Recommended maximal total serum bilirubin concentrations (mg/dl)*†

Birth weight category (grams)‡	Uncomplicated course	Complicated course§
Less than 1250	13	10
1250-1499	15	13
1500-1999	17	15
2000-2499	18	17
2500 and up	20	18

*From Gartner, L. M., and Lee, K. S.: Jaundice and liver disease. In Behrman, R. E., editor: Neonatal-perinatal medicine: diseases of the fetus and infant, ed. 3, St. Louis, 1983, The C. V. Mosby Co.

†Direct-reacting bilirubin concentrations are not subtracted unless they amount to more than 50% of the total serum bilirubin concentration. Applicable during the first 28 days of life.

‡Equivalent gestational age categories may be used in lieu of birth weight for small-for-gestational age (SGA) infants.

§Complications include perinatal asphyxia and acidosis, postnatal hypoxia and acidosis, significant and persistent hypothermia, hypoalbuminemia, meningitis and other significant infection, hemolysis, and hypoglycemia.

ilar to those described for the larger infants. In them the signs of brain damage caused by periventricular-intraventricular hemorrhage, metabolic disorders, and by fluid and electrolyte imbalances are identical to those of bilirubin encephalopathy. Kernicterus is unrecognizable during life in small premature infants. It is almost always an autopsy diagnosis. Actually, the extent to which bilirubin is bound to albumin is probably more important than its concentration in the serum. Bilirubin encephalopathy is caused by the migration of unbound bilirubin into brain substance. Therefore it may not occur at high serum bilirubin levels if the pigment is albumin bound. Conversely, it can occur at serum levels considerably below 20 mg/dl if significant quantities of bilirubin are not albumin bound. The causes of diminished albumin binding have been described on p. 319. Respiratory or metabolic acidosis, drugs, and hypothermia are impediments to albumin binding. Kernicterus has been reported in small premature infants at serum bilirubin levels below 10 mg/dl, but more often between 10 and 15 mg/dl. Yet despite these variables and the importance of unbound bilirubin, total serum bilirubin determination rather than assessment of albumin binding capacity is currently the most practical guide for evaluating the need for exchange transfusion. This guide to treatment has been used for decades and is still the most reliable group of parameters. Although several laboratory procedures that assess the status of albumin binding capacity have been described in recent years, none has been shown to be sufficiently predictive of clinical course to warrant routine application. Should these tests be used, results must be interpreted in conjunction with serum bilirubin levels, gestational age, and type and severity of illness. *There is as yet no single test that can identify the bilirubin levels that will produce damage to a neonatal brain*. Table 10-2 presents general guidelines for these bilirubin levels according to birth weight and presence of illnesses that are thought to potentiate the toxicity of bilirubin to brain tissue.

THERAPY FOR HYPERBILIRUBINEMIA
Exchange transfusion

Exchange transfusion is the classic therapeutic procedure for hyperbilirubinemia of any etiology. The two-volume exchange removes approximately 85% of the infant's red blood cells. In the case of erythroblastosis the offending cells are thus eliminated. In cases of drug toxicity the circulating drug may be largely removed. Exchange transfusion is less effective for the removal of total body bilirubin, although it remains the most valuable form of therapy for this purpose. Whereas most of the bilirubin in plasma is indeed withdrawn by the procedure, pigment in extravascular tissue rapidly migrates back into the blood after the transfusion. As a rule, serum bilirubin at the end of an exchange transfusion is approximately 50% of preexchange levels, sometimes lower. However, as a result of the diffusion of bilirubin from tissues, these levels promptly rise to 70% or 80% of their previous values, and the process may continue so that bilirubin concentrations soon equal or surpass preexisting levels. The rapidity and extent of this rebound phenomenon depend on the amount of pigment stored in tissues and the remaining vigor of the hemolytic process that caused hyperbilirubinemia. Serum bilirubin may thus reaccumulate after the first transfusion, so that one or more additional transfusions are frequently necessary. (Exchange transfusion is also discussed in more detail on p. 293.)

Administration of albumin

Since albumin binding capacity is a crucial determinant of the development of kernicterus, it would seem rational to enhance it. The use of albumin before or during the exchange transfusion is thought by some to increase binding capacity and therefore remove larger amounts of bilirubin. Presumably this occurs because the additional circulating protein pulls bilirubin out of extravascular tissue to bind it. Intravenous administration of albumin in a 25% salt-poor preparation 1 or 2 hours before exchange transfusion in a dose of 1.0 g/kg of body weight seems to exert a measurable effect. Reports that demonstrated the usefulness of albumin were soon followed by others that did not. Although albumin is given at a number of facilities, later studies diminished enthusiasm for its use.

Phototherapy

The use of intense fluorescent light to reduce serum bilirubin gained widespread acceptance in the United States after a decade of general use abroad. Blue light decomposes bilirubin by photooxidation. When light is applied to jaundiced infants, shielded skin remains more icteric, which suggests that decomposition transpires in the skin. The products formed in the breakdown of bilirubin are not toxic. There is no doubt that serum unconjugated bilirubin concentrations are reduced by phototherapy. Numerous precautions have been urged by investigators whose experience with lights is extensive. Long-term outcomes have not been completely evaluated, nor have the theoretic effects of intense light on a wide spectrum of biologic processes been assessed. Many of the objections that have been raised are hypothetical, but significant immediate adverse effects have not been demonstrated, nor have any long-term adverse effects. The etiology of jaundice must be sought before phototherapy is applied. In the presence of a mild hemolytic process, hemoglobin determination is essential at frequent intervals because anemia may develop despite diminishing bilirubin levels.

The effectiveness of phototherapy is in the blue segment of the light spectrum. This is 425 to 475 nanometers (nm). The commonly used fluorescent bulbs (daylight or cool white) deliver relatively little energy from blue light. Fluorescent bulbs, specially designed for phototherapy (for example, Vitalite) deliver more blue light, while special blue bulbs (designated BB by manufacturers) deliver the most blue light within a narrow spectrum. Incandescent light, transmitted through an appropriate filter, delivers satisfactory quantities of blue light. Fluorescent lights mounted overhead on a hood over radiant warmers have been shown to be inadequate sources of phototherapy.

The adequacy of blue light intensity can be demonstrated only by measuring energy in the 400 to 500 nm range. Special instruments are available at modest cost for this purpose. The units of energy are expressed as microwatts per square centimeter per nanometer ($\mu W/cm^2/nm$). Footcandle meters are of no value for these energy measurements. Currently, a minimum of 4 $\mu W/cm^2/nm$ is considered necessary for effective phototherapy. This will vary, however, depending on the rate of bilirubin production. There is a linear relationship between effectiveness and dose of light between 4 and 14 $\mu W/cm^2/nm$.

Phototherapy should not be used for routine prophylaxis against hyperbilirubinemia in any infant, term or premature. In ABO incompatibility, it is useful for infants who are candidates for exchange transfusion but in whom there is as yet no clear indication for its performance. Phototherapy has been used for Rh disease, and the data indicate that fewer early (first 12 hours of life) and late transfusions are necessary. One must be mindful that in removing bilirubin with phototherapy, the vulnerable red cells remain in circulation for ultimate hemolysis. The result is progressive anemia at safe levels of serum bilirubin. There is frequent prolongation of hospital stay for close observation of precipitous decline in hemoglobin. In our experience, a need arises for multiple simple transfusions because of progressive anemia. We still believe it best *in Rh disease* to observe for hyperbilirubinemia, perform the first exchange transfusion, and then apply phototherapy.

For hyperbilirubinemia from any cause, lights should never be used to delay an exchange transfusion once the serum bilirubin approaches levels that require it. If indicated, phototherapy should be instituted when the bilirubin concentration reaches 10 mg/dl in premature infants and sometimes at even lower levels in smaller babies. The response to phototherapy, assuming delivery of appropriate doses of light, will depend on the rate of bilirubin production. Rapid increases in ABO incompatibility will respond less extensively to the same dose of light than the increments that characterize physiologic hyperbilirubinemia. The effect of lights is probably immediate even though decreases in bilirubin may not be evident during the first 24 hours of therapy. Phototherapy minimizes or eliminates any increase in bilirubin that otherwise occurs without it. Rebound elevations of several milligrams per deciliter are the rule after therapy is discontinued.

In the day-to-day management of infants, the most important immediate untoward effects of phototherapy include increased metabolic rate, hyperthermia, loose stools, and significantly increased loss of water through the skin. Metabolic rate increases, and the caloric requirement thus rises. There may be difficulty in meeting caloric needs if intestinal transit time is increased to cause loose stools. Hyperthermia (and the loose stools) increases water losses. Urine may darken because photodegradation products are water soluble and are thus excreted by the kidneys.

The effect of phototherapy on growth of premature infants during the neonatal period has been assessed, and the data negate the previous conclusion (from the same investigator) that long-term growth is impaired. There is indeed diminished growth during the period of phototherapy, but there is also a catch-up period during the second and third weeks of life. It is probable that phototherapy causes increased metabolic demands and decreased intestinal absorption of milk (because intestinal transit time is increased), thus stealing calories for growth in the first instance, and diminishing their intake in the second.

That natural light conditions affect serum bilirubin levels has been demonstrated in a study from Finland, where, through the year, seasonal daily duration of daylight varies from 3 to 22 hours. Premature babies born during the "light" half of the year had significantly lower bilirubin levels than those born during the "dark" half of the year. None of them received phototherapy. Environmental light undoubtedly also influences the effect of phototherapy. Factors such as the number of windows in a nursery, the light they admit, the position of the baby in relation to windows, and the geographic location of the hospital all must be considered in evaluating the results of light therapy.

A warning issued by the Food and Drug Administration called attention to the protective effect of a plastic barrier between phototherapy lights and babies. Without a plastic shield, ultraviolet light from fluorescent bulbs has caused skin erythema. Commercial lights have Plexiglas shields built into the apparatus. The plastic walls of an incubator are also protective. Phototherapy should be used only with plastic interposed between the light and the baby. The erythematous skin caused by ultraviolet light suggests that the retina would also be jeopardized in the absence of a surface that filters out the ultraviolet light.

Because blue light is the effective segment of the spectrum that acts on bilirubin, narrow-spectrum blue lights have been used for phototherapy. Reduction of serum bilirubin levels was greater than with the usual fluorescent bulbs. However, as one might anticipate, it was impossible to detect cyanosis or pallor. Furthermore, we have also noted nausea and dizziness in a few nurses who care for infants in blue lights. Many centers mix blue fluorescent and daylight bulbs.

The "bronze baby syndrome" has received wide attention. It occurs in light-treated babies with liver disease whose hyperbilirubinemia has a significant direct component. A gray-brown discoloration of skin, serum, and urine was observed. The discoloration clears 3 weeks after therapy is discontinued. "Tanning" of black infants has been also reported. This is distinct from the "bronzing" effect. The skin simply becomes more deeply pigmented during exposure to the lights. A maculopapular rash has also been noted as one of the side effects of therapy.

The infant's eyes are shielded from the intense light he receives during phototherapy. No evidence from human eyes has indicated that the light is injurious, but microscopic injury to retinal cells has been observed in monkeys exposed to phototherapy (without shielding eyes) for 3 to 7 days. The extent of the damage was well correlated with duration of exposure. *There is thus strong evidence to justify conscientious maintenance of eye patches during treatment.* The nurse should be certain that the lids are closed when the blindfold is applied. It should be removed periodically to inspect the eyes for conjunctivitis. Failure to change the eye shields has resulted in unsuspected severe purulent conjunctivitis.

Phenobarbital

Phenobarbital has been shown to lower peak bilirubin levels of physiologic jaundice by approximately 50%. It exerts its effect by increasing activity of glucuronyl transferase and ligandin, thus increasing hepatic capacity to conjugate and take up bilirubin. There was at first widespread hope that phenobarbital therapy would materially diminish the incidence of hyperbilirubinemia. It is now apparent that its beneficial use is restricted for several reasons. It is effective when given to mothers several days to 2 weeks before delivery. Thus large numbers of mothers would receive the drug before anticipated delivery that at best could only be estimated. There would also be no method by which the need for therapy in the neonate could be identified prenatally. Postnatal administration is of limited effect for the term baby and is of little or no benefit to the premature infant. Administered to the mother, phenobarbital may precipitate withdrawal symptoms in the neonate. Thus the drug is not generally used to diminish bilirubin levels. It is of no value in combination with phototherapy. Its application is rather specific, such as in type II glucuronyl transferase deficiency.

TRANSCUTANEOUS ESTIMATION OF SERUM BILIRUBIN CONCENTRATION

Jaundice occurs in approximately 50% of term infants, imposing a responsibility of some magnitude for monitoring rising bilirubin levels in term infants who are otherwise well. A substantial volume of laboratory work is thereby entailed, all of which is performed in anticipation of toxic bilirubin levels that may cause kernicterus. It has not mattered that there is no evidence to validate the notion that high serum concentrations are more likely to cause encephalopathy. It is nevertheless a fact that bilirubin concentrations are monitored in large populations of well infants, lack of rationale notwithstanding.

A device called the "jaundice meter" bids well to diminish the laboratory hours spent in bilirubin determinations on well infants. It has thus far been useful *only to indicate whether there is a need for laboratory determination of serum bilirubin.* Although the device is commonly referred to as a "transcutaneous bilirubin meter," *it does not measure serum bilirubin.* Rather it estimates degree of skin jaundice by measuring the light reflected from the skin.

This small device weighs 9 oz. It is pressed to the skin, preferably at the forehead or the upper sternum, to trigger an emission of light similar to that used in flash photography. The light is reflected back to the instrument, and the degree of yellowness is measured by an internal meter. The device then displays a "transcutaneous bilirubin index" (tcBI) that *corresponds to the depth of skin jaundice.* The jaundice meter does not measure serum bilirubin concentration like transcutaneous oxygen and carbon dioxide monitors measure partial pressures.

Usefulness of the instrument depends on a predictable linear relationship between the extent of bilirubin storage in skin (jaundice) and the concentration of bilirubin in serum. The ratio of bilirubin concentrations at each of these sites may be altered by several factors that are intrinsic to an infant's clinical status. These factors may produce variable results from one infant to another. Furthermore, results also vary from one jaundice meter to another.

The correlation of skin and blood bilirubin content may change as a function of skin characteristics such as thickness, vascularity, and pigmentation. Thus far, data from premature infants is meager. The transcutaneous reflectance meter is not intended for use on sick infants. It is also not intended for the screening of premature infants, ill or well.

Since phototherapy diminishes the concentration of yellow pigment in skin, one must anticipate that the ratio between skin and serum will also be altered. Thus transcutaneous screening is not practical for infants under phototherapy. Monitoring after an exchange transfusion is also impractical because the concentration of bilirubin has been lowered in serum while that of skin is relatively unchanged.

Racial variations of skin color affect results. Whereas the monitor has been useful in oriental, caucasian, and black infants, specific standards of references must be developed for each race by individual hospitals.

Varying results have been observed among instruments. One cannot assume that the reading from one jaundice meter will be similar to that of another.

While there is some disagreement, most investigators have found that the transcutaneous jaundice meter is a useful screening device, but *only to identify infants who require laboratory determination of serum bilirubin*. Each nursery must construct its standard of reference for each instrument it uses, and for each of the racial components of its population. The meter is usually used to identify infants whose serum bilirubin concentration exceeds 13 mg/dl, but reference standards can be altered so that the meter identifies higher or lower serum concentrations. Occasional false-positive results are inevitable; that is, an occasional infant will be identified for a laboratory determination that is unnecessary. On the other hand, the incidence of a false-negative result is less frequent; in some studies it was rare. The transcutaneous meter does not often miss a high serum bilirubin. The instrument is a potential labor-saving device. By avoiding numerous heel sticks, it is also a pain-sparing device.

BIBLIOGRAPHY

Anttolainen, I., Simila, S., and Wallgren, E. I.: Effect of seasonal variation in daylight on bilirubin level in premature infants, Arch. Dis. Child. **50**:156, 1975.

Boggs, T. R., and Bishop, H.: Neonatal hyperbilirubinemia associated with high obstruction of the small bowel, J. Pediatr. **66**:349, 1965.

Bonta, B. W., and Warshaw, J. B.: Importance of radiant flux in the treatment of hyperbilirubinemia: failure of overhead phototherapy units in intensive care units, Pediatrics **57**:502, 1976.

Broughton, P. M. G.: The effectivness and safety of phototherapy. In Bergsma, D., Hsia, D. Y-Y, and Jackson, C., editors: Birth defects: bilirubin metabolism in the newborn, vol. VI, no. 2, White Plains, N.Y., June, 1970, National Foundation—March of Dimes.

Cashore, W. J., Gartner, L. M., Oh, W., and Stern, L.: Clinical application of neonatal bilirubin-binding determinations: current status, J. Pediatr. **93**:827, 1978.

Diamond, L. K.: A history of jaundice in the newborn. In Bergsma, D., Hsia, D. Y-Y, and Jackson, C., editors: Birth defects: bilirubin metabolism in the newborn, vol. VI, no. 2, White Plains, N.Y., June, 1970, National Foundation—March of Dimes.

Ennever, J. F., Sobel, M., McDonagh, A. F., and Speck, W. T.: Phototherapy for neonatal jaundice: in vitro comparison of light sources, Pediatr. Res. **18**:667, 1984.

Food and Drug Administration (HEW): Comment: hazard of ultraviolet radiation from fluorescent lamps to infant during phototherapy, J. Pediatr. **84**:145, 1974.

Gartner, L. M.: Breast milk jaundice. In Levine, R. L., and Maisels, M. J.: Hyperbilirubinemia in the newborn: report of the eighty-fifth Ross conference on pediatric research, Columbus, Ohio, 1983, Ross Laboratories.

Gartner, L. M., Lee, K. Vaisman, S., et al.: Development of bilirubin transport and metabolism in the newborn rhesus monkey, J. Pediatr. **90**:513, 1977.

Gellis, S. S.: Biliary atresia, Pediatrics **55**:8, 1975.

Gitzelmann-Cumarasamy, N., and Kuenzle, C. C.: Commentaries: bilirubin binding tests: living up to expectations? Pediatrics **64**:375, 1979.

Goldman, S. L., Penalver, A., and Penaranda, R.: Jaundice meter: evaluation of new guidelines, J. Pediatr. **101**:253, 1982.

Hodgman, J. E., and Teberg, A.: Effect of phototherapy on subsequent growth and development of the premature infant. In Bergsma, D., Hsia, D. Y-Y, and Jackson, C., editors: Birth defects: bilirubin metabolism in the newborn, vol. VI, no. 2, White Plains, N.Y., June, 1970, National Foundation—March of Dimes.

Kapitulnik, J., Horner-Mibashan, R., Blondheim, S. H., et al.: Increase in bilirubin-binding affinity of serum with age of infant, J. Pediatr. **86**:442, 1975.

Karp, W. B.: Biochemical alterations in neonatal hyperbilirubinemia and bilirubin encephalopathy: a review, Pediatrics **64:**361, 1979.

Keenan, W. J., Perlstein, P. H., Light, I. J., and Sutherland, J. M.: Kernicterus in small sick premature infants receiving phototherapy, Pediatrics **49:**652, 1972.

Kopelman, A. E., Brown, R. S., and Odell, G. B.: The "bronze" baby syndrome: a complication of phototherapy, J. Pediatr. **81:**466, 1972.

Lau, S. P., and Fung, K. P.: Serum bilirubin kinetics in intermittent phototherapy of physiological jaundice, Arch. Dis. Child. **59:**892, 1984.

Lester, R., Jackson, B. T., and Smallwood, R. A.: Fetal hepatic function. In Bergsma, D., Hsia, D. Y-Y, and Jackson, C., editors: Birth defects: bilirubin metabolism in the newborn, vol. VI, no. 2, White Plains, N.Y., June, 1970, National Foundation—March of Dimes.

Lucey, J. F.: The unsolved problem of kernicterus in the susceptible low birth weight infant, Pediatrics **49:**646, 1972.

Lucey, J. F.: Comment: another view of phototherapy, J. Pediatr. **84:**145, 1974.

Lucey, J. F., Ferreiro, M., and Hewitt, J.: Prevention of hyperbilirubinemia of prematurity by phototherapy, Pediatrics **41:**1047, 1968.

Maisels, M. J.: Transcutaneous bilirubin measurements in full-term infants, Pediatrics **70:**464, 1982.

Maisels, M. J.: Clinical studies of the sequelae of hyperbilirubinemia. In Levine, R. L., and Maisels, M. J.: Hyperbilirubinemia in the newborn: report of the eighty-fifth Ross conference on pediatric research, Columbus, Ohio, 1983, Ross Laboratories.

Maisels, M. J., and Lee, C.: Transcutaneous bilirubin measurements: variation in meter response, Pediatrics **71:**457, 1983.

Marcus, J. C.: The clinical syndromes of kernicterus. In Levine, R. L., and Maisels, M. J.: Hyperbilirubinemia in the newborn: report of the eighty-fifth Ross conference on pediatric research, Columbus, Ohio, 1983, Ross Laboratories.

Messner, K. H., Leŭre-Dupree, A. E., and Maisels, M. J.: The effect of continuous prolonged illumination on the newborn primate retina (abstr.), Pediatr. Res. **9:**368, 1975.

Mims, L. C., Estrada, M., Gooden, D. S., et al.: Phototherapy for neonatal hyperbilirubinemia—a dose:response relationship, J. Pediatr. **83:**658, 1973.

Modi, N., and Keay, A. J.: Phototherapy for neonatal hyperbilirubinemia: the importance of dose, Arch. Dis. Child. **58:**406, 1983.

Moller, J., and Ebbesen, F.: Phototherapy in newborn infants with severe rhesus hemolytic disease, J. Pediatr. **86:**135, 1975.

Morecki, R., Gartner, L. M., and Lee, K-S.: Jaundice and liver disease. In Fanaroff, A. A., and Martin, R. J., editors: Behrman's neonatal-perinatal medicine, ed. 3, St. Louis, 1983, The C. V. Mosby Co.

Naiman, J. L.: Erythroblastosis fetalis. In Oski, F. A., and Naiman, J. L.: Hematologic problems in the newborn, ed. 3, Philadelphia, 1982, W. B. Saunders Co.

Nakai, H., and Margaretten, W.: Protracted jaundice associated with hypertrophic pyloric stenosis, Pediatrics **29:**198, 1962.

Odell, G. B.: Neonatal hyperbilirubinemia, New York, 1980, Grune and Stratton.

Odell, G.B., Storey, B., and Rosenberg, L. A.: Studies in kernicterus, III. The saturation of serum proteins with bilirubin during neonatal life and its relationship to brain damage at five years, J. Pediatr. **76:**12, 1970.

Osborn, L. M., Reiff, M. I., and Bolus, R.: Jaundice in the full-term neonate, Pediatrics **73:**520, 1984.

Osborn, L. M., Lenarsky, C., Oakes, R. C., and Reiff, M. I.: Phototherapy in full-term infants with hemolytic disease secondary to ABO incompatibility, Pediatrics **74:**371, 1984.

Poland, R. L., and Odell, G. B.: Physiologic jaundice: the enterohepatic circulation of bilirubin, N. Engl. J. Med. **284:**1, 1971.

Shennan, A. T.: The effect of phototherapy on the hyperbilirubinemia of rhesus incompatibility, Pediatrics **54:**417, 1974.

Sisson, T. R. C., Kendall, N., Shaw, E., and Kechavarz-Oliai, L.: Phototherapy of jaundice in the newborn infant. II. Effect of various light intensities, J. Pediatr. **81:**35, 1972.

Strange, M., and Cassady, G.: Neonatal transcutaneous bilirubinometry, Clin. Perinatol. **12:**51, 1985.

Tan, K. L., and Lim, S. C.: Clinical and laboratory observations, J. Pediatr. **103:**471, 1983.

Watchko, J. F., and Oski, F. A.: Bilirubin 20 mg/dl = vigintiphobia, Pediatrics **71:**660, 1983.

Woody, N. C., and Brodkey, M. J.: Tanning from phototherapy for neonatal jaundice, J. Pediatr. **82:**1042, 1973.

Wu, P. Y. K., Lim, R. C., Hodgman, J. E., et al.: Effect of phototherapy on growth in preterm infants in the neonatal period, J. Pediatr. **85:**563, 1974.

Zuelzer, W. W., and Brown, A. K.: Neonatal jaundice, Am. J. Dis. Child. **101:**113, 1961.

CHAPTER 11

Disorders of glucose, calcium, and magnesium metabolism

GLUCOSE DISORDERS
The fetus: glucose and other sources of energy

The fetus receives glucose continuously across the placenta from maternal blood. At term, neonatal cord blood glucose is 70% to 80% of the maternal level. Glucose is the primary source of fetal energy, but to what extent it predominates among other substances is still unsettled. Investigators have estimated that glucose provides 50% to 100% of fetal energy. From presently available data, it appears that other substances such as amino acids, lactate, and perhaps ketones and free fatty acids also provide fuel, but that glucose is the preponderant factor in total energy requirement. It passes across the placenta by facilitated diffusion, a process that itself requires expenditure of energy. Lactate appears to be normally generated in the placenta, and it may well provide 25% of fetal oxidative metabolism.

The fetal uptake of glucose depends on maternal blood glucose levels. Fetal blood glucose is generally 25% to 30% lower than maternal levels. When denied glucose by virtue of maternal deprivation, the fetus may use ketones as a substitute. On the other hand, when maternal hyperglycemia exists (as in diabetic mothers), fetal blood glucose is elevated. Early in gestation fetal insulin production is negligible in response to maternal hyperglycemia, but as gestation proceeds, the beta cells in the pancreatic islets respond more vigorously. Fetuses of diabetic mothers who are recurrently hyperglycemic respond with insulin production with increasing vigor. At term or near term, the insulin-producing islet cells are hyperplastic and have been shown to contain more than normal quantities of the hormone. Normally, however, there is no need for a significant fetal insulin response because glucose is constantly fed and regulated from the mother's blood. Maternal insulin does not cross the placenta. The continuous supply of glucose also eliminates any need for the fetus to synthesize glucose from glycogen or from other noncarbohydrate sources (fluconeogenesis). It also eliminates any need for the fetus to regulate its own blood glucose level since the mother does so by regulating her levels. Fetal glucose is thus largely derived transplacentally from maternal blood. Normally this exogenous source of glucose suffices. The fetus can, however, generate glucose independently (endogenously) by gluconeogenesis and by synthesizing glucose from carbohydrate sources. The fetus utilizes glucose in two distinct pathways: (1) it may be dissipated by energy requirements or (2) it may be converted into protein, glycogen, or fat for storage.

While fuel supplied to the fetus is used for the ongoing needs of growth and development, it must also be stored for availability during the inevitable exigencies of birth and immediate postnatal life.

During the weeks that precede term birth, the storage of glycogen and adipose tissue for postnatal energy assumes major importance in preparation for the neonate's separation from the placental supply line. Glycogen content of liver and muscle, and triglycerides in adipose tissue, are at their highest levels at term. Once born, the neonate must supply his own fuel until external sources are well established. Thus something like a neonatal energy crisis transpires when the maternal source of substrate is literally cut off. Now the neonate needs fuel to survive the asphyxia of normal birth, to withstand the cold stress caused by entry into the world of air, to perform the work of initial breathing, and to sustain vigorous muscle activity. Furthermore, fuel stores must be available for unanticipated perinatal asphyxia during which glycogen stores are extravagantly dissipated. In the asphyxiated baby, myocardial survival itself is directly related to the quantity of accumulated cardiac glycogen, for with greater quantities of glycogen in storage, the survival period during asphyxia is known to be more protracted.

Glucose is stored as glycogen in fetal tissues beginning in the ninth or tenth week. Glycogen storage in the liver increases continuously to term, at which time there is about 80 to 120 mg of glycogen per gram of wet hepatic weight. This is approximately twice the adult concentration. Cardiac glycogen is also continuously accumulated so that at term its concentration is ten times that of the adults, whereas in skeletal muscle, three to five times adult concentrations have been demonstrated.

These glycogen stores are also available to the fetus at any time intrauterine stress occurs. During fetal asphyxia, glycogen is rapidly broken down by anaerobic glycolysis with a resultant sizable accumulation of lactate in blood and tissues.

The fetus synthesizes protein from amino acids that are derived transplacentally. Amino acids are probably not a direct source of energy. Triglycerides are generated from the ongoing input of glucose and are stored in fat depots. Fat deposits are not quantitatively significant until the last trimester, particularly in the latter half. Like glycogen stores, accumulations of adipose tissue serve as energy reservoirs that can be drawn on immediately after birth. As glycogen supplies are depleted and less glucose is generated, the free fatty acids derived from these fat stores become a metabolic fuel.

The neonate: glucose metabolism and the postnatal "energy crunch"

The storage of energy-yielding substrate throughout gestation, particularly during the last trimester, seems directed toward sustaining the neonate during his first postnatal days because at birth an "energy crunch" is created by amputation of the maternal supply line and by an abrupt demand for increased energy. The increased energy requirements are imposed by entry into the extrauterine environment. Specifically, substrate is consumed more rapidly because of the normal asphyxia of birth, the work of initiating extrauterine breathing, the loss of heat on exposure to cold, and the activation of muscle tone and activity. These events are ordinarily well managed by normal term neonates. In abnormal infants who are stressed for a variety of reasons, the instant switch from total maternal nurture to total, but transient, independence is often troublesome and threatening to intact survival.

After birth the infant's caloric needs must be supplied from external sources, and it may be hours or days before expended glycogen is even partially replenished. In the meantime there is abrupt diminution of glycogen stores. It follows then that intrauterine malnutrition, and the low stores of glycogen that it involves, poses a serious threat to the asphyxiated infant in terms of depleted carbohydrate. Even in normal infants, approximately 90% of liver glycogen may be consumed by the end of the third hour after birth, rising gradually thereafter to attain adult concentrations by the end of the third week. The effects of a respiratory distress on energy expenditure are well illustrated by the virtually complete depletion of glycogen stores found in postmortem analysis of the heart, liver, and diaphragm. The normal newborn infant can tolerate a relatively short period of fasting without chemical derangement. Carbohydrate stores are consumed during the first 2 or 3 days; later, fat is probably a principal source of energy.

The first defense against the fall in blood glucose after the cord is cut is activation of *glycogen breakdown (glycogenolysis)*. Within 2 hours the normal neonate's blood glucose falls from its cord blood level of approximately 70 or 80 mg/dl to 50 mg/dl. To prevent further decline, pancreatic islet cells respond to this stimulus by increasing the production of glucagon from alpha cells and diminishing the secretion of insulin from beta cells. Glucagon is one of several factors that promotes glycogenolysis, while the diminished presence of insulin does likewise. Not only is glycogen breakdown increased, but by several changeovers in the activity of hepatic enzymes, glycogen formation is inhibited as well. The net effect of these

activities is an increased release of hepatic glucose and a restoration of blood glucose to near cord blood levels. If restoration of higher levels is not accomplished, at the very least, the postnatal decline in blood glucose is reversed for the time being.

Gluconeogenesis is another source of hepatic glucose that first becomes active immediately after birth. This process involves the conversion of noncarbohydrate substances (principally amino acids) to glucose. Gluconeogenesis is not normally active in the fetus because the contransplacental supply makes activation unnecessary. The fetus can generate glucose via gluconeogenesis if the need arises. At birth it is stimulated by appearance of the hormones and hepatic enzymes required for its activation. In sheep, gluconeogenesis is initiated within 3 minutes after birth. It seems likely that in the human neonate the process also begins soon after delivery.

The restoration of blood sugar is accomplished at a cost of hepatic glycogen reserves. These are depleted rapidly during the first few hours after birth and more gradually in the ensuing 2 to 3 days. The neonate turns increasingly to fat as a fuel, and as a result, blood glucose is spared. Thus free fatty acids (FFA) are released to the blood to meet tissue energy requirements. Soon after birth, blood levels of FFA increase threefold as a consequence of the breakdown of fat deposits (lipolysis) that were accumulated in utero largely during the last trimester. Lipolysis is triggered at birth by the release of catecholamines, principally norepinephrine. The most vigorous stimulus to the secretion of norepinephrine is the low temperature of room air that is encountered at birth and perceived by the thermal receptors in the skin. This mechanism, and the effects of norepinephrine secretion, are discussed in Chapter 4.

The "energy crunch" of the immediate postnatal period is thus temporarily alleviated by release of glucose from the liver (glycogenolysis and gluconeogenesis) and by the use of FFA as an alternative fuel that is derived from the breakdown of fat stores (lipolysis). Ultimately, the provision of external nutrition must maintain adequate energy levels. With these normal events in mind, the reader can appreciate the limited capacity of some infants to cope with the perinatal "energy crunch." The premature infant, for example, stores less hepatic glycogen and less fat than he would had he gone to term. He is thus vulnerable to hypoglycemia. The more immature the infant, the smaller the stores of energy substrate. Similarly, the malnourished fetus cannot accumulate adequate stores of substrate—neither glycogen nor fat. He, too, is vulnerable to hypoglycemia. Whether normal, premature, or undergrown, the fetus who is asphyxiated will rapidly dissipate glycogen stores because he must resort to anaerobic glycolysis as a major source of energy. The effect of asphyxia on energy deprivation is even more profound when it is chronic (placental insufficiency) and when it occurs in immature or malnourished fetuses. These babies also are predisposed to hypoglycemia.

The liver has a unique capacity to convert blood glucose to hepatic glycogen for storage and to convert glycogen back to glucose for release to the blood when levels are low. Blood glucose taken up by skeletal muscles is converted to glycogen and is ultimately utilized as glucose at that site; there is no release of glucose to the blood from any organ except the liver. Adipose tissue takes up blood glucose and converts it to triglycerides; it, too, does not release glucose to the blood. At any given moment, blood sugar concentration is a reflection of two principal balancing functions: hepatic release of glucose and utilization of glucose by tissues. In the liver, glucose is primarily produced by breakdown of glycogen and production from noncarbohydrate substances (gluconeogenesis). Normal output of glucose from the liver also depends on adequate glycogen stores and effective activity of enzymes and hormones concerned with its production. Utilization of glucose by tissues is abnormally increased by the metabolic response to cold stress, acidosis, and hypoxia.

Hypoglycemia in the neonate

The diagnosis of hypoglycemia must be based on serum (or blood) glucose concentrations because hypoglycemic infants are either asymptomatic or are affected by clinical signs that are not specific to hypoglycemia. Normal glucose levels previously referred to whole blood concentrations, but now virtually all laboratories report plasma concentrations. Normal plasma values are approximately 15% higher than those of whole blood. During the first 72 hours of life in babies of birth weight >2500 g, the diagnosis of hypoglycemia is established when plasma glucose is <35 mg/dl (whole blood glucose <30mg/dl). In low birth weight infants, regardless of gestational age, the lower limit of normal for plasma glucose during the first 72 hours of life is 25 mg/dl (blood glucose <20 mg/dl). After 72 hours hypoglycemia occurs at plasma glucose concentrations <45 mg/dl in all infants regardless of birth weight. A diagnostic requirement of two consecutive and closely spaced low determinations is necessary because blood sugar levels normally fluctuate widely. The restriction of diagnostic criteria to laboratory data is unavoidable because the symptoms of hypoglycemia occur with similar frequency in normoglycemic infants with unrelated disorders. We do not play the "numbers game" with these prescribed normal levels of glucose. With or without symptoms, if blood sugar values are close to the designated low levels in an infant who is at known risk for hypoglycemia, we begin treatment.

The symptoms attributable to hypoglycemia from any cause may also occur in infants with central nervous system disorders, septicemia, hypomagnesemia, cardiorespiratory disorders, and a multiplicity of other abnormalities. There are no pathognomonic clinical signs of hypoglycemia. The signs associated with low blood sugar include apnea, cyanosis, rapid and irregular respirations, tachypnea, tremors, jitters, twitches, convulsions, lethargy, coma, abrupt pallor, sweating, upward rolling of the eyes, weak cry, and refusal to

Table 11-1. Causes of neonatal hypoglycemia

Clinical entity	Mechanism	Duration
Intrauterine malnutrition	Low liver glycogen store	Transient
Fetal asphyxia	Glycogen depletion	Transient
Cold stress	Glycogen depletion	Transient
CNS hemorrhage	Unknown	Transient
CNS malformation	Unknown	Transient
Adrenal hemorrhage, insufficiency	Ineffective catecholamine response	Transient
Infants of diabetic mothers	Increased plasma insulin activity	Transient
Erythroblastotic infants	Increased plasma insulin activity	Transient
Maternal tolbutamide, chlorpropamide	Hyperinsulinism	Transient
Abrupt stop of intravenous glucose, $\geq 10\%$	Hyperinsulinism	Transient
Glycogen storage disease (types I and II)	Defective glycogen breakdown	Protracted
Galactose intolerance (galactosemia)	Defective conversion of galactose to glucose	Protracted
Islet cell tumor	Hyperinsulinism	Protracted
Cyanotic congenital heart disease with congestive failure	Unknown	Transient
Hypopituitarism	Adrenal insufficiency	Protracted
Septicemia	Unknown	Transient

feed. The etiologic relationship of these signs to hypoglycemia is credible if they clear within a short time after intravenous glucose administration; if they do not clear, a cause other than hypoglycemia is undoubtedly operative.

Blood sugar falls to abnormally low levels if glycogen stores are suboptimal, gluconeogenesis (glucose from lipids and protein) in the liver is diminished, available insulin is excessive, or carbohydrate-regulating hormones such as cortisol, epinephrine, and glucagon are insufficient. In rare circumstances, enzyme deficiencies in the liver impair the release of glucose, thus causing hypoglycemia.

These pathophysiologic mechanisms are responsible for four broad clinical categories. Small-for-dates infants who were subjected to intrauterine malnutrition constitute one of these categories. Another category includes infants of diabetic mothers and erythroblastotic infants. Another group includes infants with birth weights

below 1250 g who are subjected to such severe stress that their metabolic requirements exceed their glycogen stores. These infants are often asymptomatic. The last group includes infants with rare developmental and genetic disorders such as glycogen storage disease, galactosemia, and tumors of the pancreatic islets (insulinomas). In any of these clinical groupings an additive hypoglycemic effect may be exerted by severe respiratory distress, hypoxia, and hypothermia. Table 11-1 lists the most important clinical entities associated with hypoglycemia and the mechanisms involved.

Hypoglycemia and intrauterine malnutrition. Hypoglycemia occurs in approximately 20% of infants with intrauterine growth retardation. The incidence is higher in males (twice as frequent as in females) and in the smaller of twins if the birth weight discrepancy exceeds 25% and the weight of the affected infant is less than 2000 g. Symptoms occur in 50% to 90% of hypoglycemic infants. Small-for-dates babies have diminished stores of hepatic glycogen and diminished capacity for gluconeogenesis. They also possess a relatively increased mass of glucose-consuming tissue because the brain is least affected by growth retardation and is closest to normal weight compared with other organs, especially the liver. In normally grown neonates the liver, which is the principal glucose supplier, weighs one third as much as the brain, which is an active glucose consumer. In malnourished infants the liver weighs only one seventh as much as the brain. The hepatic source of glucose is thus reduced in malnourished babies. Most glycogen-depleted hypoglycemic infants are below the tenth percentile on the Colorado growth charts. Other hypoglycemic infants are affected for unknown reasons, although many seem to be subjected to excessive metabolic demands resulting from some type of stress. In addition to glycogen depletion, these infants have considerably reduced fat deposits for the provision of free fatty acids as a fuel substitute for glucose.

Symptoms usually appear between 24 and 72 hours of age; occasionally they begin as early as 3 hours and as late as 7 days of age. Severely hypoxic, hypothermic small-for-dates infants are most likely to become hypoglycemic within 6 hours after birth.

Monitoring blood sugar is thus important in small-for-dates infants and in any other stressed baby. Infants who place below the tenth percentile should have blood sugar assessment at least twice during the first 24 hours and at least three times daily thereafter until 4 days of age. Screening for low values is feasible with Dextrostix. A laboratory determination for blood sugar should be requested if the Dextrostix color change indicates a level less than 45 mg/dl. The Dextrostix is exquisitely sensitive, and because it is such a simple procedure it is commonly performed inaccurately. The blood must remain on the reactive tip for precisely 1 minute. Shorter periods do not permit a complete reaction; longer periods allow too much reaction. The blood must be rinsed off by a forceful stream of water from a plastic squeeze bottle. Care must also be exercised in touching the strip to the capillary blood flowing from a heel prick because the delicate membrane that covers the tip is easily disrupted by contact with the skin. Treatment of hypoglycemia is discussed later in this chapter.

Infants of diabetic mothers (IDM). Before the introduction of insulin over 40 years ago, few diabetic women conceived, and among those who did, the outcome of pregnancy was often catastrophic. Pregnancy in diabetic women is now commonplace, and in recent years screening during pregnancy has also identified women whose gestational diabetic tendencies were unsuspected in the nonpregnant state. As a result of more effective management of diabetes, particularly during gestation, the offspring of diabetic mothers are now numerous, constituting a significant problem and a major challenge to the caretakers of high-risk infants. One in 500 to 1000 pregnant women is diabetic. The incidence of gestational diabetes is considerably higher—one in 120 pregnancies. Perinatal infant mortality and morbidity rates are inordinately high among infants of diabetic mothers. There is general agreement that diabetic pregnancies should be interrupted between the thirty-sixth and thirty-seventh weeks because earlier deliveries are associated with a high rate of neonatal mortality, whereas later ones are associated with a higher incidence of stillbirth. Fetal monitoring in diabetic and other high-risk pregnancies is discussed in Chapter 1.

The classification of diabetes during pregnancy that was introduced by Dr. Priscilla White is a universal reference for grading the severity of the maternal disease (Table 11-2). It differentiates severity according to duration of diabetes before pregnancy, age at onset, and extent of vascular involvement. Class A is the most common type; it includes gestational diabetes. Gestational diabetes is characterized by an abnormal glucose tolerance curve in an asymptomatic mother, which reverts to normal within 6 weeks after delivery. Whereas mortality in babies born of class A mothers is higher than in those of nondiabetic mothers, it is the lowest of all the groups in White's clas-

Table 11-2. White's classification of diabetes in pregnancy

Class A	Highest probability of fetal survival
	No insulin, little dietary regulation
	Includes gestational diabetes and pre-diabetes
Class B	Onset at age 20 or more
	Duration less than 10 years before pregnancy
	No vascular disease
Class C	Onset between 10 and 19 years of age
	Duration between 10 and 19 years
	Minimal vascular disease (retinal arteriosclerosis, calcification of vessels in the legs only)
Class D	Onset before age 10 years
	Duration 20 years or more
	Moderately advanced vascular disease (diabetic retinopathy, transient albuminuria, and hypertension)
Class E	Characteristics of class D plus calcification of pelvic vessels
Class F	Characteristics of class D plus nephritis
Class R	Active retinitis

sification. The most unfavorable neonatal outcomes occur in classes D through F. Toxemia of pregnancy is more likely to occur in women with vascular disease (classes D through F), and this is probably an additional contributory factor to poor pregnancy outcome. Class A and B mothers give birth to large-for-dates babies; mothers in class C and below deliver small-for-dates babies (Chapter 5).

There is no well-defined explanation for all the abnormalities in infants of diabetic mothers. The hypoglycemia that commonly occurs within hours after birth is associated with increased insulin activity in the blood. Furthermore, hyperplasia and increased insulin content of the pancreatic islet cells are demonstrated at necropsy in virtually all these infants. Current consensus holds that fetal hyperglycemia, which results from high maternal levels of blood sugar, provides a relentless stimulus to the islets for insulin production, as evidenced by their hyperplasia. Sustained fetal hyperinsulinism and hyperglycemia ultimately lead to excessive growth and deposition of fat. This may explain the high incidence of infants who are large for gestational age. When the generous supply of maternal glucose is eliminated after birth, continued islet cell hyperactivity leads to hyperinsulinism and depletion of blood glucose. Within 2 to 4 hours hypoglycemia occurs. Although this hypothesis is plausible, it does not explain the obesity of offspring from mothers who are prediabetic, that is, those who are genetically predisposed to diabetes but have none of the characteristic abnormalities; nor does it explain the multiplicity of other abnormalities in infants of diabetic mothers.

The disorders that befall infants of diabetic mothers include macrosomia, respiratory distress, hypoglycemia, hypocalcemia, hyperbilirubinemia, hyaline membrane disease (as a function of prematurity), renal vein thrombosis, and a considerably higher incidence of congenital anomalies than in infants of nondiabetic mothers.

If maternal blood glucose levels are well controlled during pregnancy, most infants are appropriate for gestational age (AGA), but about 25% to 35% are large for gestational age (LGA). Macrosomia is more severe and more common in infants of mothers whose diabetes was not successfully managed during pregnancy, particularly during the third trimester. These LGA infants have a characteristic appearance. The face is round and red, having been classically described as a "tomato face." The infant is obviously obese and is usually inactive. Hypotonia is common at rest, but paradoxically the infant is extremely irritable and tremulous when disturbed. The excessive weight of macrosomic IDM is largely attributable to copious deposits of white fat throughout the body, primarily in the subcutaneous layers. Viscera are enlarged by virtue of increased cell number and hypertrophy of individual cells. The liver, heart, and adrenals are most conspicuously affected. Some studies have shown that infants of diabetic mothers are oversized in girth, but that their length and head circumferences are usually normal for gestational age. In other studies, universal overgrowth is attributed to increased weight, length, and head circumference. In either event, increased fat deposits are prominent and are associated with diminished total body water, particularly in the extracellular compartment. Infant size at birth is related to control of maternal glucose levels. Poor maternal control results in larger babies. Skinfold thickness, which indicates the extent of subcutaneous adipose deposition, is greatest among infants of mothers whose blood glucose is inadequately managed, especially during the third trimester.

Advanced maternal diabetes is associated with vascular involvement that causes nephropathy, hypertension, retinopathy, and calcification of vessels, particularly in the pelvis. Offspring of mothers so affected are SGA rather than oversized, and they are vulnerable to the hazards of intrauterine undergrowth and malnutrition.

Respiratory distress is common. If the infant is premature, hyaline membrane disease is regularly the cause. In the IDM, hyaline membrane disease is often more severe than in non-IDM infants of equal gestational age. Delayed lung maturation is characteristic of infants of diabetic mothers. Hyaline membrane disease seems paradoxical in babies born at 34 to 36 weeks who are macrosomic, and thus appear to be at term. Abnormalities of breathing in the IDM who is born at term are most often caused by RDS type II.

At birth, blood glucose concentration is 80% or more of the maternal level. Within an hour in normal infants, it falls to a mean of 40 to 50 mg/dl, but in infants of diabetic mothers, hyperinsulinism causes a greater decline. Levels below 20 and 30 mg/dl whole blood (25 and 35 mg/dl serum) usually occur from 2 to 4 hours after birth, sometimes sooner, occasionally later. This decline is followed by a spontaneous rise between 4 and 6 hours of age. Approximately half the infants of treated diabetic mothers (classes B through F) develop plasma glucose levels below 30 mg/dl. Among infants of gestational diabetic mothers (class A), approximately 20% are affected. Occa-

sionally hypoglycemia is protracted. Rarely it appears as late as 12 to 24 hours of age. Hypoglycemia in the IDM is rarely symptomatic.

Hypocalcemia (<7 mg/dl) occurs in the IDM in the presence or absence of hypoglycemia. Hypocalcemia may occur in 50% of the offspring of insulin-dependent mothers. Diminished parathyroid hormone production in the infant is considered the primary cause of hypocalcemia. Severity and frequency of low serum calcium concentrations are considerably greater in babies of poorly controlled mothers. Hypocalcemia is a common occurrence in non-IDM babies, particularly in asphyxiated neonates at any gestational age, and in prematures whether or not asphyxiated. In studies that have excluded the influence of asphyxia and prematurity, the frequency of hypocalcemia has been shown to be significantly increased solely by virtue of maternal diabetes and its effects on the fetus. The relationship of clinical signs to hypocalcemia has not been documented. Convulsions apparently do not occur in hypocalcemic infants (IDM or non-IDM) *during the first 3 days of life*. Tremors are often attributed to low serum calcium levels, but they usually persist despite calcium therapy. Tremors are more likely caused by cerebral irritability due to factors other than hypocalcemia.

Hyperbilirubinemia is more frequent among infants of diabetic mothers than in babies of like gestational age who are born of nondiabetic mothers. The characteristics and treatment of this disorder are identical in all premature infants.

Renal vein thrombosis is a rare occurrence. It is usually unilateral and is sometimes associated with radiologic evidence of calcification. The involved kidney is palpably enlarged, and hematuria and proteinuria are the rule. The survival of affected infants is often in doubt. Nephrectomy has been recommended in the past, but numerous instances of successful medical therapy have been reported.

Congenital anomalies have evolved as the major problem of infants of diabetic mothers. Effective management of maternal diabetes during pregnancy has diminished fetal and neonatal morbidity and mortality resulting from metabolic disorders and prematurity, thus imposing increased prominence to persistent teratogenic problems. It has been estimated that 10% of diabetic pregnancies culminate in neonates who have major malformations. Congenital heart disease is probably the most frequent.

Cardiomyopathy occurs in 10% to 20% of IDM. A hypertrophied ventricular septum is frequently associated with ventricular walls of normal thickness. Occasionally left and right ventricular walls are also thickened either diffusely or irregularly. Hypertrophy of the ventricular septum and walls is associated with hypoglycemia. Severe thickening of the ventricular septum and wall obstructs outflow of blood from the left ventricle into the aorta. Clinical evidence of congestive heart failure appears within the first 7 days after delivery. Because subaortic obstruction characterizes this disorder, digoxin is contraindicated because it increases obstruction to the outflow of blood. Propranolol is currently the preparation of choice because it decreases ventricular contractility. Cardiomyopathy resolves gradually over a period of weeks, and the heart is eventually normal.

Whether or not they are overtly ill, infants of diabetic mothers should usually be managed in an intensive care facility. More than half of them have an uneventful course, but careful observation is necessary nevertheless. The severity of the maternal diabetes should be known and recorded as early as the first prenatal visit. The nursery should be notified when a diabetic woman begins labor.

The schedule for blood glucose monitoring of infants of diabetic mothers is different from that of small-for-dates infants because the timing of hypoglycemia differs. Since the lowest blood glucose levels in infants of diabetic mothers occurs at 2 to 4 hours of age, blood glucose determinations should be done on cord blood at birth and at 1, 2, 4, and 6 hours of age.

Hypoglycemia and erythroblastosis fetalis. For years the danger of hypoglycemia in erythroblastotic infants was obscured by a preoccupation with the dramatic hematologic, cardiopulmonary, and central nervous system aspects of the disease.

Low blood glucose levels may occur in almost a third of moderately or severely affected infants and in 5% of all erythroblastotic infants, regardless of severity. When cord hemoglobin is less than 10 g/dl, the incidence of hypoglycemia is comparable to that in small-for-dates infants (20%). As in the latter group, symptoms are often absent. When present, they are identical to those of hypoglycemia from other causes. Blood sugar levels may fall transiently before or after exchange transfusion, most often during the first day of life but occasionally later. Islet cell hyperplasia and increased insulin content of the islets and blood are similar to those of infants or diabetic mothers. Their cause is unknown. Erythroblastotic hypoglycemia has become infrequent since the introduction of Rhogam and a resultant diminution of Rh disease. Hypoglycemia has not been reported in association with ABO incompatibility. Blood glucose levels should be monitored every 4 to 6 hours during the first day and regularly for the ensuing 3 days. Therapy is the same as for all forms of hypoglycemia.

Hypoglycemia in very small premature infants. Low blood sugar levels are not uncommon in infants whose birth weight is less than 1250 g. Hypoglycemia may occur during the hours after birth and during the days that follow. Intravenous 10% dextrose is given routinely after birth and for variable periods thereafter. Presumably liver glycogen stores are low in these very immature infants, and the increased metabolic demands imposed by extrauterine life deplete glycogen supplies rapidly. The process is accentuated by cold stress, asphyxia, and respiratory difficulty, all of which are frequent in these small infants. Blood sugar data should be followed every 4 to 8 hours for the first 2 days of life and periodically thereafter. Since pH and blood gas determinations are usually necessary at frequent intervals, it is advisable to obtain glucose determinations simultaneously.

Iatrogenic hypoglycemia. The most frequent iatrogenic cause of hypoglycemia is the sudden discontinuation of intravenous infusions containing glucose. This usually occurs when a peripheral intravenous infusion has infiltrated and difficulty is encountered in restarting a new one. If the umbilical vein is still patent, catheterization for a temporary intravenous infusion of glucose is effective until another peripheral vein can be used. If the umbilical vein is not available, we have, on some occasions, successfully maintained normal glucose levels by administering 10% glucose by nasogastric tube. The absorption of glucose when given by the enteral route is unpredictable. Hypoglycemia has also been observed approximately 2 hours after the cessation of an exchange transfusion. The preservative used in whole blood (acid citrate dextrose or citrate phosphate dextrose) contains a relatively high concentration of glucose. The exchange transfusion thus entails the administration of a relatively high glucose load over a short period of time. The secretion of insulin in response to resultant hyperglycemia may cause hypoglycemia approximately 2 hours after termination of the exchange transfusion when blood glucose levels decline abruptly. In many hospitals, whole blood now comprises a mixture of fresh-frozen plasma and frozen erythrocytes. This reconstituted blood also requires a preservative that contains a significant amount of glucose. The preservative is CPD-Al; the 63 ml in a unit of reconstituted blood contains 2 g of glucose.

Neonatal hypoglycemia and maternal drugs. Tocolytic therapy utilizes beta-adrenergic drugs, and in the past when several of these preparations were in use, neonatal hypoglycemia was reported to be associated with virtually all of them. The preparations included isoxsuprine and terbutaline. Neonatal hypoglycemia is an infrequent occurrence in association with ritodrine, which is the tocolytic in current exclusive use.

Oral hypoglycemic agents (tolbutamide, chlorpropamide) are not used to control diabetes during pregnancy. When they were in use, severe and protracted neonatal hypoglycemia was reported. Tolbutamide has a particularly protracted half-life in the neonate, and concentrations of the drug are higher in the baby's blood than in the mother's. These preparations cross the placenta and stimulate pancreatic beta cell activity, which results in severe hyperinsulinism.

Treatment of hypoglycemia. Hypoglycemia requires treatment with intravenous glucose, whether symptoms are present or not. The method for administering glucose is identical for the hyperinsulinemic (infants of diabetic mothers, erythroblastotic infants) and the glycogen-depletion types of hypoglycemia (small-for-dates infants, smaller of twins).

Symptomatic infants who are at known risk for hypoglycemia, and whose Dextrostix indicates low blood glucose, require immediate treatment after the collection of blood for verification of the Dextrostix by plasma glucose determination. Immediately after collection of blood we administer a glucose bolus that contains 200 mg/kg in 15 ml of a 15% solution over a period of 3 to 5 minutes. Assuming verification of hypoglycemia by laboratory determination of plasma glucose, a continuous infusion of glucose is begun at a rate of 8 mg/kg/min. If normoglycemia is not restored after 15 to 20 minutes, the dose of glucose is increased to 10 mg/kg/24 h or perhaps more, depending on the severity of hypoglycemia demonstrated by another plasma glucose determination. In the absence of a satisfactory response, the dose of glucose may be increased to 14 mg/kg/24 h. If this does not result in normoglycemia after 20 minutes of infusion, steroid therapy is indicated. Hydrocortisone is usually used for this purpose, given as 5 mg/kg/*dose* every 12 hours in an intravenous infusion into muscle or by mouth. Prednisone may be used alternatively as 1 mg/kg/*dose* orally every 12 hours. Steroids stimulate glucose production from noncarbohydrate sources, mostly amino acids (gluconeogenesis).

In *asymptomatic infants* whose hypoglycemia is identified by a low Dextrostix value, two consecutive and closely spaced laboratory determinations of plasma glucose are necessary to establish the diagnosis prior to therapy because blood sugar levels normally fluctuate unpredictably. Glucose is then administered as prescribed in the preceding paragraph for symptomatic infants.

A strong case must be made for initially calculating the actual quantities of glucose required, rather than random selection of a percent solution. It is as inappropriate to arbitrarily raise or lower percent concentrations of dextrose solutions for desired changes in glucose dosage as it is to change inspired oxygen concentrations by varying flow rates in liters per minute. Both practices are anachronistic. The procedure that should be followed requires that the appropriate quantity of glucose is determined first, according to a dose that is calculated per minute. Then the appropriate 24-hour fluid requirement is determined. The percent dextrose solution to be administered is calculated based on the absolute quantity of glucose required for therapy and fluid required for water balance. The past practice of arbitrarily choosing a solution strength has disregarded the precise quantity of glucose that must be delivered over a specific time interval to restore normoglycemia.

Prognosis of neonatal hypoglycemia. Untreated symptomatic hypoglycemia in the neonate may cause death. Later in childhood the incidence of central nervous system dysfunction varies from 30% to 60% of untreated symptomatic small-for-dates infants. The incidence of later neurologic abnormality in asymptomatic infants may be considerably lower, but nevertheless significant. The destiny of asymptomatic small-for-dates babies with hypoglycemia is not known, since there are no well-controlled follow-up studies available. Clearly defined outcomes of well-treated hypoglycemic small-for-dates babies are also wanting. Data from a recent well-planned inquiry suggest that these infants still do not fare as well as normoglycemic controls, but many other unanswered questions have left the issue clouded. Outcome of the asymptomatic hypoglycemic infant has not been clarified. Until it is, the recommendation to treat such infants rapidly is virtually universal.

CALCIUM DISORDERS
Physiology

Calcium circulates in blood in three forms: (1) ionized; (2) combined with anions such as phosphate, citrate, and bicarbonate; and (3) bound to protein. Only ionized calcium is physiologically active. The calcium levels reported from most laboratories include all three forms, comprising total calcium content of plasma. Normally, ionized calcium constitutes 50% of the total calcium content in blood. Although total and ionized calcium generally correlate in the newborn, one cannot assume an ionized calcium level based on concentrations of total calcium. Thus, in the presence of metabolic alkalosis, ionized calcium may be significantly diminished, whereas in an occasional infant, total calcium levels are normal. In another example, exchange transfusion that utilizes blood with citrate preservative may cause a significant reduction of ionized calcium that combines with the citrate. Total calcium concentration is usually lowered, but it could be normal in some babies.

Calcium homeostasis is intertwined with several factors that include phosphorus, magnesium, acid-base, parathyroid hormone, vitamin D, and calcitonin. The effects of these factors on serum calcium (Ca) and phosphorus (P) are shown in Table 11-3.

During gestation, calcium is actively transported across the placenta from maternal sources. Fetal calcium requirements are but a fraction of maternal stores, and there is relatively little maternal depletion. The serum-ionized calcium concentration in the fetus is significantly higher than in the mother. At birth, and for several days there-

Table 11-3. Biochemical and hormonal effects on calcium and phosphate level

Factors	Usual effect on serum Ca	Usual effect on serum P
Biochemical		
Ca	Increase	—
P	Decrease	Increase
Mg	Increase	—
Alkalosis	Decrease	—
Hormonal		
Parathyroid hormone	Increase	Decrease
Vitamin D	Increase	Increase
Calcitonin	Decrease	Decrease

after, while calcium intake is insignificant, the neonate mobilizes needed calcium by mechanisms that release it from bone. Neonates who need intensive care often receive intravenous fluids that contain no calcium, and in sick infants calcium levels are likely to be lower than in well babies at term. This is particularly noteworthy in premature infants (30% affected), asphyxiated infants (30% affected), and half the infants of insulin-dependent diabetic mothers, who are particularly prone to hypocalcemia.

Elevated levels of serum *phosphorus* tend to depress calcium concentrations by promoting the deposition of calcium in bone. Several phenomena are normally contributory to high serum phosphorus concentrations. First, the neonate's phosphorus levels are elevated as a continuum of the high fetal levels that are significantly greater than the mother's. Second, immediately after birth the rapid breakdown of glycogen in tissues entails release of phosphorus into serum. Third, phosphorus is poorly excreted by the neonatal kidney, and it thus accumulates in serum to some extent. Fourth, diminished activity of the neonatal parathyroids elevates serum phosphorus. These factors, operative in normal term infants, are exaggerated in asphyxiated and premature infants and in the infants of diabetic mothers, all of whom are peculiarly susceptible to hypocalcemia.

Parathyroid hormone is the most significant controller of calcium equilibrium. The hormone elevates serum calcium levels largely by promoting *release of calcium from bone,* provided adequate supplies of vitamin D are on hand. To further enhance calcium levels, parathyroid hormone *diminishes renal calcium excretion* while it *enhances absorption from the intestine.* Parathyroid hormone reduces serum phosphate, and this mitigates the hypocalcemic effects of hyperphosphatemia. The hormone reduces phosphorus levels by *increasing renal phosphorus excretion.* Beyond the neonatal period the parathyroid gland is very sensitive to reductions in serum-ionized calcium concentrations. It is also sensitive to abrupt decreases of serum magnesium. Hormone secretion increases within minutes after a fall in ionized calcium. However, in the neonate, parathyroid activity is diminished for several days after birth as a continuum of intrauterine hypoactivity, because chronically elevated maternal calcium concentration toward the end of gestation is reflected in the fetus and, as a result, fetal parathyroid activity is suppressed.

Acid-base equilibrium influences the concentration of serum-ionized calcium. A low pH increases the concentration of ionized calcium; an abnormally high pH decreases it. These phenomena are rarely of clinical significance, save for those few reported instances in which bicarbonate therapy has diminished ionized calcium concentrations.

The metabolites of *vitamin D* are indispensable to the maintenance of calcium and phosphorus homeostasis. The most active metabolite of vitamin D is 1-alpha, 25-dihydroxycholecalciferol. Vitamin D metabolites promote the absorption of calcium and phosphorus from the intestine, the mobilization of calcium and phosphorus from bone into extracellular fluid, and the inhibition of calcium and phosphorus excretion through the kidney.

Calcitonin is a substance produced by specific cells (C cells) in the thyroid gland. It opposes the action of parathyroid hormone by limiting the amount of calcium released from bone and by promoting renal excretion. It exerts the same effects on phosphorus and therefore tends to decrease serum concentrations of both these elements. The level of calcitonin increases after birth, but its role in hypocalcemia is conjectural.

Hypocalcemia

The causes of neonatal hypocalcemia are multiple, and for the most part the mechanisms by which it is produced have not been unequivocally defined. Normal serum calcium levels vary from 8 to 10 mg/dl (4 to 5 mEq/L). Calcium levels below 7 mg/dl are considered abnormally depressed. The etiologic association of clinical signs with hypocalcemia, as with hypoglycemia, is difficult to establish because the symptoms occur in other unrelated disorders, and they are often nonexistent in hypocalcemic infants.

Two peaks of incidence occur, one between the first 24 and 48 hours and another between the fifth and tenth days of life. Typically the infant with early hypocalcemia is premature, either AGA or SGA. Perinatal asphyxia increases the probability of hypocalcemia. The early type is thought to be related to temporary neonatal hypoparathyroidism, diminished renal excretion of phosphorus, tissue release of phosphorus to cause hyperphosphatemia, and negligible calcium intake. Serum calcium is low, phosphorus is high, and magnesium is often diminished. Serum calcium is also related to gestational age: the shorter the gestation, the lower the calcium. Infants of diabetic mothers are often hypocalcemic. A history of abruptio placentae or placenta previa is not unusual. The symptoms of this early form of hypocalcemia, if any are discernible, often do not include neuromuscular involvement. Rather, they may be characterized by apnea, cyanotic episodes, edema, high-pitched cry, and abdominal distention; even these manifestations, however, have not been proved to be of hypocalcemic origin. Hypocalcemia does not cause seizures during the 48 to 72 hours that follow birth.

The form of hypocalcemia that begins during the fifth to tenth days is called *neonatal tetany*. It occurs in well-nourished infants who are fed evaporated milk formula that contains diminished concentrations of calcium in relation to phosphorus (decreased Ca:P ratio), compared with concentrations in human milk. An increase in serum phosporus follows several days of feeding, and the resultant hyperphosphatemia drives calcium into bone. Parathyroid activity increases in an attempt to counteract the tendency to lower serum calcium caused by increased serum phosphorus. Most proprietary brands of milk formula now contain a ratio of calcium to phosphorus closely simulating that of human milk. Neonatal tetany is rare in areas in which evaporated milk is not a prevalent formula. The signs of neonatal tetany are characterized by neuromuscular irritation—twitching, tremors, jitters, and focal or generalized convulsions. Convulsions frequently begin as the infant is taken up for a feeding. They vary in duration from a few seconds to as long as 10 minutes. Minor stimuli often provoke tremors or convulsive episodes, whereas in the undisturbed interim only restlessness may be apparent.

Maternal hyperparathyroidism is rare, but when it exists, the infant is quite likely to be hypocalcemic. A number of reports describe the diagnosis of maternal hyperparathyroidism only after identification of hypocalcemia in her newborn infant. Mothers of hypocalcemic infants should be investigated for this possibility. The pregnant woman with chronic hyperparathyroidism is hypercalcemic as a result of overactivity of that endocrine gland. Parathyroid hormone does not cross the placenta in either direction, but maternal calcium is actively taken up by the placenta; the fetus thus becomes hypercalcemic like the mother. Hypercalcemia depresses activity of the fetal parathyroid glands. At birth, with disappearance of the maternal oversupply of calcium, the neonate is left with a rapidly diminishing serum calcium level and with parathyroid glands that were depressed in utero. Parathyroid hormone is essential to calcium balance. It mobilizes calcium and increases serum levels. The neonate now has transient hypoparathyroidism and, as a result, is hypocalcemic.

Hypocalcemia is treated initially with intravenous injection of 10% calcium gluconate, 2 ml/kg of body weight (18 mg/kg of elemental calcium). The injection must be given slowly over a period of at least 10 minutes because sudden bradycardia frequently occurs during rapid administration. The heart rate should be monitored electronically or by auscultation. If it drops rapidly, the injection should be discontinued immediately. It may be resumed after a normal cardiac rate is maintained for approximately 30 minutes. Intramuscular administration of calcium gluconate is contraindicated because calcium precipitates rapidly; a calcified mass and necrosis result. Caution is also required during intravenous infusion because accidental escape to extravascular tissue produces local calcification and sloughing. Calcium gluconate thus should not be administered through scalp veins. Orally administered calcium, added to formula, is begun as soon as feasible. Following the initial dosage, calcium gluconate should be added to intravenous fluids in a daily dose of 800 mg/kg (72 mg of elemental calcium). As normal serum levels are attained, the daily dose should be lowered gradually by half each day. Abrupt discontinuation may cause rebound hypocalcemia. If oral feedings are tolerated, calcium gluconate can be fed in amounts identical to those recommended parenterally, even after the initial "push" dose.

If hypomagnesemia is coexistent, it must be corrected before a response to calcium therapy can occur.

MAGNESIUM DISORDERS
Hypomagnesemia

Normal serum magnesium concentration in the neonate is 1.2 to 1.8 mg/dl. Hypomagnesemia often accompanies hypocalcemia. It occurs during or after exchange transfusions because magnesium becomes bound to the citrate in donor blood. For unknown reasons, it may also occur in infants of diabetic mothers. Serum magnesium determinations are essential for proper evaluation of babies with signs of neuromuscular excitability. They are especially important in hypocalcemic infants who do not respond to calcium therapy. If the signs are caused by magnesium deficiency, tetany and convulsions disappear promptly after appropriate therapy. An intramuscular dose of 50% magnesium sulfate (0.2 ml/kg of body weight) is given every 4 hours for the first day. The need for subsequent therapy is determined by serial serum magnesium determinations.

Hypermagnesemia

Magnesium sulfate is a preparation of choice for the treatment of preeclampsia. When it is administered by either the intramuscular or intra-venous routes, serum magnesium levels in maternal and cord blood are higher than normal. The maternal normal range is 1.2 to 2.2 mEq/L; normal values in cord blood are 0.9 to 2.6 mEq/L. Most cases of neonatal hypermagnesemia reported to date have not been associated with clinical abnormalities, and there is some doubt that high magnesium levels are responsible for abnormal signs. However, there are several instances of severe neonatal illness associated with high serum magnesium concentrations. The correlation of clinical signs and elevated serum magnesium levels is not a good one, perhaps because the curare-like effect is more dependent on *tissue magnesium content* than on serum concentrations. The shorter the duration of maternal magnesium therapy, the less the likelihood that tissue magnesium content has had time to increase. If maternal therapy has involved high doses of magnesium but over a short time period, the neonate will probably be hypermagnesemic and asymptomatic. At high levels magnesium causes peripheral neuromuscular block (curare-like effect) and central nervous system depression as well. Clinical abnormalities in the neonate include hypotonia, weak or absent cry, and severe respiratory depression with apnea and cyanosis. The respiratory difficulty has necessitated mechanically assisted ventilation. Several investigators have used intravenous calcium in attempts to antagonize the depressive effects of excessive magnesium, but with little evidence of benefit. The consensus is that calcium therapy is not effective. However, a dramatic response to exchange transfusion has been well documented. Magnesium toxicity should be suspected in a symptomatic infant whose mother was treated vigorously with magnesium sulfate for preeclampsia.

BIBLIOGRAPHY

Anderson, J. M., Milner, R. D. G., and Strich, S. J.: Pathological changes in the nervous system in severe neonatal hypoglycemia, Lancet 2:372, 1966.

Avery, M. E., Oppenheimer, E. H., and Gordon, H. H.: Renal-vein thrombosis in newborn infants of diabetic mothers, N. Engl. J. Med. 265:1134, 1957.

Ballard, F. J.: Carbohydrate metabolism and the regulation of blood glucose. In Stave, U., editor: Perinatal physiology, New York, 1978, Plenum Medical Book Co.

Barrett, C. T., and Oliver, T. K.: Hypoglycemia and hyperinsulinism in infants with erythroblastosis, N. Engl. J. Med **278:**1260, 1968.

Brady, J. P., and Williams, H. C.: Magnesium intoxication in a premature infant, Pediatrics **40:**100, 1967.

Brazy, J. E., and Pupkin, M. J.: Effects of maternal isoxsuprine administration on preterm infants, J. Pediatr. **94:**444-448, 1979.

Breitweser, J. A., Meyer, R. A., Sperling, M. A., et al.: Cardiac septal hypertrophy in hyperinsulinemic infants, J. Pediatr. **96:**535-539, 1980.

Clarke, P. C. N., and Carre, I. J.: Hypocalcemic, hypomagnesemic convulsions, J. Pediatr. **70:**806, 1967.

Cornblath, M.: Hypoglycemia in infancy and childhood, Pediatr. Ann. **10:**356-362, 1981.

Cornblath, M., and Schwartz, R.: Disorders of carbohydrate metabolism in infancy, ed. 2, Philadelphia, 1976, W. B. Saunders Co.

Cottrill, C. M., McAllister, R. G., Jr., Gettes, L., and Noonan, J. A.: Propranolol therapy during pregnancy, labor, and delivery: evidence for transplacental drug transfer and impaired neonatal drug disposition, J. Pediatr. **91:**812, 1977.

Cowett, R. M., and Schwartz, R.: The role of hepatic control of glucose homeostasis in the etiology of neonatal hypo- and hyperglycemia, Sem. Perinatol. **3:**327-340, 1979.

Craig, W. S.: Clinical signs of neonatal tetany; with especial reference to their occurrence in newborn babies of diabetic mothers, Pediatrics **22:**297, 1958.

Craig, W. S., and Buchanan, M. F. G.: Hypocalcemic tetany developing within 36 hours of birth, Arch. Dis. Child. **33:**505, 1958.

Davis, J. A., Harvey, D. R., and Yu, J. S.: Neonatal fits associated with hypomagnesemia, Arch. Dis. Child. **40:**286, 1965.

Dodson, W. E.: Neonatal metabolic encephalopathies, hypoglycemia, hypocalcemia, hypomagnesemia, and hyperbilirubinemia, Clin. Perinatol. **4:**131-148, 1977.

Dorchy, H., and Loeb, H.: Correlation of Dextrostix values with true glucose in the range less than 50 mg/dl (editorial correspondence), J. Pediatr. **88:**692, 1976.

Epstein, M. F., Nicholls, E., and Stubblefield, P. G.: Neonatal hypoglycemia after beta-sympathomimetic tocolytic therapy, J. Pediatr. **94:**449-453, 1979.

Ertel, N. H., Reiss, J. S., and Spergel, G.: Hypomagnesemia in neonatal tetany associated with maternal hyperparathyroidism, N. Engl. J. Med. **280:**260, 1969.

Fischer, G. W., Vazquez, A. M., Buist, N. R. M., et al.: Neonatal islet cell adenoma: case report and literature review, Pediatrics **53:**753, 1974.

Fisher, D. A.: Insulin and carbohydrate metabolism. In Smith, C. A., and Nelson, N. M., editors: The physiology of the newborn infant, Springfield, Ill., 1976, Charles C Thomas, Publisher.

Fletcher, A. B.: Clinical and biochemical aspects of the infant of the diabetic mother. In Young, D. S., and Hicks, J. M., editors: The neonate: clinical biochemistry, physiology and pathology, New York, 1976, John Wiley & Sons.

Frantz, I. D., III, Medina, G., and Taeusch, H. W., Jr.: Correlation of Dextrostix values with true glucose in the range less than 50 mg/dl, J. Pediatr. **87:**417, 1975.

From, G. L. A., Driscoll, S. G., and Steinke, J.: Serum insulin in newborn infants with erythroblastosis fetalis, Pediatrics **44:**549, 1969.

Gentz, J., Persson, B., and Zetterstrom, R.: On the diagnosis of symptomatic neonatal hypoglycemia, Acta Paediatr. Scand. **58:**449, 1969.

Griffiths, A. D.: Association of hypoglycaemia with symptoms in the newborn, Arch. Dis. Child. **43:**688, 1968.

Gutberlet, R. L., and Cornblath, M.: Neonatal hypoglycemia revisited, 1975, Pediatr. **58:**10, 1976.

Habib, A., and McCarthy, J. S.: Effects on the neonate of propranolol administered during pregnancy, J. Pediatr. **91:**808-811, 1977.

Haworth, J. C.: Neonatal hypoglycemia: how much does it damage the brain? Pediatrics **54:**3, 1974.

Haworth, J. C., and McRae, K. N.: The neurological and developmental effects of neonatal hypoglycemia: a follow-up of 22 cases, Can. Med. Assoc. J. **92:**861, 1965.

Hetenyi, G., and Cowan, J. S.: Glucoregulation in the newborn, Can. J. Physiol. Pharmacol. **58:**879-888, 1980.

Jacobs, R. F., Nix, R. A., Paulus, T. E., et al.: Intravenous infusion of diazoxide in the treatment of chlorpropamide-induced hypoglycemia, J. Pediatr. **93:**801, 1978.

Jarai, I., Mestyan, J., Schultz, K., et al.: Body size and neonatal hypoglycemia in intrauterine growth retardation, Early Human Develop. **1:**25-38, 1977.

Keen, J. H.: Significance of hypocalcemia in neonatal convulsions, Arch. Dis. Child. **44:**356, 1969.

Lee, F. A., and Gwinn, J. L.: Roentgen patterns of extravasation of calcium gluconate in the tissues of the neonate, J. Pediatr. **86:**598, 1975.

Lilien, L. D., Grajwer, L. A., and Pildes, R. S.: Treatment of neonatal hypoglycemia with continuous intravenous glucose infusion, J. Pediatr. **91:**779-782, 1977.

Lilien, L. D., Pildes, R. S., Srinivasan, G., et al.: Treatment of neonatal hypoglycemia with minibolus and intravenous glucose infusion, J. Pediatr. **97:**295-298, 1980.

Lipsitz, P. J.: The clinical and biochemical effects of excess magnesium in the newborn, Pediatrics **47:**501, 1971.

Lubchenco, L. O., and Bard, H.: Incidence of hypoglycemia in newborn infants classified by birth weight and gestational age, Pediatrics **47:**831, 1971.

Lucey, J. F., Randall, J. L., and Murray, J. J.: Is hypoglycemia an important complication in erythroblastosis fetalis? Am. J. Dis. Child. **114:**88, 1967.

Milley, J. R., and Simmons, M. A.: Metabolic requirements for fetal growth, Clin. Perinatol. 6:365-376, 1979.

Milner, R. D. G.: Fetal fat and glucose metabolism. In Beard, R. W., and Nathanielsz, P. W.: Fetal physiology and medicine, ed. 2, New York, 1984, Marcel Dekker.

Miranda, L. E. V., and Dweck, H. S.: Perinatal glucose homeostasis: The unique character of hyperglycemia and hypoglycemia in infants of very low birth weight, Clin. Perinatol. 4:351-365, 1977.

Mizrach, A., London, R. D., and Gribetz, D.: Neonatal hypocalcemia: its causes and treatment, N. Engl. J. Med. 278:1163, 1968.

Naeye, R. L.: Infants of diabetic mothers; a quantitative, morphologic study, Pediatrics 35:980, 1965.

Neligan, G. A., Robson, E., and Watson, J.: Hypoglycemia in the newborn: a sequel of the intrauterine malnutrition, Lancet 1:1282, 1963.

Nusbacher, J.: Transfusion of red blood cell products. In Petz, L. D., and Swisher, S. N., editors: Clinical practice of blood transfusion, New York, 1981, Churchill Livingstone.

O'Sullivan, J. B.: Gestational diabetes: unsuspected, asymptomatic diabetes in pregnancy, N. Engl. J. Med. 264:1082, 1961.

Pedersen, J.: The pregnant diabetic and her newborn, Baltimore, 1967, The Williams & Wilkins Co.

Pildes, R. S., Forbes, A., and Cornblath, M.: Studies of carbohydrate metabolism in the newborn infant. IX. Blood glucose levels and hypoglycemia in twins, Pediatrics 40:69, 1967.

Pildes, R. S., Cornblath, M., Warren, I., et al.: A prospective controlled study of neonatal hypoglycemia, Pediatrics 54:5, 1974.

Pildes, R., and Lilien, L. D.: Metabolic and endocrine disorders: carbohydrate metabolism in the fetus and neonate. In Fanaroff, A. A., and Martin, R. J., editors: Behrman's neonatal-perinatal medicine, ed. 3, St. Louis, 1983, The C. V. Mosby Co.

Raivio, K. O.: Neonatal hypoglycemia. II. A clinical study of 44 idiopathic cases with special reference to corticosteroid treatment, Acta Paediatr. Scand. 57:540, 1968.

Raivio, K. O., and Osterlund, K.: Hypoglycemia and hyperinsulinemia associated with erythroblastosis fetalis, J. Pediatr. 43:217, 1969.

Reisner, S. H., Forbes, A. E., and Cornblath, M.: The smaller of twins and hypoglycemia, Lancet 1:524, 1965.

Rivers, R. P. A.: Adaptation of the newborn to extrauterine life. In Beard, R. W., and Nathanielsz, P. W., editors: Fetal physiology and medicine, ed. 2, New York, 1984, Marcel Dekker.

Robert, M. F., Neff, R. K., Hubbell, J. P., et al.: Association between maternal diabetes and the respiratory-distress syndrome in the newborn, N. Engl. J. Med. 294:357, 1976.

Saville, P. D., and Kretchmer, N.: Neonatal tetany; a report of 125 cases and review of the literature, Biol. Neonate 2:1, 1960.

Tsang, R. C., Ballard, J., and Braun, C.: The infant of the diabetic mother: today and tomorrow, Clin. Obstet Gynecol. 24:125-147, 1981.

Tsang, R. C., Chen, I., Hayes, W., et al.: Neonatal hypocalcemia in infants with birth asphyxia, J. Pediatr. 84:428, 1974.

Tsang, R. C., Chen, I-W., Friedman, M. A., et al.: Parathyroid function in infants of diabetic mothers, J. Pediatr. 86:399, 1975.

Tsang, R. C., Kleinman, L. I., Sutherland, J. M., and Light, I. J.: Hypocalcemia in infants of diabetic mothers, J. Pediatr. 80:384, 1972.

Tsang, R. C., Light, I. J., Sutherland, J. M., and Kleinman, L. I.: Possible pathogenetic factors in neonatal hypocalcemia of prematurity, J. Pediatr. 82:423, 1973.

Tsang, R. C., and Oh, W.: Neonatal hypocalcemia in low birth weight infants, Pediatrics 45:773, 1970.

Tsang, R. C., and Steichen, J. J.: Metabolic and endocrine disorders: disorders of calcium and magnesium metabolism. In Fanaroff, A. A., and Martin, R. J., editors: Behrman's neonatal-perinatal medicine, ed. 3, St. Louis, 1983, The C. V. Mosby Co.

Wald, M. K.: Problems in metabolic adaptation; glucose, calcium, and magnesium. In Klaus, M. H., and Fanaroff, A. A., editors: Care of the high-risk neonate, Philadelphia, 1979, W. B. Saunders Co.

Yeung, C. Y., Lee, V. W. Y., and Yeung, C. M.: Glucose disappearance rate in neonatal infection, J. Pediatr. 82:486, 1973.

Zucker, P., and Simon, G.: Prolonged symptomatic neonatal hypoglycemia associated with maternal chlorpropamide therapy, Pediatrics 42:824, 1968.

CHAPTER 12

Nutrition for the low birth weight infant

PERSPECTIVE

During the past decade, smaller infants have survived in larger numbers; cardiorespiratory support, fluid and electrolyte therapy, and the provision of a physiologic thermal environment have become more effective. With improved management of the life-threatening problems that follow birth, a need arose for protracted nutritional support of a growing population of tiny survivors. The more premature the infant, the more prominent the role of cell multiplication in the growth process (see Chapter 5). Realization that inadequate nutrition may result in a permanent paucity of brain cells has created a sense of urgency. Cell proliferation falters in the absence of adequate nutrition; an irremediable dearth of brain cells ensues.

Premature birth imposes a sizable expenditure of energy. The baby emerges from a thermoneutral and metabolically regulated intrauterine environment to one that requires metabolic autonomy, while simultaneously incurring energy expenditures for difficult breathing and for compensation of heat loss. Rapid replenishment of depleted energy stores is impossible. The premature infant is not equipped for enteral feeds. The gut has been exposed solely to amniotic fluid, which is isotonic and low in protein. Yet the gut must quickly absorb fluid feedings of far greater complexity in order to regain energy stores. Because this is not feasible, the widely utilized alternative is intravenous nutrition.

The need for nutrients is urgent because energy stores are minimal or virtually nonexistent. There was little opportunity to accumulate lipid, and the small store of glycogen was quickly depleted at birth. There was also insufficient gestational time to generate albumin, iron, and calcium. In addition, the preterm infant's renal function is limited, transepidermal water losses are copious, and the volume of enteral feeding is severely restricted by a small stomach and a limited mucosal surface in the intestine.

There is uncertainty about what to feed, when to start feeding, and how to assess success. Attempts are made to mimic intrauterine growth, but this is infrequently feasible. Furthermore, the desirability of resuming the fetal growth rate post-

351

natally is not established. There are glaring intrinsic differences between the fetus and neonate. Body composition and energy requirements change rapidly on entry into the extrauterine environment. It is possible that something less than the fetal growth rate may be better for the neonate. Inability to define optimal postnatal growth in the absence of an acceptable point of reference is compounded by difficulties in measurement. Weight, length, and head circumference, are commonly utilized parameters. Weight is often misleading; it reflects retention and loss of water, as well as tissue mass. Linear growth is a realistic parameter of tissue accretion, but accurate measurement is difficult. Head circumference is a good indication of brain growth, thus confirming the adequacy of nutrition, but assessment is delayed because growth rate is slow. Despite these uncertainties, there is agreement on them and on several additional parameters for judging nutritional status. In essence, low birth weight infants are doing well nutritionally if they grow at approximately the fetal rate, and if they have no identifiable nutritional deficiencies. The deficiencies are hypoalbuminemia, rickets, free fatty acid deficiency, vitamin E deficiency, and zinc and copper deficiencies.

Delivery of nutrition to a low birth weight infant is a real challenge. For the first few days, sometimes longer, most sick babies do not tolerate intragastric feeds. Gastric emptying time is delayed, and abdominal distention often follows feedings. Delivery of formula directly into the duodenum through a transpyloric catheter was a widespread practice a few years ago, but malabsorption and difficulties with tube placement made it impractical.

The currently established alternative to intragastric feeding is parenteral nutrition. Preparations that contain varying concentrations of glucose and fixed concentrations of crystalline amino acids are given into a peripheral vein for a few days at changing sites, or into a central vein for more protracted periods. Intravenous lipids have been added to the parenteral regimen. The use of peripheral veins for parenteral nutrition is often an overwhelming task by virtue of difficulty in initiating and maintaining an open line. The infant is often exposed to cold stress during the process of starting the IV; inoculation of bacteria is likely. Cholestatic jaundice is a relatively frequent complication of parenteral nutrition. Also, little is known about optimal amino acid concentrations in the premature infant's plasma, especially for infants less than 1000 g.

Several controversies persist. They include the superiority of preterm breast milk versus formula, the composition of artificial formula that best supports growth, the ideal protein requirement, and the long-term outcomes of various feeding modalities.

ENERGY REQUIREMENTS

The principal determinants of caloric needs are the need for energy for growth and the expenditure of energy to maintain body temperature and metabolism. Energy is also required for the infant's spontaneous activity, for metabolism of ingested food (specific dynamic action), storage of new tissue, and for losses in feces. Basal metabolism ("resting caloric expenditure") requires about 50 cal/kg/day. Accurate measurements in the preterm infant are not feasible because the required fasting period would be unsafe. Spontaneous activity costs 5 to 15 cal/kg/day; short, infrequent periods of cold stress consume about 10 cal/kg/day. Approximately 20 cal/kg/day are spent for specific dynamic action and fecal losses. Thus, in the absence of growth, maintenance calories add up to 75 to 95 cal/kg/day. Caloric needs are significantly enhanced by needless impositions of cold stress. Energy loss may diminish or even preclude growth.

The premature infant is usually inactive for at least 75% of the day; the energy cost of spontaneous activity may thus be insignificant. In such circumstances, feeding no less than 50 to 60 cal/kg daily may preserve energy stores and existing tissue, but there will be no growth; cell hyperplasia may be precluded or impaired. At the other extreme, the price of intrauterine growth rate is 140 cal/kg/day. The minimal energy required for the status quo (50 to 60 cal/kg/day) plus the energy required for maximal rate of growth (140 cal/kg/day) are sensitively influenced by severity of illness, degree of immaturity, and appropriateness of size for gestational age. An intake of 140 cal/kg/day is usually difficult to achieve during the first few weeks of postnatal life. Efforts to provide maximum calories for growth are triggered by a realistic need, but constant restraint is in order if the hazards of overfeeding small babies are to be averted. Some growth is usually attainable with an intake of 70 cal/kg/day appropriately proportioned between protein, carbohydrate, and fat, assuming the presence of an adequate thermal milieu.

REQUIREMENTS FOR SPECIFIC NUTRIENTS: ENTERAL FEEDING

The primary constituents (protein, carbohydrate, fat) should provide appropriate fractions of total caloric intake. The recommended caloric percent distribution is protein (4 cal/g) 7% to 15%, carbohydrate (4 cal/g) 40% to 60%, fat (9 cal/g) 45% to 55% (Table 12-1).

Protein requirements

Optimal intake of protein is not established, but there is sufficient evidence to indicate that 2.5 to 3.5 g/kg/day are required. Protein should provide 10% to 15% of total calories. Commercial formulas that are designed for *term infants* usually contain a caloric density of 67 cal/dl and a protein concentration of 1.5 to 2.0 g/dl. In recent years formulas for *premature infants* have been designed to offer higher caloric density (approximately 80 cal/dl) and a higher protein content (between 1.8 and 2.4 g/dl) than term infant preparations. The "humanized" preterm formulas mimic the breast milk from mothers who deliver prematurely. In relation to caloric density, the formulas provide adequate quantities of protein when caloric requirements are met. There is good evidence that protein intakes over 4.5 g/kg/day often create metabolic difficulties such as high plasma concentrations of certain amino acids, azotemia, metabolic acidosis, and hyperammonemia.

The controversy over appropriate quantitative intake of protein originated over 50 years ago. In those years the range of recommended intakes was wide, and though it is considerably narrower today, a precise recommendation for optimal

Table 12-1. Daily requirements for low birth weight infants

Total nutrients per kilogram		Total vitamins per day	
Calories	100-140	A	1500-2500 IU
Protein	2.5-4 g (10%-15%)	Thiamine	0.4 mg
Carbohydrate	10-15 g (45%-55%)	Ribloflavin	0.5 mg
Fat	5-7 g (30%-45%)	Pyridoxine	0.25 mg
Sodium	2-4 mEq	B_{12}	1.0 µg
Chloride	0.5-2.0 mEq	C	30-50 mg
Potassium	0.5-2.0 mEq	D	400 IU
Calcium	4.0-6.0 mEq	E	25 IU
Phosphorus	2.0-4.0 mEq	Niacin	6.0 mg
Magnesium	0.5-1.0 mEq	Folic acid	0.35 mg
Iron	6 mg per day	K	1.5 mg

Modified from Fanaroff, A. A., and Klaus, M. H.: The gastrointestinal tract—feeding and selected disorders. In Klaus, M. H., and Fanaroff, A. A.: Care of the high-risk neonate, ed. 2, Philadelphia, 1979, W. B. Saunders Co.

growth cannot be made. Appropriate quantity is no more significant than optimal quality. Casein is the predominant source of protein; a much smaller amount is in whey. These formulas contain a whey:casein ratio of 18:82, whereas in human milk the whey:casein ratio is 70:30. "Humanized" cow's milk formulas now contain a ratio of 60:40, more closely imitating breast milk composition. The altered protein base in commerical formulas is a significant forward step. Casein-based protein is more likely to cause the metabolic imbalances previously mentioned, especially if protein intake exceeds 4.5 g/kg/day. Whey protein has no such disadvantage.

Carbohydrate requirements

Carbohydrates should provide 40% to 50% of total caloric intake. There is no standard recommendation for specific quantities of carbohydrates. The type of carbohydrate varies from one formula to another. Lactose, sucrose, glucose, and any combination of them have been used satisfactorily.

Of the gut enzymes that promote absorption of carbohydrates, *lactase* is the latest to appear prenatally. It becomes fully active at term, but may be stimulated in premature infants when lactose-containing formulas are fed. Lactose is important for the development of normal intestinal bacterial flora. It promotes the growth of *Lactobacillus*, which apparently suppresses growth of the pathogenic gram-negative organisms known to cause serious infections in the neonate.

Fat requirements

Fat has the highest caloric density (9 cal/g). It should provide approximately 50% of total caloric intake. Linoleic acid is the only concrete recommendation for intake of a simple fat. Linoleic acid should provide approximately 3% of the total caloric intake. Certain polyunsaturated fatty acids are required at all ages (linoleic, linolenic, arachidonic acids), but linolenic and arachidonic acids are synthesized from linoleic acid, which is

therefore inflexibly required in the human diet. In premature infants, intestinal absorption of fat is inefficient; over 30% of ingested fat fails to be absorbed. Absorption is a function of the nature of the fat, and the intestinal content of bile salts and pancreatic lipase. Vegetable fats and human milk fat are more easily absorbed. Medium-chain triglycerides, which are constituents of commercial formulas, are better absorbed than long-chain triglycerides, but this enhanced absorption has not been regularly associated with better weight gain. Intestinal absorption of fat in low birth weight infants is impaired by a paucity of bile salts and pancreatic lipase in the intestine. Fat is important because of its high caloric value and because it facilitates absorption of the fat-soluble vitamins A, D, E, and K.

BREAST MILK FOR THE LOW BIRTH WEIGHT INFANT

The use of human milk for low birth weight infants has increased considerably in recent years. Several studies have compared the effects of human milk from mothers at term with milk from mothers who deliver prematurely, and with formulas that are specially modified for premature infants. Term breast milk does not support growth as well as preterm milk or preterm formula. In most studies, human milk is pooled and banked. Term milk is inadequate for premature infants because of its low protein concentration. The protein concentration in preterm milk is about 20% higher. The great disadvantage of preterm milk is the unpredictability of its content; particularly when pooled in milk banks. Milk that has been expressed has twice the protein content of "dripped" milk.

Human milk has two advantages for low birth weight infants: (1) it provides a degree of protection against infection by virtue of its secretory IgA content and its phagocytic cells, and (2) it allows active maternal contribution to infant care. Only freshly expressed milk can protect against infection; milk that is banked and pooled does not.

A recent study compared frozen banked breast milk (term) with commercial preterm formula in a population of infants less than 1500 g. Those who were fed term breast milk grew more slowly in weight, length, and head circumference; their nursery stay was significantly longer. The caloric density and protein content of term breast milk were considerably lower than the formula. Another study compared rates of growth and biochemical status in three groups of preterm infants: one was fed preterm human milk, another received term breast milk, and a third was given commercial preterm formula. The responses of infants who received preterm human milk and commercial formula were similar. Infants who were fed term breast milk required a longer time to regain birth weight; they also gained less weight thereafter. Average increments in body length and head circumference were significantly diminished in these same infants. The study concluded that infants who were fed preterm breast milk or preterm commercial formula grew more rapidly than those who were given term breast milk.

To date there is general agreement that term human milk is not an adequate source of nutrition for premature infants. It also appears that human preterm milk and preterm commercial formulas both promote better growth than term breast milk. Whether pooled, banked preterm milk provides better nutrition than preterm formulas is not known. However, there is little question that caloric and protein content of pooled preterm breast milk are unpredictable, and that commercial formulas provide adequate growth.

Widespread use of human milk for low birth weight babies now raises the question of maternal drug secretion into milk. Ingestion of some drugs may result in toublesome side effects; premature infants may be particularly vulnerable. Tables 12-2 through 12-5 are reproduced here from a 1983 report by the Committee on Drugs of the American Academy of Pediatrics. The committee state-

Text continued on p. 360.

Table 12-2. Drugs contraindicated during breastfeeding

Drug	Reported sign or symptom in infant or effect on lactation
Amethopterin*	Possible immune suppression; unknown effect on growth or association with carcinogenesis
Bromocriptine	Suppresses lactation
Cimetidine†	May suppress gastric acidity in infant, inhibit drug metabolism, and cause CNS stimulation
Clemastine	Drowsiness, irritability, refusal to feed, high-pitched cry, neck stiffness
Cyclophosphamide*	Possible immune suppression; unknown effect on growth or association with carcinogenesis
Ergotamine	Vomiting, diarrhea, convulsions (doses used in migraine medications)
Gold salts	Rash, inflammation of kidney and liver
Methimazole	Potential for interfering with thyroid function
Phenindione	Hemorrhage
Thiouracil	Decreased thyroid function; does not apply to propylthiouracil

From Committee on Drugs—American Academy of Pediatrics: The transfer of drugs and other chemicals into human breast milk, Pediatrics **72**:375, 1983. Reproduced by permission of Pediatrics.
*Data not available for other cytotoxic agents.
†Drug is concentrated in breast milk.

Table 12-3. Drugs requiring temporary cessation of breastfeeding

Drug	Recommended alteration in breastfeeding pattern
Metronidazole	Discontinue breastfeeding 12-24 h to allow excretion of dose
Radiopharmaceuticals	Radioactivity present in milk, consult nuclear medicine physician before performing diagnostic study so that radionuclide which has shortest excretion time in breast milk can be used; prior to study the mother should pump her breast and store enough milk in freezer for feeding the infant; after study the mother should pump her breast to maintain milk production but discard all milk pumped for the required time that radioactivity is present in milk.
Gallium 69 (^{69}Ga)	Radioactivity in milk present for 2 wks
Iodine 125 (^{125}I)	Risk of thyroid cancer; radioactivity in milk present for 12 days
Iodine 131 (^{131}I)	Radioactivity in milk present 2-14 days, depending on study.
Radioactive sodium	Radioactivity in milk present 96 h
Technetium 99m (^{99m}Tc), ^{99m}Tc macroaggregates, ^{99m}Tc O$_4$	Radioactivity in milk present 15 h to 3 days

From Committee on Drugs—American Academy of Pediatrics: The transfer of drugs and other chemicals into human breast milk, Pediatrics **72**:375, 1983. Reproduced by permission of Pediatrics.

Table 12-4. Maternal medication usually compatible with breastfeeding

Drug	Reported sign or symptom in infant or effect on lactation
Anesthetics, sedatives	
Alcohol	Drowsiness, diaphoresis, deep sleep, weakness, decrease in linear growth, abnormal weight gain; maternal ingestion of 1 g/kg daily decreases milk ejection reflex
Barbiturate	None; see antiepileptic drugs
Bromide	Rash, weakness, absence of cry with maternal intake of 5.4 g/day
Chloral hydrate	Sleepiness
Chloroform	None
Halothane	None
Magnesium sulfate	None
Methyprylon	Drowsiness
Secobarbital	None
Anticoagulants	
Bishydroxycoumarin	None
Warfarin	None

From Committee on Drugs—American Academy of Pediatrics: The transfer of drugs and other chemicals into human breast milk, Pediatrics **72**:375, 1983. Reproduced by permission of Pediatrics.

Table 12-4. Maternal medication usually compatible with breastfeeding—cont'd

Drug	Reported sign or symptom in infant or effect on lactation
Antiepileptics	
Carbamazepine	None
Ethosuximide	None
Phenobarbital	Methemoglobinemia (1 case); decreased responsiveness, decreased weight gain, excessive sleeping if mother's plasma level $\geq$30 µg/ml
Phenytoin	Methemoglobinemia (1 case)
Primidone	None
Thiopental	None
Valproic acid	None
Antihistamines, decongestants, and bronchodilators	
Dexbrompheniramine maleate with *d*-isoephedrine	Crying, poor sleeping patterns, irritability
Diphenhydramine	None
Dyphylline*	None
Iodides	Affects thyroid activity; see miscellaneous iodine
Theophylline	Irritability
Trimeprazine	None
Tripelennamine	None
Antihypertensive and cardiovascular drugs	
Atenolol	None
Captopril	None
Digoxin	None
Disopyramide	None
Guanethidine	None
Hydralazine	None
Methyldopa	None
Metoprolol*	None
Nadolol*	None
Propranolol	None
Quinidine	None
Reserpine	Galactorrhea
Antiinfective drugs (all antibiotics transfer into breast milk in limited amounts)	
Amantadine	Urinary retention, vomiting, and skin rash
Cefadroxil	None
Cefazolin	None
Cefotaxime	None
Chloramphenicol	None
Chloroquine	None

*Drug is concentrated in breast milk.   *Continued.*

Table 12-4. Maternal medication usually compatible with breastfeeding—cont'd

Drug	Reported sign or symptom in infant or effect on lactation
Antiinfective drugs—cont'd	
Clindamycin	None
Ethambutol	None
Isoniazid	None
Nalidixic acid	Hemolysis in infant with glucose-6-phosphate deficiency (G-6-PD)
Nitrofurantoin	Hemolysis in infant with G-6-PD
Pyrimethamine	None
Quinine	None
Rifampin	None
Salicylazosulfapyridine (sulfasalazine)	None
Sulfapyridine	Caution in infant with jaundice or G-6-PD, and ill, stressed, or premature infant
Sulfathiazole	None; nonabsorbable by mother
Sulfisoxazole	Caution in infant with jaundice or G-6-PD, and ill, stressed, or premature infant
Tetracycline	None; negligible absorption by infant
Trimethoprim	None
Antithyroid drugs	
Carbimazole	Goiter
Propylthiouracil	None
Cathartics	Abdominal cramping, colic-like syndrome
(drugs that cause abdominal cramping in mother)	
Danthron	Increased bowel activity
Diagnostic agents	
Iodine	Goiter; see miscellaneous, iodine
Iopanoic	None
Metrizamide	None
Diuretics	
Bendroflumethiazide	Suppresses lactation, thrombocytopenia (1 case)
Chlorothiazide	May suppress lactation, therefore avoid prescribing in first month of lactation; this may also apply to other thiazides; questionably dose related
Chlorthalidone	Excreted slowly
Methyclothiazide	None
Spironolactone	None
Hormones	
Chlorotrianisene	None
^{3}H-norethynodrel	None
19 norsteroid	None
Contraceptive pill with estrogen/progesterone	Breast enlargement, dose related; decrease in milk production and protein content
Estradiol	Withdrawal, vaginal bleeding

Table 12-4. Maternal medication usually compatible with breastfeeding—cont'd

Drug	Reported sign or symptom in infant or effect on lactation
Muscle relaxants	
Baclofen	None
Carisoprodol	Drowsiness, intestinal upset
Methocarbamol	None
Narcotics, non-narcotic analgesics, antiinflammatory agents	
Acetaminophen	None
Butorphanol	None
Codeine	None
Flufenamic acid	None
Heroin	None
Ibuprofen	None
Indomethacin	Seizure (1 case)
Mefenamic acid	None
Meperidine	None
Methadone	None if mother receiving ≤20 mg/24 h
Morphine	None
Naproxen	None
Phenylbutazone	None
Prednisolone, prednisone	None
Propoxyphene	None
Salicylates	Metabolic acidosis (dose related); may affect platelet function, rash
Psychotropic agents	
Antianxiety	
Chlordiazepoxide	Conflicting reports of drowsiness
Clorazepate	
Diazepam	
Meprobamate*	
Oxazepam	
Prazepam*	
Antidepressants	
Amitriptyline	None
Amoxapine	
Desipramine	
Dothiepin	
Imipramine	
Lithium	
Tranylcypromine	
Antipsychotic	
Chlorpromazine	Galactorrhea in adult; drowsiness and lethargy in infant
Haloperidol	None
Mesoridazine	None

*Drug is concentrated in breast milk.

Continued.

Table 12-4. Maternal medication usually compatible with breastfeeding—cont'd

Drug	Reported sign or symptom in infant or effect on lactation
Psychotropic agents—cont'd	
Antipsychotic—cont'd	
Piperacetazine	
Prochlorperazine	
Thioridazine	
Trifluoperazine	
Other	
Marijuana*	Unknown, only one report in literature
Stimulants	
Amphetamine	Irritability, poor sleeping pattern
Caffeine	Irritability, poor sleeping pattern, excreted slowly
Nicotine (excess)	Shock, vomiting, diarrhea, rapid heart rate, restlessness; decreased milk production
Vitamins	
B_1	None
B_{12}	None
D	Increased calcium levels
Folic acid	None
K_1	None
Pyridoxine	None
Riboflavin	None
Thiamin	None
Miscellaneous	
Atropine, scopolamine	None
Bethanechol	Abdominal pain, diarrhea
Diphenoxylate with atropine	None
Iodine (povidone-iodine/ vaginal douche)	Elevated iodine levels in breast milk, odor of iodine on infant's skin
Tolbutamide	Jaundice

*Drug is concentrated in breast milk.

ment is based on an extensive literature available to the interested reader in the original publication (Pediatrics **72:**375-383, 1983).

PARENTERAL NUTRITION

Low birth weight infants cannot survive more than 7 days of total starvation, or more than 21 days of severe partial starvation. Their illnesses during the days following birth preclude enteral feeding, and when finally initiated, the feedings are often intolerable. Parenteral nutrition, introduced in the 1960s for postoperative infants, provides an effective alternative to gastrointestinal feedings. Until the 1970s, infusions were administered solely through a deep central vein. Later, a number of reports described successful experiences with peripheral veins.

Parenteral nutrition is administered today via two routes: a deep central vein and a peripheral vein. Deep vein administration is generally re-

Table 12-5. Food and environmental agents: effect on breastfeeding

Agent	Reported sign or symptom in infant or effect on lactation
Aspartame	Caution in patient carrier of phenylketonuria
Bromide (photographic laboratory)	Potential absorption and bromide transfer into milk; see "Anesthetics, Sedatives"
Chlordane	None reported
Chocolate	Irritability or increased bowel activity if excess amounts (16 oz/d) consumed by mother
Cyclamate	None
DDT, benzenehexachlorides, dieldrin, aldrin, hepatachlorepoxide	None
Fava beans	Hemolysis in patient with glucose-6-phosphate deficiency (G-6-PD)
Fluorides	None
Hexachlorobenzene	Skin rash, diarrhea, vomiting, dark urine, neurotoxicity, death
Hexachlorophene	None; contamination of milk from nipple washing
Lead	Neurotoxicity
Methyl mercury	Affects neurodevelopment
Monosodium glutamate (MSG)	None
Polychlorinated biphenyls and polybrominated biphenyls	Lack of endurance, hypotonia, sullen expressionless facies
Saccharin	None
Tetrachlorethylene (cleaning fluid)	Obstructive jaundice, dark urine
Vegetarian diet	Signs of B_{12} deficiency

From Committee on Drugs—American Academy of Pediatrics: The transfer of drugs and other chemicals into human breast milk, Pediatrics **72**:375, 1983. Reproduced by permission of Pediatrics.

served for surgical patients whose GI tract is incapacitated.

Parenteral nutrition via deep vein

Intravenous nutrition begun soon after birth is intended to forestall catabolism. Thus at least the existing stores of energy and tissue can be preserved. The effectiveness of parenteral nutrition is well established; most babies respond with satisfactory growth. Deep vein feeds of 70 cal/kg/day satisfy requirements for basal metabolism and spontaneous activity. Nitrogen retention and growth will occur at intakes above 70 cal/kg/day. When caloric intake exceeds 100 cal/kg/day, infants can be expected to gain 15 to 20 g/kg/day.

The solution used for parenteral nutrition, whether deep vein or peripheral vein, contains essential and nonessential amino acids, glucose, electrolytes, vitamins, and trace elements. Intravenous lipids (see later) are administered from a separate source. Fluid administered via deep vein is more hypertonic than fluid given through peripheral veins. Glucose concentrations of the former infusates vary between 20% and 25%; amino acid content is 2.5 g in 125 ml of fluid.

Infusions for low birth weight infants should initially contain approximately 10 g of glucose/kg/day. During the days that follow, the glucose content is raised to attain full concentration between the seventh and tenth days of therapy. The concentration of amino acids remains unchanged.

Complications of deep vein infusions include septicemia resulting from bacteria and *Candida* organisms, thrombosis at the catheter tip, and aberrant catheter position. Metabolic complications are caused by infusate contents. The most frequently encountered is hyperglycemia. Hyperammonemia occurs occasionally; cholestatic jaundice is fairly common. Deep vein nutrition supports adequate growth. With several exceptions, the deep vein route is not the one of choice. In most instances, low birth weight infants are maintained on peripheral vein infusions. We sometimes administer parenteral nutrition through a central vein in very low birth weight infants between 500 and 750 g because they require protracted periods of intravenous nutrition.

Parenteral nutrition via peripheral vein

Peripheral veins are used far more frequently. Their most serious limitation is the relatively short life of infusion sites, necessitating frequent reinitiation in alternate veins. Another limitation is in the need to restrict glucose concentration to 12% or 13%. Peripheral vein solutions must be less hypertonic than deep vein solutions in order to minimize the occurrence of thrombophlebitis and venous occlusion.

The effectiveness of peripheral vein nutrition is well established. As utilized today, these solutions are embellishments of the glucose solutions that have traditionally been administered after birth. The peripheral vein solution contains glucose, amino acids, electrolytes, vitamins, and trace elements. Intravenous lipids must be administered from a separate source. The tubing that contains lipid is connected into the amino acid system at a point that is as close to the skin as is feasible. Caloric requirements for basal metabolism, spontaneous activity, nitrogen retention, and growth are the same as previously described for deep vein infusion.

Intravenous fat

Intravenous lipid is a principal contributor to nonprotein calories. It is available in a preparation that contains 10 g of lipid/dl. Each milliliter provides 1.1 calories. The high caloric density of intravenous fat has virtually eliminated the need for central vein infusions that provided adequate cal-

ories only because high glucose concentrations could be infused into large, deep veins. The high caloric density of the lipid permits minimum fluid volume. It prevents essential fatty acid deficiency, which often occurs after several days of parenteral nutrition with fat-free solutions.

The metabolism of intravenous lipids resembles naturally fed fats. Clearance of serum lipids requires lipoprotein lipase, which hydrolyzes plasma triglyceride bound to protein. Free fatty acids are thus released; they permeate fat depots and they are reconverted to triglycerides for storage.

The administration of intravenous fat requires a separate intravenous administration system attached by a Y-connector to the amino acid infusion tubing close to the skin. The fat emulsion disintegrates when mixed with a hypertonic solution, and it must therefore be separated from the amino acid–glucose solution.

Intravenous lipid is initiated at 0.5 g/kg/day, administered over a period of 18 to 24 hours. Daily increase should not exceed 1 g/kg/day, usually culminating at a maximum rate of 2.0 g/kg/day in preterm infants. Hyperlipemia is identified by the presence of milky plasma. Mild plasma turbidity, identified by visual inspection, is grossly unreliable. At some centers, lipid dosage is monitored by plasma triglyceride determinations. Concentrations exceeding 200 mg/dl require reduction of lipid infusion.

Term infants clear lipids from plasma as effectively as adults. They thus tolerate maximum lipid doses of 3.5 g/kg/day. Premature and SGA infants do not clear plasma lipid effectively. Clearance is slower; lipid levels are considerably higher than term infants given equal quantities of lipid. The peak rate of lipid infusion for premature and SGA infants is 2 g/kg/day.

CONCLUSION

Inadequate provision of nutriment, if only for a few days, rapidly culminates in a subacute nutritional emergency. Jeopardy is worst in the smallest babies. Their reserves are so negligible, and their growth is so nutriment-dependent, they can ill afford feedings that are too little and too late. The semi-starved infant is feeble, often to an extent that impairs respiration for want of muscle power to expand stiff lungs. The most sinister penalty of undernutrition is unseen; impaired cellular hyperplasia restricts sizes of all organs, but it is most injurious to the brain.

In only a few years, advances in intravenous nutrition, artificial formula composition, and knowledge of human milk have made it possible to avoid suboptimal states of nutrition. While much is unknown, there are sufficient data on hand for rational management and for gratifying outcomes. No matter how premature the viable baby is, we can usually provide nutrition for adequate growth.

BIBLIOGRAPHY

Brooke, O. G.: Nutrition in the preterm infant, Lancet **I:**514, 1983.

Committee on Drugs—American Academy of Pediatrics: The transfer of drugs and other chemicals into human breast milk, Pediatrics **72:**375, 1983.

Committee on Nutrition—American Academy of Pediatrics: Commentary on parenteral nutrition, Pediatrics **71:**547, 1983.

Fanaroff, A., and Klaus, M.: The gastrointestinal tract—feeding and selected disorders. In Care of the high-risk neonate, ed. 2, Philadelphia, 1979, W. B. Saunders Co.

Gross, S. J.: Growth and biochemical response of preterm infants fed human milk or modified infant formula, N. Engl. J. Med. **308:**237, 1983.

Heird, W. C., Okamoto, E., and Anderson, T. L.: Nutrition, body fluids, and acid-base homeostasis. Pt. 1. Nutritional requirements of the low birth weight infant. In Fanaroff, A. A., and Martin, R. J., editors: Behrman's neonatal-perinatal medicine, ed. 3, St. Louis, 1983, The C. V. Mosby Co.

Heird, W. C., and Anderson, T. L.: Nutrition, body fluids, and acid-base homeostasis. Pt. 2. Methods of nutrient delivery for the low birth weight infant. In Fanaroff, A. A., and Martin, R. J., editors: Behrman's neonatal-perinatal medicine, ed. 3, St. Louis, 1983, the C. V. Mosby Co.

Lucas, A., and Hudson, G. J.: Preterm milk as a source of protein for low birthweight infants, Arch. Dis. Child. **59:**831, 1984.

Reynolds, J. W.: Nutrition of the low birth weight infant. In Walker, W. A., and Watkins, J. B., editors: Nutrition in pediatrics: basic science and clinical application, Boston, 1985, Little, Brown & Co.

Tyson, J. E., Lasky, R. E., Mize, C.E., et al.: Growth, metabolic response, and development in very-low-birth-weight infants fed banked human milk or enriched formula. I. Neonatal findings, J. Pediatr. **103:**95, 1983.

Widdowson, E. M.: Nutrition. In Davis, J. A., and Dobbing, J., editors: Scientific foundations of paediatrics, ed. 2, Baltimore, 1982, University Park Press.

Perinatal infection

Although of diverse etiology, perinatal infections have many attributes in common that distinguish them from infections in later life. Whether of bacterial, viral, or protozoan causation, the tissue damage wrought by these infections and the patterns of disease they produce are remarkably different from those observed in more advanced age groups. For instance, the bacteria generally implicated in fetal and neonatal disease are not ordinarily pathogenic in older children. Conversely, organisms that cause serious disease in mature patients, such as pneumococci, group A streptococci, and meningococci, are rarely encountered during the perinatal period. Diseases caused by rubella virus, cytomegalovirus, herpesvirus, and *Toxoplasma* organisms are usually mild or asymptomatic in later life, but in the fetus and neonate these organisms produce extensive devastation of tissue, often resulting in death or dysfunctional survival.

In the pathogenesis of antepartal or intrapartal infection, maternal involvement, usually asymptomatic, always precedes fetal disease. The fetus may acquire disease from infected amniotic fluid, from the maternal bloodstream across the placenta, or by direct contact with infected maternal tissue in the birth canal. After birth the neonate must contend with the possibility of acquiring infection from other infants or from personnel or objects that surround him, particularly the equipment designed to save his life. The neonate's vulnerability to these hazards is determined by a number of variables, of which prematurity is clearly the most significant.

Another distinctive feature of perinatal infection is the immunologic response it stimulates. Special procedures are necessary to differentiate antibodies generated by the fetus and neonate from those received through the placenta from the mother. Serologic techniques that diagnose infections in older children are of little value in the newborn infant.

Physical signs of infectious disease, if any are indeed perceptible, are unique in their subtlety and their lack of specificity. Early in the course of infection one may not be aware of any disturbance, yet the disorder soon becomes rapidly fulminant and uncontrollable. Thus a severely septicemic premature infant may merely be hypoactive and refuse feeding. Furthermore, fever, the hallmark of infectious disease later in life, is often absent in the infected newborn. Coughing, which is almost universal in older children with pneumonia, is rare.

The choice of therapeutic antibiotics must usually be made before results of cultures are known. Such choices must be influenced by knowledge of the bacterial organisms most likely to cause disease. Their incidence is unique to the neonate. Equally important in the choice of therapy is an understanding of the immature pharmacologic response of the newborn infant. During the first 2 or 3 weeks of life, the absorption, metabolism,

and excretion of drugs vary considerably from those observed in older patients, and the uninformed use of some drugs may have serious results. The disastrous consequences of neglecting these differences were exemplified years ago by the widespread use of sulfisoxazole (Gantrisin) and chloramphenicol, which were administered in complete ignorance of the special hazards they imposed on the neonate. Sulfisoxazole caused an unexpectedly high incidence of kernicterus, and chloramphenicol caused numerous deaths.

This chapter discusses the salient aspects of perinatal infection, the fundamental reasons for its uniqueness, and the characteristics of its most important clinical entities.

ETIOLOGY
Bacterial agents

Most bacterial infections are caused by organisms comprising the flora of the mother's genital and intestinal tracts; beyond early infancy these agents are rarely pathogenic. Although varying lengthy lists of etiologic agents have emerged from numerous studies; a rather uniform pattern is apparent for the three major clinical entities: pneumonia, septicemia, and meningitis. Before the emergence of group B streptococci in the early 1970s as the most frequent etiologic agent, gram-negative rods produced 75% to 85% of these bacterial infections; *Escherichia coli* was predominant among them. *Pseudomonas aeruginosa* was the next most common agent. It is usually acquired postnatally; nursery equipment is a major source of its propagation. Staphylococci cause septicemia and pneumonia. Staphylococcal infection is virtually always acquired postnatally in the nursery, rarely from the mother during birth. Staphylococci are infrequently implicated in meningitis. During the worldwide nursery epidemics of the late 1950s and early 1960s, they were a prominent cause of pneumonia, and although still an important factor, they are now encountered with less frequency (see later). *Listeria monocytogenes* is a maternally derived gram-positive rod that also causes septicemia and meningitis. Most

Table 13-1. Vertically transmitted viruses implicated in fetal and neonatal infection*

Virus	Fetal/neonatal disorders
Rubella virus	Microcephaly, meningoencephalitis (chronic), cataracts, microphthalmia, glaucoma, deafness, hepatitis, jaundice, hepatosplenomegaly, pneumonitis, cardiovascular anomalies, myocardial necrosis, thrombocytopenia, anemia, purpura, inguinal hernia
Cytomegalovirus	Microcephaly, cerebral calcification, hydrocephalus, encephalitis, chorioretinitis, hepatitis, jaundice, hepatosplenomegaly, pneumonitis, cardiac anomalies, thrombocytopenia, purpura, anemia, inguinal hernia
Herpesvirus hominis	Meningoencephalitis, microcephaly, cerebral calcification, herpetic rash, hepatitis, jaundice, pneumonitis, thrombocytopenia, anemia, coagulopathy, keratoconjunctivitis, chorioretinitis
Coxsackievirus group B	Meningoencephalitis, myocarditis, hepatitis, jaundice, thrombocytopenia
Varicella-zoster	Chickenpox rash, pneumonitis, hepatitis
Variola poxvirus	Smallpox rash, pneumonitis, hepatitis, meningoencephalitis
Vaccinia virus	Vaccinia rash, pneumonitis, hepatitis, stillbirth
Poliomyelitis	Spinal or bulbar polio similar to adult, myocarditis, pneumonitis, stillbirth, abortion
Rubeola	Measles as in later life (usually benign), stillbirth, abortion
Western equine encephalomyelitis	Meningoencephalitis
Myxovirus (mumps)	Congenital parotitis, ? congenital malformations
Hepatitis virus B	Neonatal hepatitis

*Modified from Sever, J. L., and White, L. R.: Annual Rev. Med. **19:**471, 1968.

pediatric infections from this organism occur during the newborn period.

Viral agents

Viral diseases in the fetus and neonate are far less frequent than bacterial diseases, but they are an important cause of morbidity and mortality. They are generally transmitted from the mother but may also be acquired postnatally. Data on postnatally acquired viral disease are relatively meager, but considerable interest has been focused on infections acquired in utero. Thirteen viral agents are known to be vertically transmitted (from mother to fetus). These are listed in Table 13-1, accompanied by the prominent clinical findings for each. The importance of these perinatal viral diseases lies not only in the mortality they produce but in the more numerous infants who survive them with varying degrees of central nervous system damage.

Protozoan agent

Toxoplasma gondii is the most important protozoan agent involved in perinatal infection. Toxoplasmosis is discussed in detail later in this chapter.

PATHOGENESIS
Bacterial infections

Bacterial infections are acquired in utero, during descent through the birth canal, and after birth in the delivery room or nursery.

Intrauterine bacterial infection acquired by the ascending route. With few exceptions, bacterial infections are acquired prenatally by the ascending route; that is, organisms from the perineum and vagina gain entry into the uterine cavity through the cervix. Amniotic fluid is infected after passage of bacteria through a ruptured amniotic membrane, but sometimes the organisms permeate an intact one. They then gain entry into the fetus through the oral cavity and move to the lungs, gastrointestinal tract, and middle ear. Occasionally they enter the bloodstream from these sites.

The presence of organisms in amniotic fluid triggers an inflammatory response in the membranes consisting of infiltrates of polymorphonuclear leukocytes, which ultimately enter the amniotic fluid. Interestingly, the reaction begins in the maternal tissue and then spreads to the amniotic membrane, which is a fetal structure. The resultant lesion is known as chorioamnionitis. Benirschke and Driscoll have aptly pointed out that this is a unique example of response by one organism (maternal) to infection in another (fetal). The presence of bacteria in amniotic fluid thus produces chorioamnionitis and an outpouring of leukocytes into amniotic fluid. Chorioamnionitis and infected amniotic fluid do not always cause fetal disease. They merely expose the fetus to intrauterine infection. Based on the development of chorioamnionitis, several diagnostic procedures have been devised to identify exposure to intrauterine bacterial infection.

Rupture of membranes and prolonged labor. There is general agreement that early rupture of amniotic membranes predisposes to chorioamnionitis and umbilical vasculitis (inflammation of the cord and its vessels) and that the possibility of fetal infection is thus enhanced. Most investigators consider that membrane rupture is early if it occurs at least 24 hours before delivery. Beyond this time the risk of infection increases as the interval between rupture of membranes and birth is prolonged. However, for reasons as yet unknown, numerous infections occur even when membranes rupture closer to delivery than 24 hours. Length of labor is not as clearly correlated with the incidence of infection. There is little doubt that the hazard is most serious when early membrane rupture and prolonged labor are combined. For the nurse, this type of information is valuable in anticipating and detecting the signs of infection. When an infant with a history of exposure to infection in utero is admitted to the nursery, cultures should be taken. The best sites for specimen collection are the throat, axillae, inguinal folds, and external auditory canals. If these cultures are taken within 1 or 2 hours after birth, the results reveal organisms to which the infant was exposed. If signs of illness appear subsequently, the results of cultures provide some basis for the selection of therapeutic antibiotics.

The usefulness of information from skin cultures soon after birth is based on numerous studies of bacterial colonization. The skin of infants delivered by cesarean section is sterile. After vaginal delivery, *Staphylococcus epidermidis* predominates. Streptococci and coliform organisms are also present, but in far fewer number. Although *S. epidermidis* is present in large numbers, particularly in the axillae, these organisms are joined by a variety of other species soon after 12 hours of age. Approximately 25% of babies delivered vaginally are colonized by maternal vaginal flora at birth. After a week of age, most infants are colonized by coagulase-negative staphylococci. Gram-negative bacilli are not often isolated from normal infants; they are more often cultured from those who are ill or of low birth weight.

In one study, approximately 85% of infants had a sterile umbilicus for the first 24 hours of life. By the third day, *S. epidermidis* was predominant in most babies, while *Klebsiella-Enterobacter* and *E. coli* were next most numerous. Colonization varies widely depending on environment, modalities of management, and population base. Thus, in another study, *S. aureus* was cultured from the umbilicus of 22% of infants on the first day of life.

Results of cultures from the ear canal have also varied. Positive cultures soon after birth are reported in 7% to 30%, rising to 70% over the ensuing 4 days. At present, coagulase-negative staphylococci are predominant, but a few years hence other organisms will undoubtedly predominate according to experience with recurrent changes in decades past. For instance, in the early 1970s a study of 50 infants whose ear canals were cultured immediately after birth revealed 92% positive cultures of either coliform or group B streptococcal organisms, reflecting maternal vaginal flora. Fifteen years earlier, group B streptococci were rarely cultured from any site.

The pharynx is a reliable indicator of colonization status. At birth, and for several days afterwards, the nose and mouth of normal infants are usually sterile. By the end of the first week, nasal colonization has appeared in three fourths of infants. Gram-negative rods are rarely identified in normal babies, but are relatively frequent in small and ill infants. Administration of antibiotics immediately after birth diminishes rates of early colonization, but later there is a high incidence of gram-negative bacilli. Infants hospitalized in intensive care units are far more likely to be colonized with gram-negative rods. A study in New York City demonstrated that oropharyngeal culture often identifies infants at significant risk of infection and also predicts the organism that will be involved.

While culture of the blood is occasionally indicated immediately after birth, the known pathogenesis of intrauterine bacterial infection and the accumulated data on colonization both clearly indicate that cultures of the oropharynx or skin are more likely to be informative about exposure to bacterial disease in utero and during the birth process.

Gestational age and fetal infection. A strong positive association between short gestational age and increased incidence of chorioamnionitis, umbilical vasculitis, and neonatal infection has been cited universally. The shorter the gestational age, the higher their incidence. The incidence of septicemia, meningitis, and pneumonia is considerably higher among premature than among term infants.

Intrauterine bacterial infection acquired transplacentally. Syphilis and occasionally *Listeria monocytogenes* are transmitted across the placenta. Fetal tuberculosis is a rare infection, but when it occurs, it too is acquired through the placenta. Fetal infection from transplacentally derived *Pneumococcus*, *Streptococcus*, *Staphylococcus*, and *Salmonella* organisms is also rare. Before antibiotics were available, maternal septicemia due to these organisms was more frequent, and fetal infection by the placental route was an occasional sequel.

Bacterial infection acquired postnatally. Nursery personnel, infant cohorts, fixtures, and equipment utilized for care of the neonate are important sources of postnatal infection. In this respect the lessons learned from the worldwide scourge of staphylococcal epidemics are important to recall. Causative strains of staphylococci were repeatedly cultured from attendants, from other infants, and from articles in the environment such as airborne particles, linen, diapers, and blankets. An exchange between infants and environmental components was postulated by numerous investigators, and indeed the general pattern that emerged from most studies indicated as much. However, disagreement arose about the relative importance of each of these factors, and more fundamentally, about the original source of organisms. The bitter experience with staphylococcal epidemics over a period of several years led to a multiplicity of stringent hygienic measures and isolation techniques, some of which have been relaxed considerably because epidemiologic strains of staphylococci seemed to disappear from the nursery. The influence exerted by these stringent nursery practices is impossible to estimate. It is possible that a phase in the long-term natural life cycle of staphylococci has passed, largely unrelated to our feverish efforts to eliminate them. Infection control practices in the nursery are discussed later in this chapter.

Commensurate with the decline of staphylococcal disease, there was a rise in the incidence of postnatally acquired gram-negative rod infections. The increased use of mechanical equipment for the care of high-risk neonates has certainly been a factor in the upsurge of these infections. Epidemics caused by organisms such as *Pseudomonas aeruginosa*, *Serratia marcescens*, *Klebsiella*, *Aerobacter*, *Proteus*, *Achromobacter*, *Flavobacterium*, and *Alcaligenes faecalis* have been traced to a variety of unsuspected sources in the environment. Most of these organisms proliferate and thrive in water alone, and for this reason Wheeler has aptly dubbed them "water bugs." Epidemics of septicemia, meningitis, pneumonia, and conjunctivitis due to these organisms have arisen from one or more of the following sources:

Suction machines
Face masks
Resuscitation apparatus
Humidifying systems in incubators
Plastic sleeves on incubator portholes
Aerators on sink faucets
Dripping sink taps
Submerged water supply inlets in sinks
Cross connections between water inlets and waste lines
Dirty soap dispensers and soap trays
Bathing pans
Solutions used for eye irrigation
Benzalkonium (Zephiran) and other solutions used for cold sterilization

The early studies of skin and oropharyngeal colonization usually demonstrated a predominance of *S. epidermidis*. These organisms had been considered "nonpathogenic." So firmly entrenched was the concept of their innocuousness, they were considered to be markers of contaminated blood cultures. Year after year, recurrent studies have demonstrated that *S. epidermidis* is the most ubiquitous organism in the environment. Since the inception of intensive neonatal care, and even for a number of years antecedent, antibiotics were given to virtually all infants thought to be ill from any cause, whether infectious or not. At that time, *S. epidermidis* was sensitive to multiple antibiotics; it was a "benign" organism. In recent years, however, it has become resistant to virtually every available antibiotic. Infections, both deep and superficial, previously characteristic of *S. aureus*, are now also caused by *S. epidermidis*. In the past, it was a gift of nature that this ubiquitous organism rarely caused disease, but now the situation is altered. Probably as a result of years of widespread overuse of antibiotics in intensive care nurseries, coagulase-negative staphylococci now resist most antimicrobial agents.

The lesson from the experience in recent years is clear—vigilance in maintaining cleanliness of the physical environment is indispensable to the survival of all neonates.

Viral and protozoan infections

Fetal viral disease and toxoplasmosis are transmitted from the mother across the placenta. The only known exceptions are herpesvirus and cytomegalovirus infections, which are often acquired by the ascending route. Cytomegalovirus is also acquired transplacentally. The viruses listed in Table 13-1 have a presumed or proved capacity to permeate the placenta and enter the fetal bloodstream. Fetal infections may occur at any time during pregnancy. Rubella begins during the first trimester, occasionally slightly later. Cytomegalovirus infection may begin at any time during pregnancy, and in most cases herpesvirus disease is acquired in the third trimester.

Host defenses: the immune response

The mechanisms that comprise the host defenses against invasion by infectious agents are multiple and interdependent. The factors involved are regarded as nonspecific and specific. The former essentially include surface protection afforded by skin and mucous membranes, activity of phagocytic cells, and the inflammatory response. These factors are protective; they are not immune responses. Immune responses are reactions to specific antigens. The two types are called *cell-mediated immunity* and *antibody-mediated immunity*. Cell-mediated immunity is derived from a population of T lymphocytes that exist in several forms, each having a different function. Antibody-mediated immunity is derived from B lymphocytes, which give rise to plasma cells that secrete circulating antibodies.

Cell-mediated immunity. The T and B lymphocytes have a common origin. They originate from stem cells in embryonic mesenchyme, and they subsequently appear in the embryonic yolk sac. Further development involves migration to the fetal liver, and later to the bone marrow, where they remain throughout life. T lymphocytes, unlike B lymphocytes, are transferred from the fetal liver to the thymus. In the thymus, T cells differentiate into their respective functional types. At approximately 30 weeks of gestation, T lymphocytes circulate in the blood in numbers characteristic of the adult.

T cells mobilize at sites of specific antigenicity, and they then elaborate substances to recruit other cells (macrophages, neutrophils, other lymphocytes) to these sites of activity. They can react to specific antigens, but only after initial sensitization. That is, they must have been previously exposed to an antigen to which they will thereafter react. Clustering of T cells at the site of an antigen, and the aggregation of other cells attracted to that site, are responsible for the familiar reaction to a tuberculin (PPD) skin test. This and other intradermal reactions are examples of cell-mediated immunity. The positive tuberculin reaction occurs in individuals who have been previously exposed to the tubercule bacillus or to BCG vaccine. This is delayed hypersensitivity; it develops several days after intradermal injection of antigen.

Sensitized T lymphocytes are antigenically stimulated to divide and increase their population at the site of reaction. They then elaborate substances that recruit other cells to that site. The result is a local inflammatory reaction stimulated by a specific antigen. The term *cell-mediated immunity* thus refers to the pivotal function of T cells in this process.

T cells also play an indirect role in the elaboration of circulating antibodies (immunoglobulins). In this instance they stimulate activity of helper B lymphocytes which proceed to form plasma cells.

Antibody-mediated immunity; the immunoglobulins. Circulating antibodies are secreted by plasma cells, which are derived from B lymphocytes. The B lymphocyte ancestry is traced to the same stem cell from which the T lymphocyte arises. The differentiation of B cells into plasma cells occurs in the bone marrow and lymphoid tissue (lymph nodes, spleen) after the B cell has matured in the fetal liver. At 15 gestational weeks B lymphocytes circulate in the fetus in numbers that approximate those of the adult. B cells differentiate into plasma cells in the presence of both antigen and a type of T lymphocyte called the *helper cell*. It is the primary function of helper B cells to develop into plasma cells when antigenically stimulated so that specific antibody can then be elaborated. Specific antibodies exist within the several classes of immunoglobulins that are secreted by plasma cells. An antibody is a protein produced by plasma cells in response to stimulation by an antigen; an antigen is a substance of any kind that stimulates production of antibodies. Humoral antibodies circulate in plasma; they comprise the immunoglobulins. The three principal classes of immunoglobulins are IgG, IgM, and IgA. An important subclass of IgA is known as *secretory IgA*.

IgG. The IgG fraction contains antibodies to the majority of bacterial and viral organisms previously encountered by the mother. Of the three major immunoglobulins, only IgG crosses the placenta from the maternal to the fetal circulation. Maternally derived IgG first appears in the fetus during the third gestational month, accumulating progressively thereafter. Placental transfer is markedly increased during the last trimester. Length of gestation is thus a significant determinant of the IgG level at birth, which is lower in premature infants than in term infants. At 32 weeks, for example, a premature infant's cord blood contains only 400 mg/dl of IgG. In term infants the IgG concentration is at least equal to maternal levels, approximately 1000 mg/dl. Since most of the mother's circulating antibodies to bacterial and viral agents are in the IgG fraction, the fetus receives an ample supply of them from her. These antibodies are, in effect, an imprint of her own lifetime experience with infections. The uninfected neonate has virtually no other IgG at birth.

After birth, maternal IgG antibodies are catabolized, with resultant depletion over the first 3 months of life. The infant's synthesis of IgG increases gradually during the same period, and at approximately 3 months of age it is sufficient to supplant the loss of maternal IgG. The premature infant's IgG level reaches its lowest point much sooner because there was a low concentration at birth. There is thus a longer period of lower IgG levels until such time as the infant can generate significant amounts of the immunoglobulin. The fact that levels of protection are lower over a longer period may be a significant cause of the premature infant's greater susceptibility to infections and the high incidence of rehospitalization they require during the early months of the first year. Total IgG concentration in term babies thus falls from about 1000 mg/dl at birth to 400 mg/dl at 3 months, at which time a gradual increase begins as a result of the infant's accelerated synthesis. The mother's protection against infection is thus bestowed on her baby, and these protective effects are extended well beyond intrauterine life. IgG contains specific antibodies against most of the common infectious agents, including gram-positive cocci (*Pneumococcus*, *Streptococcus*), *Meningococcus*, and *Haemophilus influenzae*, the viruses, and the toxins of diphtheria and tetanus bacilli. This extended protection may explain partially, at least, the low incidence of these infections during the neonatal period, since most mothers possess antibodies to them. It should be noted in this connection that IgG does not contain antibodies against the enteric gram-negative rods; thus the infant is not protected against these infections by maternal antibody.

IgM. The fetus can produce significant amounts of IgM at about the thirtieth gestational week. Since IgM does not cross the placenta, concentrations detected in the neonate clearly represent his own synthesis of it. At birth the normal serum IgM concentration is below 20 mg/dl. Normal adult levels are 75 to 150 mg/dl. Intrauterine infections of all sorts may produce an immunologic response in the fetus that often results in higher levels. Measurement of IgM has therefore been used to establish the presence of infection. However, IgM determinations are nonspecific indi-

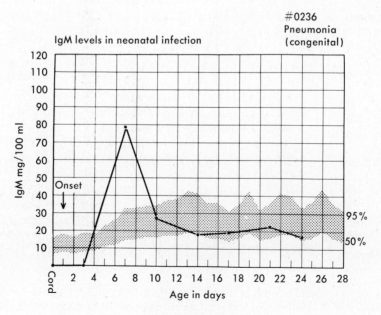

Fig. 13-1. See text.

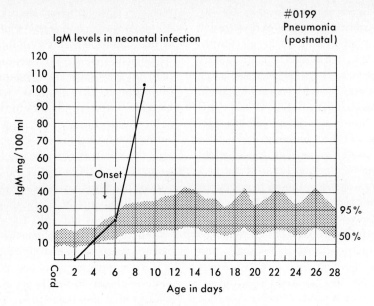

Fig. 13-2. See text.

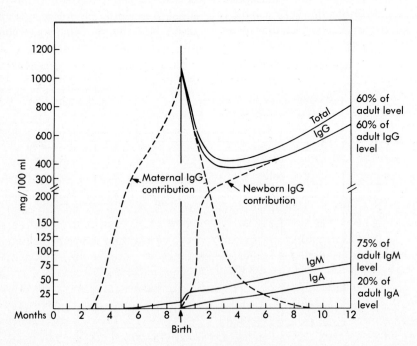

Fig. 13-3. Immunoglobulin levels in the fetus and the infant through the first postnatal year. (From Miller, M. J.: Immunology and resistance to infection. In Remington, J. S., and Klein, J. O.: Infectious disease of the fetus and newborn infant, ed. 2, Philadelphia, 1983, W. B. Saunders Co.

cators; they are no more specific for a particular type of infection than the erythrocyte sedimentation rate in older individuals. Identification of infection by elevated IgM levels is also limited by the time of appearance of such elevations as related to the onset of clinical disease. Elevations of IgM are not usually demonstrable for 5 to 10 days following the appearance of clinical disease. Our IgM determinations are performed twice weekly for at least 2 weeks following the onset of suspected infection. If within that interval IgM has not risen, we consider that an infectious process was unlikely. The onset time of clinical disease and the time of IgM elevation in a baby with congenital pneumonia is illustrated in Fig. 13-1. Abnormal signs were identified on the day of birth, yet an elevation was not evident until the fourth day of life. The stippled area represents the limits of normal IgM levels. In Fig. 13-2 a baby with postnatally acquired pneumonia became ill on the fifth day of life, yet an IgM level a day later was still normal. However, another determination on the ninth day was considerably above normal. Thus, although IgM determinations are useful for confirmation of suspected infection, *they are useless as a primary screening procedure for the early identification of bacterial infection because the appearance of elevations is so delayed*. In the mother, IgM contains antibodies against gram-negative bacteria and a scattered variety of other antigens. In the neonate, IgM production is stimulated during the initial immunologic response to virtually all infectious agents. Regardless of an infant's gestational age at birth, IgM synthesis is significant by the end of the first week of extrauterine life. IgM is the principal immunoglobulin elaborated during the early months of life. Its levels increase rapidly during the first month, more gradually thereafter. At 6 months of age a level that approximates half that of the adult's is attained; at 1 year the infant's level is 80% of the adult's (Fig. 13-3).

IgA. IgA does not cross the placenta and is not detectable in most normal infants at birth. The fetus and neonate are slower to generate IgA than

IgM, and it is thus found less regularly in serum of infected infants at birth. Normal adult levels are 200 to 400 mg/dl. IgA is also found over surfaces of intestinal and respiratory mucosa, as well as over renal epithelial surfaces in a form called "secretory IgA." The *secretory IgA* fragment is an addition to the IgA molecule. This fragment, called the secretory component, is generated by the epithelium, upon which the secretory IgA molecule ultimately resides. At these sites it is notably active as an antibody because, unlike circulating IgA, secretory IgA resists enzymatic and pH sources of destruction. The role of secretory IgA in the intestine is best known. It is present in breast milk in significant concentrations, and since it resists enzymatic digestion, it provides protection to intestinal mucosa. Thus oral polio vaccine depends for its effectiveness on multiplication of the attenuated virus in the intestinal tract. The vaccine virus fails to immunize infants on breast milk that contains a significant quantity of maternal antibody to poliovirus because the antibody inactivates vaccine virus multiplication in the gut. Secretory IgA in breast milk protects the neonate against several intestinal infections. The neonate begins to generate secretory IgA in the intestinal mucosa approximately 4 weeks after birth.

Neonatal handicaps in specific immunity. Most neonates, particularly those born at term, escape infections. At term an infant can reasonably manage minor microbial onslaughts. Passage through flora in the birth canal is not followed by infection unless the flora are sufficiently numerous to constitute a large inoculum. If the neonate is managed with aseptic nursery technique, postnatal inocula are not a problem. Maternal antibodies transferred across the placenta usually afford protection against a variety of bacterial and viral agents, but protection from gram-negative bacteria is not effective because maternal antibodies to them are in the IgM fraction, which does not cross the placenta to the fetus. Besides the transplacental IgG antibodies, a supply of antibodies is derived from secretory IgA in breast milk.

Although these protective factors are effective for most neonates, there are several handicaps in the immune system that are. The elaboration of antibodies by plasma cells, and the activity of T cells depend on initial sensitizing contact with antigen, but normally the fetus is not exposed to antigens. Initial sensitization must then await postnatal contact with antigen. A diminished capacity to respond immediately to some antigens is a distinct handicap. Thus children below 18 months of age are incapable of a vigorous response to antigenic polysaccharides in *Pneumococcus* and *Haemophilus* bacteria. The development of immunocompetence to specific antigens thus must occur over a varying period of time beyond the neonatal period. Still another handicap is the distribution of T cell types. There are larger numbers of *suppressor T cells* relative to *helper T cells* in the neonate, and there is therefore diminished conversion of B cells to plasma cells. Both delayed epidermal hypersensitivity and inflammation are also suppressed in neonates. Immune deficiencies in the term infant are exaggerated in the preterm infant, especially below 32 gestational weeks.

SPECIFIC BACTERIAL INFECTIONS
Pneumonia

Pneumonia is the most common of the serious neonatal infections. It has been cited as a cause of death in 10% to 20% of autopsies. Its peak incidence occurs during the second and third days of life. Pneumonia may be acquired in utero (congenital pneumonia) or from the nursery environment.

Congenital pneumonia is often, but not always, associated with obstetric abnormalities such as early rupture of membranes, prolonged duration of labor, maternal infection, and uncomplicated premature delivery. The bacteria most frequently involved are *E. coli* and other enteric organisms and group B streptococci. Symptoms are evident at birth or within 48 hours thereafter. When affected infants are in distress at birth, they are flaccid, pale, or cyanotic. Resuscitation is often necessary. Once respirations are established, they

are rapid and shallow. Slight retractions may be present, but they may not be as striking as those of hyaline membrane disease. If the infection is severe, repeated apneic episodes occur. Crepitant rales are sometimes audible. Temperature elevation is more likely in full-sized infants. Premature infants often have subnormal body temperature.

Postnatally acquired pneumonia is generally caused by *Pseudomonas aeruginosa*, penicillin-resistant staphylococci, and enteric organisms. Clinical signs usually appear after 48 hours of life. A substantial number of infants are hypoxic at birth for reasons unrelated to infection. The most common presenting signs are rapid respiration, poor feeding, or aspiration during feeding. Vomiting and aspiration sometimes occur during feeding because previously unsuspected pneumonia is already present. The chest film in such instances reveals densities that cannot be attributed with certainty to effects of aspirated formula or to preexisting pneumonia. Recovery from postnatal pneumonia is more frequent than from congenital pneumonia.

Antibiotic therapy for pneumonia and other bacterial infections is discussed on p. 381.

Septicemia

Septicemia is a generalized infection characterized by the proliferation of bacteria in the bloodstream. The incidence of septicemia has not diminished since the introduction of antibiotics, but the etiologic agents have changed and survival has increased. Before the antibiotic era, group A streptococci were predominant. Currently, coliform organisms and group B streptococci are the most frequent etiologic agents.

S. epidermidis is fast becoming the most common etiologic agent in neonatal septicemia. During the first 9 months of 1984 in one neonatal intensive care unit (NICU), the organism was involved in 42% of 33 cases of neonatal septicemia. In the meantime, the incidence of group B streptococci septicemia seems to be declining in many nurseries. In New York, *S. epidermidis* is reported as the most frequent cause of bacteremia during a 17-month period in 1981-1982. Among the 23 episodes of septicemia, 10 were associated with colonized vascular catheters, and 4 occurred in infants with necrotizing enterocolitis. Most of the strains of *S. epidermidis* were resistant to all antibiotics except vancomycin.

Since the introduction of antibiotics for the treatment of septicemia, mortality has decreased remarkably from over 90% to a range of 17% to 45%, depending on the reporting investigator. Premature infants are most commonly involved; males are affected twice as often as females. The incidence of neonatal septicemia varies from one institution to another. Bacterial infections of all sorts have been observed in 25% of admissions to a neonatal intensive care unit. Superficial infection was involved in 40% of the total. Septicemia was documented in 14%. Another facility has noted a 16.9% incidence of all bacterial infections. In England, 13.8% of infants admitted to intensive care had major infections. The older literature describes incidence of infection before the advent of neonatal intensive care. The incidence of septicemia must necessarily increase as smaller infants are maintained for longer periods of time, and as invasive procedures are performed more frequently.

The early symptoms are vague and nonspecific. One expects chills, fever, and prostration in older infants, but the neonate may merely lose vigor, refuse feedings, or lose weight. The nurse may simply note that he is "doing poorly." Other abnormal signs are less subtle and as wide ranging as the bloodstream itself. Vomiting and diarrhea occur in approximately 30% of patients. Abdominal distention may be prominent. Abnormal respiration (apnea, tachypnea, and cyanosis) occurs in 20% to 30% of affected infants. Jaundice is a frequent finding. Hyperbilirubinemia may involve a high concentration of conjugated (direct) bilirubin, mostly in infants over 1 week of age. Hypoglycemia is not uncommon, being associated with gram-negative rod infection almost exclusively. It responds to increased concentrations of

intravenous glucose, as described on p. 344. We have found that *hyperglycemia* is at least as frequently associated with septicemia as hypoglycemia. In sick babies who are not receiving excessive quantities of intravenous glucose, hyperglycemia has been a surprisingly strong indication of bacterial infection—usually septicemia. A wide variety of skin lesions occur. Pustules, furuncles, and subcutaneous abscesses are most often associated with streptococcal and staphylococcal infections, and less often with *E. coli* and *P. aeruginosa*. The latter organism also produces localized purplish cellulitis that breaks down into a black, gangrenous ulcer. Petechiae and ecchymoses are not common.

Meningitis occurs in a third of septicemic infants, although clinical signs are evident in only half the infants with this complication. The symptoms include convulsions, altered state of consciousness, irritability, spasticity, and fullness of the anterior fontanelle (see later).

The diagnosis of septicemia can be unequivocally documented only by recovery of organisms from blood culture, which requires at least 24 hours for growth. Since organisms are also present in the spinal fluid, lumbar taps are essential components of the diagnostic approach. By applying Gram's stain to centrifuged spinal fluid, the morphologic identify of the bacteria may be established, thus affording a rational basis for immediate choice of antibiotics. Cultures of blood and spinal fluid must be taken before treatment is begun. If there is nothing to suggest the identity of the offending organism, kanamycin (Kantrex) or gentamicin (Garamycin) plus ampicillin are given immediately.

The total leukocyte count alone is of little value in assessing the likelihood of bacterial infection. Instead, three other characteristics of the white blood cells are important: (1) the total *neutrophil* count, (2) the percent of the total neutrophils that are immature forms (bands), and (3) the presence of toxic granulations in neutrophils. Among infants with documented bacterial infections in one study, at least one of these three factors was abnormal. Furthermore, if all three were normal, the presence of bacterial disease was very unlikely. In the first week of life, neutropenia is primarily caused by septicemia (or other bacterial disease). It is also associated with maternal hypertension, severe asphyxia, and periventricular hemorrhage even in babies who are not infected. In the absence of the latter disorders, septicemia is a very likely diagnosis in the presence of a low total neutrophil count. By 72 hours, the minimum total neutrophil count is 1750/mm³. Less than that number is highly suggestive of infection in the absence of the other associated disorders mentioned above. Furthermore, infection is probable when the *percent of bands to total neutrophils* exceeds 16% during the first 24 hours and approximately 12% thereafter. The sensitivity of these neutrophil indices has since been confirmed in other studies. Thrombocytopenia (platelet count less than 150,000 mm³) with or without associated evidence of disseminated intravascular coagulation (p. 311) is a common hematologic abnormality. IgM (p. 370) determination often reveals elevated levels (over 20 mg/dl in the first week of life). Usually the elevation is not evident for 3 to 7 days after onset of symptoms. High IgM levels generally confirm a diagnosis of bacterial infection days after the decision to treat with antibiotics has been made.

Once symptoms of illness are evident in a neonate, it becomes a matter of urgency to determine the need for antibiotic therapy. One is faced with the necessity of demonstrating the likelihood of bacterial infection or, alternatively, to simply administer antibiotics to any infant who appears to be ill. The latter alternative is practiced in many estimable neonatal intensive care units.

Several laboratory tests bid well to reliably select infants likely to be infected, thus sparing the uninfected ones needless therapy. There are dangerous disadvantages in the widespread use of antibiotics, and these have been described repeatedly since their introduction. The most sinister aftermath of indiscriminate use is the emergence of resistant strains. This phenomenon has been noted recurrently, and it is apparently achieving new prominence with the emergence of coagulase-negative staphylococci as pathogens that have become resistant to virtually all antimicrobial drugs.

A large number of tests have been investigated in an attempt to identify septicemia as early as possible. These have included serum IgM, which is useless for early identification because of its delayed elaboration. It has also included C-reactive protein (CRP), which appears to be a promising procedure. A number of studies have demonstrated that the vast majority of infants with documented septicemia (blood cultures were positive) have significantly elevated CRP concentrations. Furthermore, successful treatment seems to be indicated by a decline of CRP concentration. Serial quantitative determinations of CRP are thus preferred. In several recent reports the presence of organisms detected by Gram stain of tracheal secretions seems to correlate with the pneumonia and perhaps septicemia. Gram stain of tracheal secretions is still an unproved predictive procedure, however. The examination of a buffy coat smear using acridine orange stain holds considerable promise for rapid identification of septicemia. The procedure is simple; a fluorescent microscope is essential. Failure to identify bacteria in the buffy coat by this method is not sufficient to exclude the possibility of septicemia. A commercially available latex agglutination assay is helpful for the rapid diagnosis of group B streptococcal infection. The test is most accurate when used for cerebrospinal fluid and urine. It is most widely used in urine.

The treatment of septicemia is complex because of the pathophysiology associated with widespread infection and because antibiotic therapy is often unsuccessful. The use of appropriate antibiotics is traditional and fundamental. Those that are commonly used in the neonate for bacterial infections are listed in Table 13-2. While efforts to eliminate the offending organism depend on antibiotics, supportive treatment seeks to prevent or alleviate shock, metabolic acidosis, and renal shutdown. Therapeutic efforts have also attempted to bolster the neonate's deficient host defense mechanism. In past years, gamma globulin has been administered to provide circulating antibodies, but to little avail. Recently human immune gamma globulin has been tried, but the results are at best equivocal. Recently, reports have indicated impressive success with irradiated granulocyte transfusions. The procedure entails administration of neutrophils that have been separated from adult donor blood by a special process in the blood bank. There is sound rationale to the procedure because the phagocytizing capacity of the neonate's neutrophil is significantly diminished compared to the adult. Furthermore, neutropenia in the presence of depleted neutrophilic reserves in bone marrow and spleen are frequent occurrences in septicemic infants. Several controlled studies report survival rates up to 100%. The sequestration of neutrophils from donor blood is a demanding process that is not yet widely available. However, the use of *fresh blood* in a double-volume exchange transfusion may accomplish the same end. As many as 15 granulocyte transfusions have been administered to a single patient; an equal number of exchange transfusions would be cumbersome and somewhat hazardous.

Meningitis

Almost half of all cases of meningitis in children occur during the first year of life, and the incidence is highest during the neonatal period. It is considerably more frequent in premature than in term infants and in males rather than in females. The causative organisms and the obstetric complications associated with meningitis are the same as those cited for septicemia.

Systemic symptoms cannot be differentiated from those of septicemia. Fullness of the anterior fontanelle is the most specific sign of meningitis. Stiffness of the neck, which is so frequent in older infants and children, is rare in the neonate. Opisthotonos occurs in one fourth of the infected infants; coma and convulsions occur in half of them.

The diagnosis must be confirmed by spinal fluid abnormalities and isolation of the organism from a cultured specimen. White cell content of spinal fluid may vary from 20 to several thousand per cubic millimeter. Polymorphonuclear leukocytes predominate. If the infection is caused by *Listeria monocytogenes*, mononuclear cells are in the majority. Sugar content is usually low, and protein is elevated. Organisms are evident on Gram-stained smears of centrifuged spinal fluid. Blood cultures yield the etiologic agent in 75% of cases. Fatality rates vary from approximately 35% to 60%, and in approximately 30% to 35% of the survivors, central nervous system handicaps persist. In only 5% have these CNS handicaps required custodial care.

Treatment of meningitis utilizes the same antibiotics as that for septicemia. Therapy should continue for 2 weeks after the first sterile spinal fluid is obtained. The addition of intrathecal gentamicin by lumbar puncture to systemic administration was shown to be no more effective than systemic therapy alone. There was no less mortality or residual central nervous system abnormality among survivors.

Group B streptococcal disease

Special mention is made of group B streptococcal infection because of its startling increase in frequency during the last decade. The major diseases it produces are septicemia, meningitis, and pneumonia, but otitis media and conjunctivitis also occur.

Group B streptococcus was previously believed to be significant only as a cause of mastitis of cattle. It behaves in humans, however, very much like the more familiar *Listeria monocytogenes*. Both organisms can be recovered from the cervices of asymptomatic pregnant women, and both are sometimes recovered from the urethras of asymptomatic male partners of such women. Maternal colonization during pregnancy may result in spontaneous abortion, severe neonatal septicemia, or a normal baby.

Two clearly defined syndromes occur, depending on their time of onset. The early-onset disease (so-called septicemic form), in which meningitis can nevertheless occur, is seen in the first few days after delivery. It is apparently acquired by the ascending route in utero or by contact with infected tissue during birth. It often progresses rapidly and relentlessly to cause death in 1 or 2 days. The lungs are heavily involved, and septicemia is almost the rule. In most instances meningitis is absent. The most frequent symptoms are respiratory distress, coma, shock, and jaundice. The organism can be cultured from any number of sites, including the nasopharynx, skin, external ear canal, meconium, and blood. Mortality ranges from 25% to 100%. The late-onset, or meningitic, form occurs several days to 3 months after discharge from the nursery. It almost invariably involves the meninges; its onset is not as abrupt as the early form, and its prognosis for survival is better. Mortality is approximately 20%.

From 4% to 6% of asymptomatic pregnant women have cervical cultures positive for group B streptococci. Cultures of the vulva and vagina have been positive more frequently, with up to 14% of vaginal cultures having been reported as positive. About 1% to 2% of all neonates are colonized with the organism, but colonization does not necessarily lead to disease. Approximately one in ten colonized babies becomes diseased. The organisms recovered from babies are usually identical to those grown from their mothers.

Group B infection departs from the usual pattern of perinatal infections in two ways: maternal complications are not necessarily increased (although in some uncontrolled series complications were said to be increased), and the term infant may be as vulnerable as the premature infant. In fact, in some series the incidence of the disease was higher in the term infants.

The organism is sensitive to penicillin and ampicillin. Group B disease has thus not been a problem in which the appropriate drug is not available. Most authors agree that the early form is an example of vertical transmission (mother to baby). The epidemiology of the late form is not yet clar-

ified, but there are data suggestive of the role of nursery personnel in transmission of the late variety of the disease. Mother-to-infant transmission may also play a role, or the colonized infant may leave the hospital in health only to become ill later. This phenomenon is common in staphylococcal disease.

Diarrhea

Several bacterial agents can produce primary diarrhea. The most important is *enterotoxigenic* or *enteropathogenic E. coli* (EEC). *Salmonella*, *Shigella*, and staphylococci are infrequent causes. Serologic techniques have identified 140 groups of *E. coli;* somewhat over a dozen have been implicated in nursery epidemics of diarrhea.

Regardless of etiology, the early signs of infection consist of refusal to feed, weight loss, and hypoactivity. These may precede the diarrhea itself by a day or two. Blood and pus in the stool are rare, except in shigellosis, which itself is rare. As diarrhea continues, the infant becomes toxic, dehydrated, and acidotic (metabolic acidosis). These signs may appear abruptly during the early phase of explosive diarrhea. Dehydration is even more rapid if vomiting is also present. An ashen gray color, or pallor, is indicative of vasomotor collapse and impending death. Rapid correction of metabolic acidosis and dehydration is therefore crucial. Milder forms of the disease are not unusual, being characterized by protracted diarrhea with fewer stools and a refusal to feed.

Institutional outbreaks are almost inevitable if an infected infant is in the nursery. The disease spreads from one bassinet to the next. Feces of infected babies contain an enormous quantity of organisms, and contamination occurs easily, mostly from unwashed hands of personnel and from gowns. Enteropathogenic *E. coli* has been cultured from the nasopharynx, thus suggesting that airborne spread occurs in some instances.

Diarrheal stools must be cultured as soon as they are evident. Most often a bacterial agent is not causative, and the microbiology laboratory will report that no pathogens are identifiable.

When viral cultures are performed, they, too, are often negative. Enteropathogenic *E. coli* may cause explosive epidemics. For this reason oral neomycin or polymyxin, which constitutes effective therapy, is administered even before the results of cultures are returned. If these are positive, the infant should be removed from the nursery, and all other babies should be cultured and treated with the same antibiotics. An indication that diarrhea is of bacterial etiology may be gained from a smear of stool for polymorphonuclear leukocytes (pus cells). If the diarrhea is of bacterial etiology, pus cells are usually demonstrable. These cells are not present if diarrhea is caused by a virus or by any other agent.

Urinary tract infection

Neonatal urinary tract infections have been observed to occur as frequently as septicemia. For unknown reasons, renal infection in the neonate has received relatively scant attention. It is far more common in males than in females, the reverse of sex distribution in later childhood. Furthermore, its occurrence in a male does not strongly suggest underlying anomaly, as it does in older children.

Suspicion of infection should be aroused if more than 10% of body weight is lost during the first 5 days in an infant who is not especially ill. Fever is not unusual, particularly if the onset of symptoms is later than 5 days. A significant number of babies appear gray or cyanotic; abdominal distention and jaundice occur in relatively few. During the second week of life, however, jaundice with a high level of direct bilirubin is commonly associated with renal infection, almost always in males. Convulsions, in the absence of meningitis, occur in a small number of infants.

The organisms are gram-negative enteric rods with few exceptions. Blood cultures may be positive in up to 30% of affected babies. Two consecutive urine cultures, obtained by suprapubic aspiration, are diagnostic. Treatment is effective with appropriate antibiotics. Death occurs from complications of septicemia such as meningitis.

Sometimes clinical symptoms, bacteriuria, and pyuria all disappear spontaneously, before treatment is begun.

Conjunctivitis

Infection of the conjunctivae may be acquired during birth or from the nursery environment. Bacterial conjunctivitis is usually due to *Staphylococcus*, *P. aeruginosa*, and enteric organisms. Clinical signs include swelling and redness of the conjunctiva, with varying amounts of purulent exudate. In its mildest form, conjunctivitis causes "sticky eyes," with little or no swelling.

Gonorrheal infection causes the most serious form of conjunctivitis. It is acquired during delivery by direct contact with infected maternal tissue. Initial symptoms are noted between the second and fifth days of life, sometimes later. Severe conjunctival redness, swelling of the eyelids, and copious pus are typically evident. Untreated, the infection may spread to the eyes, causing panophthalmitis and extensive destruction of ocular tissue. It also causes severe arthritis. Rapid diagnosis is possible from a Gram-stained smear of exudate from the eye, which reveals gram-negative cocci within pus cells.

Gonorrheal infection is treated with intramuscular penicillin. Conjunctivitis caused by other organisms is effectively controlled by local instillation of an eye ointment containing polymyxin, bacitracin, and neomycin.

Omphalitis

Severe infection of the umbilical stump causes edema, redness, and purulent exudate in the region of the umbilicus. In milder infections there is no visible exudate, but redness and induration of the periumbilical skin are evident. Extension of erythema upward from the umbilicus is particularly significant. Slight periumbilical erythema without induration is not pathologic. Inflammation of the umbilical stump may herald septicemia. Culture of the blood and the umbilicus is indicated, and treatment for septicemia should be started immediately.

Necrotizing enterocolitis (NEC)

Bacterial infection plays a prominent role in the pathogenesis of necrotizing enterocolitis, but there is no real evidence that it initiates the disease process. The disorder involves segmental or diffuse necrosis of the small or large intestine. An isolated patch of bowel wall may be involved in the mildest form of the disease; the most severe form involves the entire length of intestine from the stomach through the large bowel. Necrosis may superficially involve mucosa and submucosa, or in the extreme it may extend through the entire thickness of the intestinal wall. Perforation of the gut is not uncommon; it invariably leads to peritonitis that may or may not be grossly purulent.

Necrotizing enterocolitis occurs in 1% to 3% of infants admitted to intensive care units. It has been estimated that 3500 to 5000 babies are affected in the United States annually. Reported mortality has ranged from less than 10% to 55%.

The smaller the baby, the more likely is the occurrence of necrotizing enterocolitis. Thus overall incidence statistics, based on live births or numbers of admissions to intensive care units, may be misleading. Among the smallest babies (1.0 to 1.49 kg) the incidence is fifty-fold greater than in term infants (over 2.5 kg). The majority of affected infants are preterm; a preponderance of infants are less than 33 weeks of gestational age and below 1500 g at birth.

Associated clinical factors, often referred to as risk factors, are numerous. They have thus far defied interpretation for purposes of establishing etiologic factors. Etiologic factors have not been identified because there are a number of circumstances that influence appearance of the disease. Virtually every hazard of prematurity and intensive care has been cited as a possible precipitating cause of the disease process. There is, however, pervasive agreement that the process begins with diminished perfusion of the gut wall. Ischemia and hypoxia of intestine leads to necrosis and gangrene in the extreme. Invasion of susceptible tissue by a variety of microorganisms is probably secondary to the initial diminution of microcirculatory perfusion.

Necrotizing enterocolitis is known to occur in clusters of infants over relatively short periods of time. The pattern of incidence, the season, and the disease-free interval are variable in different institutions. The pattern is suggestive of a primary infectious disease; and the clustered incidence may indicate an epidemic. The organisms implicated have been numerous. They are known to occur in normal intestinal flora of unaffected infants. Successful control of apparent outbreaks following stringent isolation techniques has been reported, but this may be mere happenstance. Controlled studies are not available. The disease appears sporadically; it is known to come and go spontaneously.

NEC becomes apparent in most infants during the first 5 to 10 days of life. The onset occurs after feedings are begun. Only a few affected infants have been unfed. Necrotizing enterocolitis appears as late as 6 weeks of age, but this is uncommon. As a rule, onset is earlier in the larger babies.

The disease usually begins while infants are fed by nasogastric tube. The earliest signs include inordinate quantities of gastric formula retention, which is sometimes bile-stained. Bile-stained gastric contents are generally associated with serious disease. Soon thereafter, abdominal distention becomes obvious. Vomiting occurs in a minority of instances. The disease is unique in that affected infants are often in obvious pain. Furthermore, those who seem comfortable at rest react to the severe discomfort caused by palpation of the abdomen. Stools may be grossly or microscopically bloody; they are usually free of blood. Diarrhea is not characteristic.

In some infants the onset is abruptly stormy. Recurrent apnea is a frequent presenting sign. Respiratory distress, requiring supplemental oxygen or mechanical ventilatory support, is not uncommon. In the extreme the baby is in shock soon after onset appearance of abnormal signs. Profoundly affected infants are pale because of poor perfusion; they are flaccid and immobile. In essence, they appear septic. In fact, blood cultures are positive in approximately 30% of these infants. A variety of organisms, usually gram-negative rods, are cultured from the blood.

Metabolic acidosis is the rule in very sick infants. An occasional baby is hyperglycemic early in the course of the disease. Hyperglycemia is most often associated with positive blood cultures. Routine examination of the blood may indicate no abnormalities, but leukopenia and neutropenia are frequent. Thrombocytopenia (less than 200,000 platelets) occurs in at least two thirds of affected infants. It is not unusual, in following platelet counts, to observe levels that fall below 50,000/mm³. In the most severe cases, disseminated intravascular coagulation is identified.

The clinical diagnosis is largely dependent on the radiologic appearance of the intestine. Perhaps the earliest sign of intestinal disease is segmental distention of the small bowel. This may occur in the absence of the cardinal x-ray sign of the disease, intestinal intramural air. Segmental or loop distention of the intestine is stage one of the disease. Intramural air is present in several characteristic contours. The radiolucency may be linear or roughly circular. In either case the radiolucency is seen as a thin line, often difficult to discern with certainty. The appearance of radiolucencies in the intestinal wall is stage two. Intestinal perforation occurs in a minority of infants, and it is readily identified by the presence of free air in the abdomen. This is stage three. Free air is seen in the peritoneal space, and it can be visualized most reliably on x-ray examination of the abdomen taken in the left lateral decubitus position.

Suspicion of necrotizing enterocolitis requires cessation of feedings. Blood cultures should be taken and antibiotics (gentamicin and ampicillin) administered. Other therapy is supportive. Respiratory distress and hypoxia require appropriate support. Metabolic acidosis, dehydration, and thrombocytopenia require specific remedial measures. We have been impressed with the pain that most infants experience. We usually administer meperidine (Demerol), which apparently makes the infant more comfortable.

ANTIMICROBIAL TREATMENT

The antibiotics of choice for neonatal infections are listed in Table 13-2. In most instances they must be chosen before results of cultures are available. It is thus essential that they be effective against most of the organisms likely to infect the neonate. Major consideration must be given to the bacterial infections acquired in utero and during birth; they are derived from normal maternal intestinal flora (coliforms, group B streptococci). Penicillin-resistant staphylococci and *P. aeruginosa* are more likely to be etiologic in postnatally acquired infections than in congenital ones. When onset of symptoms occurs after 48 to 72 hours, additional consideration must be given to these possibilities.

The overall effectiveness of some antibiotics has diminished through the years. About three decades ago streptomycin was highly active against coliform infections, but it ultimately lost its effectiveness and was replaced by kanamycin (Kantrex). Now the activity of kanamycin against *E. coli* has begun to decline significantly. In the years immediately following its introduction, kanamycin was active against 90% to 95% of *E. coli* strains; currently it eliminates approximately 60% or less in some hospitals. In the early phases of their use both streptomycin and kanamycin were also effective against staphylococci, and this effectiveness, too, was soon lost. Diminished activity of these drugs is related to their widespread use. At present, gentamicin is a satisfactory alternative to kanamycin. Gentamicin is also effective against *P. aeruginosa*, thus offering a decided advantage in the treatment of bacterial infection.

For over two decades penicillin has remained useful against most strains of staphylococci that are not hospital acquired, streptococci, syphilis,

Table 13-2. Antibiotics of choice (1986)

Antibiotics	Routes of administration	Dosages (mg/kg/day) and intervals of administration			
		Body weight < 2000 g		Body weight > 2000 g	
		Age 0-7 days	>7 days	Age 0-7 days	>7 days
Amikacin	IM, IV	15 div q12h	30 div q8h	20 div q12h	30 div q8h
Ampicillin,	IV, IM				
Meningitis		100 div q12h	150 div q8h	150 div q8h	200 div q6h
Other diseases		50 div q12h	75 div q8h	75 div q8h	100 div q6h
Cefazolin	IV, IM	40 div q12h	40 div q12h	40 div q12h	60 div q8h
Cefotaxime	IV, IM	100 div q12h	150 div q8h	100 div q12h	150 div q8h
Cephalothin	IV	40 div q12h	60 div q8h	60 div q8h	80 div q6h
Chloramphenicol	IV, PO	25 once daily	25 once daily	25 once daily	50 div q12h
Erythromycin	PO	20 div q12h	30 div q8h	20 div q12h	30-40 div q8h
Gentamicin	IM, IV	5 div q12h	7.5 div q8h	5 div q12h	7.5 div q8h
Kanamycin	IM, IV	15 div q12h	30 div q8h	20 div q12h	30 div q8h
Methicillin	IV, IM				
Meningitis		100 div q12h	150 div q8h	150 div q8h	200 div q6h
Other diseases		50 div q12h	75 div q8h	75 div q8h	100 div q6h
Mezlocillin	IV, IM	150 div q12h	225 div q8h	150 div q12h	225 div q8h
Moxalactam	IV, IM	100 div q12h	150 div q8h	100 div q8h	150 div q8h
Oxacillin	IV, IM	50 div q12h	100 div q8h	75 div q8h	150 div q6h
Nafcillin	IV	50 div q12h	75 div q8h	50 div q8h	75 div q6h
Penicillin G	IV				
Meningitis		100,000 U div q12h	150,000 U div q8h	150,000 U div q8h	200,000 U div q6h
Other diseases		50,000 U div q12h	75,000 U div q8h	50,000 U div q8h	100,000 U div q6h
Penicillin G	IM				
Benzathine		50,000 U (one dose)	50,000 U (one dose)	50,000 U (one dose)	50,000 U (one dose)
Procaine		50,000 U once daily	50,000 U once daily	50,000 U once daily	50,000 U once daily
Ticarcillin	IV, IM	150 div q12h	225 div q8h	225 div q8h	300 div q6h
Tobramycin	IM, IV	4 div q12h	6 div q8h	4 div q12h	6 div q8h
Vancomycin	IV	30 div q12h	45 div q8h	30 div q12h	45 div q8h

From McCracken, G. H., Jr., and Nelson, J. D.: Antimicrobial therapy for newborns, New York, 1983, Grune & Stratton. By permission.

Listeria monocytogenes, and gonorrheal organisms. However, ampicillin has largely replaced penicillin because it is active against the same organisms and a majority of *E. coli* strains as well. The staphylococci resistant to penicillin must be treated with nafcillin or a similar type of drug specifically active against penicillin-resistant strains.

Infections manifest during the first 48 hours are best treated with gentamicin plus ampicillin. Onset at a later age implies that hospital-acquired organisms may be etiologic. For these infections ticarcillin with gentamicin plus nafcillin may be used.

SPECIFIC VIRAL INFECTIONS

The viruses implicated in perinatal infections are listed in Table 13-1. They are transmitted across the placenta from mother to fetus, except for herpesvirus, which is usually acquired by the ascending route, and cytomegalovirus, which is sometimes acquired similarly. Maternal transmission may occur early in pregnancy, causing chronic intrauterine infections such as rubella or cytomegalovirus, or closer to delivery, causing postnatal onset of infections such as herpesvirus, Coxsackievirus, varicella, and smallpox. One of several consequences may befall the fetus or neonate as a result of maternal infection: (1) death may occur in utero or after birth as a result of fetal disease, (2) intrauterine death may follow severe maternal toxicity, (3) survival may occur despite infection but with congenital malformations or destruction of tissue (brain and liver), or often with no apparent aftermath, or (4) the virus may not be transmitted to the fetus.

The intrauterine infections of primary importance are rubella, cytomegalovirus infection, and herpesvirus infection.

Rubella

The congenital rubella syndrome is a chronic virus infection of the fetus and neonate that begins during the first trimester of pregnancy and usually persists for months after birth. The virus has been recovered from abortuses, placentas, and amniotic fluid. At autopsy it has been grown from virtually every organ of the body. In life it has been cultured from the throat, urine, meconium, conjunctival secretion, and spinal fluid, from surgically removed segments of the ductus arteriosus, from cataractous lenses, and from liver specimens. The majority of infants may harbor virus as long as 3 months. In some infants the virus persists for several months or years longer. Virus has been recovered from the lens of a 3-year-old child. Persistently infected infants may be a source of contagion; small epidemics among hospital personnel have been traced to them. Pregnant women are thus at risk when exposed to these infants.

Approximately 10% to 20% of gravid women are susceptible to rubella. Estimates of the risk of fetal disease after maternal infection have varied through the years from one epidemic to the next. In general, maternal infection during the first gestational month causes disease in 33% to 50% of exposed fetuses; during the second month 25% are affected, and during the third month 9% are affected. There is a distinct but smaller risk during the fourth month of pregnancy; 4% of exposed fetuses may be affected, primarily by lifelong hearing impairment.

Whether positive or negative, a history of infection is unreliable because at least half the infected older children and adults are asymptomatic. Furthermore, the clinical signs of rubella are difficult to interpret during nonepidemic periods, since they mimic several other virus infections. During the extensive epidemic of 1964, half the mothers of diseased infants were unaware of infection during pregnancy. Fetal disease is no less severe in the asymptomatic mother than in the symptomatic one.

The cardinal clinical signs are intrauterine growth retardation, congenital heart disease, and cataracts. The organs of growth-retarded infants are hypoplastic because rubella virus impairs the proliferative (mitotic) phase of growth (Chapter 5). Several types of cardiac malformation have been noted; the most common are patent ductus arteriosus and stenosis of the peripheral pulmonary arteries. Severe myocardial degeneration also occurs in a few infants. Cataracts may be bilateral or unilateral; they are usually present at birth, but occasionally they develop days or weeks later. Other eye abnormalities include microphthalmia, glaucoma, and a pigmented retinopathy. Thrombocytopenia and petechiae are present in 40% to 80% of infected neonates. Enlargement of the liver and spleen is common, and unconjugated hyperbilirubinemia, largely resulting from hemolysis, is also frequent. When hepatitis occurs, it further contributes to the retention of unconjugated bilirubin, but it also causes elevations of direct bilirubin as well (obstructive jaundice). Occasionally rubella hepatitis progresses to cirrhosis. Interstitial pneumonia is not uncommon, the virus having been recovered from affected lungs. Neurologic abnormalities are present in a minority of neonates; they usually appear later in infancy. Microcephaly, for instance, ordinarily develops after the newborn period. Spinal fluid abnormalities consist of elevated protein concentration and increased white cells, usually lymphocytes. In the neonate they are more frequent than clinical neurologic abnormalities.

The diagnosis of congenital rubella is strongly suggested by the combined presence of cataracts and congenital heart disease. Elevated IgM levels are usually detectable at birth. Serologic documentation is possible by demonstrating rubella antibody in serum IgM. Other serologic tests are not helpful because they measure maternal IgG antibody, which may be present as a result of an infection that preceded pregnancy by many years.

The immune status among nursery personnel of childbearing age should be determined at the onset of employment. If serologic tests indicate susceptibility, attenuated rubella virus vaccine should be administered. Infected infants are contagious; susceptible personnel who are exposed while unknowingly pregnant are at risk of having an infected fetus.

Cytomegalovirus (CMV) infection

The cytomegaloviruses are ubiquitous agents that cause infections in populations of all ages throughout the world. Perinatal infections are acquired transplacentally from asymptomatic mothers. In the presence of primary acute maternal infection, 50% of fetuses are affected. The acutely infected mother is more likely to transmit the disease early in pregnancy than later. Early gestational transmission also seems to be associated with greater severity of fetal disease. Beyond the neonatal period, acquired cytomegalovirus infections are usually asymptomatic; the excretion of virus in urine (viruria) is thus required for the identification of infected individuals. Maternal viruria at the time of delivery has been noted in 3% to 4% of apparently normal women. Positive cultures from the cervix at the time of delivery have been demonstrated in 4.5% of women in Pittsburgh and as many as 28% in Japan. Similar studies have identified viruria in 1% of randomly selected newborns, most of them apparently normal, in whom viruria often persists through the first year of life. Cytomegalovirus has been recovered from an abortus as early as the twelfth gestational week. The fate of apparently healthy viruric neonates has not been documented, but estimates of later central nervous system damage range from 10% to 25%. The only report of postnatal acquisition of the disease in the nursery concerns two premature infants who may have become infected from blood transfusions.

The results of congenital infection range from widespread tissue damage that is incompatible with life, to survival associated with extensive brain damage, and to complete absence of signs during the neonatal period. Diseased infants are often small-for-dates and hypoplastic. The principal target organs are the blood, brain, and liver, although virtually every organ of the body can be affected. Hemolysis causes anemia and unconjugated hyperbilirubinemia. Thrombocytopenia with petechiae and ecchymoses in the skin is frequent. Obstructive jaundice (direct hyperbilirubinemia) is a consequence of liver damage. Enlargement of the liver and spleen are common. Cytomegalovirus also produces encephalitis; the resultant clinical signs vary from lethargy and hypoactivity to convulsions. Microcephaly may be present at birth, or it may develop over the ensuing few months. Skull x-ray examinations may reveal calcification in the brain, which is also present in infants with toxoplasmosis. Chorioretinitis is discernible in 10% to 20% of symptomatic infants; this lesion, too, is similar to the eye findings in infants with toxoplasmosis. Pneumonia occurs occasionally.

The diagnosis is best established in babies with typical clinical signs by recovery of virus from urine. There is considerable diagnostic value in the demonstration of elevated IgM levels, but these are not specific for CMV. Specific identification of cytomegalovirus antibodies within the IgM fraction is the most accurate serologic method. Although several antiviral drugs have been utilized for treatment, their efficacy has not been clearly established.

Herpesvirus infection

Herpesvirus is classified into type 1 and type 2 varieties, each with distinctive serologic attributes and clinical implications. Type 1 causes the common, and often recurrent, lesions in the lips of older children and adults. It also produces gingivostomatitis and skin lesions above the waist. Type 2 causes the vast majority of lesions in the cervix, vagina, and external genitalia. Most neonatal infections are due to type 2 virus. The fetus acquires herpesvirus by the ascending route from infected genitalia or by direct contact with these tissues during the birth process. Neonatal herpesvirus is thus a venereal disease acquired by the infant in a manner similar to gonorrhea. Transplacental acquisition probably occurs, but it is apparently rare, having been reported in only a few suggestive cases. Delivery by cesarean section has been recommended for infants whose mothers are known to have genital herpes. The value of this prophylactic approach is not established, but most authorities recommend it nevertheless. If membranes rupture 6 hours or more before section is performed, ascent of virus may infect the fetus. A number of instances have been reported in which herpes infection followed delivery by cesarean section.

Like most other infectious agents that affect the neonate, herpesvirus produces a broad spectrum of clinical signs. The neonatal disease exists in disseminated and nondisseminated forms. The disseminated variety is fatal to 96% of affected infants. Although microscopic lesions may be found in every organ of the body, the most extensive involvement occurs in the adrenals, liver, brain, blood, and lung. Initial symptoms may be present at birth, or they may not appear until 3 or 4 weeks of age. Fever is detectable in approximately one third of infected infants. Other common signs include hepatosplenomegaly, hepatitis with jaundice (associated with direct hyperbilirubinemia), bleeding diathesis, and neurologic abnormalities. These neurologic signs are described later. Vesicular skin lesions are almost pathognomonic, but unfortunately they occur in only one third of the patients. They are usually sparsely distributed over the entire body; occasionally they appear in clusters. Sudden bleeding from the gastrointestinal tract, needle punctures, and circumcision sites portends death within 48 hours. Most infants so affected have been shown to have disseminated intravascular coagulation.

Several nondisseminated forms are composed of central nervous system, skin, and eye abnormalities, which occur singly or in combination. In none of them is there visceral involvement. These varieties of the disease cause death in 25% of the infants, but over half the survivors have residual damage to the brain and eyes. Neurologic abnormalities are the most frequent. They include convulsions (focal or generalized), abnormal muscle tone, opisthotonos, bulging fontanelle, and lethargy or coma. The spinal fluid contains an elevated protein concentration and increased leukocytes (predominantly lymphocytes). The eye signs include cloudy corneas (keratitis), conjunctivitis, and chorioretinitis. In a substantial proportion of infants with nondisseminated infection, skin involvement is the sole manifestation. As a rule they survive, but psychomotor damage is residual in some. New skin lesions continue to appear for several days; occasionally they recur sporadically up to 2 years of age. These recurrences may be associated with routine immunizations, unrelated febrile disease, or trauma. Most often the lesions appear for no known reason.

The most seriously disabling sequelae among surviving infants are neurologic. They consist of microcephaly or hydrocephalus and varying degrees of psychomotor retardation. Ocular residua may cause total or partial blindness as a result of scars in the cornea (from keratitis) and retina (from chorioretinitis).

In the absence of skin lesions, the diagnosis is elusive because the symptoms are otherwise nonspecific, most often being confused with septicemia. Cultures of virus from skin vesicles and the throat or identification by electron microscopy are the most reliable diagnostic procedures. Positive culture results are observable within 24 to 48 hours.

Several studies have demonstrated the effectiveness of *adenine arabinoside* (ara-A, vidarabine). Mortality of disseminated herpes is diminished by half while mortality of central nervous system herpes has been decreased from 50% in untreated babies to 10% in those who are treated. Ara-A is immunosuppressive, and it suppresses hematopoiesis. *Acyclovir* is an effective antiherpesvirus drug that has not yet been documented for treatment of neonates. Preliminary results indicate reasonable efficacy and less toxicity than ara-A.

PROTOZOAN INFECTION
Toxoplasmosis

Toxoplasmosis, caused by the protozoan *Toxoplasma gondii*, is usually an asymptomatic infection in older individuals. It is widespread to varying degrees among different populations over the world. In the United States it occurs in 1 to 4 per 1000 live births—approximately 3000 infected infants annually. It is an important perinatal infection, being transmitted across the placenta from an apparently healthy, but infected, mother. The acutely infected mother is more likely to transmit the organism to her fetus in late rather than early pregnancy. Fetal infection from maternal illness is 17%, 24%, and 62% in the first, second, and third trimesters, respectively. The reasons for this phenomenon are unknown. Symptoms appear in the infant at birth or soon thereafter, but many infants are asymptomatic for the first several weeks of life. The organism has been found in every cell type in the body except the red blood cell, and the resultant clinical signs are thus variable. An array of neurologic abnormalities includes convulsions, coma, severe generalized hypotonia, microcephaly, or hydrocephalus. Skull films may reveal diffuse, comma-shaped intracranial calcifications. Chorioretinitis occurs in most symptomatic infants; microphthalmia is also common. Other signs include hepatosplenomegaly, jaundice (direct and indirect hyperbilirubinemia), petechiae and ecchymoses of the skin (thrombocytopenia), and pallor (anemia). The fatality rate among diseased neonates is 12%. Neurologic deficits are extremely common in survivors.

Serologic diagnosis is feasible immediately after birth by demonstration of specific toxoplasma IgM antibodies. Other serologic procedures, if they reveal sufficiently high titers, also establish the diagnosis (hemagglutination inhibition).

CONTROL OF NURSERY INFECTION

Because of continuous presence in the nursery and involvement with hour-by-hour care, the nurse is the baby's most supportive caretaker. However, a lack of concern for hygienic practices can become a serious threat to the infant's survival. The prenatal acquisition of bacterial infection is in large measure unpreventable, but with few exceptions postnatally acquired infectious disease can indeed be avoided. Aside from the strict sterility that is obviously required during administration of parenteral fluids and medications or during performance of invasive procedures, the practices of nursery personnel need only be predicated on a few simple rules of hygiene. Realistically there is nothing aseptic about these practices; rather, they are clean to the utmost. The provision of a continuously germ-free environment is impossible, even in most sophisticated nurseries; nor does it seem desirable when one considers that animals maintained in such environments experience a significant delay in their capacity to produce antibodies because of the absence of antigenic stimuli.

Traditionally the practices advocated for prevention of infections have also tended to make the nursery a forbidding place to enter. Such an atmosphere is particularly inadvisable for neonatal intensive care units because the infants in them require greater attention from more people than any other type of patient in the hospital. Surgeons, cardiologists, neurologists, hematologists, anesthesiologists, x-ray technicians, laboratory technologists—all these individuals, besides the nursery staff itself, must regularly converge on sick infants. The resultant traffic if often something to behold. This type of care requires unimpeded access to the nursery, but careful hygienic demeanor is mandatory for all concerned. The simpler and more rigid the rules, the more consistently they are followed. A number of studies have provided a scientific basis for discarding needless and obstructive so-called aseptic techniques. The nurse's role in all this is pivotal. Daily practices must protect patients from exposure to infection, and, in addition, the nurse should be the most effective and vociferous promulgator of established rules of hygienic technique.

Infections are propagated by people and by things. In addition to a predisposition to infection because of illness, the sick neonate is also at great risk because a large cohort of personnel must use a multiplicity of objects in giving care. Furthermore, the nature of a special care nursery is such

that it attracts referrals from other institutions. As a consequence, a relatively large number of profoundly ill infants are housed in one facility for extended periods, thus increasing the hazard of cross-contamination. The practices to be described are applicable to any nursery—routine or special care. The risks they are designed to minimize are greater in special care facilities.

Propagation of infection by personnel

Personnel carriers of various organisms have been studied extensively, and their role in epidemics has been conjectural. There is some evidence that they may spread infection by the airborne route, but the current consensus is that direct contact by contaminated hands is the principal modality.

Most published studies concern the spread of staphylococci and their colonization among infant cohorts. Colonization of staphylococci occurs when organisms settle on the skin, in the nose, and in the throat without producing disease. The colonized infant is at considerably higher risk of subsequent disease than the noncolonized one. For instance, staphylococcal skin infection has been noted in 20% of infants who become colonized in the first 2 days of life, whereas only 1.4% of noncolonized infants are similarly afflicted. Colonization has been noted in as many as 100% of infants in a single nursery during epidemic years, but high rates also occur during nonepidemic periods. The significance of staphylococcal colonization is not restricted to the diseases that may subsequently appear during the nursery stay; discharged infants often become ill at home. They may also spread the organism to cause household epidemics, even though they remain healthy.

It thus follows that the effects of various procedures for minimizing nursery infections can be gauged from colonization rates and the incidence of overt disease. A number of excellent studies have in fact utilized this approach, and they are in general agreement on the validity of some of the procedures. In each instance the investigators caution that the conclusions reached are directly applicable to conditions in their respective facilities and that universal adoption of their practices may or may not be valid.

Failure to wash hands properly between handling of different infants is undoubtedly the principal mode of spread of infection by any organism. Nothing is more fundamental to proper nursery hygiene than handwashing. On first entering the nursery, personnel should wash to a level above the elbows for at least 2 minutes. Between patients, washing for 15 seconds should be adequate. Currently the use of any type of soap or an iodinated detergent is recommended. The iodinated preparations are preferable, at least for the initial 2-minute scrub, because they are active against gram-positive cocci and gram-negative rods as well, but they sometimes cause skin sensitivity.

In December 1972, statements from the Food and Drug Administration and the American Academy of Pediatrics recommended that routine total body bathing of infants, utilizing hexachlorophene-containing detergents, be discontinued. Although clinical signs of toxicity in human infants had not been documented, diffuse cystic lesions were observed in the brains of monkeys who were bathed daily for 90 days with a detergent containing hexachlorophene. Furthermore, blood levels of hexachlorophene in human newborns had been demonstrated, presumably absorbed from the skin. Several weeks after these statements were issued, the Center for Disease Control reported approximately 60 nursery outbreaks of staphylococcal disease throughout the nation. Whether these outbreaks were related to the discontinuation of hexachlorophene bathing is still conjectural. The temporal relationship between the two events suggests as much, although documentation is lacking. The original statements of the Food and Drug Administration and the American Academy of Pediatrics were subsequently modified to recommend that hexachlorophene bathing may be utilized in the presence of a staphylococcal outbreak, but it is unlikely to halt the spread of infection. The modified statements also emphasized the fundamental importance of handwashing and the necessity to investigate all nursery practices to determine the sources of staphylococcal colonization and disease. The preferred method of skin care is now "dry skin care" (see Skin Care of Newborns, Statement, Fetus and Newborn Committee, American Academy of Pediatrics).

Nursery personnel should wear short-sleeved scrub dresses to accommodate washing to the elbows. At some facilities the use of gowns by physicians and other personnel has been discontinued if infants are not removed from incubators. However, long-sleeved gowns should be worn and changed between handling infants if they are taken from an incubator or bassinet, whether to feed or to perform a procedure (individual gown technique). Caps, masks, and hairnets are no longer recommended.

Isolation and suspect nurseries are not considered essential, but infants with diarrhea and draining infections must be removed from the nursery. Infants with bacterial meningitis, septicemia, and pneumonia need not be isolated, nor is there a need to remove infants if amniotic membranes have ruptured early (even if the fluid is purulent), if there is a history of antepartum or postpartum maternal fever, or if the baby was born anywhere outside the delivery room.

Several studies have revealed that colonization rates and the incidence of infectious disease are not increased when parents are permitted in the nursery. This development is particularly important in light of the recent realization that the mother is profoundly affected by protracted separation from her sick newborn; it may significantly alter her attitude for some time afterward (Chapter 15). The precautions regarding handwashing and gowning for personnel are similarly applicable to parents.

Details of nursery techniques and measures for the management of nursery epidemics are fully presented in a recent revision of *Guidelines for Perinatal Care (1983)*, published by the American Academy of Pediatrics and the American College of Obstetricians and Gynecologists. A copy of this publication should be available at every facility that cares for newborn infants.

Infection from equipment and fixtures

The widespread use of indwelling catheters at the umbilical site and in peripheral veins has added another potential source of serious infection. The risk of infection involved in umbilical vessel catheters is well known. It is not generally appreciated, however, that catheters in peripheral veins cause a considerably higher incidence of bacteremia and local infections. These catheters must be placed with meticulously aseptic technique. They should be managed in the same fashion as the deep vein catheters that are used for total parenteral alimentation.

A group of gram-negative organisms, aptly dubbed by Wheeler as "water bugs," has been identified as an important cause of individual and epidemic infection. These organisms are spread primarily from contaminated equipment. Infants are infected by an enormous inoculum of bacteria capable of proliferating in clear water. Illness usually begins several days after birth or some time later if the nursery stay is protracted.

Pseudomonas is the most prevalent of these organisms. Other frequent offenders are *Aerobacter, Alcaligenes, Achromobacter, Flavobacterium, Serratia*, and *Erwinia* (implicated in contaminated caps on bottles of intravenous fluids). The epidemics caused by these bacteria may be widespread in the nursery during a short period, or the infections may occur sequentially in one or a few infants over a protracted interval. They emanate from any piece of equipment, particularly those associated with high humidity or moisture of any kind. Plumbing fixtures are also important sources of contamination. A list of these objects is presented on p. 369.

Regularly obtained cultures from most of these articles are an essential component of bacteriologic surveillance. Furthermore, autoclaving or gas sterilization is indicated for all items that lend themselves to these processes. Water in the reservoirs of incubators has been discontinued in many nurseries. Oxygen humidifiers are changed daily, and the water within them is changed every 8 hours. Disposable plastic tubes from oxygen outlets are discarded every 24 hours. Mist generators that provide clouded moisture in incubators for infants in respiratory distress are avoided because such treatment is useless, and it increases the incidence of "water bug" infections. Sterile distilled water from previously unopened bottles that is used in ultrasonic nebulizers is changed every 8 hours. Cotton balls are not stored in solutions of benzalkonium chloride (Zephiran) because in these circumstances *Pseudomonas* has been repeatedly recovered from the disinfectant. It is disconcerting to realize that bacteriologists use compounds related to benzalkonium chloride in their media to encourage the growth of *Pseudomonas* by impairing proliferation of other organisms.

The sources of infection in the nursery have multiplied commensurate with recent advances in the care of sick infants. It is essential for the nurse supervisor to execute a program of bacteriologic surveillance and sterilization of equipment. The staff nurse must be certain that equipment has been cleaned or sterilized in accordance with this program. These programs must be planned in conjunction with the physician in charge of the nursery, an infectious disease expert, an epidemiologist, and a representative from the hospital bacteriology laboratory.

The spread of organisms from people and from things must be eliminated, or at least minimized, by applying sensible techniques of proved value. As in so many other aspects of newborn care, the nurse can assure or destroy the success of infection control procedures better than any other staff member. Close and continuous contact with the babies qualifies the nurse as a perceptive monitor of the incidence of infection, and repeated contacts with physicians and other personnel provide the opportunity to appraise and regulate their demeanor in regard to infection control.

BIBLIOGRAPHY

Ablow, R. C., et al.: A comparison of early-onset group B streptococcal neonatal infection and the respiratory distress syndrome of the newborn, N. Engl. J. Med. **294:**65, 1976.

Ainbender, E., Cabatu, E. E., Guzman, D. M., and Sweet, A. Y.: Serum C-reactive protein and problems of newborn infants, J. Pediatr. **101:**438, 1982.

Alford, C. A., Neva, F. A., and Weller, T. H.: Virologic and serologic studies on human products of conception after maternal rubella, N. Engl. J. Med. **271:**1275, 1964.

Alford, C. A., et al.: A correlative immunologic, microbiologic and clinical approach to the diagnosis of acute and chronic infections in the newborn infant, N. Engl. J. Med. **277:**437, 1967.

Anderson, G. S., et al.: Congenital bacterial pneumonia, Lancet **2:**585, 1962.

Baker, C. J., Barrett, F. F., Gordon, R. C., and Yow, M. D.: Suppurative meningitis due to streptococci of Lancefield group B: a study of 33 infants, J. Pediatr. **82:**724, 1973.

Barnard, J. A., Cotton, R. B., and Lutin, W.: Necrotizing enterocolitis: variables associated with the severity of disease, Am. J. Dis. Child. **139:**375, 1985.

Barrie, D.: Incubator-borne *Pseudomonas* pyocyanea infection in a newborn nursery, Arch. Dis. Child. **40:**555, 1965.

Barton, L. L., Feigin, R. D., and Lins, R.: Group B beta-hemolytic streptococcal meningitis in infants, J. Pediatr. **82:**719, 1973.

Bell, W. E., and McGuiness, G. A.: Suppurative central nervous system infections in the neonate, Sem. Perinatol. **6:**1, 1982.

Benirschke, K.: Routes and types of infection in the fetus and the newborn, Am. J. Dis. Child. **99:**714, 1960.

Benirschke, K., and Driscoll, S. G.: The pathology of the human placenta, New York, 1967, Springer-Verlag New York.

Benuck, I., and David, R. J.: Sensitivity of published neutrophil indexes in identifying newborn infants with sepsis, J. Pediatr. **103:**961, 1983.

Bergstrom, R., Larson, H., Lincoln, K., and Winberg, J.: Studies of urinary tract infections in infancy and childhood. XII. Eighty consecutive patients with neonatal infection, J. Pediatr. **80:**858, 1972.

Blanc, W. A.: Pathways of fetal and early neonatal infection, viral placentitis, bacterial and fungal chorioamnionitis, J. Pediatr. **59:**473, 1961.

Brown, E. G., and Sweet, A. Y., editors: Neonatal necrotizing enterocolitis, New York, 1980, Grune and Stratton.

Cabrera, H. A., and Davis, G. H.: Epidemic meningitis of the newborn caused by flavobacteria. I. Epidemiology and bacteriology, Am. J. Dis. Child. **101:**289, 1961.

Cairo, M. S., Rucker, R., Bennetts, G. A., et al.: Improved survival of newborns receiving leukocyte transfusions of sepsis, Pediatrics **74:**887, 1984.

Davies, P. A., and Gothefors, L. A.: Bacterial infections in the fetus and newborn infants, Philadelphia, 1984, W. B. Saunders Co.

Davis, L. E., et al.: Cytomegalovirus mononucleosis in a first trimester pregnant female with transmission to the fetus, Pediatrics **48:**200, 1971.

Desmond, M. M., et al.: Congenital rubella encephalitis, J. Pediatr. **71:**311, 1967.

Eichenwald, H. F.: Congenital toxoplasmosis: a study of 150 cases, Am. J. Dis. Child. **94:**411, 1957.

Eickhoff, T. C., Klein, J. O., Daly, A. K., et al.: Neonatal sepsis and other infections due to group B beta-hemolytic streptococci, N. Engl. J. Med. **271:**1221, 1964.

Evans, H. E., Akpata, S. O., and Baki, A.: Bacteriologic and clinical evaluation of gowning in a premature nursery, J. Pediatr. **78:**883, 1971.

Foley, J. F., et al.: *Achromobacter* septicemia—fatalities in prematures, Am. J. Dis. Child. **101:**279, 1961.

Franciosi, R. A., Knostman, J. D., and Zimmerman, R. A.: Group B streptococcal neonatal and infant infections, J. Pediatr. **82:**707, 1973.

Friedman, C. A., Wender, D. F., and Rawson, J. E.: Rapid diagnosis of group B streptococcal infection utilizing a commercially available latex agglutination assay, Pediatrics **73:**27, 1984.

Gitlin, D., Kumate, J., Urrusti, J., et al.: The selectivity of the human placenta in the transfer of plasma proteins from mother to fetus, J. Clin. Invest. **43:**1938, 1964.

Gluck, L., and Wood, H. F.: Staphylococcal colonization in newborn infants with and without antiseptic skin care; a consideration of epidemiologic routes, N. Engl. J. Med. **268:**1265, 1963.

Hanshaw, J. B., Dudgeon, J. A., and Marshall, W. C.: Viral diseases of the fetus and newborn, ed. 2, Philadelphia, 1985, W. B. Saunders Co.

Hanson, L. A., Jodal, U., Sabel, K-G., and Wadsworth, C.: The diagnostic value of C-reactive protein, Pediatr. Infect. Dis. **2:**87, 1983.

Hardyment, A. F., et al.: Observations on the bacteriology and epidemiology of nursery infections. I. Staphylococcal skin infections, Pediatrics **25:**907, 1960.

Harris, M. C., and Polin, R. A.: Neonatal septicemia, Pediatr. Clin. North Am. **30:**243, 1983.

Hildebrandt, R. J., et al.: Cytomegalovirus in the normal pregnant woman, Am. J. Obstet. Gynecol. **98:**1125, 1967.

Hindocha, P., Campbell, C. A., Gould, J. D. M., et al.: Serial study of C-reactive protein in neonatal septicaemia, Arch. Dis. Child. **59:**435, 1984.

Hoffman, M. A., and Finberg, L.: *Pseudomonas* infections in infants associated with high humidity environments, J. Pediatr. **46:**626, 1955.

Horn, K. A., Zimmerman, R. A., Knostman, J. D., and Meyer, W. T.: Neurological sequelae of group B streptococcal neonatal infection, Pediatrics **53:**501, 1974.

James, L. S.: Hexachlorophene, Pediatrics **49:**492, 1972.

Kleiman, M. B., Reynolds, J. K., Schreiner, R. L., et al.: Rapid diagnosis of neonatal bacteremia with acridine orange-stained buffy coat smears, J. Pediatr. **105:**419, 1984.

Kohen, D. P.: Neonatal gonococcal arthritis: three cases and review of the literature, Pediatrics **53:**436, 1974.

Kopelman, A. E.: Cutaneous absorption of hexachlorophene in low-birth-weight infants, J. Pediatr. **82:**972, 1973.

Korones, S. B., Ainger, L. E., Monif, G. R., et al.: Congenital rubella syndrome: new clinical aspects with recovery of virus from affected infants, J. Pediatr. **67:**166, 1965.

Korones, S. B., Roane, J. A., Gilkeson, M. R., et al.: Neonatal IgM response to acute infection, J. Pediatr. **75:**1261, 1969.

Kresky, B.: Control of gram-negative bacilli in a hospital nursery, Am. J. Dis. Child. **107:**363, 1964.

Light, I. J., and Linnemann, C. C., Jr.: Neonatal herpes simplex infection following delivery by cesarean section, Obstet. Gynecol. **44:**496, 1974.

Light, I. J., Brackvogel, V., Walton, R. L., and Sutherland, J. M.: An epidemic of bullous impetigo arising from a central admission-observation nursery, Pediatrics **49:**15, 1972.

Lockhart, J. D.: How toxic is hexaclorophene? Pediatrics **50:**229, 1972.

Manroe, B. L., Weinberg, A. G., Rosenfeld, C. R., and Browne, R.: The neonatal blood count in health and disease. I. Reference values for neutrophilic cells, J. Pediatr. **95:**89, 1979.

McCracken, G. H.: Changing pattern of the antimicrobial susceptibilities of *Escherichia coli* in neonatal infections, J. Pediatr. **78:**942, 1971.

McCracken, G. H., Hardy, J. B., Chen, T. C., et al.: Serum immunoglobulin levels in newborn infants. II. Survey of cord and follow-up sera from 123 infants with congenital rubella, J. Pediatr. **74:**383, 1969.

McCracken, G. H., Jr., and Nelson, J. D.: Antimicrobial therapy for newborns, New York, 1983, Grune and Stratton.

Miller, D. R., Hanshaw, J. B., O'Leary, D. S., and Hnilicka, J. V.: Fatal disseminated herpes simplex virus infection and hemorrhage in the neonate: coagulation studies in a case and a review, J. Pediatr. **76:**409, 1970.

Miller, M. E., and Stiehm, R.: Immunology and resistance to infection. In Remington, J. S., and Klein, J. O., editors: Infectious diseases of the fetus and newborn infant, ed. 2, Philadelphia, 1983, W. B. Saunders Co.

Monif, G. R. G., Avery, G. B., Korones, S. B., et al.: Postmortem isolation of rubella virus from three children with rubella-syndrome defects, Lancet **1:**723, 1965.

Monif, G. R. G., Egan, E. A., Held, B., and Eitzman, D. V.: The correlation of maternal cytomegalovirus infection during varying stages in gestation with neonatal involvement, J. Pediatr. **80:**17, 1972.

Nahmias, A. J., Alford, C. A., and Korones, S. B.: Infection of the newborn with herpesvirus hominis, Adv. Pediatr. **17:**185, 1970.

Noel, G. J., and Edelson, P. J.: *Staphylococcus epidermidis* bacteremia in neonates: further observations and the occurrence of focal infection, Pediatrics **74:**832, 1984.

Olding, L.: Bacterial infection in cases of perinatal death, a morphological and bacteriological study based on 264 autopsies, Acta Paediatr. Scand. **171**(supp.):1, 1966.

Overall, J. C., Jr.: Neonatal bacterial meningitis: analysis of predisposing factors and outcome compared with matched control subjects, J. Pediatr. **76:**499, 1970.

Overbach, A. M., Daniel, S. J., and Cassady, G.: The value of umbilical cord histology in the management of potential perinatal infection, J. Pediatr. **76:**22, 1970.

Peter, G., Lloyd-Still, J. D., and Lovejoy, F. H., Jr.: Local infection and bacteremia from scalp vein needles and polyethylene catheters in children, J. Pediatr. **80:**78, 1972.

Philip, A. G. S.: Acute-phase proteins in neonatal infection, J. Pediatr. **105:**940, 1984.

Powell, H., Swarner, O., Gluck, L., and Lampert, P.: Hexachlorophene myelinopathy in premature infants, J. Pediatr. **82:**976, 1973.

Prod-hom, L. S., Choffat, J. M., Frenck, N., et al.: Care of the seriously ill neonate with hyaline membrane disease and with sepsis (sclerema neonatorum), Pediatrics **53:**170, 1974.

Sann, L., Bienvenu, F., Binevenu, J., et al.: Evolution of serum prealbumin, C-reactive protein, and orosomucoid in neonates with bacterial infection, J. Pediatr. **105:**977, 1984.

Sever, J. L.: Possible role of humidifying equipment in spread of infections from the newborn nursery, Pediatrics **24:**50, 1959.

Sever, J. L.: Perinatal infections affecting the fetus and newborn, Proceedings of a Conference on Mental Retardation Through Control of Infectious Diseases, June 9-11, 1966, Public Health Service Publication no. 1962, Washington, D.C., 1966, Government Printing Office.

Sherman, J. D., et al.: Alcaligenes faecalis infection in the newborn, Am. J. Dis. Child. **100:**212, 1960.

Sherman, M. P., Chance, K. H., and Goetzman, B. W.: Gram's strains of tracheal secretions predict neonatal bacteremia, Am. J. Dis. Child. **138:**848, 1984.

Shuman, R. M., Leech, R. W., and Alvord, E. C., Jr.: Neurotoxicity of hexachlorophene in humans. II. A clinicopathological study of 46 premature infants, Arch. Neurol. **32:**320, 1975.

Siegel, J. D.: Neonatal sepsis, Sem. Perinatol. **9:**20, 1985.

Silverman, W. A., and Homan, W. E.: Sepsis of obscure origin in the newborn, Pediatrics **3:**157, 1949.

Silverman, W. A., and Sinclair, J. C.: Evaluation of precautions before entering a neonatal unit, Pediatrics **40:**900, 1967.

Snowe, R. J., and Wilfert, C. M.: Epidemic reappearance of gonococcal ophthalmia neonatorum, Pediatrics **51:**110, 1973.

South, M. A.: Enteropathogenic *Escherichia coli* disease: new developments and perspectives, J. Pediatr. **79**:1, 1971.

Sprunt, K., Redman, W., and Leidy, G.: Antibacterial effectivenss of routine hand washing, Pediatrics **52**:264, 1973.

Starr, J. G., and Gold, E.: Screening of newborn infants for cytomegalovirus infection, J. Pediatr. **73**:820, 1968.

Starr, S. E.: Antimicrobial therapy of bacterial sepsis in the newborn infant, J. Pediatr. **106**:1043, 1985.

Stern, H., and Tucker, S. M.: Prospective study of cytomegalovirus infection in pregnancy, Br. Med. J. **2**:268, 1973.

Swartzberg, J. E., and Remington, J. S.: Transmission of toxoplasma, Am. J. Dis. Child. **129**:777, 1975.

Tanner, M. S., and Stocks, R. J.: Neonatal gastroenterology—contemporary issues, Newcastle upon Tyne (England), 1984, Intercept.

Wasserman, R. L.: Neonatal sepsis: the potential of granulocyte transfusion, Hosp. Pract. **17**:95, 1982.

Watson, D. G.: Purulent neonatal meningitis: a study of forty-five cases, J. Pediatr. **50**:352, 1957.

Weller, T.: The cytomegaloviruses: ubiquitous agents with protean clinical manifestations, I and II, N. Engl. J. Med. **285**:203, 1971.

Wheeler, W. E.: Water bugs in the bassinet, Am. J. Dis. Child. **101**:273, 1961.

Wilson, M. G., et al.: New source of *Pseudomonas aeruginosa* in a nursery, J.A.M.A. **175**:1146, 1961.

Yeung, C. Y.: Hypoglycemia in neonatal sepsis, J. Pediatr. **77**:812, 1970.

Zuckerman, A. J.: The problem and control of hepatitis B infection in the fetus and the newborn. In Krugman, S., and Gershon, A. A., editors: Infections of the fetus and the newborn infant, New York, 1975, Alan R. Liss.

CHAPTER 14

Central nervous system disorders of perinatal origin

Concern for survival of sick neonates is surpassed only by an anxiety to avoid residual brain damage. Although the incidence of residual neurologic impairment has diminished considerably since the advent of fetal medicine and neonatal intensive care, there remains an unacceptable number of infants whose lives are destined to be of limited quality and longevity. Our success in avoiding these tragic sequelae is substantial but partial, and the implications of our failures are diffuse. The lives of the immediate family of the affected infant are disrupted. Also, those who are responsible for management of these sick infants are beset with ethical considerations that usually remain unresolved, largely as a function of our inability to predict long-term effects. There is also a concern about the potential number of handicapped survivors and the resulting fiscal liabilities.

This chapter is devoted to a discussion of the principal forms of noninfectious brain damage that are identifiable during the perinatal period, their etiologies insofar as these are known, the possibilities of prevention, and the available modes of therapy. Discussion will focus on those central nervous disorders that are largely attributable to asphyxia; those resulting from birth trauma are discussed in Chapter 2.

THE CENTRAL NERVOUS SYSTEM SEQUELAE OF PRENATAL AND POSTNATAL ASPHYXIA AND ISCHEMIA

The occurrence of damage to a previously normal brain during the antepartum and intrapartum periods is most often the result of oxygen deprivation. This may occur either as a result of diminished blood oxygen content in the presence of normal perfusion or as a result of diminished perfusion (ischemia) even if oxygen content is normal. The prenatal causes of hypoxia-ischemia are usually a consequence of the chronic fetal distress associated with maternal toxemia, other causes of placental insufficiency, severe postmaturity, and occasionally maternal diabetes. The other causes of protracted fetal distress are listed in Table 2-1. Acute hypoxia is more likely to occur during labor and delivery. The causes of these acute episodes, such as abruptio placentae, placenta previa, and prolapsed cord, are also listed in the same table. Hypoxia-ischemia that occurs postnatally is generally a result of severe cardiorespiratory distress and vascular collapse (hypotension) from severe infection.

Other causes of damage to the brain include infections acquired prenatally and postnatally, maternal drug habits and drug therapy, postnatal metabolic disorders such as hypoglycemia, and congenital malformations.

We are concerned here with the aftermath of hypoxic-ischemic episodes, whether these occur before or after birth. Ninety percent of them occur prenatally. A variety of lesions may be produced, depending on the severity of the insult and the gestational age. In term infants the most common consequence of hypoxia-ischemia is *cerebral necrosis*. In the premature infant, *periventricular necrosis (periventricular leukomalacia) and intraventricular hemorrhage* are most frequent. Another hemorrhagic consequence of hypoxia (and sometimes of trauma) is *primary subarachnoid hemorrhage* in both premature and term infants.

Perinatal hypoxic-ischemic injury results in lesions that are distributed throughout the brain according to its vascular pattern. Lesions thus occur in relation to gestational age at the time of the injury because the vascular pattern changes radically as gestation proceeds. Vascular supply is profuse in the deeper brain structures early in gestation. As the vascular pattern approaches term, blood supply to the more peripheral structures (the cortex) increases. At term, or in the two or three weeks that precede it, the lesions are thus generally confined to the cerebral cortex. In premature infants, those below 35 or 36 weeks, lesions are located in the deeper structures close to the ventricles (periventricular region).

Cerebral blood flow and autoregulation

The rate of cerebral vascular blood flow is lower during the perinatal period than it is in older children and adults. Blood flow is intimately related to metabolic rate in the brain, which in the perinate is approximately 60% lower than in adults. The perinate's cerebral blood flow is thus lower by approximately equal magnitude. *Autoregulation* is a mechanism by which an uninterrupted and relatively unwaivering blood supply to the brain is maintained despite fluctuations in systemic blood pressure. Steady cerebral perfusion continues within fairly wide fluctuations of systemic blood pressure. Autoregulation is operative in preterm infants as well as in term infants. It is impaired or eliminated as a result of asphyxia. In such circumstances, systemic hypotension or hypertension cause diminished or increased blood flow, respectively, because systemic arterial pressure is transmitted to the cerebral blood vessels in the absence of the modulating influence of autoregulation. The capacity to regulate flow by changing vascular resistance becomes impaired in the presence of a high $PaCO_2$, low PaO_2, and acidosis. These biochemical abnormalities additionally impose injury on capillaries, disrupting normal structure of endothelium tight junctions, and basement membranes. It is in this setting that intraventricular-periventricular hemorrhage seems to occur in preterm infants.

In human neonates brain damage is a function of diminished cerebral blood flow. In two excellent independent studies, mean cerebral blood flow has been found to be 37 to 40 ml/100 g/min. There is also good evidence that at a flow rate below 20 ml/100 g/min, survivors are dysfunctional because of cerebral atrophy.

It has long been known that immature brains are more resistant to hypoxia-ischemia than mature brains. This phenomenon has been demonstrated repeatedly in a variety of animal species. Newborn rats tolerate hypoxia-ischemia for periods that are 25 times longer than adults. Infant monkeys survive periods 5 to 10 times longer. Precise data for humans are not available, but clinical observations indicate that the same phenomenon is operative. The explanation in animals is not in enhanced capacity for energy production in the brain as formerly proposed. Rather, survival of a hypoxic insult is related to the diminished metabolic rate in the brain that has been demonstrated in neonatal animals and humans. In humans, the metabolic rate is 60% that of the adult brain, and there is a commensurate diminution in cerebral blood flow. The aftermath of increased capacity to survive is enhancement of residual brain damage. In other words, the experimental evidence suggests that the ability to survive longer periods of asphyxia is associated with an increased likelihood of permanent brain damage.

Hypoxic-ischemic encephalopathy in term infants

Damage is incurred as the result of hypoxemia or the diminished cerebral perfusion that accompanies systemic hypotension. Usually, both of these factors are operative. Varying degrees of cellular necrosis occur in selected areas of the cerebral cortex, basal ganglia, brain stem, and cerebellum. Often the initial insult is followed shortly by edema of the brain. These changes occur to a varying extent, according to the severity of the hypoxic-ischemic episode. If the infant survives, cerebral atrophy is demonstrable by computerized tomographic (CT) scan several months later. The long-term sequelae of major concern include seizures, motor deficits, choreoathetosis and ataxia, and mental retardation. This combination of clinical signs is often referred to as "ce-

rebral palsy." It should be understood, however, that cerebral palsy does not necessarily include mental retardation.

Clinical course of profound asphyxia. The clinical course of affected term infants has been followed by a number of investigators whose findings have been presented in terms of time intervals following birth. The major abnormalities involve the sensorium, muscle tone, seizure activity, and abnormal eye findings. As a rule, the fewer the symptoms or the more rapid the recovery from those that are present, the better the long-term outcome.

In light of present knowledge, *it is inadvisable to predict the quality of life based on a particular clinical course*. Persistence of abnormalities immediately after birth is usually associated with long-term neurologic impairment, but the precise extent of this impairment is generally unpredictable. The earlier the disappearance of an abnormal sign, the better the outlook. The description of abnormalities that follows is applicable to term infants who begin with serious asphyxia. The description that follows this one (p. 396) concerns *stages of involvement* (Table 14-1) without allusion to timing of manifestations.

Sensorium. Alertness is diminished to the point of lethargy, or in the extreme, to stupor. Some improvement usually occurs within 12 to 24 hours, even in severely affected babies. Those who are mildly affected may progress to alertness within a shorter period. Following the period of improvement, the more severely affected infants relapse into stupor or coma between 24 and 72 hours after birth. In most infants, alertness may be regained in a few days, but stupor persists for weeks in the most severely affected babies.

Eyes. During the first 12 to 24 hours the pupils are reactive to light. Frequently, coordinated (conjugate) roving eye movements occur. Abnormal extraocular movements appear some time between 24 and 72 hours after birth in moderately and severely affected infants. Thus "bobbing" eye movements may be in evidence. They are characterized by conjugate, but random, vertical motion. Skew deviation may also occur. Vertical position of the eyes is disparate; one eye is lower than the other.

Muscle tone. During the first 12 to 24 hours most infants are flaccid; their spontaneous movements are absent or markedly diminished. During the next 12 to 24 hours, muscle tone improves along with consciousness, and spontaneous movement appears. Between 24 and 72 hours, severely affected infants become markedly hypotonic again; their spontaneous movements disappear. Beyond 72 hours they remain hypotonic for protracted periods.

Seizures. Some form of seizure activity is identifiable in approximately 50% of affected infants. The seizure activity is not often discernible before 6 hours of age. Early manifestations include sustained horizontal conjugate eye deviation; repeated blinking of the lids; sucking, smacking, and tongue thrusting movements; and swimming motions of the limbs. Apneic episodes are frequent. Tonic and clonic convulsive movements are multifocal. It is a peculiarity of the neonate that the tonic and clonic movements occur at random, not in the ordered sequence so characteristic of older children and adults. These blatant convulsive movements sometimes accompany the very early subtle signs of convulsions, but more frequently they follow them within hours. Within 6 to 24 hours, seizure activity may worsen. Tonic and clonic movements are predominant. These convulsions are difficult to control pharmacologically. Apneic episodes become more frequent and protracted. The most profoundly injured infants have status epilepticus. Severe seizure activity may continue for 48 to 72 hours and then disappear. In some infants, convulsions recur sporadically over the next few weeks. Sometimes jitteriness occurs between convulsive episodes when these are sporadic. Jitteriness is not always a benign sign, even if it occurs in the absence of convulsions.

Anterior fontanelle. Since the response to hypoxia often involves swelling of brain cells, water content is increased and intracranial pressure is elevated. Often, between 24 and 48 hours after birth, tight bulging of the anterior fontanelle and separation of the sutures of the skull first appear. These findings may persist for several days, and they are usually associated with the *syndrome of inappropriate secretion of antidiuretic hormone* (Chapter 7).

In the extreme, infants who are most profoundly damaged remain lethargic or stuporous and are unable to feed, thus requiring nasogastric feedings. Feeding difficulty generally improves over a few days or occasionally over a period of several weeks. Beyond the first 72 to 96 hours after birth, many infants who will have long-term effects remain hypotonic and cannot take feedings.

Asphyxial encephalopathy: degrees of involvement. Table 14-1 summarizes clinical signs that indicate varying degrees of hypoxic injury to the brain. These clinical signs are largely determined by severity and duration of an asphyxial insult, whether in utero, during the birth process, or immediately after delivery. Although overlapping of these degrees of involvement is inevitable, the clinical signs that delineate them are usually distinguishable with reasonable clarity.

Mild involvement of full-term infants does not depress sensorium. Rather, affected infants are alert or occasionally excessively alert. The latter state is characterized by widened palpebrae and by an intense facial expression that suggests explorative curiosity. Muscle tone is normal or perhaps moderately increased; these changes, when present, are most prominent in the upper extremities. Deep tendon reflexes are normal or exaggerated; the grasp, suck, and rooting reflexes are undisturbed. The Moro response is also normal. Doll's eye, gag, and pupillary reflexes are intact.

With moderate involvement, lethargy and hypotonia are characteristic. Reactions to sensory stimulation (light, acoustic, pain) are identifiable but obviously depressed. The deep tendon reflexes are usually hyperactive and correspondingly, ankle clonus is demonstrable. Pupils react normally to light. Seizures occur in a substantial num-

Table 14-1. Postasphyxial encephalopathy: Degrees of involvement

Factor	Mild	Moderate	Severe
Level of consciousness	Alert	Lethargy	Coma
Muscle tone	Normal	Hypotonia	Flaccidity
Tendon reflexes	Increased	Increased	Depressed or absent
Myoclonus	Present	Present	Absent
Complex reflexes			
Sucking	Active	Weak	Absent
Moro response	Exaggerated	Incomplete	Absent
Grasping	Normal to exaggerated	Exaggerated	Absent
Oculocephalic (Doll's eyes)	Normal	Overreactive	Reduced or absent
Autonomic function			
Pupils	Dilated	Constricted	Variable or fixed
Respiration	Regular	Variations in rate and depth, periodic	Ataxic, apnea
Heart rate	Normal or tachycardia	Bradycardia	Bradycardia
Seizures	None	Common	Uncommon
EEG	Normal	Low voltage, periodic and/or paroxysmal	Periodic or isoelectric

From Sarnat, H. B. and Sarnat, M. S.: Arch. Neurol. **33**:696-705, 1975. Copyright 1975, American Medical Association. As modified by Voorhies, T. M. and Vannucci, R. C.: Perinatal cerebral hypoxia-ischemia: diagnosis and management. In Sarnat, H. B., editor: Topics in neonatal neurology, Orlando, Fla., 1984, Grune & Stratton.

ber of these moderately asphyxiated babies. Convulsions first appear between 6 and 12 hours after birth, but sometimes sooner.

The *severely asphyxiated* infant is comatose and unresponsive. Flaccidity is extreme; deep tendon reflexes and other reflexes are markedly depressed or absent. The pupillary response to light is absent or extremely sluggish. Systemic signs are generally prominent in this group of profoundly affected infants. Bradycardia, abnormal respirations, and hypotension are generally present. During this comatose stage, with its absence of spontaneous movements and severe flaccidity, seizures do not occur. If the infant improves to involvement described above for moderate asphyxia, seizures are likely as improvement progresses.

Treatment. Since cerebral edema is such a common manifestation of this type of brain injury, fluids are restricted in infants who are thought to have experienced intrauterine asphyxia. Thus we administer approximately 50 ml/kg/24 h to affected babies. The treatment of seizures is described later in this chapter.

A number of attempts are under way to evaluate several agents for the alleviation of cerebral edema. The use of hyperosmotic agents such as mannitol and glycerol is under study. Diuretics such as furosemide are also being investigated. Corticosteroids have been advocated on a trial basis because of their salutary effect in older patients, particularly those with cerebral edema following trauma. The protracted type of cerebral edema that follows hypoxic-ischemic injury apparently does not respond similarly. The status of corticosteroid therapy is thus far undetermined.

Periventricular leukomalacia

Periventricular leukomalacia occurs in premature infants. It is largely the result of diminished blood flow and is thus an area of infarction. The affected regions of the brain are adjacent to the lateral ventricles. Most often the lesion does not include a hemorrhagic component. Many affected infants are not symptomatic during the neonatal period, but they may be simply lethargic and hypotonic. The motor fibers that descend from the cortex to the extremities run through the infarcted area of brain. Thus injury to these fibers results in the long-term abnormality known as *spastic diplegia*, which does not necessarily include mental retardation. Spastic diplegia is grouped with the other abnormalities that constitute "cerebral palsy." It is a permanent abnormality that is unique to premature infants. Although all four limbs may be affected by spastic paralysis, the lower limbs are characteristically more involved. A remarkable diminution in the incidence of spastic diplegia has been observed in numerous centers since the advent of neonatal intensive care.

Intraventricular-periventricular hemorrhage (IVH/PVH)

Intraventricular hemorrhage is a common consequence of hypoxia-ischemia that is peculiar to premature infants. It has been reported in a few term infants, but as a rule, the shorter the gestational age, the higher the incidence of hemorrhage. The term *intraventricular* implies that the hemorrhage bursts into the cerebral spinal fluid to circulate within the ventricular system. This does in fact occur, but the hemorrhage occurs first in the tissue immediately adjacent to the ventricular wall and it may occasionally remain there, never to burst into the cerebral spinal fluid in the ventricles.

The incidence of intraventricular hemorrhage is difficult to estimate. Just a few years past, the only methodology available for the diagnosis of these lesions was examination of cerebral spinal fluid extracted by lumbar puncture. The lumbar puncture was performed only after the appearance of clinical neurologic abnormalities. With the use of CT scanning, new clinical correlations with the appearance of intraventricular hemorrhage

have come to light. Thus in a survey of 46 infants who weighed less than 1500 g, 20 of them (43%) had evidence of intraventricular hemorrhage as demonstrated by the CT scan. Later studies, also utilizing CT scans, confirmed this percent incidence. Among the infants with hemorrhage who survived, seven were identified by the scanning technique *even though they were apparently asymptomatic*. Furthermore it was possible to grade the severity of the lesions according to the CT scan appearance. We have entered an era in which the relationship of perinatal clinical events to long-term outcome will be identified and etiologic factors that are applicable to prevention will be demonstrated. In the study previously mentioned, the frequency of intraventricular hemorrhage among infants who weighed less than 1500 g (43%) was astonishing. Previous studies have demonstrated at *autopsy* that intraventricular (periventricular) hemorrhage was identifiable in 50% to 70% of infants *who died*. In another recent study, a follow-up of fifteen infants who survived intraventricular hemorrhage demonstrated that six (40%) were normal between 12 and 36 months of age. Moderate or severe neurologic handicaps were identifiable in only three of the fifteen babies (20%). In the remaining six (40%), neurologic handicaps were of minor significance. We have come to the realization that this lesion is far more frequent than previously suspected, and that intact survival, or survival with minor impairment, is common. The contemporary difference in this new outlook is the result of an ability to detect these hemorrhages by surveillance techniques that do not depend on the appearance of clinical signs. It appears that the incidence of survival, and its quality, approximates that which has been reported for neonatal bacterial meningitis. Furthermore, based on CT scan appearance, the extent (severity) of these lesions can be graded. Grade I (the mildest) through grade IV (the most severe) seem to correlate with the severity of residual handicap and with the appearance of hydrocephalus.

The use of CT scans for identification of intraventricular-periventricular hemorrhage was no sooner introduced than it became historic. It is now commonplace in most intensive care units to survey infants whose birth weight is less than 1500 g for IVH/PVH with intracranial ultrasonography. Real-time ultrasound does not require ionizing radiation, and it can be performed at the bedside. It is a noninvasive procedure that affords serial and multiple images of the brain, obtainable in a very short period of time. The beam of ultrasound is applied by placing a probe over the anterior fontanelle. Views are routinely recorded in longitudinal and coronal planes. The presence of periventricular or intraventricular hemorrhage and other abnormalities is clearly visible. CT scan, because of the inconvenience and difficulties in transporting a baby to the apparatus, has been replaced by intracranial ultrasonography for the purpose of visualizing the brain during the nursery stay. With widespread use of cranial ultrasound, the incidence of IVH/PVH has been observed to be higher than observed by CT scan. An incidence as high as 90% of infants less than 1500 g was described in one study, but most studies estimate the incidence between 30% and 50%. Ultrasonography has demonstrated a large number of hemorrhagic lesions that are asymptomatic, and are apparently of no consequence in long-term outcome. Four grades of hemorrhage have been described.

Grade I refers to subependymal bleeding, restricted to the area of the germinal matrix, that does not enter the ventricles. This is the most common type of hemorrhage. By serial ultrasound examinations it appears to resolve in most instances, leaving no abnormal structural residua.

Grade II refers to bleeding into the lateral ventricles. In this category the ventricles do not dilate.

Grade III describes ventricular bleeding associated with dilatation of the ventricles.

Grade IV includes intraventricular hemorrhage, dilatation of the ventricles, and bleeding into the surrounding brain tissue. This is the most serious form of hemorrhage.

Clinical signs. IVH/PVH rarely, if ever, occurs after the fifth postnatal day. Most episodes become apparent within 48 hours following birth. Clinical signs are variable. At one extreme, these lesions occur in infants who are asymptomatic, while on the other, a catastrophic sequence of events results in death within minutes or hours. The catastrophic course is characterized by worsening of existing respiratory difficulty (apnea, hypercapnia, hypoxemia) despite previously adequate mechanical ventilatory support. The blood pressure drops precipitously. Normal body temperature is difficult or impossible to maintain. Cyanosis persists despite vigorous attempts to provide optimal respiratory support. Hypotonia is severe. Within a few hours the anterior fontanelle is tight and bulging. Seizures occur soon after the onset or within several hours. Opisthotonic posture, coma, and fixed, dilated pupils are frequent. The hematocrit falls at least 20% from its previous level, often by as much as 50% or 60%. Metabolic acidosis is severe and persistent, presumably as a result of vascular instability and poor general perfusion. The cerebral spinal fluid is bloody, but this is usually difficult to distinguish from the bloody fluid of a traumatic lumbar puncture. However, if the infant survives at least 24 hours, lumbar puncture later yields dark red-brown fluid that represents old blood.

Before the routine use of intracranial ultrasound imaging, this, to us, was the most reliable indication of an IVH. Otherwise, fresh blood in spinal fluid was too often the result of a traumatic tap. Furthermore, the spinal fluid was often normal in the presence of an IVH.

A less severe clinical course is probably most frequent. These signs are usually milder or evanescent. In some instances they are virtually undetectable, while biochemical data is highly suggestive. Thus a number of infants may manifest jaundice that is otherwise unexplained, while abnormal neurologic signs are barely discernible. Persistent metabolic acidosis or the sudden appearance of hyperglycemia or hypoglycemia may similarly suggest an intraventricular hemorrhage in which clinical signs are difficult to detect. More often, such infants become lethargic and hypotonic; they may also have intermittent opisthotonos. Focal seizures may occur and often disappear rapidly. In other instances subtle clinical signs, the significance of which cannot be determined, may be followed in 1 to 2 weeks by enlargement of the head, tightness of the anterior fontanelle, and separation of sutures. The use of the CT scan has revealed numerous instances of ventricular dilatation that has preceded enlargement of head circumference by a considerable period. The symptoms of intraventricular hemorrhage may appear, disappear, and reappear intermittently prior to ultimate cessation, or they may persist for several days and then disappear only to be followed by enlargement of the head. Of all the mild clinical signs, lethargy and hypotonia are most frequently encountered. The critical importance of clinical diagnosis has disappeared because ultrasound imagery is so reliable.

Pathogenesis. IVH/PVH occurs in an area of the brain called the *germinal matrix*. The germinal matrix is located adjacent to the walls of the ventricles; its capillary blood supply is copious. The germinal matrix is an early developmental structure that is not present in the term infant. Therefore hemorrhage in this area is unique to the premature infant. The capillaries in the germinal matrix are extremely fragile; they are almost devoid of supportive connective tissue. They are thus vulnerable to rupture with relative ease. Furthermore, the capillaries become particularly vulnerable to disruption because hypoxic-ischemic events damage their walls. In premature infants whose gestational age is below 32 or 33 weeks, hemorrhage occurs in the deeper structures of the brain because of incomplete development of vascular supply. Before this time, a preponderance of blood flows to the central (deep) brain structures. As gestation proceeds, blood vessels extend centrifugally, and at term, a preponderance of the circulation is in the cerebral cortex. Thus in preterm babies most insults in-

volve deep structures; in term infants involvement is closer to the surface of the brain in the cortical region. In some instances of hemorrhage into the germinal matrix, blood breaks through the ependymal wall into the ventricles and circulates in the cerebral spinal fluid. Obstruction to the flow of cerebral spinal fluid often occurs as a result, and the ventricles dilate in response to accumulating pressure. *This ventricular dilatation progresses for at least 1 to 2 weeks before enlargement of the head is clinically perceptible.* Ventriculomegaly and severe enlargement of the head has been reported at birth in an infant whose IVH/PVH had occurred in utero. Hydrocephalus was previously thought to occur in approximately 80% of infants with intraventricular hemorrhage. More recently the incidence of hydrocephalus is cited in 20% to 25% of such affected infants.

The role of coagulopathy has been investigated. Disturbed hemostasis is more frequent in babies with IVH/PVH, but a causative role cannot be ascribed to impaired clotting. Some believe that coagulopathy contributes to severity of hemorrhagic episodes.

Treatment. Supportive treatment to remedy hypoxemia, acidosis, and hypotension is the highest priority. Following stabilization of the baby, the most promising regimen involves daily lumbar punctures to relieve the pressure within the ventricular system. Removal of spinal fluid also serves to remove the blood therein and probably diminishes the possibility of obstruction to flow. From preliminary data, it appears that this regimen may diminish the incidence of hydrocephalus. Hyperosmotic agents such as glycerol have been used in an attempt to minimize the accumulation of fluid within the ventricles, but they are not conclusive.

Primary subarachnoid hemorrhage

Hemorrhage into the subarachnoid space may be primary or it may occur secondarily as an extension of bleeding that originated elsewhere (intraventricular hemorrhage or subdural hematoma). *Primary subarachnoid hemorrhage involves* bleeding into the subarachnoid space that does not involve other areas. The most common cause of such hemorrhage is hypoxia; birth trauma is a less frequent etiologic factor. Three fourths of the affected infants are premature.

In most instances, symptoms of primary subarachnoid hemorrhage are absent or mild. In a substantial number of infants, however, seizure activity occurs—particularly in term infants. These seizures characteristically appear on the second day of life; they are sporadic and persist for several days. This disorder is unique in that infants who convulse repeatedly seem to be well in the interim. In premature infants, primary subarachnoid hemorrhage is an infrequent cause of recurrent apnea in the absence of seizures.

Sequelae of this lesion are rare. Hydrocephalus may result from obstructed flow or impaired absorption of cerebral spinal fluid over the convex surfaces of the cerebral hemispheres. Massive subarachnoid hemorrhage is even more infrequent. It is usually associated with severe hypoxia or trauma and rarely culminates in death.

NEONATAL SEIZURES

Neonatal seizures may be subtle and barely discernible or blatant and life-threatening. They are nonspecific symptoms caused by a variety of serious disorders. Recognition of their significance and identification of their causes are prerequisite to effective therapy.

The signs of seizure activity are frequently subtle and are most likely to escape the attention of inexperienced observers. These signs include sustained horizontal deviations of the eyes, paroxysms of horizontal or vertical nystagmus, blinking, chewing, sucking or vigorous tongue thrusting, transient abrupt loss of muscle tone, and vasomotor instability that is manifested by evanescent mottling or blotching. A number of less subtle signs are more likely to attract attention, including rowing motions of the upper extremities and bicycle movements of the lower ones, sudden assumption of a rigid posture, and fist clenching so forceful that it blanches the hand. Apnea has also

been identified as a component of seizure activity, but rarely by itself. More frequently, apnea occurs in association with one or several of the more subtle manifestations.

The progressive tonic-clonic seizure that occurs in older infants is not observed in the neonate. Rather, convulsive episodes are usually one or the other, tonic or clonic. Tonic convulsions may involve the entire body. The infant stiffens; the back may arch. The lower extremities are in rigid extension; the toes point upward. The upper extremities are also stiff as they extend outward or forward. Occasionally, tonic postures are restricted to one or more of the extremities. Clonic activity consists of repetitive jerks at a rate of one to three per second. It is multifocal, migrating from one extremity to another in a disorganized fashion. In addition, facial twitches may be prominent. In a minority of instances, clonic seizures are focal; that is, they are restricted to one extremity, while unaccompanied by an altered state of consciousness. The distribution of localized tonic or clonic seizure activity bears no relationship to the location of lesions in the brain. Localized seizures are usually the result of diffuse cerebral disturbance.

Myoclonic seizures, rare in the neonate, are characterized by discrete gross jerks of one or more extremities. They are sometimes associated with abnormal eye movements and blinking.

Jitteriness is a rather frequent occurrence that must be differentiated from true seizures. Jitteriness is often benign and is most commonly associated with hyperactive and agitated states that are precipitated by hunger, thirst, or discomfort. If the infant's neurologic status is otherwise normal, jitteriness is not indicative of neurologic abnormality. However, jitters may be a sign of serious disorders such as hypocalcemia, hypoglycemia, drug withdrawal, and hypoxic-ischemic encephalopathy. Jitteriness is characterized by rapid alternating movements of equal amplitude in both directions. In contrast, clonic movements during true seizures have a fast and slow component and are not usually so rapid. Jitteriness can be stimulated by a disturbance of any kind and it can be eliminated by gently touching or flexing an involved extremity. Seizures are rarely initiated by disturbances. Furthermore, jitteriness is not associated with any of the subtle signs of seizure activity such as blinking or abnormal ocular motion.

Once the infant's abnormal movements are identified as seizures, the need to demonstrate etiologic factors becomes urgent. The clinical entities that produce seizures are numerous, but they can be grouped into five categories:

Perinatal difficulties (asphyxia, trauma)
Metabolic disorders
Infectious diseases
Drug withdrawal
Congenital malformations of the brain

Perinatal difficulties, primarily those that occur during labor and delivery, are the most frequent causes of neonatal seizures. Intrauterine asphyxia is responsible for most cases of hypoxic-ischemic encephalopathy. In most instances prenatal asphyxia is caused by maternal difficulties or placental abnormalities. In a minority, traumatic labor and delivery is causative, such as occurs from prolonged labor with transverse arrest, high forceps extraction, breech presentation, or difficult manual extraction. Low Apgar scores of infants who have experienced intrauterine asphyxia reflect a continuation of the misadventure that began in utero. Trauma generally causes cerebral contusion, which is most frequent in term infants. Subarachnoid hemorrhage and skull fractures occur less frequently; subdural hematoma is now rare. Intraventricular hemorrhage is virtually always a disorder of premature infants. It is a sequel to asphyxia, and seizures appear approximately 6 hours after the hemorrhage (Chapter 2).

Hypoglycemia and hypocalcemia are the principal metabolic disorders that produce seizures. Others that occur less frequently are the aminoacidurias, bilirubin encephalopathy (kernicterus), hypernatremia or hyponatremia; and drug withdrawal (narcotics and alcohol). Hypoglycemia is usually defined as a blood glucose level less than 20 mg/dl in premature babies and less than 30 mg/dl in term infants. However, most hospital laboratories perform glucose determinations in serum rather than whole blood, and hypoglycemic levels in serum are higher. Hypoglycemia occurs at serum levels of 25 mg/dl in premature infants and at 35 mg/dl in term infants. The longer the duration of hypoglycemia, the more likely is seizure activity. Most hypoglycemic infants are asymptomatic. Among symptomatic babies, approximately 20% manifest some type of seizure activity. Immediate diagnosis by Dextrostix is the method of choice, but laboratory determination of glucose levels must be performed to verify the results of the Dextrostix.

Hypocalcemia is defined by a serum calcium less than 7 mg/dl. The incidence of hypocalcemia clusters around the first 2 or 3 days and again at 6 to 10 days of age. The latter group of infants are usually born at term and are given milk preparations that contain an inappropriate calcium-phosphorus ratio. In recent years, late onset hypocalcemia has become infrequent because of widespread use of proprietary formulas that contain a higher calcium-phosphorus ratio. Early onset hypocalcemia occurs in infants who have experienced perinatal stress. In them, low serum calcium concentrations are associated with other factors such as asphyxia, trauma, and hypotension. In such circumstances the role of hypocalcemia in the causation of seizures can be established only if seizures disappear within minutes following intravenous administration of calcium solution. Such is rarely the case in early onset hypocalcemia.

The infectious diseases that produce neonatal seizures (Chapter 13) are those that include meningitis and encephalitis. Bacterial infections predominate and among them *E. coli* and group B streptococcal septicemia with meningitis are the most common. Both these organisms are usually acquired by the fetus from the mother during the birth process. Thus clinical signs of disease usually appear within 5 days of age. However, bacterial meningitis may begin at any time during the nursery stay if the infant is inoculated from the environment or by personnel carriers. Other etiologic agents of infectious disease include the nonbacterial group (toxoplasma, rubella virus, cytomegalovirus, and coxsackievirus). Seizures occur in affected babies by virtue of the encephalitis produced by these agents.

The two underlying disorders that most urgently require specific diagnosis are hypoglycemia and bacterial infection. Dextrostix for blood sugar will adequately determine the presence of the former; immediate examination of spinal fluid for cells and organisms will demonstrate the latter. Hypoglycemic levels demonstrated by Dextrostix should be verified by laboratory determination of calcium, sodium, potassium, and magnesium. Variations in the infant's history and physical findings may indicate additional determinations or delete others.

Management of the convulsing infant is composed of specific therapy for metabolic disorders (hypoglycemia, hypocalcemia, hypomagnesemia) and for bacterial infection. It is also composed of anticonvulsant medication and supportive therapy for adequate respiratory function, hydration, electrolyte balance, and body temperature. When seizures first appear, we determine the presence of hypoglycemia by Dextrostix and draw blood for glucose, calcium, phosphorus, and magnesium. If the Dextrostix indicates normoglycemia, we administer phenobarbital as described below.

For hypoglycemia we infuse 2 to 4 ml of 25% glucose intravenously over a period of approximately 5 minutes. This is followed by continuous administration of a solution that provides 0.5 g to 0.8 g/kg of glucose per hour, depending on the results of repeated Dextrostix and laboratory determinations of glucose levels. Anticonvulsant medication is not indicated for treatment of hypoglycemia.

Specific therapy for hypocalcemia is instituted only after serum calcium levels are known. We administer 150 mg to 200 mg/kg of calcium gluconate intravenously (3 to 4 ml/kg of a 5% solution) over a period of approximately 10 minutes. Heart rate is monitored by a cardiotachometer during the infusion of calcium. A sudden fall in heart rate requires that calcium administration be halted. *Hypocalcemia rarely, if ever, causes seizures during the 48 to 72 hours following birth.* If seizures are severe and continuous, we use phenobarbital when calcium administration cannot be continued. Late onset hypocalcemia is frequently associated with hypomagnesemia which, if untreated, will cause persistence of the convulsive state despite calcium therapy. Magnesium sulfate is given intramuscularly in a dose of 0.2 ml/kg/24 h as a 50% solution. Overdoses of magnesium may produce severe muscle paralysis by virtue of the curare-like effect that the magnesium ion produces.

Phenobarbital is the anticonvulsant drug of choice. In the absence of hypoglycemia or hypocalcemia, we give an initial intravenous dose of 15 to 20 mg/kg. If seizures have not subsided in 30 minutes, the same dose is repeated. Thereafter, phenobarbital is maintained at 5 mg/kg/24 h in divided doses every 12 hours. Convulsions caused by perinatal asphyxia are notoriously difficult to control; maintenance doses of phenobarbital up to 10 mg/kg may be required. Phenobarbital is often ineffective.

We do not use diazepam to control seizures because phenobarbital is effective, the effect of diazepam is relatively transient, and diazepam may cause vascular collapse, particularly when used with phenobarbital. Furthermore, the vehicle in which the drug is administered contains sodium benzoate, which displaces bilirubin from its albumin binding sites. The result is a vulnerability to kernicterus because of the increased quantity of free bilirubin that has become unbound from albumin.

HYDROCEPHALUS

Hydrocephalus is an abnormal physical finding that is produced by a number of underlying disorders. It is characterized by the accumulation of cerebrospinal fluid (CSF) within the ventricular

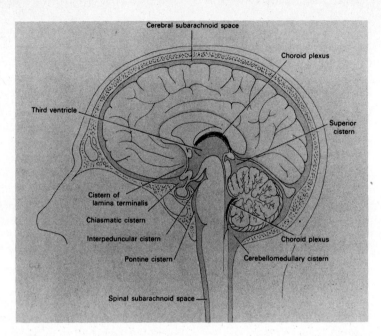

Fig. 14-1. Midline view of the brain showing the ventricles and the subarachnoid space in the shaded area. The two choroid plexuses are in the third (uppermost) and fourth ventricles. Spinal fluid flows from the choroid plexus into the ventricles within the brain to the subarachnoid space that envelops its external surfaces. (From Carpenter, M. B.: Human neuroanatomy, Baltimore, 1976, The Williams & Wilkins Co.)

system secondary to an obstruction of normal flow. Intraventricular pressure rises; the ventricles become distended. Ultimately, distention of the ventricles progresses, and within days or weeks enlargement of the head is obvious. At this point the anterior fontanelle is tight and bulging; the skull sutures are widened.

Cerebrospinal fluid is generated by the choroid plexus and by the brain substance as well. It is produced at an average rate of 0.4 ml/min, ranging from 0.26 to 0.65 ml/min. Normally, fluid flows from the lateral ventricles into the third ventricle after passing through the foramen of Monro. From the third ventricle it enters the aqueduct and proceeds to the fourth ventricle, from which it leaves the ventricular system by passing through the foramina of Luschka and Ma-

gendie. Fluid next flows over the convex surfaces of the cerebral hemispheres within the subarachnoid space and is returned to the sagittal sinus to reenter the bloodstream (Figs. 14-1 and 14-2).

Obstruction to the flow of spinal fluid may occur anywhere along the pathway just described. The obstruction may be caused by tumor, blood clot, adhesions, or congenital malformations, and it may be located within the ventricles or outside them. In the neonate, hydrocephalus occurs most frequently as a sequel to intraventricular hemorrhage and bacterial meningitis. In both instances the obstruction is a result of residual adhesions from the initial disease process. Ventricular dilatation following IVH is most often a *communicating hydrocephalus*. The points of obstruction are diffusely distributed in the subarachnoid space

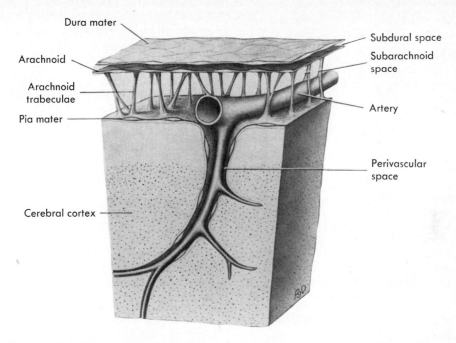

Fig. 14-2. The subarachnoid space is shown in relationship to the external surface of the brain, the blood vessels, and the meninges. (From Carpenter, M. B.: Human neuroanatomy, Baltimore, 1976, The Williams & Wilkins Co.)

rather than the ventricles, foramina, or aqueduct of Sylvius.

Hydrocephalus produces only one early clinical sign—enlargement of the head. If other neurologic abnormalities are evident, they are the result of the underlying disorder that caused the hydrocephalus. Head enlargement is also produced by a number of other entities such as subdural hematoma, porencephaly, hydranencephaly, and achondroplasia. The spurt in growth that occurs following adequate feeding of a malnourished infant is often characterized by transient rapid enlargement of head.

The most reliable diagnostic procedure is the CT scan. Ultrasound scans at the bedside will in the future provide a more convenient and rapid method for demonstration of ventricular enlarge-

ment. If the remaining cerebral cortex is thin, transillumination of the skull (Chapter 6) can demonstrate the accumulated fluid.

The treatment of hydrocephalus is generally unsatisfactory. Pharmacologic therapy, whether aimed at diminishing the production of cerebrospinal fluid or withdrawing it from the ventricular system into the bloodstream, has not been successful. Surgical treatment is currently the most acceptable approach, despite its difficulties. It consists of the placement of a shunt from the ventricles into the peritoneal space or the heart. This provides an ongoing run-off for excessive intraventricular fluid. Shunts in small infants must generally be revised later as their growth proceeds. The shunting catheters frequently become obstructed, and they also may become infected at either the intracranial or distal end. Despite these complications, there is unfortunately no better method available for the management of hydrocephalus.

There is equivocal evidence that in the presence of communicating hydrocephalus, repeated lumbar punctures, performed every other day, prevent or ameliorate ventricular dilatation. The efficacy of this therapy is not firmly established at present.

BIBLIOGRAPHY

Beverley, D. W., Chance, G. W., Inwood, M. J., et al.: Intraventricular haemorrhage and haemostasis defects, Arch. Dis. Child. **59**:444, 1984.

Brann, A. W., Jr., and Schwartz, J. F.: Central nervous system disturbances. In Fanaroff, A. A., and Martin, R. J.: Behrman's neonatal-perinatal medicine, ed. 3, St. Louis, 1983, The C. V. Mosby Co.

Elliott, D.: Ultrasonography of the neonatal brain. In Sarnat, H. B., editor: Topics in neonatal neurology, Orlando, Fla., 1984, Grune and Stratton.

Fitzhardinge, P. M.: Complications of asphyxia and their therapy. In Gluck, L., editor: Intrauterine asphyxia and developing fetal brain, Chicago, 1977, Year Book Medical Publishers.

Hill, A., and Rozdilsky, B.: Congenital hydrocephalus secondary to intrauterine germinal matrix/intraventricular haemorrhage, Dev. Med. Child. Neurol. **26**:524, 1984.

Horwitz, S. J., and Amiel-Tison, C.: Neurologic problems. In Klaus, M. H., and Fanaroff, A. A., editors: Care of the high risk neonate, Philadelphia, 1979, W. B. Saunders Co.

Krishnamoorthy, K. S., Shannon, D. C., DeLong, G. R., et al.: Neurologic sequelae in the survivors of neonatal intraventricular hemorrhage, Pediatrics **64**:233, 1979.

Levene, M. I., and DeVries, L.: Extension of neonatal intraventricular haemorrhage, Arch. Dis. Child. **59**:631, 1984.

McDonald, M. M., Johnson, M. L., Rumack, C. M., et al.: Role of coagulopathy in newborn intracranial hemorrhage, Pediatrics **74**:26, 1984.

McGuinness, G. A., and Smith, W. L.: Head ultrasound screening in premature neonates weighing more than 1,500 g at birth, Am. J. Dis. Child. **138**:817, 1984.

Ment, L. R., Duncan, C. C., Ehrenkranz, R. A., et al.: Intraventricular hemorrhage in the preterm neonate: timing and cerebral blood flow changes, J. Pediatr. **104**:419, 1984.

Mitchell, W., and O'Tuama, L.: Cerebral intraventricular hemorrhages in infants: a widening age spectrum, Pediatrics **65**:35, 1980.

Palma, P. A., Miner, M. E., Morriss, F. H., et al.: Intraventricular hemorrhage in the neonate born at term, Am. J. Dis. Child. **133**:941, 1979.

Papile, L.-A., Burstein, J., Burstein, R., and Koffler, H.: Incidence and evolution of subependymal and intraventricular hemorrhage: a study of infants with birth weights less than 1500 gm, J. Pediatr. **92**:529, 1978.

Seay, A. R., and Bray, P. F.: Significance of seizures in infants weighing less than 2500 grams, Arch. Neurol. **34**:381, 1977.

Szymonowicz, W., Schafler, K., Cussen, L. J., and Yu, V. Y. H.: Ultrasound and necropsy study of periventricular haemorrhage in preterm infants, Arch. Dis. Child. **59**:637, 1984.

Szymonowicz, W., and Yu, V. Y. H.: Timing and evolution of periventricular haemorrhage in infants weighing 1250 g or less at birth, Arch. Dis. Child. **59**:7, 1984.

Szymonowicz, W., Yu, V. Y. H., and Wilson, F. E.: Antecedents of periventricular haemorrhage in infants weighing 1250 g or less at birth, Arch. Dis. Child. **59**:13, 1984.

Vannucci, R. C., and Voorhies, T. M.: Perinatal cerebral hypoxia-ischemia: pathogenesis and neuropathology. In Sarnat, H. B., editor: Topics in neonatal neurology, Orlando, Fla., 1984, Grune and Stratton.

Volpe, J. J.: Perinatal hypoxic-ischemic brain injury, Pediatr. Clin. North Am. **23**:383, 1976.

Volpe, J. J.: Observing the infant in the early hours after asphyxia. In Gluck, L., editor: Intrauterine asphyxia and the developing fetal brain, Chicago, 1977, Year Book Medical Publishers.

Volpe, J. J.: Neonatal intracranial hemorrhage: pathophysiology, neuropathology, and clinical features, Clin. Perinatol. **4**:77, 1977.

Volpe, J. J.: Neonatal periventricular hemorrhage: past, present, and future, J. Pediatr. **92**:693, 1978.

Voorhies, T. M., and Vannucci, R. C.: Perinatal cerebral hypoxia-ischemia: diagnosis and management. In Sarnat, H. B., editor: Topics in neonatal neurology, Orlando, Fla., 1984, Grune and Stratton.

CHAPTER 15

Impact of intensive care on the parent-infant relationship

Jean Lancaster

The development of an affectionate, nurturing, and reciprocal relationship between infant and parent is essential for a healthy psychologic outcome. Recent studies have increased our understanding of the psychologic response and emotional stresses experienced by families of newborn infants who require intensive care. The anticipated feelings and excitement at the birth of a healthy child are shattered. Parents are overwhelmed by the emotions of grief at a time when the intensification of attachment behaviors between parent and infant is expected. The purpose of this chapter is to discuss how the birth of a high-risk infant affects the family and to offer suggestions for intervention during the crisis period.

ATTACHMENT BEHAVIORS

Recent studies have increased our understanding of the early development of parent-infant relationships; however, the precise process of attachment is unknown. Attachment refers to the quality of affectional ties between parents and their infant that begin to develop early in pregnancy, appear to increase when fetal movement is felt, and are intensified with seeing, touching, and caring for the infant after birth.

Attachment behaviors are intensified immediately after birth when both parents and infant engage in reciprocal interactions. During the first hour of life, the newborn is alert, makes eye-to-eye contact, and begins to feed. The parents interact with their newborn through touch, eye-to-eye contact, and talking to the infant in high-pitched tones of voice.

Parents first use touch to become acquainted with their baby, and later use it to express love. They systematically explore the infant's body with their fingertips, gradually using palms of their hands, and finally holding him close to their body. Parents of term infants will often complete this process within 10 minutes. Parents who have sick or premature infants often express difficulty in believing that they have a child. Yet when these parents have contact with their babies, they use the same touching behaviors as those for terms infants, but proceed at a slower pace.

Reciprocal eye-to-eye contact between parents and their children is a powerful elicitor of parental affection. Similarly, the performance of caretaking activities and the derivation of satisfaction from the child both seem to be necessary preludes to the development of love.

It is apparent that the moments after birth are exquisitely sensitive for the *initiation* of attachment. In recent years the long- and short-term benefits of this encounter between parent and child have acquired a mystic aura of indispensability. Even more than that, there is a pervasive persuasion among the laity and professionals that absence of this early contact inflicts irrevocable maternal disaffection, which in turn ultimately influences the attitude of the child. It is unfortunate that a simple, understandable, and natural desire to experience the sheer joy of first contact after birth has become complicated by the idea that nothing will ever be right if for any reason these moments are missed. They are indeed missed when the neonate requires resuscitation and when separation of parent and infant is unavoidable because intensive care must be instituted. Now, the unrealistic fear of future disaffection is added to the guilt and grief of giving birth to a troubled baby. We have observed this phenomenon repeatedly in parents of premature infants. However desirable this early contact may be, we should advise parents that its absence does not preclude a normal relationship in the future. The attachment of parent and child is ongoing and dynamic. In normal circumstances it is highly resistant to permanent disruption.

GRIEF

For families who deliver an infant who requires intensive care, there is a period of time when they suffer psychological estrangement from their high-risk newborn and are overwhelmed by the emotions of a grief reaction. Their grief and subsequent pain are over the loss of the normal child they anticipated during pregnancy, and the realization that their baby is "less than perfect." This crisis period may delay, distort, or preclude parental attachment to their infant unless they are assisted in dealing with their emotional stresses.

To therapeutically assist parents in working through this grief process, health professionals must understand it and must be able to identify and interpret behavior patterns that parents should anticipate.

Grief is a normal and characteristic response to the loss of, or separation from, a significant person that occurs over time. It creates emotional and physical pain. Uncomplicated grief seems to run a predictable course; it is influenced by the abruptness of the loss, preparation for the loss, and the relationship between the survivor and the lost object. Grief includes an initial period of shock that is usually followed by either denial or panic. Essentially, the same sequence of events occurs during grief caused by death, premature birth, or birth of a severely handicapped infant.

Denial is a defense mechanism that cushions the impact of loss and has been called a "human shock absorber" to tragedy. Emotions are temporarily defused; the sense of time is suspended in an attempt to delay the impact of loss. This emotional detachment allows a bereaved individual some time to organize inner resources and to search for an appropriate response to the devastating event. Yet the expression of denial is often inconsistent. To the physician, for example, the parents may exhibit vehement denial when told their infant is critically ill. Thus, after being informed, the mother may say: "My baby will be ready to go home with me when I am discharged from the hospital." On the other hand, she may talk openly with the social worker. Apparently, grieving parents often find it inappropriate to share their hurt with the physician (or perhaps the nurse as well) who must care for their child; they fear that their own pessimism will influence the treatment that is provided. They feel safer divulging their deep feelings with staff members who are not directly involved in medical care.

In response to their loss, some parents panic. When stability is disrupted by the loss of a significant relationship, emotional expressions often have no limit. Panic is manifested by intense anxiety, excitement, or paranoid ideas. Panic can usually be minimized if calm and authoritative management is provided by a responsible professional—nurse, physician, or social worker. A person in panic is desperately seeking resources to restore order to inner chaos.

As shock and denial are replaced by awareness of reality, strong feelings of anger, guilt, shame, and helplessness emerge. Crying, sleep disturbances, loss of interest in daily activities, and somatic symptoms of distress and pain are commonly experienced. The absence of crying may well predispose the mourner to pathological grief. Crying seems to involve the recognition of the loss and allows one to be comforted. If these feelings are not openly expressed, perhaps because of strong inhibitions for any number of reasons, anger is sealed within, guilt evolves, and release from shock is experienced as severe depression. Depression is a response to loss; it is a device for coping. Depression often signals a need to verbalize suppressed fear and anxiety. Recovery is impeded when we do not interpret such behavior accurately. An environment must be provided to allow verbalization of feelings. Short-term depression is a normal response to loss. Its absence indicates an abnormal coping behavior. The grieving parents must externalize their feelings of anger, guilt, and disappointment.

Parents' attempts to make sense of their loss are often manifested in such questions as: "Why me? What did I do wrong? Why did God let my baby die?" Behind these questions are anxiety, poor self-image, and a desperate desire for someone who cares enough to listen to their real fears. We must be open and honest; we should encourage verbalization, rather than restrain it. Parents' questions must be answered to avoid further guilt, which will delay the mourning process.

Finally, the grieving person enters the phase of acceptance and recovery when grief continues, but the trauma of loss is gradually overcome and a state of equilibrium is once again established. This period of grief is trying for parents, particularly those whose infants have major abnormalities or do not survive. Many parents feel that the

grief has been resolved, only to find themselves depressed and their daily routines hampered by exhaustion. Family and friends fail to recognize that grief takes months to resolve. They often unknowingly abandon the grieving family after the initial crisis. Many parents express the fear that the revitalization of their feelings indicates that they have lost control or that they will never be able to resolve the loss. This is a time when parents need to communicate openly with each other and with close friends. Group meetings, such as "graduate parents," Parents Experiencing Perinatal Death (Memphis, Tennessee), or groups for parents of infants with specific anomalies, are extremely helpful. At such meetings, communication with parents in similar situations provides effective support. Such communication also demonstrates that the behavior they fear in themselves is actually pervasive and normal and that in time the impact of their loss will diminish.

Although grieving is painful, it is necessary for a healthy outcome. An indication that grieving has been resolved is the ability of parents to remember comfortably both pleasure and disappointments of the relationship. In the extreme, failure to mourn a significant loss is associated with long-term depression, psychosomatic illness, and other pathologic consequences.

PREMATURE BIRTH

The long-awaited physical contact with a newborn, the anticipated interaction, and the provision of nurturing care to their offspring are all fantasies of parents-to-be and are all abruptly terminated by the birth of a sick, premature infant. Fears for the survival and intactness of the child are paramount. The parents experience the loss of the perfect child of their dreams, as well as the blow to their self-esteem because the child they have created is imperfect. Their grief is different from that of parents whose infant has died. They must surrender the baby of their dreams to form a relationship with their real child, who may be normal or handicapped. If the baby's survival is in doubt, the parents may be reluctant to invest in a relationship. Anticipatory grief is evident at this time. Study and experience have documented the pervasiveness of anticipatory grieving by parents of infants transferred to a regional neonatal center. Parents prepare themselves for the death of their infant, while at the same time continuing to hope that their baby will live. In our experience the most common manifestation of anticipatory grief is delayed naming of the baby until survival is assured. In the presence of electronic monitors, catheters, and other forbidding equipment, it is understandably difficult for parents to focus on their baby; their attention is fixed on the equipment and the threatened loss that it symbolizes.

The work of anticipatory grief can be accelerated by frequent visiting and providing specific caretaking activities for the parents. Yet in many instances, initiation of a close relationship with the baby is unlikely until the parents are convinced that a favorable outcome is certain.

Working with parents of premature infants

The ultimate goals of our work with parents of premature infants are (1) to foster the development of attachment to their infant and (2) to minimize the psychosocial disorganization of the family during and after the infant's hospitalization. Since the birth of a premature infant creates a sense of loss, attachment cannot be achieved totally until the parents have resolved their grief. To facilitate the grieving process and to enhance the reality of the living child, parents must be allowed to see their infant at the earliest opportunity, preferably at the time of delivery. Parents whose infant is to be transferred to another hospital should see the infant and meet at least one member of the transport team prior to transport. They must discuss the condition of their infant with members of the health care team. Parents need compassionate and knowledgeable personnel with whom they can share their fears and concerns without fear of being judged.

Prior to the parents' first visit, the nurse must prepare them for the baby's appearance and for the equipment in use. At the bedside, the func-

tion of each item and its role in promoting recovery should be explained. Comments about the baby's individuality are particularly helpful, and statements such as "He likes to hold my finger while I feed him" or "She is very active" will help the parents see their baby beyond the equipment. Phototherapy should always be temporarily discontinued and eye patches should be removed to permit eye-to-eye contact between parents and child. If the infant is too ill to open his eyes, parents need to be told this to avoid feelings of rejection.

The nurse must be present with the parents at the beginning of the visit. Later, parents should be left alone with their baby. Constant supervision and hovering by personnel tends to inhibit parenting responses such as touch and eye-to-eye contact. Some parents can tolerate only brief visits in the beginning because of the emotional pain experienced. When they indicate a need to leave, they should be reassured that their reactions are common and normal and that they are welcome to return at will.

For the mother who has been hospitalized elsewhere, we have found it helpful to send a picture of the baby. The picture provides some visual contact that is otherwise impossible. Fathers also find these helpful when explaining the care given to the baby at a regional center. Fathers are encouraged to be open and truthful in communicating with the mother. Withholding information about the infant's condition not only creates anxiety and distrust but increases communication failures between parents. Marital difficulties, which seem to be increased after the birth of a high-risk infant, are often associated with lack of communication between parents.

Parents are encouraged to call the nursery at any time to talk with the nurse who cares for their baby. Night hours are extremely stressful for parents; we receive many telephone calls between 10 p.m. and 1 a.m.

In our center, parents are encouraged to visit their babies and touch and fondle them while they are still very ill. We tell parents that the infant thrives on being touched, caressed, and talked to. In the case of a premature infant, the nurse must prepare parents for the generalized startle reaction to touch, instead of the expected localized physical response. They must also be informed about the lack of response of a depressed infant, regardless of maturity. For example, when the premature infant who is touched by his mother simply exhibits a Moro reflex and cries, the mother may perceive the response as displeasure. She should not be allowed to believe that she is unwanted by her baby, that her attention has been repelled. She should be told of this expected response to spare her the agony of a misinformed reaction.

Mothers who wish to breast feed should be encouraged to do so. Although the premature infant may be unable to nurse at the breast, mothers can be taught to express the milk, freeze it, and bring it to the center. Breast feeding offers the mother of the hospitalized premature infant an opportunity to provide something that no one else can.

Many of our parents bring pictures of the family, which are then taped to the side of the crib. Small, washable toys and music boxes are common in our infants' cribs. Parents should be encouraged to bring toys that are black, white, medium pink, or yellow in color because the infant will attend the object longer.

Parents are encouraged to participate in selected caretaking activities for their infant soon after birth. At first these activities may only include changing a diaper or cleaning the infant's mouth with a soft, wet sponge. However menial this task appears to the health professional, it is of great significance to the parents because it lessens their feelings of helplessness and facilitates the development of their parental role. As parents become more comfortable in handling their infant, they are engaged in other caretaking activities that elicit positive reinforcement of their endeavors. They must be protected from feelings of incompetence lest they withdraw from their baby. All parents are encouraged to feed and bathe their babies repeatedly before discharge. Since a mother may interpret poor feeding, sleeping during feeds, or regurgitation as indications of her own ineptness, she should be forewarned of the normal nature of these occurrences. The nurse should not immediately take the infant who feeds poorly from the mother and then feed the baby successfully in her presence. The resultant feelings of inadequacy and resentment are thus cruelly imposed on her already existing emotional difficulties. Rather, the nurse should help by demonstrating techniques such as gentle rotation of the nipple or stroking of the infant's cheek to initiate a sucking reflex.

Diminishing the impact of psychological separation is more difficult. Some understanding of the parents' feelings is prerequisite to any attempt to alleviate them. The physician, nurse, and social worker must assist parents in their attempts to deal with grief and accept the infant so they can become involved in his care. Consistency in communication is necessary to prevent parental misunderstanding. Communication failures often lead to a less than optimal adjustment to the crisis. Effective intervention and communication with parents requires observation of behavior and identification of the stage of grieving. Parents should know that their feelings are common. As previously stated, parents usually progress through shock, a developing awareness of reality, and finally an acceptance of reality. During the period of shock, they cannot comprehend what is said to them. A frequent claim by parents is that everything is unreal or dreamlike, and they may deny the reality of their predicament. It is important to realize that parents in this phase of grief can ill afford to be overwhelmed with too much information. An honest, simple explanation is all that is needed; it is certainly all they can understand at the moment. Problems at hand should be discussed; predicting problems such as jaundice, pneumothorax, retardation, or possible death must be avoided in an attempt to prevent completion of the grief process. Once the grief process is completed, parents must reestablish a relationship with a baby who is perceived as dead and buried; frequently the reestablishment of this relationship is never accomplished.

Active intervention into the grief process by describing reality, allowing the parents to see the infant, and encouraging them to express their feelings will assist their progress. They must not be pushed into discussing their feelings. With a developing awareness of reality, the parents move into the second stage of grief. They may be overcome with feelings of anger. Anger is often turned toward self and results in depression and an increased sense of guilt and shame. Parents may lash out at those who come to their aid. The mother may berate herself or her spouse for dreadful failure. Transfer of parental guilt and anger to medical and nursing staff is common. It is a great temptation for the staff to categorize such a parent as "difficult." As a result of this categorization, personnel withdraw from the family member in question; in fact, complete abandonment is not uncommon. Yet the parent has merely grasped at anger and hostility as an immediately available mode of coping with his or her catastrophe. No greater harm can be inflicted at that moment than abandonment by the only individuals who could be supportive and who could thereby avert a potentially long-term attitudinal difficulty. Parents must be encouraged to express these negative emotions, which indicate attempts to cope with a stressful situation. Only as feelings are externalized can one begin to move toward acceptance of reality, and only then can parents begin to establish a relationship with their baby.

One indication of progress is the development of an interest in the infant and his care. However, when parents ask the same questions over and over again in their struggle to grasp the situation, those who work with them should be genuinely concerned and patient. It is during this time that parents can first be taught to care for their infant and thus relate to him. Impatience with frequent questions may impede ultimate acceptance of their baby. Several studies have shown that par-

ents who exhibit little anxiety in relation to the child's prematurity or illness, who seek little information about their baby, and who are unable or unwilling to share their own fears and concerns are destined for a difficult, if not pathologic, relationship with their child. Identification of such behavior urgently requires parental counseling by others besides the nurse. A significant correlation between lack of interest and paucity of telephone calls and visits has been observed. Furthermore, the incidence of children who are destined for parental battering increases in the face of these signs of detachment or neglect.

If survival of the infant is in doubt, parents may emotionally prepare for death while simultaneously maintaining hope for survival. They may physically withdraw from their infant during such a crisis; yet they usually maintain contact by phone. They must begin to accept the reality of an uncertain prognosis. It is important for both parents to be accurately informed about the baby's condition. Cautious optimism must be used in counseling parents about their infant's condition. Informing them that death is a certainty or that mental retardation is a likelihood will be detrimental to the establishment of an acceptable relationship should the baby survive. Parents must not be allowed to develop unrealistic optimism, but close contact should nevertheless be encouraged. Close early contact with an infant who later dies does not cause a dangerous increase in grief among mothers with no history of emotional difficulty. The last stage of the grief process, acceptance of reality, may take several months and indeed may never be accomplished, particularly if the infant is handicapped.

Parents need frequent praise and reassurance as they learn to care for their baby. The nurse should guide the parent who has difficulty with a caretaking activity, rather than supplant them. The competence of the nurse may well discourage the parent from trying to learn. Mothers often express the feeling that their infants belong to them only after providing total care for the babies.

Nurses can evaluate the parents' emotional state by being alert to signs of tension, such as rapid breathing, muscle tension, perspiration, rapid or stilted conversation, and looking away from the infant. When parents are participating in care of their baby, their approach to touching and holding him often reveals a great deal about their emotional state. During the learning period, an unsure parent will handle the baby rather stiffly and awkwardly, tending to hold him away from the body. At first they prefer only to touch him with their fingertips rather than enfold him in their arms. A distant sort of handling and holding is often manifest during feeding. Parents who are at ease with their baby hold him closely, with his head resting in the crook of the elbow in proximity to, or touching, the breast. They usually hold him turned toward them, and they seek repeated eye contact with him. Both baby and parent are relaxed in a comfortable position. In contrast, the parents who are uneasy and anxious usually assume an awkward, uncomfortable position. The arm is stiff and it tires easily. In their insecurity they are preoccupied with the mechanics of the feeding process and thus make no attempt to establish eye contact with their infant. They seek reassurance from the nurse repeatedly and must receive positive responses from their baby, such as consuming all of the offered formula or sleeping postprandially. They are visibly upset if the baby fails to take all of the milk or if he regurgitates. This behavior reinforces feelings of incompetence and is often perceived as rejection. Eventually, with support from an adept nurse, these parents will develop a comfortable relationship with their baby.

An occasional parent, for one reason or another, fails to establish a firm attachment to the baby. They hold him on their knee with his head on the forearm but at a distance from the breast. The baby will likely be on his back or perhaps turned away from them. Instead of making eye contact, they gaze around the room, apathetic and disinterested. Because little attention is paid to the baby, the bottle is tilted incorrectly, so that the

nipple is filled with air rather than milk. These parents need counseling if they are ever to form a healthy relationship with their baby. Identifying such parents in the early phase of their relationship with the baby and referring them for help may prevent multiple problems in the future. It should be noted that most parents transiently exhibit some signs of discomfort with their babies; it is the predominant and persistent behavior patterns that are important.

As the parents become acquainted with their baby, they seek some indication that they are successfully meeting his needs. Relaxation, sleep, and successful feeding of the infant are the most common early signs of such success. Unfortunately, because of their biologic difficulties, high-risk babies are often at first unable to respond favorably to the parents' ministrations. Parents should thus be taught that this lack of response is not a reflection of poor parenting, so that the baby's inability to respond does not further jeopardize the relationship.

DEATH OF A NEWBORN

Until recently, few health professionals appreciated the depth of grief that is experienced by parents whose newborn infant dies. Studies indicate that parents' grief reactions from the death of a neonate are similar to those associated with the loss of an older child or adult.

The mourning response may begin immediately after death, it may be delayed, or it may be entirely absent if strong denial mechanisms exist. One long-term study demonstrated that one third of the mothers who experienced perinatal death developed severe psychiatric problems. Our personal experience suggests that mothers who do not see or touch their infant before death seem to have more difficulty in completing the grief process than those who did. The health professional's role must thus continue after death of the infant. The principal tasks are to facilitate the parents' acknowledgment of the death as a reality, to assure that grieving progresses to acceptance, and to be available to the parents during the resolution process. Several meetings with parents are usually required to accomplish these goals.

Parents should be informed of their infant's death in a quiet and private place. Privacy allows expression of emotions without inhibitions or fears of judgment by others. The events surrounding the death should be discussed in appropriate detail; parents' questions must be answered. They should be offered the opportunity to see and hold their infant after death because loss of the infant and resolution of the grief process seems to be enhanced thereby. Observations of 25 mothers who had touched, but never held, their infants have demonstrated the same behavior pattern after death that one sees when the baby is alive—touching the extremities with their fingertips, rubbing the extremities, trunk, and head, and finally embracing the infant. All these mothers, except one, embraced the infant, kissed the infant, and made very personal remarks expressing both love and sadness. At the end of the holding period, every mother remarked, "You can have him now," or "She is yours now." Apparently, as mothers hold their dead infants, their need to caress and identify is satisfied, denial is eliminated, and death becomes a reality.

Providing the family with a picture of their infant and a set of footprints is helpful for many parents in that it provides some tangible remembrance of the infant instead of just the emotional and physical pain experienced in response to loss.

Contact with parents should recur 2 to 3 weeks after the baby's death. The purpose of this visit is to answer questions concerning the death, review autopsy findings, evaluate their reaction to the loss, and help them understand their feelings and behavior. Many parents are concerned about losing control of their emotions and having feelings of impending insanity. Mere verbalization of these fears and assurance from the health professional that these are normal reactions often brings relief. The importance of encouraging ongoing communication between spouses and with their living children cannot be overemphasized. It is not unusual for husbands and wives to find themselves at different stages of grief. Marital difficulties are virtually unavoidable when husband and wife communicate poorly following the death of their baby. Parent groups are extremely helpful during the long grieving period.

The third scheduled contact with parents should occur some 2 to 3 months after the infant's death. The primary purpose of this contact is to make sure that the grieving process is moving toward acceptance. At this time, parents usually express feelings of depression, anger, and isolation. Depression indicates that death has become a reality. During this time, parents are beset with introspection regarding the meaning of life, death, religion, and the baby's care before death. Feelings of isolation are often magnified. Relatives and friends often incorrectly view parental return to routine activity as a sign of the termination of grief. The health professional who is aware of the length of the grieving process can be helpful to parents at this time by listening to their concerns and assuring them that their feelings, even though disturbing and painful, are normal in the resolution of their grief.

In some parents, pathologic grief reactions may be identified at this time. Symptoms include total denial of the loss, inappropriate hostility or cheerfulness, severe depression, psychosomatic disorders, and inability to cope. Recognition of the symptoms and referral for psychiatric assistance is indispensable.

In time, parents who have successfully worked through their anger and depression in response to their infant's loss will reach a stage of acceptance in which they are neither angry nor depressed. They simply accept the fact that the infant is dead. Periods of sadness are recurrent, particularly on special occasions such as birthdays and family holidays.

Sibling reactions

The death of a newborn infant produces a significant emotional response from siblings within a family. Behavior such as separation anxiety, enuresis, punishment-seeking, nightmares, and school problems occur in at least one child in approximately one half of all families who lose a child by death. The literature suggests that the change in parents' behavior toward the remaining children, rather than the death itself, has a greater effect on the child's response to the loss. Children often receive little help in dealing with loss because parents are so deeply concerned about their loss that they are unable to either recognize or respond to the child's feelings and behavior. Others just avoid the subject of death in an attempt to protect the child. The child senses the change in parental behavior. Failure to understand parents' reactions leaves the child with only fantasized interpretations, which can be terrifying.

Children's perceptions of death are influenced by their developmental level of abstract and concrete thinking, life experiences, and parents' response to loss. Thus it is essential that the health professional help the parents to understand how children in various age groups respond to death.

During the first three years of life, the child is relatively ignorant of death. Yet, interruptions of parents' interactions as a result of grieving will leave the child totally disorganized.

The toddler is egocentric. He is concerned with his own activity and needs. His actions and feelings reflect those of his parents because of his internalized image of his parents. When parents are anxious, the toddler is anxious and fearful. Inability to comprehend the sadness and change in parents' behavior often leaves him with his greatest fear, that of separation from his mother.

The preschool-age child (3 to 5 years of age) views death as a reversible state. It is a temporary separation, like going to sleep. He can recognize death, but believes the dead person can still breathe, eat, and has feelings. Questions such as "When will he come back?" "Can he breathe in that box?" supports the belief that the dead infant continues to have biologic function.

The preschool-age child is in a stage of development characterized by omnipotent and magical thinking. Therefore, he believes that his thoughts are sufficient to cause events. When death occurs in a newborn infant who may have been unwanted by a jealous sibling, anxiety and guilt are often manifested because the preschooler believes he had some responsibility for the infant's death.

The child is self-centered, and the whole world revolves around him. He can neither empathize with his parents' grief nor verbally express his feelings. Failure to comprehend the sadness expressed by parents and the decreased individualized attention he received prior to the baby's death threatens his security. Because death is viewed as separation from the family, the child's fears of being separated from his parents are manifested by increased crying and clinging behavior.

Children between the ages of 5 and 8 develop the concept that death is final and irreversible. Developmentally, they are sorting out impressions and discovering the laws of the universe and how they function. Their understanding of death demonstrates gradual awareness of how the universe operates. They learn that death is final. However, death is often personified in this age group. The thoughts of death are projected onto another person because the thought of himself dying is too threatening. Death is associated with evil thoughts, magical thinking, and darkness. The child may easily believe that a "death man" carried the baby away. Resentment toward his parents for spending time away from him when the baby was ill may increase his feelings of guilt and responsibility for the infant's death.

Children above the age of 9 have reached a level of understanding that death is inescapable and is the termination of life on this earth. Death becomes personal. It can happen to them as well as other people.

Implications for parents

Children of various age groups have different concepts of death. Because of the parents' emotional loss and the child's ability to understand the loss, parents find it difficult to explain the death of a neonate to the siblings. However, it is imperative that the child be helped to understand the loss, understand his parents' reactions, and to share his feelings regarding the loss.

Parents are encouraged to talk about the death and share their grief with the sibling. Children can accept reality; fantasized interpretations of parents behavior create anxiety and fears. Several studies suggest that the best explanation for children under age 8 will be those that are simple, concrete, and honest.

Correct terms should be used when talking about the death. Such terms as "the baby went to sleep" or "God took the baby to be one of his angels" creates a repertoire of confused feelings and should be avoided. The young child will be inquisitive and will want to know why or what made the baby die. A simple, honest explanation is all that is needed. After the parent talks to a sibling, he should ask the child to explain what he has been told. Open communication is essential to clear up any misconceptions concerning the death.

Unnecessary guilt and fear can be alleviated when parents tell the child that they are sad about the infant's death and not upset with them. Because a child of this age indulges in magical thinking, he must be told that no one was responsible for the baby's death.

Generous affection toward the siblings during the crisis period is essential. At a time when parents are emotionally upset, the child not only needs verbal assurance of being loved, but physical assurance as well by being hugged. The young child who cannot understand the parents' behavior certainly can understand the affection given to him. Parents often have difficulty in deciding if a child should attend a funeral service. Children need an explanation of what will happen at the funeral, and they should be encouraged to ask questions. Children should be included in this service only if they wish to attend. However, it is advisable that the child be accompanied by a person who can provide undivided attention to him. Participation in the funeral with the family not only helps to make the baby and his death real, but will help complete the grief process.

Following the death of a newborn infant, open communication, love, and affection with the siblings is essential. Without it, the family can be psychologically pulled apart.

CONGENITAL MALFORMATION

The birth of an infant with congenital malformations precipitates a major family crisis. The idealized, healthy infant has not materialized. Parental reactions are greatly influenced by the type of malformation, visibility of the malformation, social and personal values, and previous relationships with family and friends. Attitudes of health professionals toward the infant's defect also contribute to the parental response.

Mourning the loss of the "perfect" infant requires time; the process requires parents to gradually relinquish the dreams of their wished for child and to adapt to the handicapped baby who was born. Parents have little time to grieve their loss before demands are made to invest in a relationship with the imperfect child. Grief is complicated by preoccupation with demands of the child's physical care.

Parents of children with congenital anomalies need continuing support from a variety of professionals to deal with their shock and disappointment and to facilitate their long-term attachment. They should be gently informed of the infant's problems as soon as possible. Truthfulness with parents is essential to prevent increased anxiety. Allowing parents to see the infant helps to overcome denial and alleviate exaggerated and grotesque fantasies by providing the opportunity to discuss the normal characteristics of the infant. Images of the unseen are invariably worse than the actual problem. Early and frequent contact allows parents to become acquainted with the infant's features; usually the contact supports positive maternal feelings. This identification and initiation of a relationship is a major step in reducing the emotional turmoil associated with the birth of a handicapped child. Parental self-esteem is increased as they become involved in the care of their infant and as responses from the infant are appreciated.

Parents need to know the purpose of care rendered, what to expect from their infant, and community services that are available. Protracted counseling with parents is essential and is best accomplished by perinatal social workers. It is only by learning parents' fears and concerns that one can assess their stage of adaptation. Dealing with reality decreases the tendency of parents to deny their problems. Persistent denial should be avoided because it prolongs grief.

Mourning the birth of a handicapped child is an exhausting experience that cannot be hurried or denied. Parents need the opportunity to discuss all aspects of the child's condition and treatment. They should discuss their feelings in an uninhibiting environment; their role in caring for the infant must be active. With support, most parents identify many positive aspects of their infant, and they eventually provide the love and nurture that are fundamental to parent-infant attachment.

BIBLIOGRAPHY

Adler, C. S.: The meaning of death to children, Ariz. Med. **26:**266, 1969.

Averill, J. R.: Grief, its nature and significance, Psychol. Bull. **70:**721, 1968.

Barnard, M. U.: Supportive nursing care for the mother and newborn who are separated from each other, Am. J. Nurs. **1:**107, 1976.

Barnett, C. R., Leiderman, P., Grobstein, R., and Klaus, M.: Neonatal separation: the maternal side of interactional deprivation, Pediatrics **45:**197, 1970.

Beaton, J. L.: A systems model of premature birth: implications for neonatal intensive care, J.O.G.N. Nurs. **13:**173, 1984.

Benfield, D. G., Leib, S. A., and Reuter, J.: Grief response of parents after referral of the critically ill newborn to a regional center, N. Engl. J. Med. **294:**975, 1976.

Bibring, G. L.: Some considerations of the psychological processes in pregnancy, Psychoanal. Study Child. **14:**113, 1959.

Bowlby, J.: Processes of mourning, Int. J. Psychoanal. **42:**22, 1961.

Brazelton, T., Scholl, M., and Robey, J.: Visual responses in the newborn, Pediatrics **37:**284, 1966.

Cain, A. C., Fast, I., and Erikson, M. E.: Children's disturbed reactions to the death of a sibling, Am. J. Orthopsychiatry **34:**741, 1964.

Campbell, S. B. G., and Taylor, P. M.: Bonding and attachment: theoretical tissues, Sem. Perinatol. **3:**3, 1979.

Cohen, R. L.: Some maladaptive syndromes of pregnancy and the puerperium, Obstet. Gynecol. **27:**562, 1966.

Cullberg, J.: Mental reactions of women to perinatal death. In Morris, N., editor: Psychosomatic medicine in obstetrics and gynecology, New York, 1972, S. Karger.

D'Archy, E.: Congenital defects—mothers' reactions to first information, Br. Med. J. **3:**796, 1968.

Davidson, G. W.: Death of the wished-for child: a case study, Death Educ. **1:**265, 1977.

Davidson, G. W.: Living and dying, religion and medicine series, Minneapolis, 1975, Augsburg Publishing House.

De Chateau, P., and Wiberg, B.: Long-term effect on mother-infant behavior of extra contact during the first hour post partum. I. First observations at 36 hours. Acta. Paediatr. Scand. **66:**137, 1977.

De Chateau, P., and Wiberg, B.: Long-term effect on mother-infant behavior of extra contact during the first hour post partum. II. Follow-up at three months. Acta. Paediatr. Scand. **66:**145, 1977.

Deutsch, H.: The psychology of women: a psychoanalytic interpretation. II. Motherhood, New York, 1945, Grune and Stratton.

Drotar, D., Bashiewicz, A., Irvin, N., et al.: The adaptation of parents to the birth of an infant with a congenital malformation: a hypothetical model, Pediatrics **56:**710, 1975.

Dubois, D. R.: Indications of an unhealthy relationship between parents and premature infant, J. Obstet. Gynecol. Nurs. **4:**21, 1975.

DuHamel, T. R., Lin, S., Skelton, A., and Hantke, C.: Early parental perceptions and the high risk neonate, Clin. Pediatr. **13:**1052, 1974.

Eager, M., and Exoo, R.: Parents visiting parents for unequaled support, M.C.N. **5:**35, 1980.

Elliott, B. A.: Neonatal death: reflections for physicians, Pediatrics **62:**96, 1978.

Engle, G. L.: Is grief a disease? Psychosom. Med. **23:**18, 1961.

Fanaroff, A. A., Kennell, J. H., and Klaus, M.: Follow-up of low birth weight infants: the predictive value of maternal visiting patterns, Pediatrics **49:**287, 1972.

Friedman, S. B., Chodoff, P., Mason, J. W., et al.: Behavioral observations on parents anticipating the death of a child, Pediatrics **32:**610, 1963.

Funke, J., and Irby, M. I.: An instrument to assess the quality of maternal behavior, J. Obstet. Gynecol. Nurs. **7:**19, 1978.

Furman, E. P.: The death of a newborn: care of parents, Birth and Fam. J. **5:**214, 1978.

Gartley, W., and Bernasconi, M.: The concept of death in children, J. Genet. Psychol. **110:**71, 1967.

Gibson, J. J.: Observation of active touch, Psychol. Rev. **69:**477, 1962.

Giles, P. F. H.: Reactions of women to a perinatal death, Aust. N.Z.J. Obstet. Gynaecol. **10:**207, 1970.

Gilson, G. J.: Care of the family who has a lost a newborn, Postgrad. Med. **60:**67, 1976.

Green, M., and Solnit, A. J.: Reactions to the threatened loss of a child: a vulnerable child syndrome. III. Pediatric management of the dying child, Pediatrics 34:58, 1964.

Greenberg, M., and Morris, N.: Engrossment: the newborn's impact upon the father, Am. J. Orthopsychiatry 44:520, 1974.

Grollman, E. A.: Talking about death—a dialogue between parent and child, Boston, 1976, Beacon Press.

Hawkins-Walsh, E.: Diminishing anxiety in parents of sick newborns, M.C.N. 5:30, 1980.

Hersher, L., Richmond, J., and Moore, A.: Maternal behavior in sheep and goats. In Rheingold, H., editor: Maternal behavior in mammals, New York, 1963, John Wiley & Sons.

Jeffcoate, J. A.: Improving communication in a special care unit, Early Human Dev. 3/4:341, 1979.

Jewett, C. L.: Helping children cope with separation and loss, Harvard, Mass., 1982, Harvard Common Press.

Johnson, S. H., and Grubbs, J. P.: The premature infant's reflex behaviors: effect on the maternal-child relationship, J. Obstet. Gynecol. Nurs. 4:15, 1975.

Kaplan, D., and Mason, E.: Maternal reactions to premature birth viewed as an acute emotional disorder, Am. J. Orthopsychiatry 30:539, 1960.

Kennedy, J. C.: The high-risk maternal-infant acquaintance process, Nurs. Clin. North Am. 8:549, 1973.

Kennell, J. H., and Klaus, M. H.: Care of the mother of the high-risk infant, Clin. Obstet. Gynecol. 14:926, 1971.

Kennell, J. H., and Rolnick, A. R.: Discussing problems in newborn babies with their parents, Pediatrics 26:832, 1960.

Klaus, M. H., and Kennell, J. H.: Mothers separated from their newborn infants, Pediatr. Clin. North Am. 17:1015, 1970.

Klaus, M. H., Jerauld, R., Kreger, N. C., et al: Maternal attachment: importance of the first postpartum days, N. Engl. J. Med. 286:460, 1972.

Klaus, M. H., Kennell, J. H., Plumb, N., and Zuehike, S.: Human maternal behavior at the first contact with her young, Pediatrics 46:187, 1970.

Klopfer, P. H.: Mother love: what turns it on? Am. Sci. 59:404, 1971.

Lamb, M. E.: Early contact and maternal-infant bonding: one decade later, Pediatrics 70:763, 1982.

Leifer, A. D., Leiderman, P. H., Barnett, C. R., and Williams, J. A.: Effects of mother-infant separation on maternal attachment behavior, Child Dev. 43:1203, 1972.

Lindemann, E.: Symptomatology and management of acute grief, Am. J. Psychiatry 101:141, 1944.

Mandelbaum, A.: The group process in helping parents of retarded infants, Children 14:227, 1967.

Manguiten, H. H., Slade C., and Fitzsimons, D.: Parent-parent support in the care of high-risk newborns, J. Obstet. Gynecol. Nurs. 8:275, 1979.

Mason, E. A.: A method of predicting crisis outcome for mothers of premature babies, Public Health Rep. 78:1031, 1963.

McKeever, P. T.: Fathering the chronically ill child, M.C.N. 6:124, 1981.

Mercer, R. T.: Mother's response to their infants with defects, Nurs. Res. 23:133, 1974.

Minde, K. Trehub, S., et al.: Mother-child relationships in the premature nursery: an observational study, Pediatrics 61:373, 1978.

Miya, T. M.: The child's perception of death, Nurs. Forum 2:215, 1972.

Myers, B. A.: The informing interview, Am. J. Dis. Child. 137:572, 1983.

Nagy, M.: The child's theories concerning death, J. Genet. Psychol. 73:3, 1948.

Nystrom, C.: What happens when we die? Chicago, 1981, Moody Press.

O'Connor, S., Vietze, P., Hopkins, J., et al.: Post partum extended maternal-infant contact: subsequent mothering and child health, Pediatr. Res. 11:380, 1977.

Owens, C.: Parents' reactions to defective babies, Am. J. Nurs. 64:83, 1964.

Parkes, C.: Bereavement and mental illness. Part I. A clinical study of the grief of bereaved psychiatric patients, Br. Med. J. Psychol. 38:1, 1965.

Poznanski, E. O.: The "replacement child": a saga of unresolved parental grief, J. Pediatr. 81:1190, 1972.

Raphael, D.: The tender gift: breastfeeding, Englewood Cliffs, N. J., 1973, Prentice Hall.

Robson, K. S.: The role of eye-to-eye contact in maternal-infant attachment, J. Child Psychol. Psychiatry 8:13, 1967.

Rowe, J., Clyman, R., Green, C., et al.: Follow up of families who experience a perinatal death, Pediatrics 62:166, 1978.

Rubenstein, J.: Maternal attentiveness and subsequent exploratory behavior in the infant, Child Dev. 38:1089, 1967.

Rubin, R.: Basic maternal behavior, Nurs. Outlook 9:683, 1961.

Rubin, R.: Maternal touch, Nurs. Outlook 11:828, 1963.

Saylor, Rev. D. F.: Nursing response to mothers of stillborn infants, J. Obstet. Gynecol. Nurs. 6:39, 1977.

Schowalter, J. E.: How do children and funerals mix? J. Pediatr. 89:139, 1976.

Schraeder, B. D.: Attachment and parenting despite lengthy intensive care, M.C.N. 5:37, 1980.

Seigler, M.: Pascals' Wager and the hanging of crepe, N. Engl. J. Med. 293:853, 1975.

Shogan, M.: Intensively caring, Crit. Care Nurse 4:34, 1984.

Solnit, A., and Stark, M.: Mourning the birth of a defective child, Psychoanal. Study Child 16:523, 1961.

Taylor, P. M., and Hall, B. L.: Parent-infant bonding: problems and opportunities in a perinatal center, Sem. Perinatol. 3:73, 1979.

Ujhely, G. B.: Grief and depression: implications for preventive and therapeutic nursing care, Nurs. Forum 5:23, 1966.

Vredevelt, P. W.: Empty arms, Portland, Ore., 1984, Multnomak Press.

Weston, D. L., and Irvin, R. C.: Preschool child's response to death of infant sibling, Am. J. Dis. Child. 106:564, 1963.

CHAPTER 16

Organization and functions of a neonatal special care facility

PERSPECTIVE

Advanced diagnostic and therapeutic techniques have resulted in the evolution of specialized facilities for the care of sick neonates. Prior to the 1960s, infants were admitted to a term or a premature nursery. Infected babies were admitted to a separate, irregularly staffed nursery that was reserved solely for contagious disease. Uninfected sick infants were managed in the premature or term nursery to which they were originally admitted. In many hospitals an observation nursery was set aside for infants with unproved but suspected infection. Postoperative neonates were treated in surgical areas along with children of all ages and, in many instances, with adults as well.

The contemporary special care facility arose in response to an awareness of the singular characteristics of perinatal disorders. A newly acquired understanding of pathophysiologic phenomena during this period of life, and the capacity to apply this knowledge clinically, required an appropriate setting in which the severely ill baby could be managed. These developments occurred simultaneously with advances in electronics and biochemistry. Practical methods for the evaluation of numerous crucial parameters of fetal and neonatal illness were thus made available. Continuous monitoring of cardiorespiratory function became a reality. The performance of multiple biochemical determinations on minute quantities of blood was facilitated by new microtechniques. Conservation of body heat became feasible with the availability of radiant heaters and servocontrolled incubators. With confidence in improved methods for the control of infection, a direct impetus was provided for housing all medically and surgically ill infants in a common area, whether they were premature or mature, infected or noninfected. This approach revolutionized requirements of nursery architecture, fixtures, and equipment. Furthermore, a need was created for specially

419

trained personnel in several disciplines who must function cohesively if lives were to be saved.

The allocation of one nursery for prematures and another for term infants gave way to a facility in which personnel and equipment were concentrated for the treatment of all sick neonates, regardless of their maturity. Several small rooms for six to eight infants each were replaced by fewer and larger rooms or by a straightforward unicameral arrangement. Environmental considerations were primarily geared to optimal performance of personnel. Deployment of beds, cabinets, and counters were planned to accommodate lifesaving equipment and to facilitate nursing activity. The intensity and spectrum of light were aimed at undistorted visual evaluation by personnel; a neutral color for walls was recommended to avoid distortion of infants' skin tones, particularly for evaluation of cyanosis, jaundice, and pallor. Avoidance of excessive noise was considered essential because of its disturbing effect on the nursery staff.

These early considerations, still valid in the 1980s, were extended to include the direct effects of environmental factors on the infant. In addition to an interest in the tone and intensity of light for visual monitoring, there arose an added interest in the lack of circadian variation and its effect on infant behavior. To anxiety about the disturbing effect of noise on personnel was added concern for its potential to impair infant hearing (American Academy of Pediatrics, 1974). Moreover, recent observations have suggested that excessive noise is an unrecognized cause of hypoxemia. Thus the approach to physical factors in the nursery environment has evolved from a primary concern for personnel function to concern about direct effects on the infant. A single exception to this evolutionary pattern was the early interest in thermal environment and its influence on the infant's capacity to maintain body temperature.

The importance of physical factors in the environment has been further expanded to include ecologic considerations—the interplay among personnel, between personnel and babies, and between both of them and the physical environment. Thus an enlarging literature describes, analyzes, and speculates on the emotional stress experienced by caretakers in the newborn intensive care unit, particularly among nurses and, less frequently, among social workers and physician trainees. There are also reports on fatigue associated with the long working hours of physician trainees—its effect on the quality of care and on the trainees themselves.

The effects of tactile stimulation on infants have been explored during recent years. We first focused attention on the frequency with which babies were disturbed within a 24-hour period. A daily mean of 132 hands-on events among 11 infants was recorded. The results showed that sick infants were thoughtlessly disturbed more often than was necessary and certainly more often than had been the case with sick adults. A later study demonstrated the significance of frequent disturbance more concretely than we did. The disturbances in this study were associated with hypoxemic episodes. Hypoxemia was considerably more frequent as handling of the infant increased; 75% of the total time in hypoxemia was associated with handling of infants by personnel.

The paucity of stimulation from the environment of intensive care units was deplored in publications that appeared during the early 1970s. However, later more accurate assessments concluded that there was indeed an abundance of stimulation from light, noise, and touch, but that these "stimuli" were purposeless, unplanned, and disorganized. They did not stimulate; they merely disturbed.

Although survival is an obvious end point by which to gauge the success of vigorous efforts, *intact* survival is the overriding consideration. There is good reason to assume that diminished mortality and decreased incidence of central nervous system damage among survivors go hand in hand. The factors that contribute to perinatal mortality may, if present to a less severe degree, result in central nervous system dysfunction rather than death. By minimizing the effects of these factors, diminished mortality is probably associated with a decreased incidence of dysfunctional survival.

Do mortality rates decrease when intensive care is applied? In the early assessments there was excellent evidence that they did indeed. In the Province of Quebec, among hospitals with special care units or with access to them by transfer of sick infants, mortality during the first week of life was approximately half that of hospitals without such services. Similar benefits have been reported from Nova Scotia and from several large centers in the United States. In Arizona the mortality rate of babies with hyaline membrane disease who were *not* transported to an intensive care unit was 59% (1967 to 1970); among those who *were* transported the mortality rate was 32%. In the same state, in intensive care institutions themselves, the mortality rate of babies between 1000 and 2500 g fell from 11.5% in 1964 to 5.9% in 1970. At Vanderbilt University Hospital the mortality rate of babies in the same weight bracket was 11.8% before intensive care; it was 6.5% afterward. At Mount Zion Hospital in San Francisco, the mortality rate of low birth weight infants was 21.8% before intensive care and 6.6% after it was introduced. At the Robert B. Green Hospital in San Antonio, Texas, in just 2 years (1969 to 1971) the mortality rate of infants who weighed 1500 to 2500 g was reduced from 18% to 7.8%. There is little doubt that intensive care programs have indeed increased survival. In 1984, out of 1611 admissions to our unit, inborn survival was 94.1%; overall survival was 93%. Sixty-nine infants were admitted at weights between 501 and 750 g; 40% survived. There were 130 babies whose admission weights were less than 1000 g; 58% survived.

During the first year of our program at the University of Tennessee, there was a 28% decline in the mortality of low birth weight infants from the average of the preceding 8 years. We attribute this decline to the training of personnel; new equipment was not acquired until the last 5 or 6 months of that period. Although electronic monitors, mechanical respirators, and other such

items are important, they are nevertheless a secondary consideration. *The care of sick babies cannot be intensive unless personnel perform with intensity.* Without this ingredient, complex equipment is useless. The heavy staffing requirements imposed by special care units should preclude indiscriminate establishment of these facilities by hospitals that merely seek to enhance or maintain their community images.

REGIONALIZATION OF PERINATAL CARE

The advances in neonatal intensive care were like a show of fireworks—spectacular to behold, despite numerous fizzles. As the effectiveness of therapeutic modalities gained credibility, diminished neonatal mortality at the major centers began to contrast sharply with the unchanging experience of smaller hospitals. The concept of regionalization arose in response to a demonstrated need for the delivery of advanced levels of care to smaller communities and to smaller hospitals in large communities. The improved care provided by research had not yet been delivered to the bedside, except in the major centers where most of the research had transpired.

In simplest terms, regionalization is a formalized contemporary version of the pattern of medical practice that has long pervaded this country. Physicians in small communities have referred patients with complex problems to the "big city specialists" for years; they have attended conferences at medical centers habitually. Obviously, regionalization of perinatal care is a considerably more complex arrangement, but the fundamental idea is to deliver advanced levels of health care to all patients, regardless of geographic factors, and to impart new information to perinatal caretakers everywhere. The professional advice and supervision that constitute perinatal care in the 1980s should be available to every pregnant woman and newborn child. Although the vast majority of newborn babies are healthy, intact survival is jeopardized in a substantial number who require complex care for their severe illnesses. In many instances neonatal complications can be anticipated, ameliorated, or eliminated by special management of their high-risk mothers. This brand of care entails recruitment of a variety of professional personnel who are generally concentrated in densely populated communities. It is in these large communities that the full spectrum of medical consultants, nurse specialists, laboratory capabilities, and facilities with equipment are found. That perinatal mortality and morbidity are significantly reduced by the best contemporary technology has been plainly demonstrated for at least two decades. Thus there is an urgency to make the technology available to all mothers and infants, to eliminate any existing inaccessibility to complex care, and to ensure optimal quality of medical attention in every hospital, regardless of its geographic location or the complexity of care it can provide.

Optimal care can be planned for a region as a whole. The region is defined geographically according to preexisting patterns of medical referrals, commercial ties, and sociocultural bonds. Personnel and money can be allocated to avoid duplication of facilities and to ensure proper use of services. Theoretically the needs of individual patients should be met within a perinatal region, with all levels of care available. The sole determinants of the care given to mother and infant should be the severity and complexity of their illnesses. Services are best offered in facilities that are close to home, but the transfer of patients from one hospital to another is inevitable if an appropriate level of care is to be delivered.

A coordinated regional system requires designation of hospitals by the level of care that they provide. Beyond the designation of care levels, activation of effective communication for consultation and for transport of patients provides functional continuity between the diverse hospitals in a region. Fundamental to all these activities is a plan for continuing education of personnel; without it, any system will falter. Although guidelines are usually addressed to hospitals because they are institutional providers of care, the real pitch is to physicians, nurses, and other personnel as the personal providers of care.

Referral for transport

Level III units usually maintain a system of transport for mothers and infants. Alternatively, such a system may be maintained in a region by cooperative responsibility of its constituent hospitals. In either case, transport (by ground or air) requires nurses and physicians who are specifically educated for this purpose. In numerous localities, clinical nurse specialists manage the entire process of infant transfer; in most areas, physicians (often advanced trainees) are charged with this responsibility. Transport vehicles for infants vary from ambulances of standard size that carry incubators with monitors and ventilators to larger vehicles that are as fully equipped as the nursery itself. At the University of Tennessee Newborn Center we use the latter type, which is 30 feet in length with two radiant warmer beds, ventilators, monitors, blood gas apparatus, a sink with running water, and a complete supply of consumable items. Air transport (usually fixed-wing aircraft) is used in regions that are spread over a large area and in some large cities where heavy vehicular traffic creates problems that are surmountable only by helicopters. Maternal transport is the referral modality of choice. Adept screening at any hospital should predict 60% to 70% of the infants who will be in jeopardy at birth. Referral of these high-risk mothers for delivery of their babies at a tertiary care unit constitutes the best contemporary care available.

Educational programs

The regional center is responsible for the dissemination of information to the staffs of all hospitals within its region. These educational activities have been largely directed to practicing physicians and nursing staffs. Structured series of lectures and demonstrations or single sessions devoted to a specific topic are the usual formats of presentation. Instruction is usually given at the outlying hospitals but often at the regional centers as well. In Tennessee, extensive compilations of educational objectives have been circulated throughout the state for nurses, physicians, and social workers. Nurses' objectives are organized by specific care levels ("Educational Objectives for Nurses—Levels I, II, III, Neonatal Transport Nurses," 1982). The guide for physicians is directed to pediatricians and family practitioners ("Outlines of Courses for Physicians," 1982). The social workers' material is intended for level II and level III facilities ("Educational Objectives in Medicine for Perinatal Social Workers," 1982). Courses and sessions offered by each of the four regional centers in the state are based on these educational objectives. Regionalized professional education programs are emphasized throughout the country because the quality of perinatal care is ultimately dependent on the effectiveness of its educational efforts.

A regionalized system should include three types of facilities located within designated geographic perinatal care areas. They are designated by levels of care according to the *extent* of their respective capacities. *These designations do not indicate quality of available care; they refer only to the extent of care*. Table 16-1 lists the suggested functions of each of the three levels of care.

Level I facilities

The level I facility has three principal functions: (1) the management of normal pregnancy, labor, and delivery; (2) the earliest possible identification of high-risk pregnancy or high-risk neonates after birth; and (3) the provision of competent emergency care in the event of unanticipated obstetric or newborn emergencies. These facilities are generally located in small communities within hospitals that are vital to the overall health care of the area. They are defined as primary (level I) care centers only by virtue or their limited capacity to manage perinatal complications. There is little justification for hospitals in densely populated (urban) areas to offer the necessarily limited facilities that characterize level I care. Level I facilities generally deliver approximately 500 livebirths annually. Since the occurrence of complications is an infrequent event, staffing and equipment requirements are not as demanding as for level II and III care.

Level II facilities

These are larger perinatal services in hospitals that serve more densely populated areas, generally urban and suburban communities. The ideal level II facility should be capable of managing 75% to 90% of maternal and neonatal complications. However, this must necessarily vary according to the capacity of an individual hospital. In any event, a level II facility must manage a number of perinatal complications in addition to offering a full-range of maternity and newborn care in uncomplicated circumstances. As in the case of the previously described level I unit, the activities of a level II institution are assumed to be of the highest quality compatible with contemporary practice. The designation implies that a few functions are not within the capacity of a level II unit, which must therefore be obtained at a level III facility.

Level III facilities

Level III facilities, in addition to offering a complete spectrum of care for uncomplicated maternity and newborn patients, should have the capacity to manage the most complex of all perinatal disorders. Thus in the case of neonatal disorders, the level III facility has at its disposal a complete roster of pediatric subspecialists, pediatric surgeons, pediatric radiologists, geneticists, and hospital epidemiologists. This facility should deliver all the modalities of complex care that constitute sophisticated contemporary practice. In a densely populated region in which there is more than one level III unit, only one of them should be designated as a *regional center*. The regional center has the responsibility for coordinating the perinatal activities of its geographically delineated perinatal region. It is also responsible for maintaining consultative services for obstetricians, pediatricians, and the respective nursing services. It is expected that all level III units, and at regional centers in particular, a staff of *perinatal social workers* will be available to manage the multiplicity of problems that arise among families whose infants receive intensive care. The regional center must conduct ongoing continuing educa-

Table 16.1. Services provided by perinatal facilities*

Services	Level I	Level II	Level III
Complete prenatal care for maternity patients with no complications or with minor complications	X	X	X
Complete prenatal care for maternity patients with most complications		X	X
A special diagnostic and management clinic for high-risk prenatal patients			X
Risk identification scoring system	X	X	X
Management of uncomplicated labor and devlivery of normal term fetus	X	X	X
Prompt management of unexpected complications occurring during labor and delivery, including anesthesia, cesarean section, and blood administration	X	X	X
Management of complicated labor and delivery		X	X
Intrapartum intensive care			X
In-house anesthesia service		X	X
Electronic fetal monitoring	X	X	X
Physically separated facilities for obstetrics	X	X	X
Capability for resuscitation of depressed neonate at every delivery	X	X	X
Care for the healthy newborn	X	X	X
Stabilization and risk assessment of all neonates	X	X	X
Intravenous fluid administration to neonates	X	X	X
Management of most neonates who have complications up to short-term assisted ventilation		X	X
Continuous neonatal monitoring capability		X	X
Blood gases available on 24-hour basis		X	X
Neonatal intensive care including assisted ventilation and hyperalimentation			X
Neonatal surgical capability			X
Availability of pediatric subspecialists in cardiology, genetics, and hematology			X
Care of mothers with no complications postpartum	X	X	X
Management of unexpected postpartum complications including hemorrhage and sepsis	X	X	X
Management of most postpartum complications		X	X
Data collection on performance and outcome	X	X	X
Laboratory services for electrolytes, bilirubin, blood glucose, calcium on 24-hour basis	X	X	X
X-ray services with portable film capability on 24-hour basis	X	X	X
Laboratory services to assess fetal well-being and maturity		X	X
Diagnostic x-ray and ultrasound		X	X
Nutritional consultation		X	X
Social service		X	X
Respiratory therapy consultation		X	X
Sterilization and family planning services	X	X	X
Follow-up developmental assessment clinic			X

*From Graven, S. N.: The organization of perinatal health services. In Behrman, R. E., editor: Neonatal-perinatal medicine: diseases of the fetus and infant, ed. 3, St. Louis, 1983, The C. V. Mosby Co.

tion programs intramurally and in other hospitals of the region as well.

The level III unit, whether or not it is a designated regional center, must have a full-time obstetrician who is a subspecialist in maternofetal medicine and a full-time pediatrician who is a subspecialist in neonatal-perinatal medicine. Clinical nurse specialists in obstetrics and in newborn care should direct their respective nursing services in coordination with the efforts of the physicians. Staff physicians in the neonatal intensive care unit should also be subspecialists in neonatal-perinatal medicine.

PHYSIOLOGIC MONITORING AND THERAPY: ELECTRONIC AND OTHER TYPES OF EQUIPMENT

Electronic monitoring has greatly facilitated the detection of cardiovascular and respiratory difficulties. *These instruments are intended for use by skillful personnel; they are not intended to replace them.* In addition to cardiorespiratory monitoring, the control of temperature and ambient oxygen concentrations is also feasible with appropriate instrumentation. Following are the general categories of equipment required for intensive neonatal care.

I. Monitors
  A. Respiration (apnea)
  B. Heart rate
  C. Blood pressure
  D. Temperature (rectal, ambient, or skin probes), with or without controller
  E. Electrocardiogram (oscilloscopes, writers)
  F. Oxygen analyzers (ambient)
  G. Transcutaneous sensors for P_{O_2}, P_{CO_2}, and pH

II. Therapeutic equipment
  A. Incubators, with servocontrolled temperature
  B. Infusion pumps for intravenous fluid administration
  C. Phototherapy lamps
  D. Radiant heaters

III. Oxygen administration
  A. Plastic head hoods

  B. Humidifier warmers, preferably with variable temperature control
  C. Respirators (positive pressure with pressure or volume limiters; negative pressure)

IV. Resuscitation equipment
  A. Insufflation bags with masks
  B. Endotracheal tubes and adapters
  C. Laryngoscopes with premature blades
  D. Defibrillator

BIOCHEMICAL MONITORING

The special care unit should have its own laboratory staffed by technologists who are aware of the clinical significance of their efforts. At the very least, blood gas and pH determinations should be available within minutes after they are ordered for infants in respiratory distress and for periodic monitoring of other conditions such as late metabolic acidosis of prematurity. Since large units are usually located in sprawling hospital complexes whose central laboratories are at some distance from the nursery, the special care unit's laboratory should provide as many biochemical parameters as possible. Reliability and immediate availability of results are best assured when laboratory personnel are involved with newborn medicine on a full-time basis and are thus familiar with the special problems of sick infants. Blood glucose, bilirubin, and electrolyte determinations are indispensable. Hemoglobin and hematocrit determinations, stained blood smears, and Gram stains are also important.

RADIOLOGIC DIAGNOSIS

Chest films are the most frequent radiologic need in the nursery. They are best procured with minimal disturbance to the infant and thus should be taken by portable x-ray equipment, with the infant in an incubator. Films of the skull, abdomen, and extremities also can be taken with portable equipment. Gastrointestinal series and intravenous pyelograms should be performed in an x-ray room within the special care unit. If such a room is not available, the infant should be transported to the hospital radiology department only if accompanied by a nurse or a physician. A transport incubator with its own battery to provide heat, and its own portable source of oxygen, must be available for this purpose.

Ultrasound imaging is performed at the bedside. It is most frequently used to visualize the brain, particularly for hemorrhage and ventriculomegaly. It is also indispensable to cardiologic evaluations and assessment of renal morphology. Visualization of thrombi in the aorta and its immediate tributaries has become possible with use of ultrasonography.

STRUCTURAL COMPONENTS

The complete tertiary unit contains areas designed for intensive, intermediate, and minimal care. Infants are admitted directly to these areas, depending on their status, or they may be moved from one section to another according to changes in conditions. Thus an infant who was successfully treated for hyaline membrane disease, perhaps with ventilatory assistance, can be transferred with ease from the intensive care to the intermediate care area. Minimal care sections are generally devoted to convalescent growing infants.

Special care facilities should be as close as possible to the labor and delivery rooms. Currently, most new neonatal units are constructed by remodeling existing facilities, thus imposing severe limitations on optimal location, floor plan, and space. A number of notable units in the United States and in Canada are housed in children's hospitals rather than in general hospitals. These centers function solely as referral units, since they are usually at some distance from obstetric facilities.

The ideal center should accommodate infants who are distributed among the three graduated care areas. Complete units for fewer than 15 to 20 infants who are similarly distributed may be too expensive to operate. They may also fail to provide sufficient clinical material to maintain the interest and skill of personnel.

The number of bassinets and incubators within each of the three graduated care areas must be determined individually for each institution. These calculations depend on the population to be served. In some hospitals or communities the incidence of low birth weight is 7% of live births; in others, such as our own, it may be 15% to 17%. Since the principal source of infants requiring special care is the low birth weight group, the number of maximal care stations is largely determined by the incidence of small babies. The extent of referrals from the community is another important consideration in these calculations.

Current trends are toward housing all infants who need special care in a single large room, with sections organized administratively for the three levels of graduated care. Such an arrangement permits assignment of personnel according to their respective skills while providing ease of movement of patients and personnel from one area to another.

The earliest consideration in planning a neonatal unit is a determination of its location within the hospital. It should be juxtaposed to the delivery room or at least close to it. The next decision concerns the number and configuration of infant rooms. The two most prevalent floor plans utilize a single large room or smaller multiple rooms, usually two or three in number. Configuration is most often dictated by the design of the building if new construction is involved or by a preexisting arrangement if renovation is utilized. A square room is best. A number of centers have opted for a single large room.

Spacing is the single most important element of structural design; its fundamental determinant is patient census. Most publications recommend 80 to 100 sq ft per infant, but it is more effective to begin by planning for bed arrangements with respect to the *space that separates* them. In terms of operational effectiveness, bed intervals and aisles are the least amenable to compromise. Bed intervals that are less than 5 ft wide and aisles that are less than 6 ft wide will result in situations that range from inconvenience to impossibility. Intervals greater than 6 ft and aisles of more than 8 ft are impractical, particularly for nurses who must care for more than one patient. Planning for deployment of beds should begin by considering interval and aisle space requirements rather than primary assignment of square feet per bed, because a number of space-occupying variables ultimately impinge on bed spacing, including (1) the width and number of island cabinets for infant care; (2) the number and size of counters and cabinets for supplies; (3) preparation of medication; (4) clerical functions; and (5) the space that must remain unoccupied at entry ways. Furthermore, generous yet practical allocation of space between beds is essential for placing equipment and using x-ray and ultrasound machines. Because today's state-of-the-art is tomorrow's anachronism, effective planning must also provide ade-

quately for the use of equipment that has yet to be devised.

The Newborn Center at the University of Tennessee is an example of a modern special care unit (Figs. 16-1 to 16-6). It is composed of a single large room, 6600 sq ft, for 60 maximal and intermediate care babies and a number of other rooms for ancillary functions. A smaller room, adjacent to the larger one, houses 20 minimal care babies in an area of 1000 sq ft. The plan was developed to conserve nursing energy by minimizing walking distances entailed in use of the telephone, procurement of instruments and supplies, and recording of notes in charts that are otherwise stored at a central desk. The diagram of our floor plan (Fig. 16-1) shows the disposition of incuba-

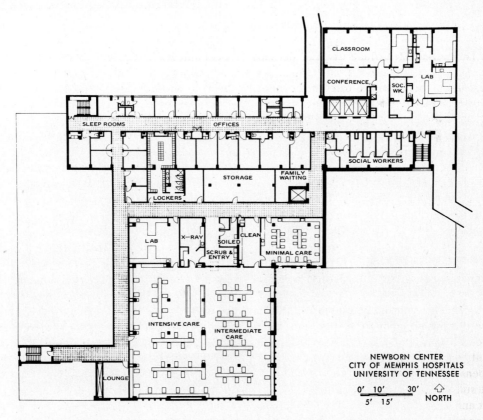

Fig. 16-1. Floor plan of the Newborn Center at the City of Memphis Hospital, University of Tennessee. (Courtesy of Yeates, Gaskill, and Rhodes, Architects, Memphis, Tennessee.)

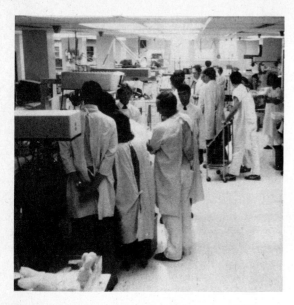

Fig. 16-2. Spaciousness accommodates two full teams during teaching rounds at the Newborn Center, University of Tennessee, Memphis.

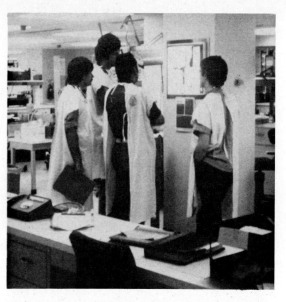

Fig. 16-3. X-ray viewing during rounds. View boxes are dispersed throughout the unit; films are stored at bedside. (Newborn Center, University of Tennessee, Memphis.)

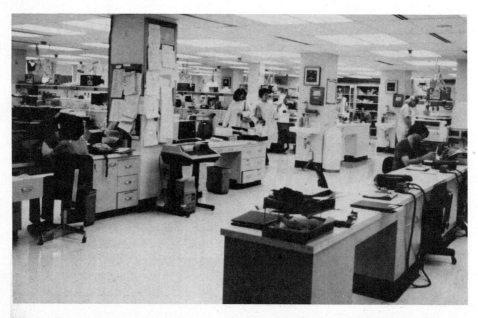

Fig. 16-4. View from entry of Newborn Center, University of Tennessee, Memphis. Ward clerk desks are in foreground.

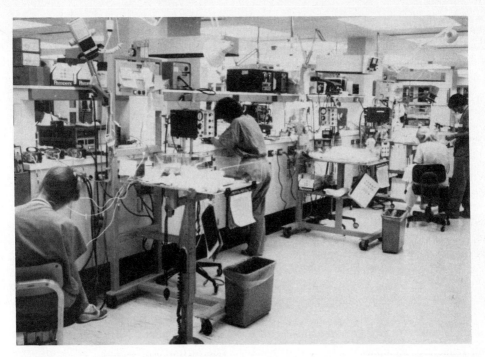

Fig. 16-5. Six-foot intervals between radiant warmers allow for multiple personnel and apparatus at bedside. (Newborn Center, University of Tennessee, Memphis.)

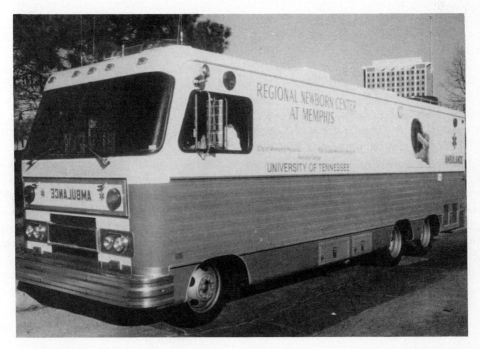

Fig. 16-6. Transport van of the Newborn Center, University of Tennessee, Memphis.

tors or bassinets and the placement of wall cabinets and other cabinets throughout the room. Supplies are stored as close to the infant as possible, permitting the nurse to remain in the area to which she is assigned. Formula in individual bottles is stored in the cabinets. Extensive work surface adjacent to each infant is provided by the counter tops. Daily notes are made at the cribside. The area contains ten sinks operated by foot pedals for convenient handwashing. Telephone extensions are placed at several points in the room. At least 10 electrical outlets are available for each care station. Two oxygen lines and a suction and two air outlets serve each incubator. In addition to copious illumination from lighting fixtures, an adjustable work light is suspended from the ceiling over each maximal care incubator. Infant stations in the intermediate care areas are provided with identical service receptacles as those in the maximal care area. Each incubator or open radiant-heated bed is placed 6 ft apart. A red light in the ceiling over each infant station is synchronized with the infant's monitor so that when the alarm sounds on the monitor, the appropriate red light flashes. These lights were installed to circumvent the frustrating lack of direction that is characteristic of the alarm sounds on most cardiorespiratory monitors.

Appropriate space for all supportive services is located on the same floor as the infant area. Thus there are six offices for each of the social workers, appropriate offices for supervising nurses, fellows, and physician faculty. The laboratory is immediately adjacent to the large infant area. An x-ray developing room is situated adjacent to the laboratory. All x-ray films are developed in the unit and remain at the infant's bedside until discharge. The radiologist reads all x-ray films in a designated area within the unit. A classroom that seats 60 individuals and a conference room that seats 20 to 30 are located on the same floor. Sleeping accommodations for physician staff and laboratory personnel are available for six individuals.

A baby-viewing area was not provided. Based on the concepts presented in Chapter 15, parents are encouraged to visit their infants in the nursery.

The delivery suite is located two floors below the special care unit. An express elevator transports infants from the delivery room directly to the nursery. The facility for normal term infants is one floor below the special care nursery.

PERSONNEL

The series of events that is triggered by the admission of a sick neonate involves a sizable group of people who are well versed in the functions they must perform. When the birth of a distressed infant is anticipated, a *physician* and a *nurse* from the intensive care unit await the baby in the delivery room. The *obstetrician* has notified the nursery of the impending admission of a severely depressed infant. The *respiratory therapist* sets up a ventilator; a *nurse* and an *aide* prepare the radiant warmer bed. Upon arrival of the baby, *three nurses* perform admission procedures, ranging from determination of blood pressure, body temperature, blood sugar, and weight, to adjustment of the warmer, starting intravenous fluids, and preparing for umbilical artery insertion. The *physician* provides manually assisted ventilation with a bag until the baby is placed on the respirator. The *ward clerk* notifies radiology and the laboratory that are needed immediately. A *blood collector* takes samples for the laboratory, and a *medical technologist* performs the tests requested. An *x-ray technologist* takes the film that was ordered, develops it, and submits it to the *radiologist*. A *social worker* visits the baby's family as soon after birth as is feasible. This typical admission, which occupies a period of approximately 1 hour, already involves 12 individuals. The ongoing care of this baby will ultimately involve more than 20 different disciplines and an even greater number of individual caretakers. In no instance can any individual, physicians, nurses, or ward clerks, be drafted abruptly from another area of the hospital to fill a gap in the neonatal intensive care unit (NICU).

A staff of physicians in the level III unit has at

its core an appropriate number of board-certified neonatologists. If the unit is an integral part of a university program, fellows in neonatal-perinatal medicine are also part of the staff. The university program provides residents who spend 5 to 6 months in the NICU during the course of their three-year training in pediatrics, and in some units, as in ours, residents in obstetrics, anesthesiology, and family medicine are also regularly present. In a large university unit, therefore, 6 to 10 physicians may be present during regular hours; most of them are trainees under the supervision of senior physicians. At most nonuniversity centers, there are fewer physicians but all are likely to be senior. Trainees are subjected to an overbearing work schedule. They are on duty every third or fourth night. In a large unit this translates into 1 or 2 hours of sleep, if any at all. A considerably reduced level of effectiveness can be expected from them as the night wears on and during the day that follows.

More so than any other type of personnel, the quality of nurses is the most critical determinant of the overall quality of an intensive care unit. The role of the registered nurse has changed dramatically during the past 15 years. In the late 1960s and even into the very early 1970s, there was a real need to decry the "handmaiden" concept of nursing that was then pervasive. Burgeoning activity and new knowledge precipitated an urgent need for increased nursing responsibility and enhanced expertise to activate it. "Handmaiden" changed to "colleague" as postgraduate courses arose for the specific education of neonatal intensive care nurses. There soon followed a movement to develop clinical nurse practitioners and specialists whose responsibilities were more like those of a physician than those of the traditional nurse. The cohort of nurses in the average level III unit of the 1980s is remarkably heterogeneous. There are instructors who deal primarily with in-service and outreach education of nurses, practitioners who manage selected babies as physicians do, transport nurses who manage infants from outlying hospitals during their

transfer, research nurses who knowledgeably assist physicians in clinical research and conduct their own as well, and staff nurses whose expertise in caring for sick infants hour by hour cannot be duplicated by others who are neither educated nor dedicated to the purpose.

A corps of registered nurses, practical nurses, and nurse assistants or technicians must be deployed to match training and skill with the level of care required for each infant. For every shift, optimal staffing should provide one nurse for two infants in the maximal care area and one nurse for three to six infants in the other sections. Nursing students and postgraduate nurse trainees are regularly present in units that are affiliated with schools of nursing and medicine.

The urgent need to alleviate the emotional crises of parents caused by the severe illness of their newborn infants became apparent early in the history of neonatal intensive care. Social and emotional support for parents is an essential component of total neonatal care. Temperamentally and professionally, no one is better equipped for this task than the neonatal social worker. In essence, social workers are compassionate activists. Their list of functions is lengthy, and the scope of nonmedical support is broad. The social worker is a parent advocate to the nursery staff, an interpreter of medical jargon and concepts to parents, a procurer of tangible necessities for parents, a coordinator of the staff's efforts at emotional support, a counselor in all forms of grief, a source of information on available community facilities, a facilitator of conferences, an arranger of postdischarge follow-up, an adviser on financial problems, and a vocal conscience on the ethical dilemmas.

Overlap of the roles of physicians, nurses, and social workers is easily identified. We consider this to be an advantage. The separate disciplines, utilizing their primary responsibilities as a focal point of parental contact, reinforce each other in the total effort. Ultimately the social worker is responsible for the coordination of psychosocial care. There is neither time nor reason for interdisciplinary friction because of overlapping functions. For instance, the nurse, who is often the first to encounter parents, briefs them about the medical situation, assesses their reactions, attempts to comprehend their attitudes, and supports them during stressful moments. The nurse functions similarly during subsequent parental visits and vigils. During these encounters the nurse has roles that ordinarily accrue to physicians or social workers. Nevertheless, these encounters are effective with few exceptions. The physician, who also plays multiple roles, draws on explanations of biologic disorders and on predictions of outcome, but effectiveness would be incomplete if these contacts with parents were devoid of psychosocial elements.

If the psychosocial concerns of physicians and nurses tend to reinforce the social worker's primary commitment, the latter's concern with medical matters is also reciprocally constructive. Neonatal social work requires sufficient knowledge of medical events to relate these to psychosocial difficulties. Without such knowledge, there is little basis for most of the social worker's counseling activities in an intensive care unit. Explanations of medical difficulties by physicians and nurses are too often replete with scientific terms that impair parental understanding. The social worker minimizes or eliminates confusion by offering explanations that are more easily understood. Also, parents are less restrained and self-conscious in the presence of the social worker; they more readily acknowledge confusion and ask more questions. The social worker is also an intermediary, relaying to the physician the parental anxieties that arise from an overtechnical explanation of an infant's biologic disorder. We have had a historic commitment to social work in our unit, having nine full-time perinatal social workers on our staff. Social work, like medicine and nursing, is indispensable to such totality.

Other disciplines are significantly active, each with a unique indispensability. The respiratory therapist has been educated to the singular characteristics of neonatal ventilatory support. The therapist whose principal responsibilities are to adults, or even to older pediatric patients, is not as expert as one who is specifically trained and experienced in tending to neonates. The same can be said for the physical therapist, who must be knowledgeable in the characteristics of infant development, the peculiarities of neonatal neuromuscular disorders, the effects of an environment that necessarily neglects psychosocial contacts during acute life-threatening illness, and the multiple aspects of infant management that indirectly influence the areas of concern to the physical therapist.

In recent years the philosopher has been summoned to the scene—not by any particular individual but rather by the well-known sequence of events that has increased the capacity to sustain the lives of smaller and more severely ill infants. This medical ethicist has brought knowledge to the bedside that is farther removed from endotracheal tubes, respirators, and catheters than any other discipline thus far recruited for the purposes of total neonatal intensive care. Added to intense anxieties for the infant's intact survival are the ethics of decisions, demeanor, and motivation. At one end of the spectrum is the question of who dies and who decides. On the other extreme is the contention that no one dies by decision and therefore no one need decide. Medical ethicists are consulted regularly in a number of centers; in some, protocols have been written requiring such consultations, and in others the ethicist is periodically present during rounds in the nursery. Many institutions are planning the establishment of an Infant Bioethics Committee that will be composed of representatives of nonmedical disciplines as well as physicians to assist in the resolution of ethical problems.

SUMMARY

The milieu of the neonatal intensive care unit is best described as "ordered chaos." Recurrent emergencies preclude a smooth routine. Situations vary from severely stressed infants (a primary concern) and emotionally stressed parents, to shortages of critical equipment and personnel, to iatrogenic misadventures that are inevitable in such a setting. Structural components thus far have proved to be appropriate means to fundamental ends. A multidisciplinary team of personnel, predominantly oriented toward intact survival, has now become aware of the environmental contributions to "intactness." The time is right for a systematic acquisition of ecologic data and observations in the nursery environment.

The patient is sensitive and fragile. Physical elements in the environment, such as excessive noise, are hazardous and should be minimized or eliminated. Psychosocial factors are significant, and their neglect is an impediment to optimal outcome. Random disturbance can be minimized, and coordinated stimulation can be enhanced. Neonates are unique, but not so unique that we can be mindless of their status as patients whose environmental needs must be met and whose human needs require thoughtful social interaction.

BIBLIOGRAPHY

Committee on Perinatal Health: Toward improving the outcome of pregnancy, White Plains, N. Y., 1976, The National Foundation–March of Dimes.

Davies, P. A., and Stewart, A. L.: Low-birth-weight infants: neurological sequelae and later intelligence, Br. Med. Bull. **31**:85, 1975.

Desmond, M. M., Rudolph, A. J., and Phitaksphraiwan, P.: The transitional care nursery: a mechanism for preventive medicine in the newborn, Pediatr. Clin. North Am. **13**:651, 1966.

Desmond, M. M., Rudolph, A. J., and Pineda, R. G.: Neonatal morbidity and nursery function, J. A. M. A. **212**:281, 1970.

Gluck, L.: The newborn special care unit: its role in the large medical center, Hosp. Pract. **3**:33, 1968.

Gottfried, A. V., Wallace-Land, P., Sherman-Brown, S., et al.: Physical and social environment of newborn infants in special care units, Science **214**:673, 1981.

Korones, S. B.: Evolution of nursery design and function: the Memphis story, Clin. Perinatol. **10**:127, 1983.

Korones, S. B.: The role of social workers in the neonatal intensive care unit—views of a neonatologist. In Davis, J. A., Richards, M. P. M., and Roberton, N. R. C., editors: Parent-baby attachment in premature infants, London/New York, 1983, Croom Helm, Ltd./St. Martin's Press.

Korones, S. B.: Physical structure and functional organization of neonatal intensive care units. In Gottfried, A. W., and Gaiter, J. L., editors: Infant stress under intensive care, Baltimore, 1985, University Park Press.

Long, J. G., Lucey, J. F., and Philip, A. G. S.: Noise and hypoxemia in the intensive care nursery, Pediatrics **65**:143, 1980.

Long, J. G., Philip, A. G. S., and Lucey, J. F.: Excessive handling as a cause of hypoxemia, Pediatrics **65**:203, 1980.

Lucey, J. F., editor: Problems of neonatal intensive care units, Report of the Fifty-ninth Ross Conference on Pediatric Research, Columbus, Ohio, March 1968, Ross Laboratories.

Lucey, J. F.: Why we should regionalize perinatal care, Pediatrics **52**:488, 1972.

Organization for perinatal care. In Gluck, L., editor: Clin. Perinatol. vol. 3, Philadelphia, 1976, W. B. Saunders Co.

Schlesinger, E. R.: Neonatal intensive care: planning for services and outcomes following care, J. Pediatr. **82**:916, 1973.

Sheridan, J. F.: The typical perinatal center: an overview of perinatal health services in the United States, Clin. Perinatol. **10**:31, 1983.

Silverman, W. A.: Intensive care of the low birth weight and other at-risk infants, Clin. Obstet. Gynecol. **13**:87, 1970.

Stewart, A. L., and Reynolds, E. O. R.: Improved prognosis for infants of very low birth weight, Pediatrics **54**:724, 1974.

Swyer, P. R.: The regional organization of special care for the neonate, Pediatr. Clin. North Am. **17**:761, 1970.

Tennessee Perinatal Care System: Educational objectives in medicine for perinatal social workers, Nashville, 1982, Tennessee Department of Public Health, Division of Maternal and Child Health.

Tennessee Perinatal Care System: Educational objectives for nurses—levels I, II, III, Nashville, 1982, Tennessee Department of Public Health, Division of Maternal and Child Health.

Tennessee Perinatal Care System: Guidelines for regionalization, hospital care levels, staffing and facilities, Nashville, 1984, Tennessee Department of Health and Environment, Division of Maternal and Child Health.

Tennessee Perinatal Care System: Outlines of courses for physicians, Nashville, 1982, Tennessee Department of Public Health, Division of Maternal and Child Health.

Index